ESSENTIAL ATLAS OF

GASTROENTEROLOGY *and* HEPATOLOGY *for* PRIMARY CARE

ESSENTIAL ATLAS OF GASTROENTEROLOGY *and* HEPATOLOGY *for* PRIMARY CARE

Editor

Mark Feldman, MD
Southland Professor and Vice Chairman
Department of Internal Medicine
University of Texas Southwestern Medical Center at Dallas
Chief, Medical Service
Veterans Affairs Medical Center
Dallas, Texas

Contributing Editors

Willis C. Maddrey, MD, MACP
Executive Vice President for Clinical Affairs
Professor and Department Administrator
Department of Internal Medicine
University of Texas Southwestern Medical Center at Dallas;
Zale Lipshy University Hospital
Aston Ambulatory Care Center (Clinic)
Dallas, Texas

C. Richard Boland, MD
Professor and Chief, Division of Gastroenterology
Department of Medicine
University of California, San Diego
La Jolla, California

Paul E. Hyman, MD
Director, Pediatric Gastrointestinal Motility Center
Children's Hospital of Orange County
Orange, California
Associate Clinical Professor of Pediatrics
University of California, Los Angeles, School of Medicine
Los Angeles, California

Roy C. Orlando, MD
Professor of Gastroenterology and Hepatology
Section Chief, Gastroenterology
Department of Gastroenterology and Hepatology
Tulane University Medical School;
Tulane University Medical Center
New Orleans, Louisiana

Nicholas F. LaRusso, MD
Professor of Medicine and Biochemistry and Molecular Biology
Chairman, Division of Gastroenterology
Mayo Foundation
Rochester, Minnesota

Lawrence R. Schiller, MD
Clinical Associate Professor
Department of Internal Medicine
University of Texas Southwestern Medical Center
Baylor University Medical Center
Dallas, Texas

Phillip P. Toskes, MD
Professor and Chairman
Department of Medicine
University of Florida College of Medicine
Gainesville, Florida

With 103 Contributors

Blackwell Science

Developed by Current Medicine, Inc.
Philadelphia

Current Medicine, Inc.
400 Market Street
Suite 700
Philadelphia, PA 19106

Managing Editor	*Lori J. Bainbridge*
Development Editor	*Scott Thomas Hurd*
Editorial Assistant	*Deborah Singer*
Art Director	*Paul Fennessy*
Design and Layout	*Robert LeBrun, Patrick Whelan*
Illustration Director	*Ann Saydlowski*
Typesetting	*Ryan Walsh*
Production	*Lori Holland and Sally Nicholson*
Indexer	*Maria Coughlin*

Library of Congress Cataloging-in-Publication Data
Essential atlas of gastroenterology and hepatology for primary care / Mark Feldman, editor
p. cm.
Abridged version of: Gastroenterology and hepatology / series editor, Mark Feldman. c1996– .
Includes bibliographical references and index.
ISBN 0-63204-394-6 (hardcover)
1. Digestive organs—Diseases—Atlases. 2. Liver—Diseases—Atlases. 3. Primary care (Medicine) I. Feldman, Mark, 1947– .
[DNLM: 1. Gastrointestinal Diseases—atlases. 2. Liver Diseases—atlases. WI. 17 E78 1997]
RC807.E87 1997
616.3′3—dc21
DNLM/DLC 97—35820
for Library of Congress CIP

©**Copyright 1998 by Current Medicine, Inc.** All rights reserved. No part of this publication may be reproduced, stored in a retrieval system or transmitted in any form by any means electronic, mechanical, photocopying, recording, or otherwise, without prior written consent of the publisher.

Library of Congress Cataloging-in-Publication Data
ISBN 0-63204-394-6

Printed in Singapore by Imago Productions (FE) Pte Ltd.

10 9 8 7 6 5 4 3 2 1

Although every effort has been made to ensure that drug doses and other information are presented accurately in this publication, the ultimate responsibility rests with the prescribing physician. Neither the publishers nor the authors can be held responsible for errors or for any consequences arising from the use of information contained herein. Products mentioned in this publication should be used in accordance with the prescribing information prepared by the manufacturers. No claims or endorsements are made for any drug or compound at present under clinical investigation.

DISTRIBUTED WORLDWIDE BY BLACKWELL SCIENCE, INC.

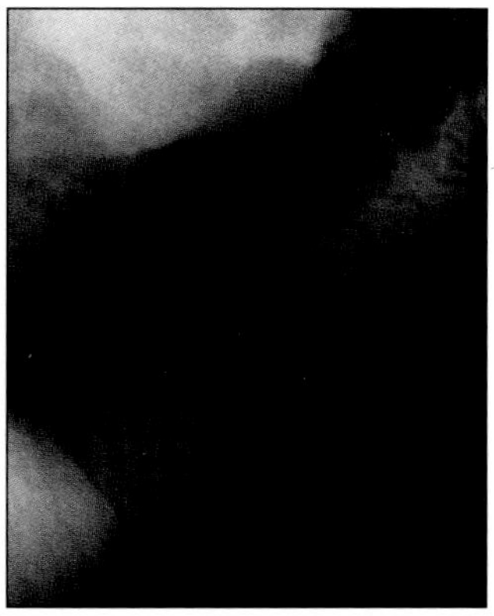

Preface

Primary care physicians frequently diagnose and treat patients with acute or chronic digestive disorders. This clinical spectrum ranges from managing acute diarrhea in children to severe constipation in the elderly; or from evaluating the cause of jaundice in pregnancy to interpreting a slightly elevated alanine aminotransferase (ALT) during a routine office visit. More and more, primary care physicians are involved in screening (and preventing) digestive diseases, such as judicious use of fecal occult blood testing to screen for colorectal cancer and hepatitis A and B vaccination.

In the past few years, there has been a staggering number of discoveries related to the etiology, diagnosis, treatment, and prevention of gastrointestinal and hepatic diseases. Examples include the role of *Helicobacter pylori* in peptic ulcer disease, the discovery of hepatitis C and the introduction of interferon in its therapy, improved understanding of the molecular biology of colorectal cancer (both familial and sporadic forms), prevention and treatment of gastrointestinal complications of AIDS, and the use of laparoscopic surgery to remove the gallbladder or appendix or to treat gastroesophageal reflux.

Essental Atlas of Gastroenterology and Hepatology for Primary Care is a collection of more than 600 images that pictorially displays the diseases of the gastrointestinal tract, liver, biliary tree, and pancreas in both adults and children. This collection has been distilled from a larger collection of more than 4000 images in an eight-volume collection entitled, *Gastroenterology and Hepatology: The Comprehensive Visual Reference*. The authors of this eight-volume collection have selected those images that they thought were most relevant to primary care physicians in clinical practice. These images include photographs, charts, tables, drawings, algorithms, and diagrams.

I wish to thank many people for their contributions to this series. The dedication and expertise of the volume editors—Willis Maddrey, Rick Boland, Paul Hyman, Nick LaRusso, Roy Orlando, Larry Schiller, and Phil Toskes—was critical and most appreciated. The nearly 100 contributing authors were both creative and generous with their time and teaching materials. Special thanks to Abe Krieger, President of Current Medicine, for recruiting me for this unique project, and to his talented associates at Current Medicine, including Lori Bainbridge, Scott Hurd, and Ira Smiley.

The images contained in this collection are available not only in print, but also in slide format and in CD-ROM. The editors and contributors hope that this collection is useful to primary care physicians whose patients suffer from gastrointestinal disorders.

Mark Feldman, MD

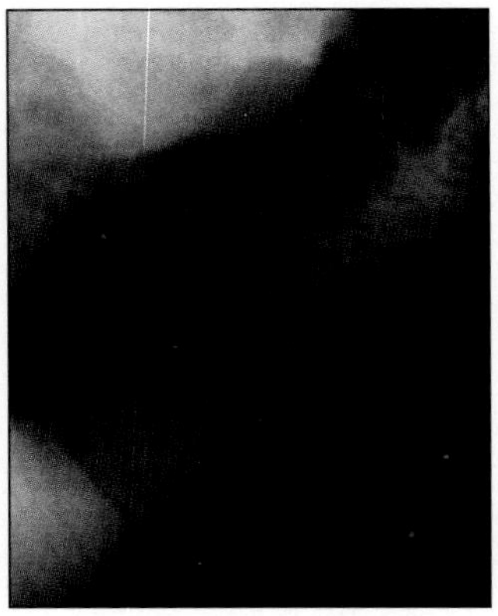

Contributors

Ignacio Aiza, MD
Fellow, Department of Hepatology
University of Miami
Miami, Florida

Matthew S.Z. Bachinski, MD
Assistant Professor of Medicine
Department of Gastroenterology
Uniformed Services University of the Health Sciences
Evans, Georgia

Bruce R. Bacon, MD
Professor of Internal Medicine
Department of Internal Medicine
Division of Gastroenterology and Hepatology
Saint Louis University School of Medicine
St. Louis, Missouri

Jeffrey L. Barnett, MD
Associate Professor
Department of Internal Medicine
University of Michigan Hospitals;
University of Michigan Medical Center
Ann Arbor, Michigan

Carlos Belmonte-Montes, MD
Visiting Fellow
Department of Surgery
University of Minnesota
St. Paul, Minnesota

David Bernstein, MD, FACB, FACP
Assistant Professor of Medicine
Department of Medicine
Health Sciences Center
State University of New York at Stony Brook
Stony Brook, New York

Carol Lynn Berseth, MD
Associate Professor
Department of Pediatrics
Baylor College of Medicine;
Texas Children's Hospital
Houston, Texas

Laurence Blendis, MD
Professor
Department of Medicine
University of Toronto;
The Toronto Hospital
Toronto, Ontario
Canada

Joseph R. Bloomer, MD
Professor, Department of Medicine
University of Alabama at Birmingham;
The Kirklin Clinic University Hospital
Birmingham, Alabama

Eugene M. Bozymski, MD
Professor of Medicine
Department of Internal Medicine
Division of Digestive Disease and Nutrition
University of North Carolina ;
Chief of Endoscopy and Attending Physician
University of North Carolina Medical Center
Chapel Hill, North Carolina

M. Stanley Branch, MD
Assistant Professor of Medicine
Department of Medicine
Duke University Medical Center
Durham, North Carolina

Robert S. Bresalier, MD
Associate Professor of Medicine
Department of Medicine
University of Michigan School of Medicine
Ann Arbor, Michigan
Director, Gastrointestinal Oncology
Henry Ford Health Sciences Center
Detroit, Michigan

Robert S. Brown, Jr., MD
Assistant Professor of Medicine
Department of Medicine
University of North Carolina;
Medical Director
Liver Transplantation Program
Chapel Hill, North Carolina

Peter C. Buetow, MD
Assistant Professor
Department of Radiology and Nuclear Medicine
Uniformed Services University of Health Sciences
Bethesda, Maryland;
Chief, Gastrointestinal Radiology
Armed Forces Institute of Pathology
Washington, District of Columbia

David L. Carr-Locke, MD
Associate Professor of Medicine
Department of Medicine
Harvard Medical School;
Director of Endoscopy
Brigham and Women's Hospital
Boston, Massachusetts

Donald O. Castell, MD
Professor
Department of Medicine
Allegheny University of the Health Sciences;
Kimbel Professor and Chairman
Department of Medicine
University of Pennsylvania
Philadelphia, Pennsylvania

Anupama Chawla, MD, DCh
Assistant Professor of Pediatrics
Department of Pediatric Gastroenterology
Cornell University Medical College
North Shore University Hospital
Manhasset, New York

Harold O. Conn, MD
Professor of Medicine (Emeritus)
Department of Internal Medicine
Yale University School of Medicine
East Haven, Connecticut;
Clinical Professor of Surgery
Liver and Bowel Transplantation
University of Miami School of Medicine
Pompano Beach, Florida

Byron Cryer, MD
Assistant Professor
Internal Medicine
University of Texas Southwestern Medical School
Department of Digestive Disease
Dallas Veterans Affairs Medical Center
Dallas, Texas

Christopher S. Cutler, MD
Fellow in Gastroenterology/Hepatology
Department of Medicine
Indiana University School of Medicine
Indianapolis, Indiana

Albert J. Czaja, MD
Professor of Medicine
Department of Medicine
Division of Gastroenterology and Hepatology
Mayo Medical School;
Consultant in Gastroenterology
Mayo Clinic
Rochester, Minnesota

Fredric Daum, MD
Professor of Pediatrics
Department of Pediatric Gastroenterology
Cornell University Medical College
North Shore University Hospital
Manhasset, New York

Wendy Z. Davis, MD
Associate Professor
Department of Medicine
Division of Gastroenterology
Duke University Medical Center
Durham, North Carolina

Daniel C. DeMarco, MD
Attending Physician
Gastroenterology Department
Baylor University Medical Center
Dallas, Texas

Rita De Vos, DSc
Professor
Department of Morphologic Imaging
Catholic University Leuven;
University Hospital at St. Raphael
Leuven University
Leuven, Belgium

Valeer J. Desmet, MD, PhD
Emeritus Professor
Department of Pathology
Leuven University
Leuven, Belgium

Adrian M. Di Bisceglie, MD
Associate Chairman
Professor of Internal Medicine
Department of Internal Medicine
St. Louis University School of Medicine
St. Louis, Missouri

Carlo Di Lorenzo, MD
Associate Professor of Pediatrics
Department of Pediatrics
University of Pittsburgh;
Associate Professor of Pediatrics
Director of Motility Center
Children's Hospital of Pittsburgh
Pittsburgh, Pennsylvania

John H. Donahue, MD
Associate Professor
Department of Surgery
Mayo Medical School;
Consultant
Department of Surgery
Mayo Clinic and Mayo Foundation
Rochester, Minnesota

Joanne M. Donovan, MD
Assistant Professor of Medicine
Department of Medicine
Harvard Medical School;
Chief, Gastroenterology Section
Brockton/West Roxbury Veterans Affairs Medical Center
Boston, Massachusetts

Peter R. Durie, BSc, MD, FRCPC
Professor
Department of Pediatrics
University of Toronto;
Head, Division of Gastroenterology and Nutrition
The Hospital for Sick Children
Toronto, Ontario
Canada

Gulchin A. Ergun, MD
Assistant Professor of Medicine
Department of Medicine
Division of Gastroenterology and Hepatology
Northwestern University Medical School;
Northwestern University Memorial Hospital
Chicago, Illinois

Christopher E. Forsmark, MD
Associate Professor
Department of Medicine
University of Florida College of Medicine
Shands Hospital at the University of Florida
Gainesville, Florida

Lawrence S. Friedman, MD
Associate Professor of Medicine
Harvard Medical School;
Associate Physician
Gastrointestinal Unit
Massachusetts General Hospital
Boston, Massachusetts

Karl Fukunaga, MD
Clinical Instructor
Department of Medicine
University of Southern California School of Medicine
Los Angeles County and University of Southern California Medical Center
Los Angeles, California

Ralph A. Giannella, MD
Mark Brown Professor of Medicine
Department of Internal Medicine
University of Cincinnati
Cincinnati, Ohio

Fiona Graeme-Cook, MD
Assistant Professor
Department of Pathology
Harvard Medical School;
Assistant Pathologist
Department of Pathology
Massachusetts General Hospital
Boston, Massachusetts

Joel K. Greenson, MD
Assistant Professor of Pathology
Department of Pathology
University of Michigan Medical Center;
University of Michigan Hospitals
Ann Arbor, Michigan

James H. Grendell, MD
Professor
Department of Medicine
Cornell University Medical College
Chief, Division of Digestive Diseases
New York Hospital-Cornell Medical Center
New York, New York

Salima Haque, MD
Assistant Professor
Department of Pathology and Laboratory Medicine
Tulane University School of Medicine
New Orleans, Louisiana

William L. Hasler, MD
Assistant Professor
Department of Internal Medicine
Division of Gastroenterology
University of Michigan Medical Center
Ann Arbor, Michigan

Bernard M. Jaffe, MD
Professor and Vice Chairman
Department of Surgery
Tulane University School of Medicine
New Orleans, Louisiana

Robert T. Jensen, MD
Chief, Digestive Diseases Branch
National Institute of Diabetes, Digestive, and Kidney Diseases
National Institute of Health
Bethesda, Maryland

Peter J. Kahrilas, MD
Professor of Medicine
Department of Medicine
Northwestern University Medical School;
Northwestern Memorial Hospital
Chicago, Illinois

Samuel Klein, MD
Professor
Department of Internal Medicine
Washington University School of Medicine
Barnes-Jewish Hospital
St. Louis, Missouri

Douglas Kliewer, MD
Fellow in Gastroenterology
Department of Internal Medicine
University of Texas Southwestern Medical School
Parkland Hospital Veterans Affairs Medical Center
Dallas, Texas

Raymond S. Koff, MD
Professor of Medicine
Department of Medicine
University of Massachusetts Medical School
Worcester, Massachusetts;
Chairman, Department of Medicine
Chief, Hepatology Section
Metrowest Medical Center
Framingham, Massachusetts

Ann M. Kools, MD
Assistant Professor
Department of Medicine
University of Minnesota
Minneapolis, Minnesota;
Park Nicollet Clinic
St. Louis Park, Minnesota

Amy M. Kusske, MD
Resident
Department of Surgery
UCLA Medical School
Los Angeles, California

John R. Lake, MD
Associate Professor of Medicine
Department of Medicine
GI Division
University of California, San Francisco;
Medical Director
Liver Transplantation Program
University of California Medical Center
San Francisco, California

Jacob C. Langer, MD
Associate Professor
Department of Surgery
Washington University Medical School;
St. Louis Children's Hospital
St. Louis, Missouri

Juan Lechago, MD, PhD
Professor
Department of Pathology
Baylor College of Medicine;
Director, Surgical Pathology
The Methodist Hospital
Houston, Texas

Edward L. Lee, MD
Professor
Department of Pathology
University of Texas Southwestern
Medical Center;
Chief, Pathology and Laboratory Medicine Service
Veterans Affairs North Texas Health Care System
Dallas, Texas

William M. Lee, MD
Professor
Department of Internal Medicine
University of Texas Southwestern
Medical School;
Director
Clinical Center for Liver Diseases
Dallas, Texas

Louis P. Leite, DO
Division of Gastroenterology
The Graduate Hospital
Philadelphia, Pennsylvania

Felix W. Leung, MD
Professor of Medicine
Department of Medicine
University of California, Los Angeles,
School of Medicine
Los Angeles, California;
Sepulveda Veterans Affairs Medical Center
Sepulveda, California

Charles S. Lieber, MD
Professor, Department of Medicine
and Pathology
Mount Sinai School of Medicine;
Director, GI-Liver Program and Alcohol
Research and Treatment Center
Veterans Affairs Medical Center
Bronx, New York

Keith D. Lindor, MD
Associate Professor of Medicine
Division of Gastroenterology and Hepatology
Mayo Medical School;
Mayo Clinic
Rochester, Minnesota

Gordon D. Luk, MD
Chief, Gastroenterology
Department of Veterans Affairs Medical Center
Dallas, Texas

R. Lee Meyers, MD
Clinical Instructor
Department of Medicine
Division of Digestive Diseases
University of North Carolina
Chapel Hill, North Carolina

Ravinder K. Mittal, MD
Associate Professor
Department of Internal Medicine
University of Virginia
Charlottesville, Virginia

Milton G. Mutchnick, MD
Professor, Department of Internal Medicine
Division of Gastroenterology
Wayne State University;
Director
Division of Gastroenterology
Harper Hospital
Detroit, Michigan

Timothy T. Nostrant, MD, FACP, FACG
Professor of Internal Medicine
Department of Internal Medicine
University of Michigan
Ann Arbor, Michigan

Thomas O'Dorisio, MD
Professor of Medicine
Department of Internal Medicine
Ohio State University College of Medicine
Ohio State University Medical Center
Columbus, Ohio

Susan R. Orenstein, MD
Professor
Department of Digestive Disorders
University of Pittsburgh School of Medicine;
Children's Hospital of Pittsburgh
Pittsburgh, Pennsylvania

Amit G. Pandya, MD
Associate Professor
Department of Dermatology
University of Texas Southwestern
Medical Center
Dallas, Texas

J. Javier Perez-Ramirez, MD
Visiting Fellow
Department of Surgery
University of Minnesota
St. Paul, Minnesota

Henry A. Pitt, MD
Professor and Chairman
Department of Surgery
Medical College of Wisconsin;
Surgeon-in-Chief
Froedtert Memorial Hospital
Milwaukee, Wisconsin

Rodney V. Pozderac, MD
Clinical Associate Professor
Radiology
Ohio State University College of Medicine
Ohio State University Medical Center
Columbus, Ohio

Eamonn M.M. Quigley, MD, FRCP
Associate Professor
Department of Internal Medicine
University of Nebraska
University Hospital
Omaha, Nebraska

Howard A. Reber, MD
Resident
Department of Surgery
UCLA Medical School
Los Angeles, California

Douglas K. Rex, MD
Professor
Department of Medicine
GI Division
Indiana University School of Medicine
Indianapolis, Indiana

Arvey I. Rogers, MD
Professor
Department of Medicine
University of Miami
Veterans Affairs Medical Center
University of Miami Hospital and Clinics
Jackson Memorial Hospital
Miami, Florida

Charles M. Rosen, MD
Instructor of Clinical Medicine
Department of Medicine
University of Miami
Mount Sinai Medical Center
Miami, Florida

Philip Rosenthal, MD
Professor of Pediatrics and Surgery
Department of Pediatrics;
Director
Pediatric Liver Transplant Program
University of California, San Francisco
San Francisco, California

Tania Roskams, MD, PhD
Assistant Professor
Department of Pathology
University of Leuven, Faculty of Medicine;
Pathologist (Staff Member)
Department of Pathology
University Hospital of Leuven
Leuven, Belgium

Alfred D. Roston, MD
Advanced Endoscopy Fellow
Brigham and Women's Hospital
Harvard Medical School
Boston, Massachusetts;
Attending Physician
White Plains Hospital Center
White Plains, New York

David A. Rothenberger, MD
Clinical Professor and Chief
Division of Colon and Rectal Surgery
University of Minnesota
Minneapolis, Minnesota;
Colon and Rectal Surgery Associates
St. Paul, Minnesota

Richard I. Rothstein, MD
Associate Professor of Medicine
Section of Gastroenterology
Dartmouth Medical School
Hanover, New Hampshire;
Dartmouth-Hitchcock Medical Center
Lebanon, New Hampshire

David B. Sachar, MD, FACP
The Dr. Burrill B. Crohn Professor of Medicine
Mount Sinai School of Medicine of the City University of New York
Director of the Dr Henry D. Janowitz Division of Gastroenterology
The Mount Sinai Hospital
New York, New York

George Sachs, MD, DSc
Professor
Departments of Physiology and Medicine
University of California, Los Angeles, School of Medicine
Los Angeles, California

Miguel Saps, MD
Colaborator
Department of Pediatrc Gastroenterology
Facultad de Medicina
Hospital Pereira-Rossell;
Gastroclinica
Montevideo, Uruguay

Robert H. Schapiro, MD
Clinical Associate Professor
Department of Medicine
Harvard University;
Director
Gastrointestinal Endoscopy Unit
Massachusetts General Hospital
Boston, Massachusetts

Ellen J. Scherl, MD
Assistant Attending
Department of Medicine
Mount Sinai Medical School
Mount Sinai Hospital
New York, New York

Eugene R. Schiff, MD
Professor
Department of Medicine
University of Miami School of Medicine;
Director
Center for Liver Diseases
Miami Medical Center
Miami, Florida

Neal E. Seymour, MD
Assistant Professor
Department of Surgery
Yale University School of Medicine;
Surgical service
Veterans Affairs Medical Center
New Haven, Connecticut

Eldon A. Shaffer, MD
Professor and Regional Clinical Department Head
Department of Internal Medicine
University of Calgary
Calgary, Alberta
Canada

Herbert J. Smith, MD
Professor of Radiology
Department of Veterans Affairs
North Texas Health Care System
University of Texas Southwestern Medical School
Dallas, Texas

William M. Steinberg, MD
Professor
Department of Medicine
George Washington University School of Medicine and Health Sciences
Washington, DC

Edward T. Stewart, MD
Professor, Department of Radiology
Medical College of Wisconsin;
Chief, GI Radiology
Froedtert Memorial Lutheran Hospital
Milwaukee, Wisconsin

Robert W. Summers, MD
Professor of Internal Medicine
Department of Internal Medicine
University of Iowa College of Medicine
University of Iowa Hospitals and Clinics
Iowa City, Iowa

Johnson L. Thistle, MD
Professor of Medicine
Department of Gastroenterology and Hepatology
Mayo Medical School;
Mayo Clinic
Rochester, Minnesota

Vasundhara Tolia, MD
Professor
Department of Pediatrics
Wayne State University;
Director
Pediatric Gastroenterology and Nutrition
Children's Hospital of Michigan
Detroit, Michigan

James Toouli, PhD, FRACS
Professor
Department of Surgery
Flinders University;
Senior Director
GI Surgical Unit
Flinders Medical Centre
Adelaide, South Australia
Australia

Mark Toyama, MD
Resident
Department of Surgery
UCLA Medical School
Los Angeles, California

Jon A. Vanderhoof, MD
Professor of Pediatrics
Department of Pediatrics
University of Nebraska
Omaha, Nebraska

Arnold Wald, MD
Professor
Department of Medicine
University of Pittsburgh;
Division of Gastroenterology and Hepatology
University of Pittsburgh Medical Center
Pittsburgh, Pennsylvania

W. Allan Walker, MD
Conrad Taff Professor of Pediatrics and Nutrition
Harvard Medical School;
Chief, Combined Program in Pediatric Gastroenterology and Nutrition
Children's Hospital
Boston, Massachusetts;
Director
Mucosal Immunology Laboratory
Massachusetts General Hospital
Charlestown, Massachusetts

C. Mel Wilcox, MD
Associate Professor
Department of Medicine;
Director of Clinical Research
Division of Gastroenterology and Hepatology
University of Alabama at Birmingham
Birmingham, Alabama

Florence Wong, MD
Assistant Professor
Department of Medicine
University of Toronto;
Staff Gastroenterologist
The Toronto Hospital
Toronto, Ontario
Canada

Roy K.H. Wong, MD
Professor of Medicine
Department of Medicine
Uniformed Services
University of the Health Sciences
Bethesda, Maryland

Wallace C. Wu, MD
Professor of Medicine
Department of Medicine
Bowman Gray School of Medicine;
Attending Physician
North Carolina Baptist Hospital
Winston-Salem, North Carolina

Russell David Yang, MD, PhD
Assistant Professor of Medicine
Department of Medicine
Baylor College of Medicine;
Los Angeles County and University of Southern California Medical Center
Los Angeles, California

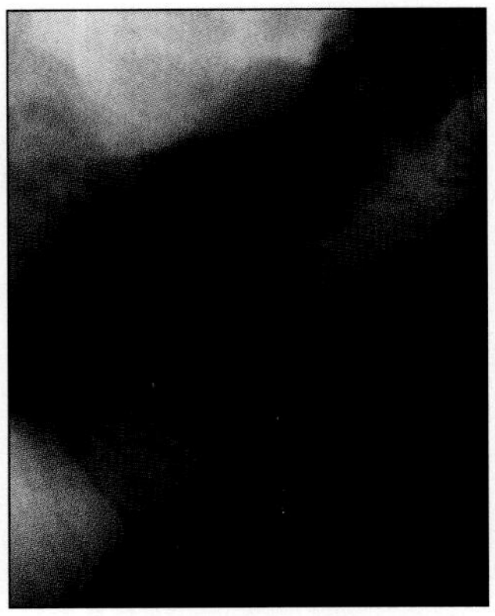

Contents

Chapter 3
Disorders of the Small Intestine
LAWRENCE R. SCHILLER

Ralph A. Giannella, Samuel Klein, Edward L. Lee, Gordon D. Luk, Amit G. Pandya, Eamonn M.M. Quigley, Francisco C. Ramirez, Arvey I. Rogers, Charles M. Rosen, David B. Sachar, Ellen J. Scherl, Herbert J. Smith, Robert W. Summers

Chapter 4
Disorders of the Colon, Rectum, and Anus
C. RICHARD BOLAND

Jeffrey L. Barnett, Carlos Belmonte-Montes, Robert S. Bresalier, Chistopher S. Cutler, Lawrence S. Friedman, Fiona Graeme-Cook, Joel K. Greenson, William L. Hasler, Timothy T. Nostrant, Amit G. Pandya, J. Javier Perez-Ramirez, Douglas K. Rex, David A. Rothenberger, Robert H. Schapiro, Edward T. Stewart, Arnold Wald

Chapter 5
Disorders of the Liver
WILLIS C. MADDREY

Ignacio Aiza, Bruce R. Bacon, David Bernstein, Laurence Blendis, Joseph R. Bloomer, Robert S. Brown Jr., Peter C. Buetow, Harold O. Conn, Albert J. Czaja, Adrian M. Di Bisceglie, Raymond S. Koff, Ann M. Kools, John R. Lake, William M. Lee, Charles S. Lieber, Milton G. Mutchnick, Eugene R. Schiff, Florence Wong

Chapter 6
Disorders of the Gallbladder and Biliary Tree

Nicholas F. LaRusso

M. Stanley Branch, David L. Carr-Locke, Wendy Z. Davis, Rita De Vos, Valeer J. Desmet, John H. Donahue, Joanne M. Donovan, Keith D. Lindor, Henry A. Pitt, Tonia Roskams, Alfred D. Roston, Eldon A. Shaffer, Johnson L. Thistle, James Toouli

Chapter 7:
Disorders of the Pancreas

Phillip P. Toskes

Christopher Forsmark, James H. Grendell, Amy M. Kusske, Thomas O'Dorisio, Rodney V. Pozderac, Howard A. Reber, William M. Steinberg, Mark Toyama

Chapter 8
Pediatric Gastroenterologic and Hepatic Disorders

Paul E. Hyman

Carol Lynn Berseth, Anupama Chawla, Fredric Daum, Carlo Di Lorenzo, Peter R. Durie, Jacob C. Langer, Susan R. Orenstein, Philip Rosenthal, Vasundhara Tolia, Jon A. Vanderhoof

Chapter 1

Disorders of the Esophagus

EDITOR

Roy C. Orlando

CONTRIBUTORS

Matthew S.Z. Bachinski
Eugene M. Bozymski
Donald O. Castell
Gulchin A. Ergun
Salima Haque
Bernard M. Jaffe
Peter J. Kahrilas
Louis P. Leite
R. Lee Meyers
Ravinder K. Mittal
Amit G. Pandya
Richard I. Rothstein
Roy K.H. Wong
Wallace C. Wu

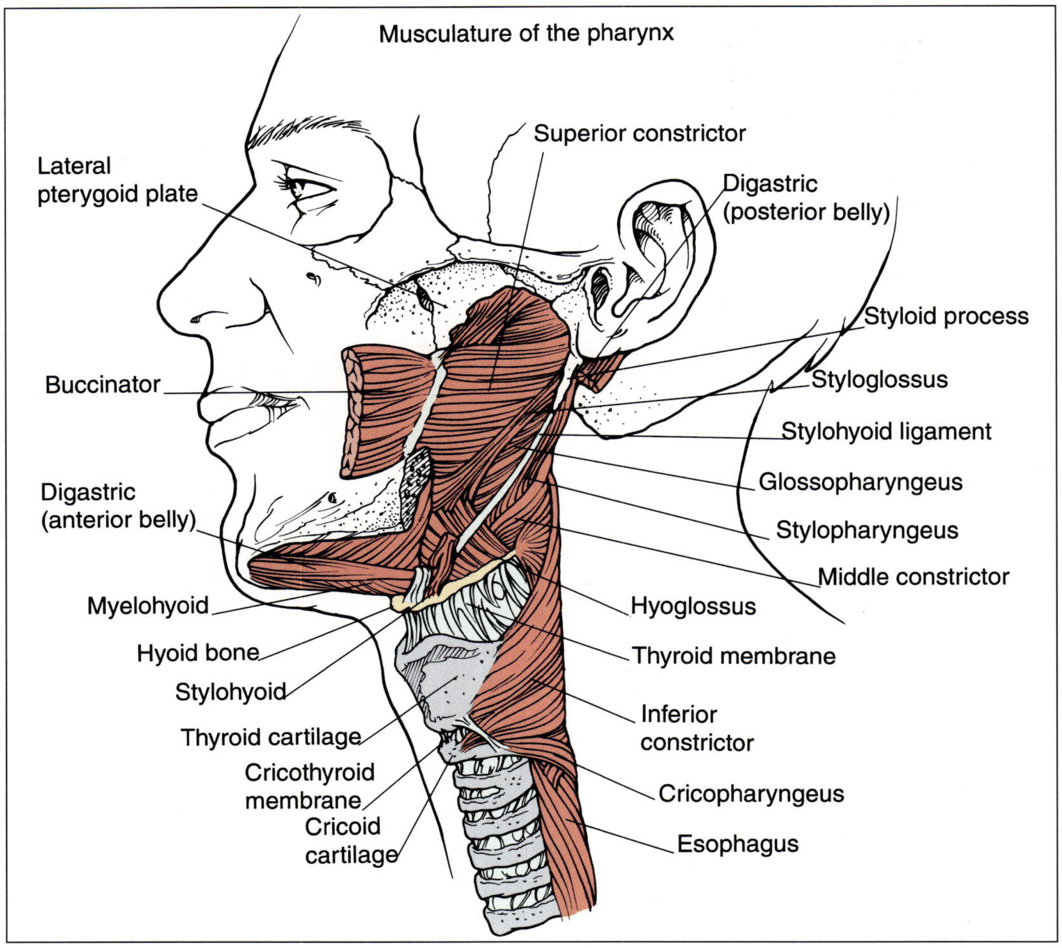

FIGURE 1-1.

Musculature of the oral cavity, pharynx, larynx, and proximal esophagus as displayed in a cutaway view. The oral cavity, pharynx, and larynx are all involved in transferring food from the mouth to the esophagus. Within the oral cavity, the lips, teeth, tongue, soft palate, mandible, and floor of the mouth serve various functions in chewing and manipulating food to create a bolus that is suitable for transfer to the pharynx. The walls of the oropharynx are composed of the superior, middle, and inferior constrictors posteriorly and the base of the tongue, which opposes constrictors anteriorly. The superior constrictor arises from the pterygoid hamulus, pterygomandibular raphe, mandible, and tongue, passes posteromedially, and inserts into the posterior median raphe. The middle constrictor arises from the hyoid bone and stylohyoid ligament, passes posteromedially, and also inserts into the posterior median raphe. The inferior constrictor is composed of the thyropharyngeus superiorly and the cricopharyngeus inferiorly. The thyropharyngeus arises from the thyroid cartilage and passes posteromedially to insert into the median raphe. The cricopharyngeus, however, has superior and inferior components that arise from both sides of the cricoid lamina such that the superior fibers course posteromedially to the median raphe and the inferior fibers loop around the esophageal inlet without a median raphe. The cricopharyngeus muscle separates the pharynx from the esophagus.

The pharyngeal walls are supported by attachments to the epiglottic, arytenoid, cuneiform, corniculate, and cricoid cartilages. The larynx and trachea are suspended in the neck between the hyoid bone superiorly and the sternum inferiorly. The laryngeal strap muscles contribute to this suspension and the intrinsic elasticity of the trachea permits the larynx to be elevated and lowered. The hyoid bone serves as the base for the tongue and is positioned as a fulcrum, crucial in directing forces anteriorly and superiorly toward the larynx, and hence, esophageal inlet. Laryngeal movement is critical in permitting the swallow response as the laryngeal inlet is closed and physically removed from the bolus path during the course of the swallow. Failure to achieve laryngeal elevation can result in aspiration of solids and liquids. (*Adapted from* Kahrilas [1].)

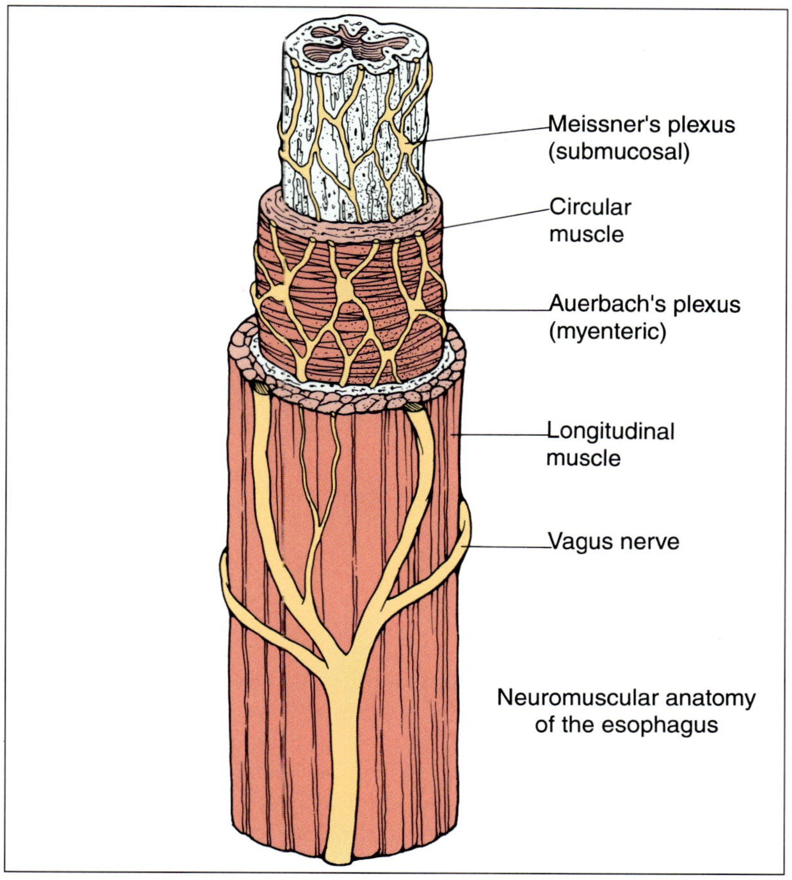

FIGURE 1-2.

Cutaway view showing anatomy of the tubular esophagus. The esophagus is a muscular tube that is composed of longitudinal and circular muscle with extensive neural network in between. Auerbach's plexus (myenteric) lies between the longitudinal and circular muscle layers. Another nerve network, Meissner's plexus (submucosal), is situated between the muscularis mucosa and the circular muscle layer. Note that there is no serosa to the esophagus and that the lumen is collapsed and empty. In fact, activity of both esophageal sphincters preserves the vacuum of the esophagus; the upper esophageal sphincter acts to exclude air during respiration and the lower esophageal sphincter excludes gastric contents from refluxing back into the esophagus. (*Adapted from* Kahrilas [1].)

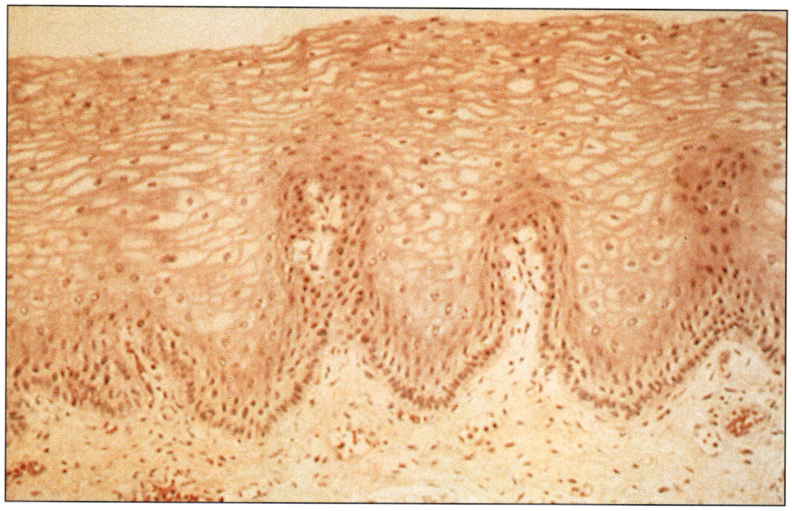

FIGURE 1-3.

Normal histology of the esophagus. The lining of the esophagus is a partially or nonkeratinized stratified squamous epithelium that overlies the connective tissue of the submucosa and the thick circular and longitudinal muscle layers (not shown). (*Courtesy of* Dr. Sambastiva Rao, Northwestern University Medical School.)

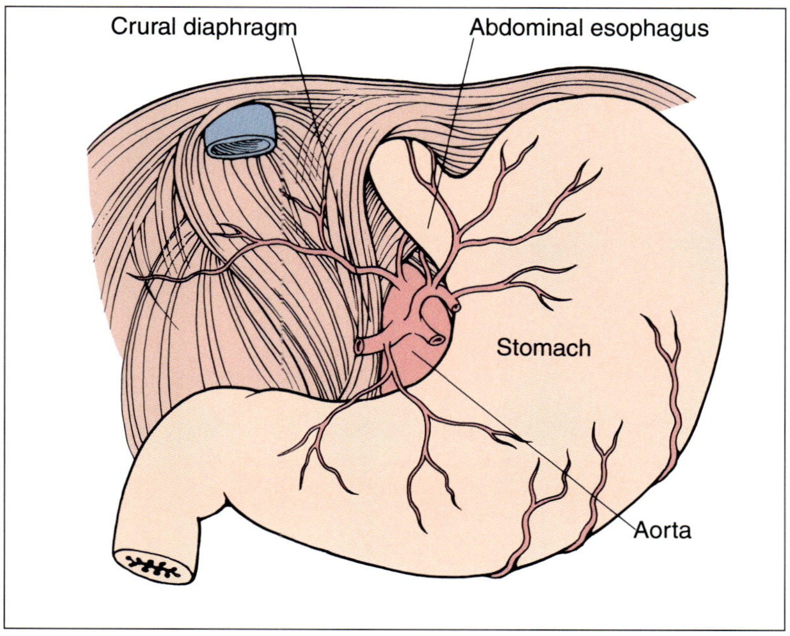

FIGURE 1-4.

Anatomy of the gastroesophageal junction highlighting the relationship between the diaphragm and the lower esophageal sphincter (LES). The esophagus, vagal trunks, and esophageal branches of the left gastric vein traverse the diaphragm through the esophageal hiatus. The crural fibers of the diaphragm encircle the esophagus in such a manner that a contraction of the muscle during inspiration constricts the esophagus.

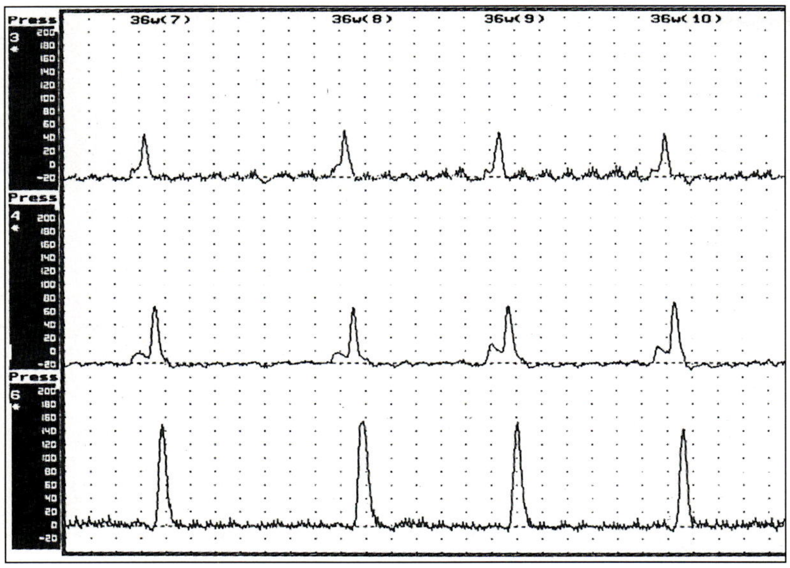

FIGURE 1-5.

Normal manometric tracing from within the esophageal body. Recording sites are located at 3 cm (bottom tracing), 8 cm (middle tracing), and 13 cm (top tracing) above the lower esophageal sphincter (LES). A series of four water swallows is illustrated, demonstrating the sequential contraction pattern of typical peristalsis in the distal esophagus. Amplitudes in the distal two recording sites vary between approximately 60 and 150 mm Hg and represent a typical average pressure of approximately 100 mm Hg.

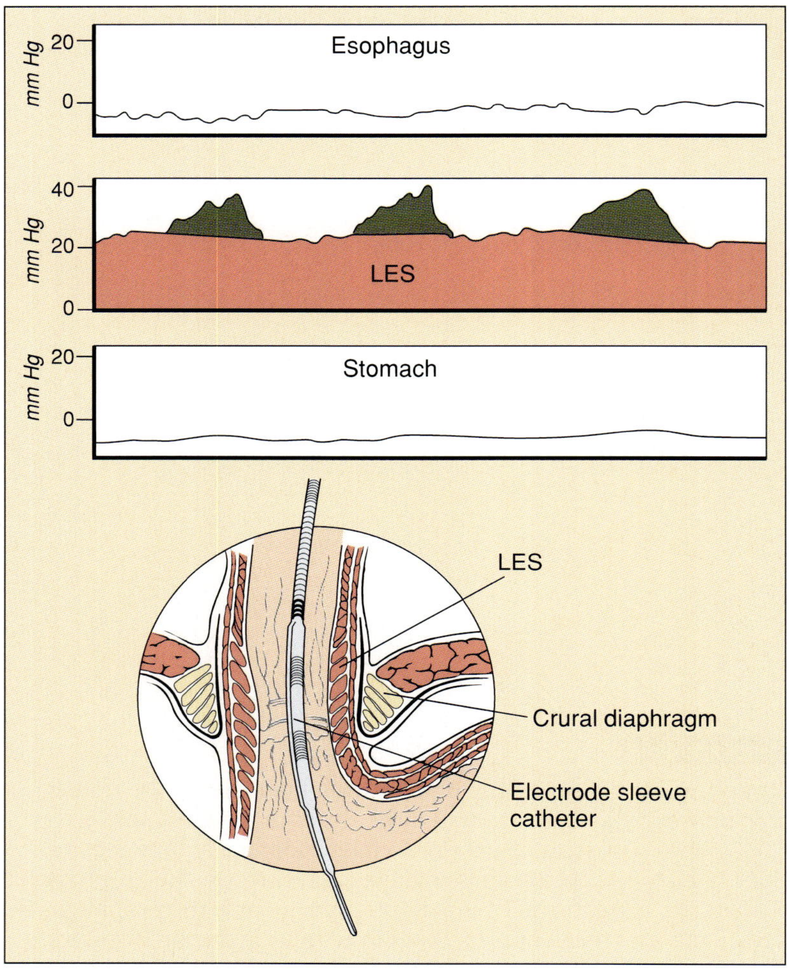

FIGURE 1-6.

Intrinsic lower esophageal sphincter (LES) pressure. The LES is a 3- to 4-cm segment of tonically contracted smooth muscle with a resting tone that varies from 10 to 30 mm Hg relative to gastric pressure. This positive pressure gradient between the stomach and the esophagus can be considered the driving force for gastroesophageal reflux, with the high pressure zone at the gastroesophageal junction considered a barrier to the prevention of reflux of gastric contents. The high pressure zone has two components: (1) a tonic pressure caused by the LES, which is believed to be caused by a combination of myogenic factors, active tonic neural excitation, and complex interactions of other neural and hormonal factors [2], and (2) superimposed phasic pressure oscillations resulting from contractions of the diaphragmatic crus that encircles the LES [3–6].

This figure shows the contribution of diaphragm contraction (green portion) to basal LES pressure (orange portion). Note that a significant component of LES pressure is contributed by the diaphragm and that augmentation of the LES pressure corresponds temporally and quantitatively with the augmentation of crural electromyographic activity. (*Courtesy of* Dr. R. Mittal, Charlottesville, VA.)

DIAGNOSIS: RADIOLOGY VS. ENDOSCOPY

RADIOLOGY VS. ENDOSCOPY IN ESOPHAGEAL DISEASES

	Radiology	Endoscopy
Oropharyngeal dysphagia	++++	—
Cervical web	++++	++
Extrinsic compression	++++	+
Esophageal diverticula	++++	+++
Carcinoma	++++	++++
Acute caustic injury	—	++++
Pill-induced injury	++	++++
Foreign body	+++	++++
Gastroesophageal reflux disease*	++	+++
Peptic stricture	++++	++++
Barrett's epithelium	++	++++
Lower esophageal mucosal ring	++++	+++
Infectious esophagitis	+++	++++
Varices	+++	++++
Achalasia	++++	++
Diffuse esophageal spasm	++	—
Nonspecific esophageal motor dysfunction	++	—

*As defined by 24-hour pH monitoring.
+—poor sensitivity; ++—fair sensitivity; +++—good sensitivity; ++++—excellent sensitivity.

Figure 1-7.

Comparison of diagnostic accuracy of radiology with that of endoscopy. Endoscopy is superb for mucosal lesions and has biopsy and therapeutic potentials. On the other hand, the role of endoscopy in the diagnosis of esophageal motor disorders is limited. For this reason, in patients with dysphagia caused by both solids and liquids, it may be more appropriate to obtain an esophagogram as the initial diagnostic procedure. An esophagogram also enables clinicians to rule out oropharyngeal causes of dysphagia that cannot be assessed with endoscopy.

INDICATIONS FOR ENDOSCOPY OF THE ESOPHAGUS

Diagnostic

- Dysphagia and odynophagia
- Certain patients with suspected gastroesophageal reflux disease
- Patients with suspected infectious esophagitis
- Cancer surveillance (eg, Barrett's esophagus)
- Abnormal results of barium esophagogram

Therapeutic

- Dilatation of strictures, both benign and malignant
- Sclerotherapy and banding of varices
- Stent placement in palliative therapy of malignant stricture
- Laser therapy of esophageal and gastroesophageal malignancies
- Removal of foreign body

Figure 1-8.

Almost all patients with esophageal symptoms should be evaluated initially with a barium esophagogram and endoscopy. Probably not all patients with suspected gastroesophageal reflux disease require endoscopy. The major advantages of endoscopy over barium esophagogram are that endoscopy not only provides biopsy capabilities but also has other therapeutic potentials. Removal of foreign bodies, esophageal dilatation with a guide wire, sclerotherapy and banding of varices, and palliative treatment of esophageal neoplasms can all now easily be done using the endoscope.

CONTRAINDICATIONS TO ENDOSCOPY

Absolute Contraindications	Relative Contraindications
Patients who are unable to cooperate	Patients with large Zenker's diverticulum
Patients who are moribund	Dysphagic patient who has not had an esophagogram recently
Patients with suspected perforated viscus	
Patients who are hemodynamically unstable	

FIGURE 1-9.

In general, endoscopy can be safely performed in almost all patients. It should, however, not be used in uncooperative and moribund patients. It should also not be performed in patients with a suspected perforated viscus because the nonsterile instrument and air insufflation needed to perform the procedure will more than likely aggravate mediastinal or peritoneal contamination. In a patient with Zenker's diverticulum the endoscope could preferentially pass through the diverticulum rather than through the esophagus. Hence, in this situation the endoscope should be passed carefully under direct vision. Perforation of a Zenker's diverticulum has been reported. It may be more appropriate to obtain an esophagogram before endoscopy in a patient with dysphagia.

ESOPHAGEAL MOTILITY DISORDERS

A. CLASSIFICATION OF PRIMARY ESOPHAGEAL MOTILITY ABNORMALITIES

Diagnosis	Motility Findings
Achalasia (the true disorder)	Absent distal peristalsis
	Incomplete LES relaxation (residual pressure > mm Hg)
	Elevated resting LES pressure (> 45 mm Hg)
	Increased baseline esophageal pressure
Abnormal Motility Patterns (nonspecific esophageal dysmotility)*	
Diffuse esophageal spasm	Simultaneous contractions (≥20% wet swallows)
	Intermittent peristalsis
	Repetitive contractions (≥3 peaks)
	Prolonged duration contractions (> 6 sec)
Hypercontracting esophagus	
Hypertensive peristalsis (nutcracker esophagus)	Increased distal peristaltic amplitude (> 180 mm Hg)
	Increased distal peristaltic duration (> 6 sec)
Hypertensive LES	Resting LES pressure > 45 mm Hg
	May be incomplete LES relaxation (residual pressure > 8 mm Hg)
Hypocontracting esophagus	
Ineffective motility†	Increased nontransmitted peristalsis (≥ 30%)
	Low distal peristaltic amplitude (< 30 mm Hg)
Hypotensive LES †	Resting LES pressure (< 10 mm Hg)
Others	Retrograde contractions
	Triple-peaked contractions
	Isolated incomplete LES relaxation (> 8 mm Hg)

*Defined as exceeding two standard deviations from the mean of normal values.
†May be "secondary" to gastroesophageal reflux disease.

FIGURE 1-10.

Classification of esophageal motility abnormalities. Traditionally, esophageal motility abnormalities have been divided into primary (occurring without associated diseases), representing abnormalities limited to the esophagus (**A**),

(continued on next page)

B. CLASSIFICATION OF SECONDARY ESOPHAGEAL MOTILITY ABNORMALITIES

Diagnosis	Motility Findings
Systemic sclerosis	Loss of distal (smooth muscle) peristalsis Weak LES pressure (< 10 mm Hg) Normal proximal esophagus and UES (striated muscle)
Chagas' disease	Identical to idiopathic achalasia (see above)
Diabetes mellitus	A variety of motility abnormalities of the esophageal body
Chronic idiopathic intestinal pseudo-obstruction	Loss of distal esophageal motility
Chronic gastroesophageal reflux disease	Ineffective motility Hypotensive LES

FIGURE 1-10. (CONTINUED) or secondary, defined as esophageal involvement in a patient with an associated systemic disease (**B**). LES—low esophageal sphincter; UES—upper esophageal sphincter.

Achalasia

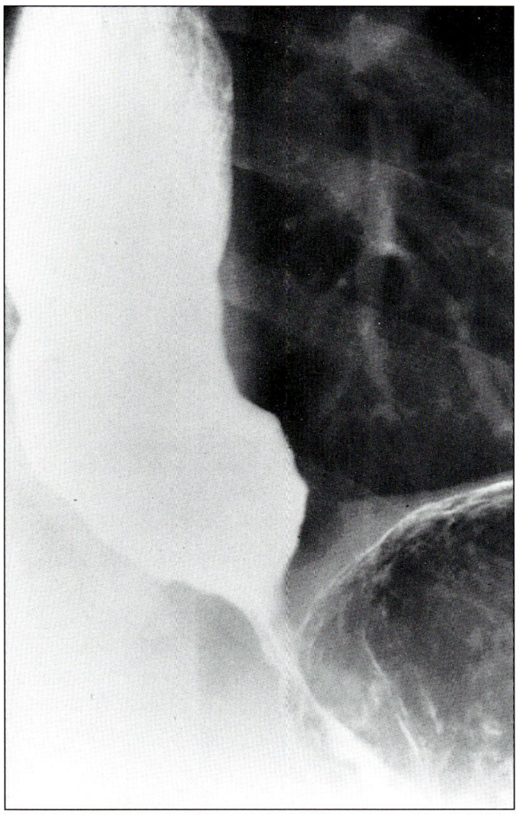

FIGURE 1-11. Barium esophagogram and endoscopy are complementary to each other in the diagnosis of esophageal diseases. This figure represents the lower esophagus of a patient with dysphagia. Esophagogram showed a bird's beak appearance of the gastroesophageal junction and total aperistalsis of the esophageal body consistent with the diagnosis of achalasia.

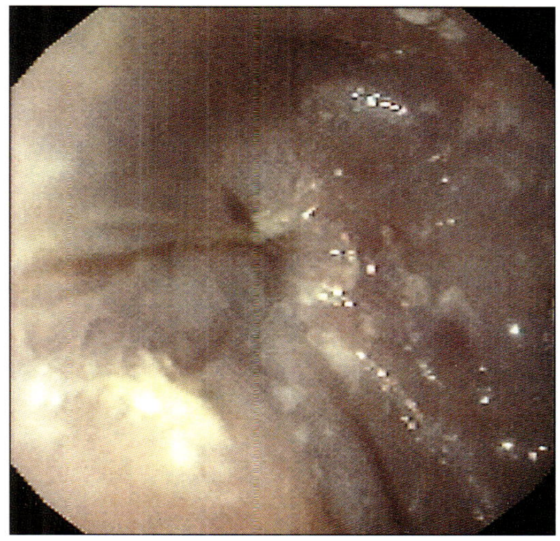

FIGURE 1-12. Classic rosette appearance of the gastroesophageal junction in a patient with documented achalasia. This finding is caused by the tightly closed lower esophageal sphincter.

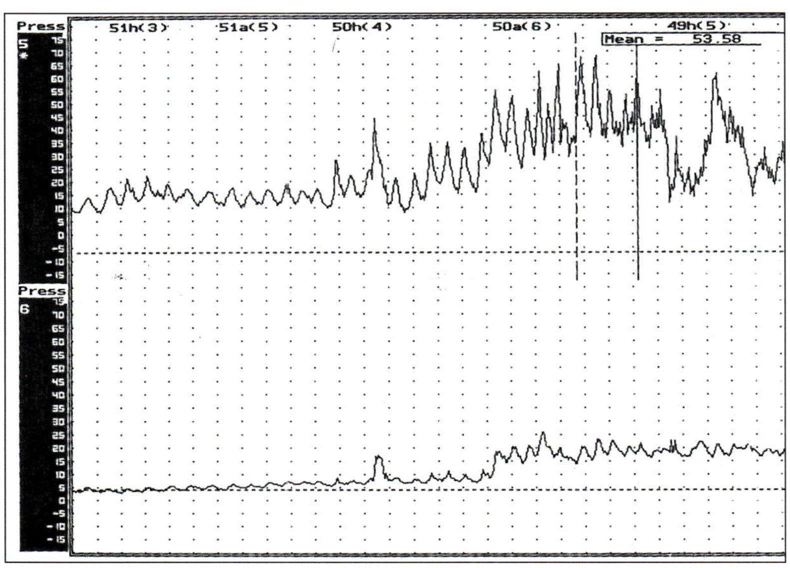

FIGURE 1-13. Manometric tracing of a pull through into the lower esophageal sphincter (LES) in a patient with achalasia. Note the high resting LES pressure of approximately 54 mm Hg. During water swallows (right side of tracing) relaxation is incomplete, with a residual pressure of approximately 20 mm Hg. The bottom tracing shows the trailing transducer moving into the LES.

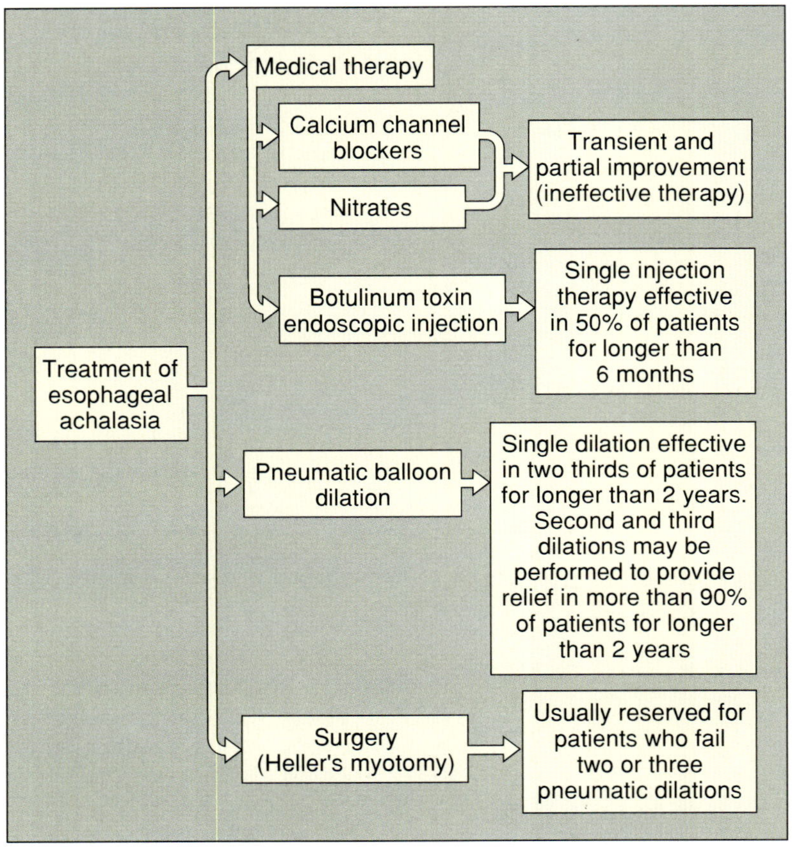

FIGURE 1-14.

Algorithm for treatment of esophageal achalasia. Achalasia of the esophagus can be treated either medically or surgically. Smooth muscle relaxants, nitrate, and calcium channel blockers reduce laser esophageal sphincter pressure and improve dysphagia symptom. Injection of botulinum toxin can also reduce sphincter pressure and improve esophageal emptying; however, standard therapy for achalasia is pneumatic dilation. Patients with recalcitrant symptoms, despite medical therapy, require surgical myotomy.

Diffuse esophageal spasm

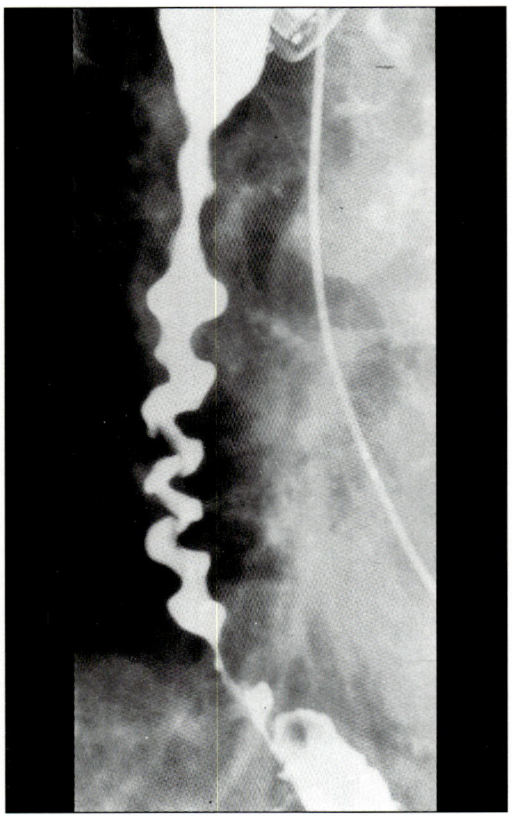

FIGURE 1-15.

Endoscopy is an excellent tool in the diagnosis of mucosal lesions. Unfortunately, it is unable to differentiate between normal and abnormal peristalsis and hence is insensitive in the diagnosis of motility disorders of the esophagus. This figure depicts the esophagogram of a patient with dysphagia and chest pain. His endoscopy is completely normal. Esophagogram shows classic changes of diffuse esophageal spasm. Esophageal manometry confirms the diagnosis.

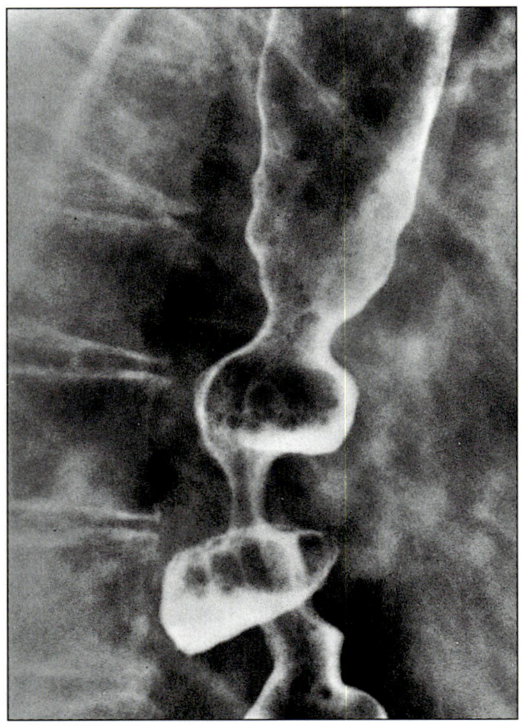

FIGURE 1-16.

Barium swallow study in another patient with diffuse esophageal spasm. Note the corkscrew or rosary-bead appearance along the length of the distal esophagus.

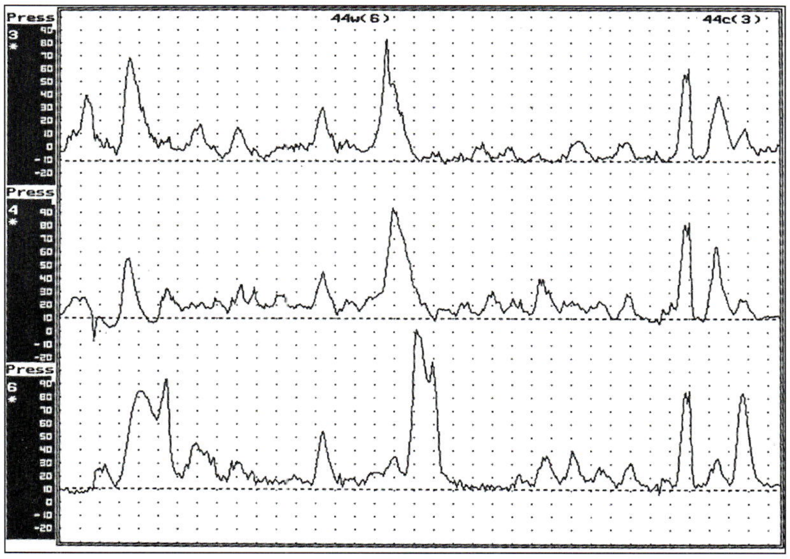

FIGURE 1-17.

Manometric tracing of a patient with diffuse esophageal spasm (DES). Recording sites are located at 3 cm (bottom tracing), 8 cm (middle tracing), and 13 cm (top tracing) above the lower esophageal sphincter. Variations in manometric responses (as shown in this patient) are quite typical of DES. On the left a spontaneously occurring simultaneous contraction is shown. This is followed by a swallow-induced peristaltic wave that appears normal. The final water swallow (on the right) shows simultaneous and repetitive contractions, which are typical of DES. This entity is characterized by increased numbers of simultaneous contractions after wet swallows (20% or more), but with intermittent normal peristaltic responses, as illustrated in this figure.

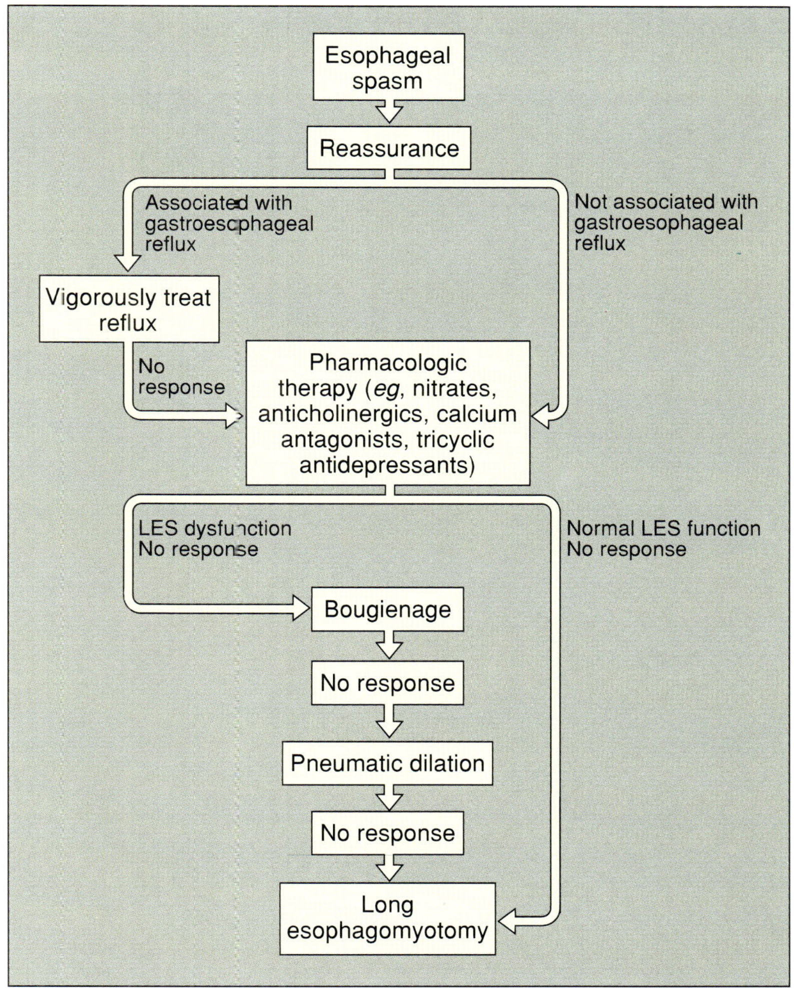

FIGURE 1-18.

Algorithm for the treatment of esophageal spasm. Infrequent symptoms caused by esophageal spasm are best treated by reassurance. Frequent symptoms require medical therapy with antireflux agents or smooth muscle relaxants. Surgical therapy is reserved for most symptomatic patients who are resistant to medical therapy.

Systemic sclerosis

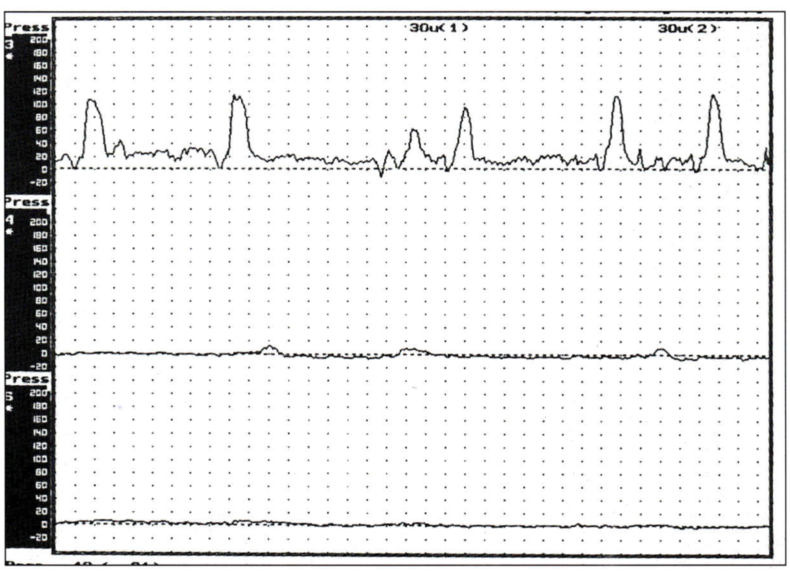

FIGURE 1-19.

Manometric tracing from a patient with systemic sclerosis. Recording sites are 1 cm (top tracing), 6 cm (middle tracing), and 11 cm (bottom tracing) below the upper esophageal sphincter. Contraction is regular in the proximal, striated muscle segment of the esophagus with each swallow, but transmission fails in the peristaltic contraction into the distal (smooth muscle) esophagus. Loss of smooth muscle peristalsis is typical of systemic sclerosis being a manifestation of the collagen replacement of the smooth muscle in this portion of the esophagus. Often the resting lower esophageal sphincter (LES) pressure is below normal. This combination of manometric events results in extreme acid reflux, often with markedly prolonged acid clearance because of the loss of peristaltic function in these patients. Skin findings are presented in Figure 1-72. (*From* Miller *et al.* [7]; with permission.)

CLASSIC SYMPTOMS OF ANGINA PECTORIS MAY BE INDISTINGUISHABLE FROM THOSE ARISING FROM ESOPHAGEAL CAUSES

Esophageal Chest Pain Usually:

Produces pressure-like squeezing or burning

Can radiate to neck, jaw, back, or arms

May persist minutes to hours

May be sharp and severe

Resolves or abates often spontaneously when treated with antacids or nitrates

Features in the History That Help to Distinguish Esophageal Pain from Cardiac Pain:

Atypical response to exercise

Pain that continued as a background ache

Retrosternal pain without lateral radiation

Pain that disturbed sleep

Presence of certain esophageal symptoms (*eg*., heartburn, regurgitation, dysphagia)

FIGURE 1-20.

Characteristics of esophageal chest pain. Consecutive patients presenting with chest pain on an emergency basis were interviewed before they were fully investigated; features tending to favor a cardiac or esophageal source were identified [8,9]. Although 83% of the esophageal group described having associated symptoms of heartburn, regurgitation, dysphagia, and vomiting, a finding confirmed by Hewson and coworkers [10], these symptoms were also experienced by 46% of patients with chest pain ultimately ascribed to a cardiac source. Although the chest pain of esophageal origin is often described as nonexertional, exercise-induced gastroesophageal reflux does occur with reproduction of angina-like chest pain in patients with normal coronary anatomy [11].

COMPARISON OF TEST RESULTS IN PATIENTS WITH NONCARDIAC CHEST PAIN (*N*=17)

	Omeprazole, 80mg	24-hr pH symptom index	Bernstein test	Placebo
Sensitivity (13)	69%	92%	46%	7.7%
Specificity (4)	75%	100%	50%	25%
Predictive value (+)	75%	100%	75%	25%
Predictive value (-)	43%	80%	78%	7.7%

FIGURE 1-21.

Single-dose omeprazole as a test for noncardiac chest pain (NCCP). In patients with either biopsy-proven esophagitis or positive symptom index to indicate an esophageal acid–related NCCP, the single-dose omeprazole test had similar efficacy to identify an acid sensitive esophagus as 24-hour pH monitoring with symptom index; it was superior to the Bernstein test [12]. A single 80-mg dose of omeprazole relieved chest pain symptoms in 10 of 17 patients with NCCP compared with 1 of 17 treated with placebo ($P < 0.015$) in this pilot study. Similar results for improvement of symptoms in patients with gastroesophageal reflux disease (GERD) and NCCP treated with high-dose ranitidine have been reported [13]. In a study of patients with nutcracker esophagus found at time of manometry, 35% had evidence of abnormal reflux and 83% of these patients obtained significant improvement of symptoms following 8 weeks of medical antireflux therapy, with less frequent pain episodes, fewer number of days with pain, and diminished pain severity [14]. (*Adapted from* Squillace *et al.* [12].)

ESOPHAGEAL MOTILITY DISORDERS IN NONCARDIAC CHEST PAIN

Achalasia
- Absent peristalsis in esophageal body*
- Incomplete LES relaxation*
- Hypertensive LES†
- Elevated intraesophageal pressures relative to gastric pressure†

Diffuse esophageal spasm
- Simultaneous contractions (>10% of wet swallows)*
- Intermittent normal peristalsis*
- Repetitive or prolonged contractions†
- High-amplitude and spontaneous contractions†
- LES hypertensive with or without incomplete relaxation†

Nutcracker esophagus
- Normal peristalsis*
- High-amplitude contractions*
- Long-duration contractions†

Hypertensive LES
- Elevated resting LES pressure*
- Normal LES relaxation*
- Normal peristalsis*

Nonspecific esophageal motility disorder (NEMD)
- Abnormal motility other than already noted*
- Nontransmitted contractions†
- Multiple-peaked contractions†
- Incomplete LES relaxation†
- Prolonged contractions†

**Required for diagnosis. †Associated findings.*

FIGURE 1-22.

Esophageal motility disorders in noncardiac chest pain. LES—lower esophageal sphincter.

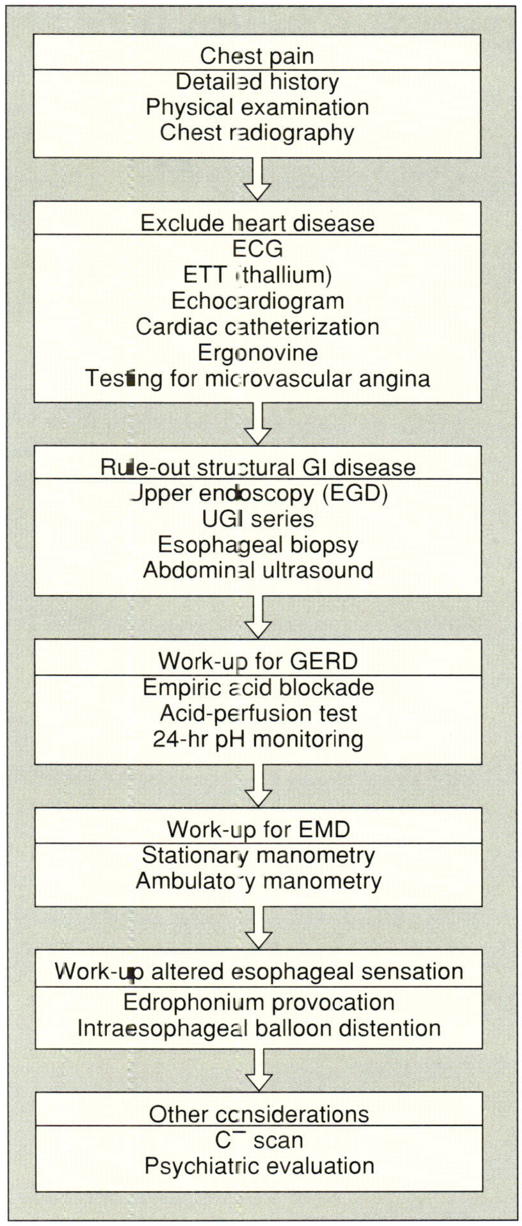

FIGURE 1-23.

Diagnostic approach to patients presenting with chest pain. CT—computed tomography; CXR—chest x-ray (radiography); EGD—esophagogastroduodenoscopy; ETT—exercise tolerance test; GERD–gastroesophageal reflux disease; GI—gastrointestinal.

UPPER ESOPHAGEAL DYSFUNCTION AND ZENKER'S DIVERTICULUM

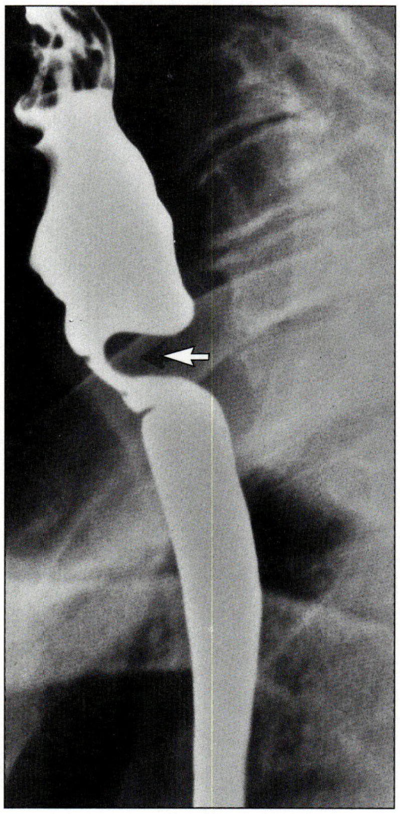

FIGURE 1-24.

Radiologic appearance of cricopharyngeal bar. The indentations (*arrow*) seen in the barium swallow, usually occurring at the level of cervical vertebra 4 or 5, represent either a nonrelaxing or a noncompliant upper esophageal sphincter. The patient usually has oropharyngeal dysphagia; however, asymptomatic individuals can have this radiologic finding.

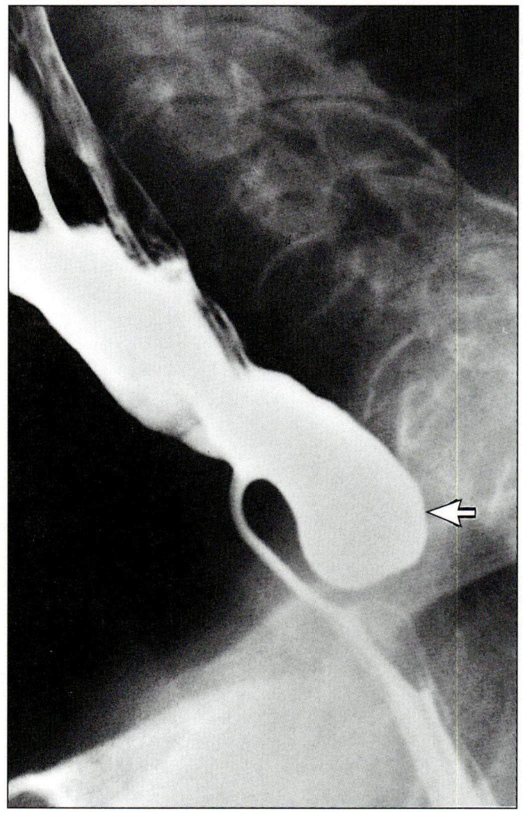

FIGURE 1-25.

Zenker's diverticulum. Radiograph of a 70-year-old patient with oropharyngeal dysphagia, coughing, choking spells, and recurrent pneumonia. Note the outpouching of the pharynx above the level of the cricopharyngeus (*arrow*). This outpouching is located in the posterior wall of the pharynx. Zenker's diverticulum is a true pulsion diverticulum and is the result of increased intrapharyngeal pressures during swallowing as a result of a noncompliant or nonrelaxing upper esophageal sphincter. There may be penetration of the barium into the laryngeal inlet and spilling into the tracheobronchial tree. The treatment of this condition in the setting of severe symptoms is usually cricopharyngeal myotomy.

GASTROESOPHAGEAL REFLUX DISEASE

Pathogenesis and epidemiology

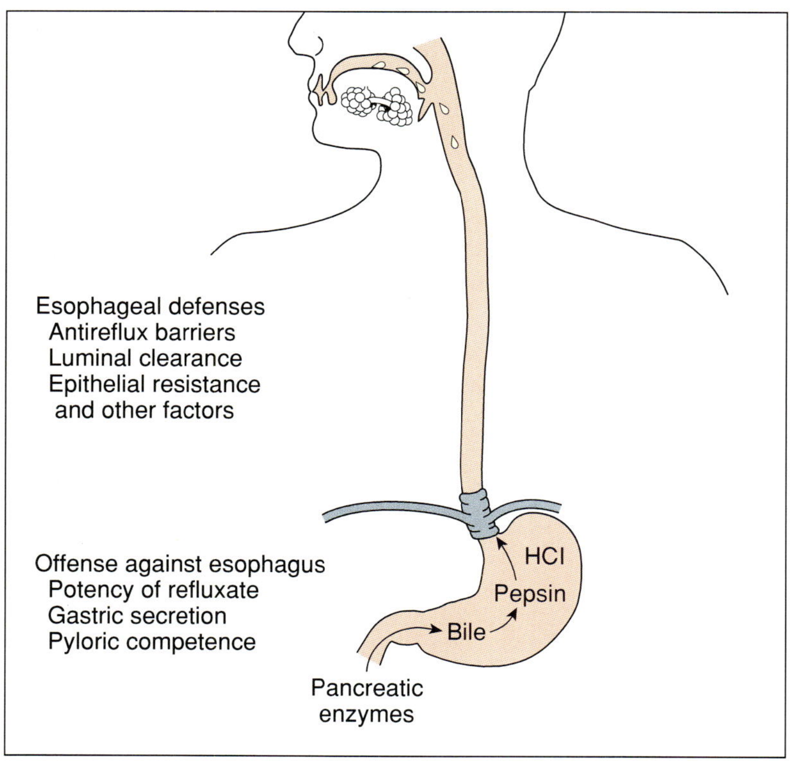

FIGURE 1-26.

Although the cause of reflux-induced esophageal disease is unknown, it involves abnormalities in one or more of the elements depicted in this figure. These elements include antireflux barriers to minimize reflux frequency, luminal clearance mechanisms to minimize duration of contact between epithelium and contents of the refluxate, and factors compromising tissue resistance to minimize damage during contact of epithelium with refluxate. HCl—hydrochloric acid. (*Adapted from* Orlando [15].)

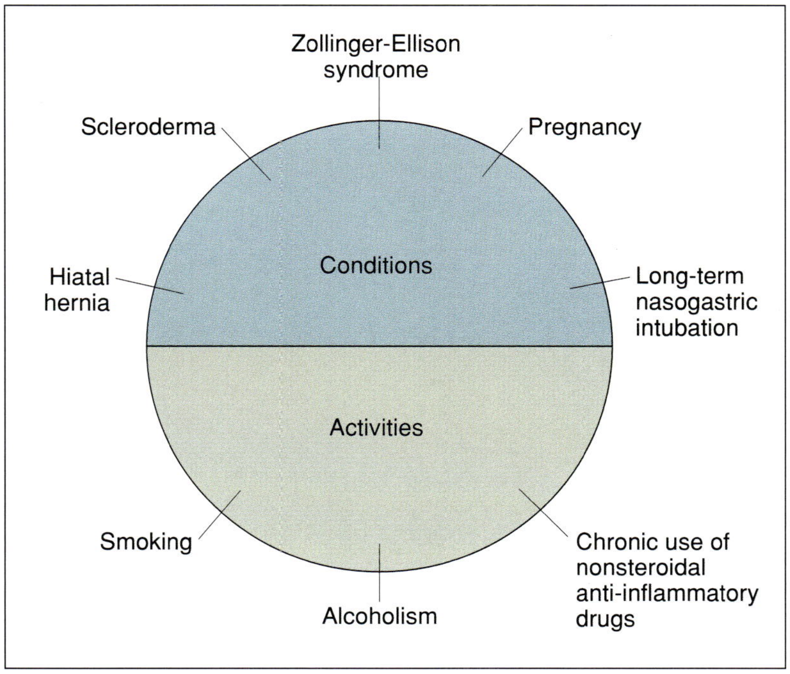

FIGURE 1-27.

Conditions and activities reported in association with reflux-induced gastroesophageal disease. This figure depicts those conditions and activities for which epidemiologic data suggest a relationship with the development of reflux esophagitis.

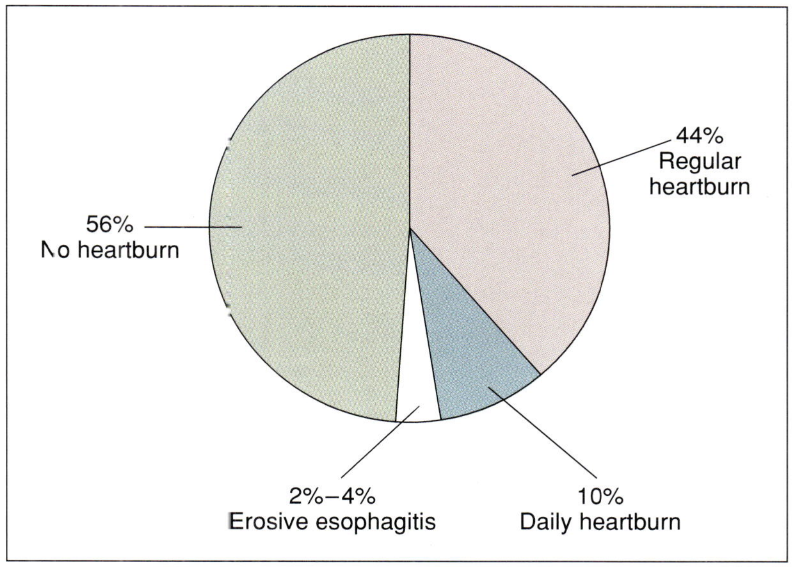

FIGURE 1-28.

The prevalence figures for symptomatic reflux (heartburn) and reflux (erosive) esophagitis for the adult U.S. population were extrapolated from data provided in the Gallup Organization National Survey, in reports by Nebel and associates, and by Rasmussen [16–18]. GERD has a 2–3:1 male:female predominance, and although common in whites, is uncommon in African Americans [19].

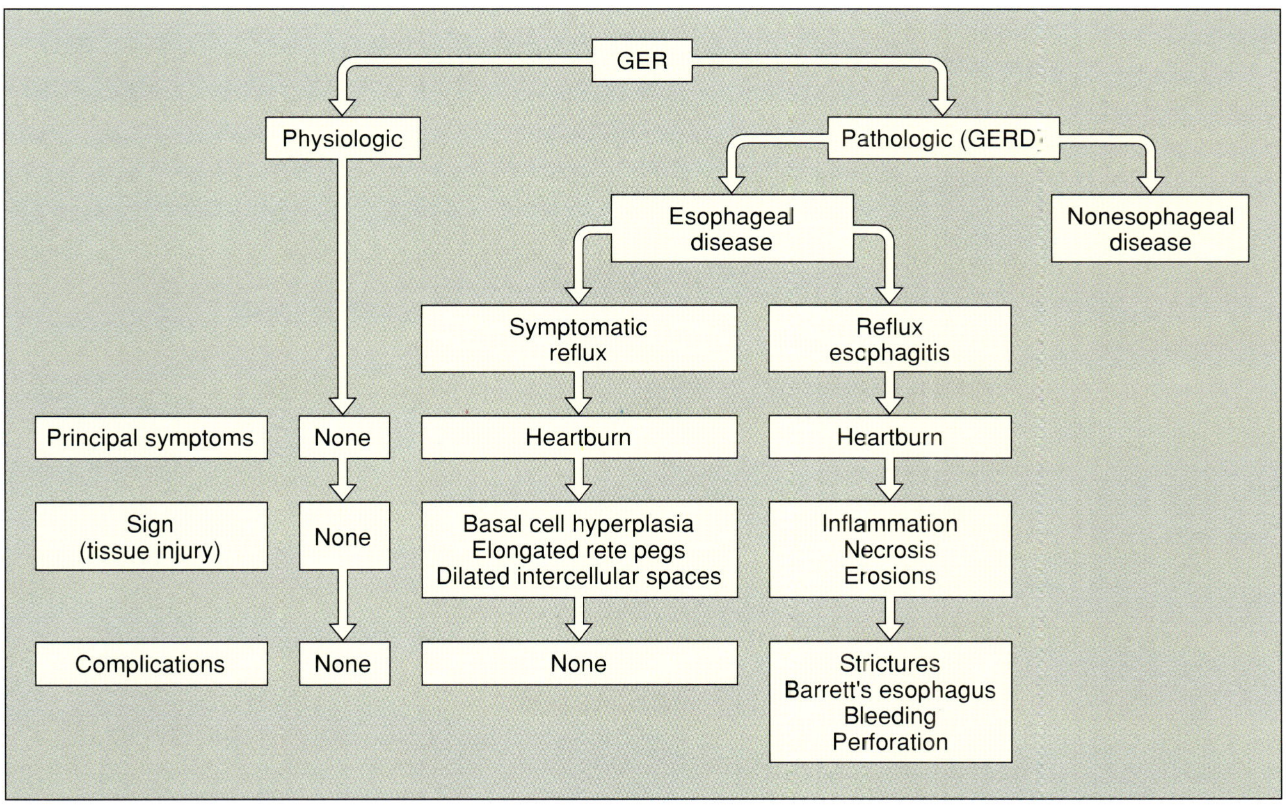

FIGURE 1-29.

The presumed relationship between the phenomenon of gastroesophageal reflux (GER) and gastroesophageal reflux disease (GERD) is depicted. GERD encompasses both nonesophageal and esophageal pathology, with esophageal pathology being subdivided into patients with "symptomatic reflux" and patients with "reflux esophagitis," based on the endoscopic or histologic demonstration of inflammation and necrosis.

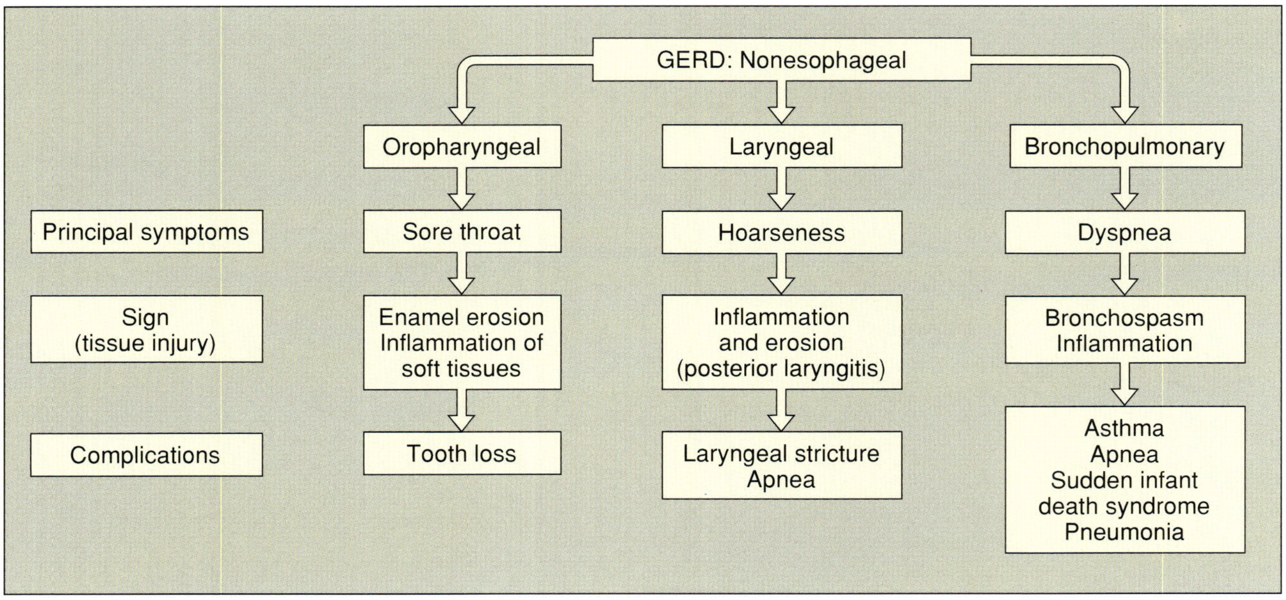

FIGURE 1-30.

The range of nonesophageal signs, symptoms, and complications attributed to GERD is depicted.

Diagnosis

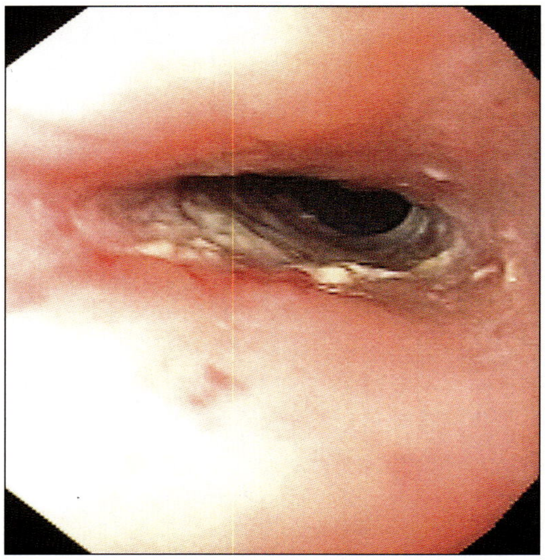

FIGURE 1-31.

Erosive esophagitis: endoscopic view. The hallmark of reflux esophagitis on endoscopy is the presence of one or more erosions within the distal esophagus [21]. Although the finding of such lesions is neither sensitive, (being found in less than 50% of those whose heartburn is explored endoscopically) nor specific (because they can occur with other esophageal injuries), the diagnosis is established by the chronicity of symptoms coupled with the typical nature of the lesions in the absence of other definable causes (*eg,* infectious or pill-induced esophagitis.)

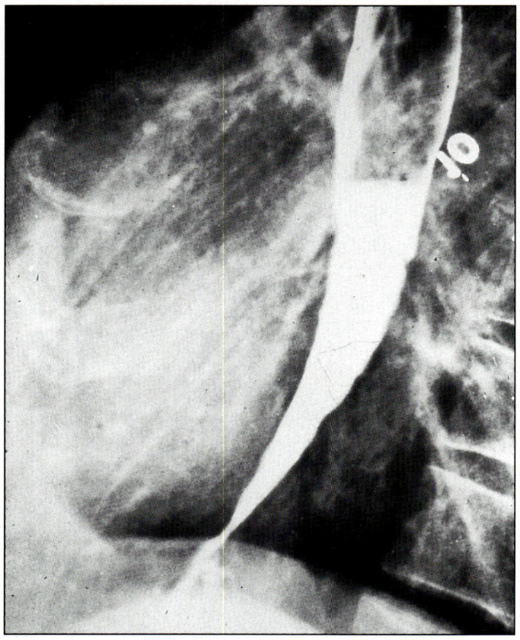

FIGURE 1-32.

Esophageal stricture. A barium esophagogram demonstrates the presence of a partially obstructing smooth-walled distal esophageal stricture secondary to reflux esophagitis. Patients with this complication may note amelioration of heartburn when a new symptom (*ie,* dysphagia for solid foods) becomes more pronounced. (*From* Orlando [15]; with permission.)

TESTS FOR DIAGNOSTIC ASSESSMENT OF GASTROESOPHAGEAL REFLUX DISEASE, ITS MECHANISMS, AND ITS CONSEQUENCES

Tests for reflux
- Upper gastrointestinal series
- Tuttle's (standard acid reflux) test
- Continuous intraesophageal pH monitoring
- Radionuclide (^{99}Tc) scintigraphy

Tests to assess symptoms
- Bernstein's (acid-perfusion) test
- Continuous intraesophageal pH monitoring

Tests to assess esophageal damage
- Barium esophagogram or upper gastrointestinal series
- Upper endoscopy
- Esophageal biopsy
- Esophageal potential difference measurement*

Tests to assess pathogenesis of esophagitis
- Acid clearance test*
- Radionuclide (^{99}Tc) scintigraphy*
- Esophageal manometry
- Gastric analysis

**Principally investigational.*

FIGURE 1-33.

Diagnostic testing in gastroesophageal reflux disease (GERD). Testing falls into four categories, depending on whether designed to document: (1) the presence and degree of reflux, (2) the relationship between reflux and atypical chest pain, (3) the type and extent of reflux-induced esophageal damage, or (4) the pathophysiology of reflux-induced disease [15]. (*Adapted from* Orlando [15].)

24-HOUR AMBULATORY pH VALUES FOR NORMAL SUBJECTS*

	Median	Range	95th percentile
Total, %	1.10	0–8.6	5.78
Upright, %	1.45	0–12.4	8.15
Supine, %	0.10	0–8.5	3.45
Total episodes (n)	18.0	0–101	46.00
Episodes > 5 min (n)	0	0–7	4.0
Longest episode, *min*	3.0	0–46	18.45

**n=110 Subjects (47 M, 63 W, mean age = 38 years).*
"%" refers to % of 24-hour pH study that distal esophagael pH dropped below 4.0 (measured 5 cm above proximal border of the manometrically located LES).

Figure 1-34.

Twenty-four-hour pH values for normal patients are shown in this table.

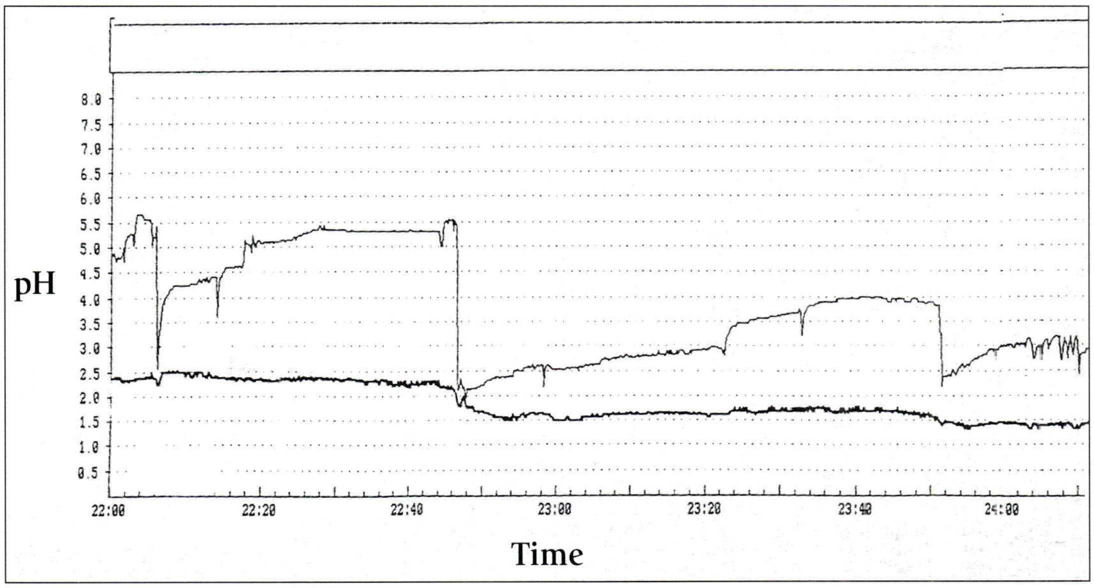

Figure 1-35.

Dual electrode pH recording on the computer screen showing esophageal (top tracing) and gastric (bottom tracing) pH in a patient with severe recumbent gastroesophageal reflux. Note the abrupt drop in pH followed by prolonged recovery, itself followed by additional episodes of reflux. This tracing demonstrates the markedly prolonged esophageal acid exposure time that occurs in patients with both recumbent reflux and prolonged acid clearance.

Barrett's esophagus

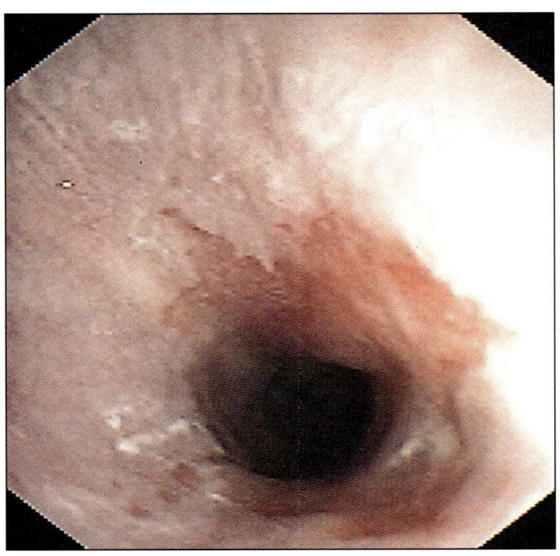

Figure 1-36.

Barrett's esophagus. The endoscopic appearance of a columnar-lined lower esophagus (*ie,* Barrett's) is shown for a patient with reflux esophagitis. The typical red coloration of the columnar epithelium is readily distinguished from the lighter pink or orange stratified squamous epithelium [20]. For a specific diagnosis, however, endoscopic biopsy is required for histologic confirmation of the nature of the epithelium lining the lower esophagus. Barrett's esophagus predisposes to esophageal adenocarcinoma, which occurs in 5% to 10% of patients.

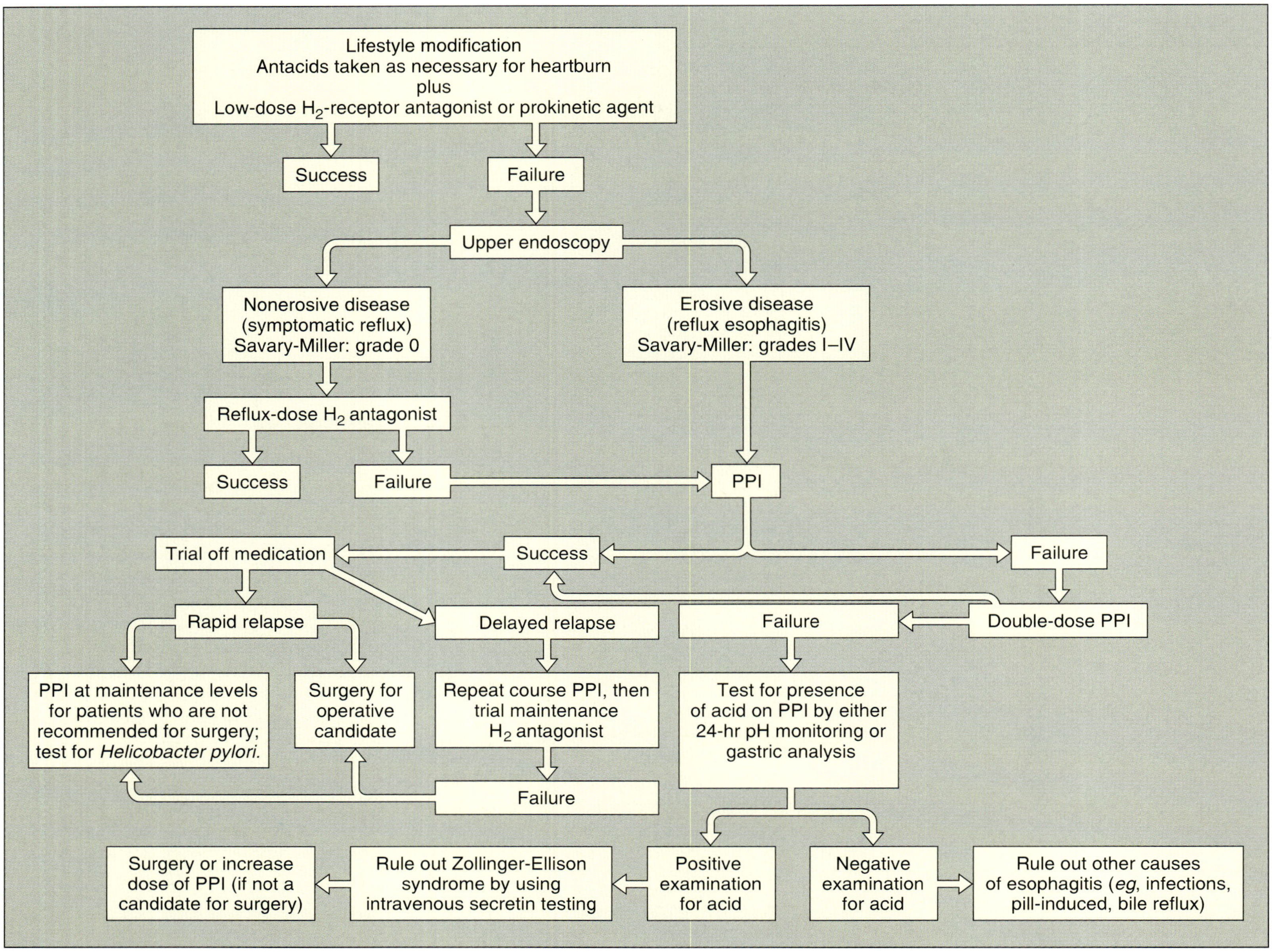

FIGURE 1-37.

Strategy for the management of esophagitis. This strategy uses a stepped approach to the treatment of heartburn. When patients require more than standard-dose H_2-receptor antagonists regularly for control of symptoms, endoscopy is recommended to evaluate for the presence of erosive disease, complications of reflux, such as Barrett's esophagus, and the presence of *Helicobacter pylori* gastric infection. Those with erosive esophagitis are treated with a proton pump inhibitor (PPI), and those without erosive disease are managed by increasing doses of the H_2-receptor antagonist. If antireflux doses of H_2-receptor antagonist are unsuccessful, a PPI is used. Failure of PPIs at twice their standard dose to control symptoms or heal lesions should prompt an assessment of whether they have effectively controlled gastric acid secretion (gastric analysis on therapy) or esophageal acidity (24-hr pH monitoring on therapy). Those that remain acid producers should have Zollinger-Ellison syndrome ruled out, and those that are achlorhydric should have other causes for esophageal disease ruled out (*eg*, infectious or pill-induced esophagitis). All patients on protracted therapy with high-potency acid suppressive medication should be evaluated for *H. pylori* infection, and if positive, therapy for its eradication should be employed to prevent the development of gastric atrophy.

MODIFICATIONS OF LIFESTYLE TO LESSEN REFLUX ESOPHAGITIS

Elevate the head of the bed 6"	Foods to avoid:	Drugs to avoid, when possible:
Stop smoking	Chocolate	Anticholinergics
Stop consuming excessive alcohol	Carminatives (spearmint, peppermint)	Theophylline
Reduce fat in diet	Coffee (caffeinated and decaffeinated)	Diazepam
Reduce size of meals	Tea	Narcotics
Avoid eating at bedtime	Cola beverages	Calcium channel blockers
Lose weight (if overweight)	Tomato juice	β-Adrenergic agonists (isoproterenol)
	Citrus juices	Progesterone (some contraceptives)
		α-Adrenergic antagonists (phentolamine)

FIGURE 1-38.

Medical management: lifestyle modifications. The commonly recommended lifestyle modifications are listed [21]. All patients will likely gain some benefit by elevating the head of the bed and by changing diet. The benefit-to-risk ratio of reducing or stopping medications prescribed for other active diseases should be carefully considered because reductions in lower esophageal sphincter pressure in most cases are modest; these agents have not been shown to produce reflux symptoms independently. (*Adapted from* Orlando [22].)

MANAGEMENT OF GASTROESOPHAGEAL REFLUX DISEASE BY PHARMACOTHERAPY

CONVENTIONAL DRUGS	DOSE	MECHANISM(S) OF ACTION*
Antacid: liquid (*eg*, Mylanta II/Maalox TC) (HCl neutralization, capacity 25 mEq/5 mL)†	15 mL/q.i.d. 1 h after meals and at bedtime	Buffer HCl ↑ LESP
Gaviscon (Al hydroxide, Mg trisilicate, $NaHCO_3$, Alginic acid)	2–4 tablets, q.i.d. after meals and at bedtime	↓ Reflux by viscous mechanical barrier Buffer HCl in esophagus
H_2-receptor antagonists		
Cimetidine (Tagamet)	800 mg b.i.d.	↓ HCl secretion, ↓ Gastric volume } by inhibiting H_2-receptor
Ranitidine (Zantac)	150 mg q.i.d./300 mg b.i.d.	
Famotidine (Pepcid)	20 mg b.i.d.	Same as cimetidine
Nizatidine (Axid)	150 mg b.i.d.	
Prokinetics		
Bethanechol (Urecholine)	25 mg q.i.d. 1/2 h before meals and at bedtime	↑ LESP ↑ Esophageal acid clearance
Metoclopramide (Reglan)	10 mg q.i.d.	↑ LESP
Cisapride	10 mg t.i.d. or q.i.d. 1/2 h before meals and at bedtime	↑ LESP, ↑ gastric emptying
Mucosa Protectant		↑ Gastric emptying
Sucralfate (Carafate)	1 g q.i.d. 1 h after meals and at bedtime	↑ Tissue resistance Buffer HCl in esophagus Bind pepsin and bile salts
Inhibitors of H^+-K^+-ATPase		
Omeprazole (Prilosec)	20 mg/day	↓ HCl secretion, ↓ gastric volume
Lansoprazole (Prevacid)	30 mg/day	↓ HCl secretion, ↓ gastric volume

**LESP—lower esophageal sphincter pressure; ↑—increase; ↓—decrease.*
†Note: Patients with reflux are generally not known to be hypersecretors of gastric acid. Therefore, therapeutic doses of antacids are based on capacity to buffer basal HCl secretion of approx. 1–7 mEq/hr (mean 2 mEq/hr) and peak meal-stimulated HCl secretion of approx. 10–60 mEq/hr (mean 30 mEq/hr).

FIGURE 1-39.

Medical management: pharmacotherapy. Commonly prescribed classes of medications used in the treatment of reflux esophagitis include antacids that act by buffering gastric acid, either within the esophageal lumen or stomach; H_2-receptor antagonists or proton pump inhibitors that act by inhibiting gastric acid secretion, thereby making the refluxate less noxious to the esophageal epithelium; prokinetics that act to increase smooth muscle contractility, thereby increasing lower esophageal sphincter pressure, amplitudes of esophageal peristaltic contractions, and the rate of gastric emptying; and mucosal protective agents that act on the epithelium to reduce the damaging action of acid and pepsin [15]. (*Adapted from* Orlando [15].)

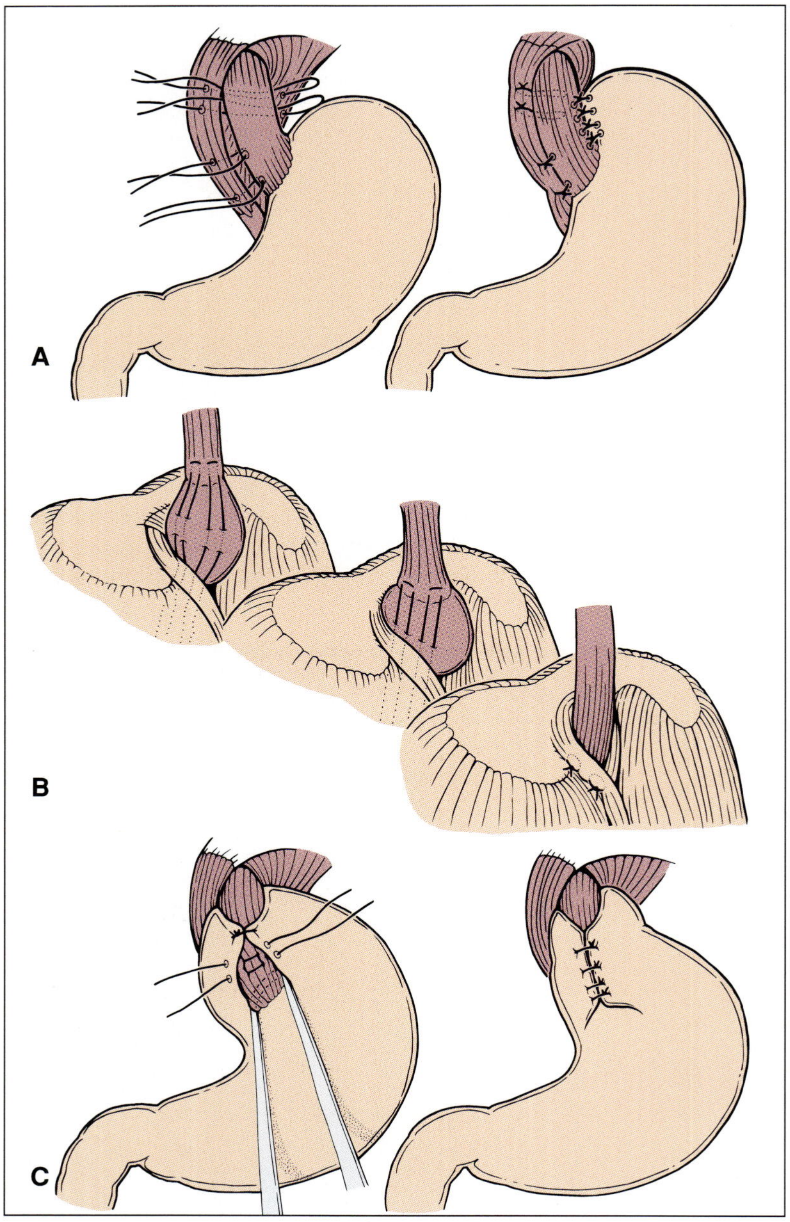

FIGURE 1-40.

Surgical management. The most commonly performed surgical procedures for gastroesophageal reflux disease include Hill's gastropexy (**A**), Belsey's fundoplication (**B**), and Nissen fundoplication (**C**) [20]. The Nissen procedure can be performed either as an open procedure or using a laparoscopic approach. (*Adapted from* Pope [23].)

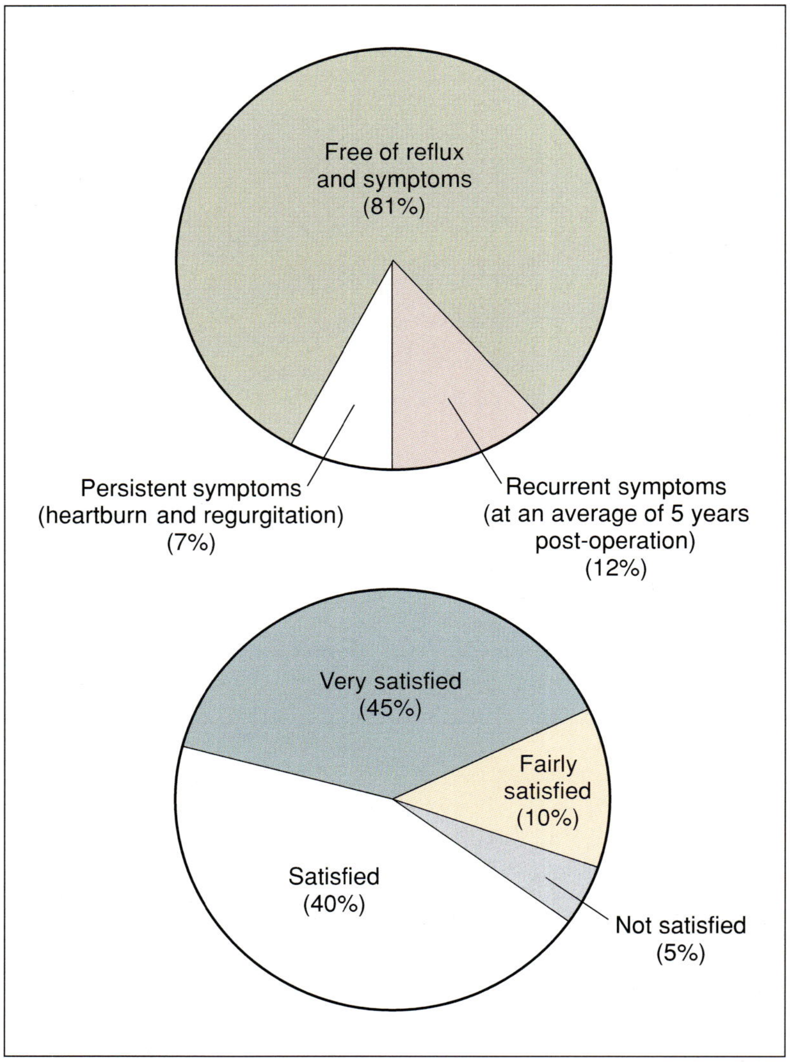

FIGURE 1-41.

Results of Nissen fundoplication 10 years after surgery. The results of transabdominal fundoplication for gastroesophageal reflux are excellent [24]. The most frequent postoperative side effects are change in mastication (food is chewed more completely), excessive flatus, and difficulty in belching. When the operation is performed using a 40-Fr bougie, dysphagia is a rare complication.

Candida

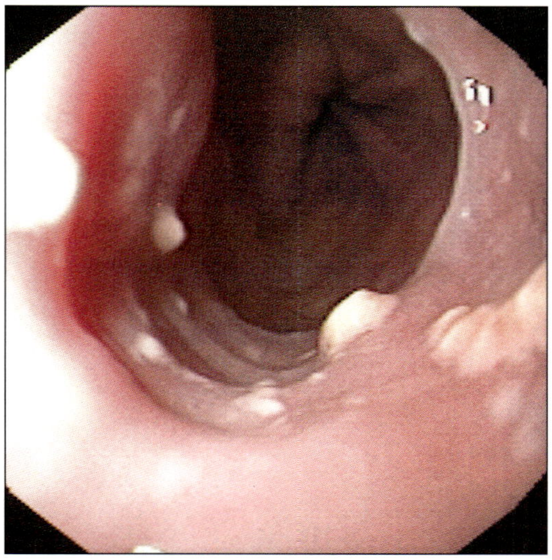

FIGURES 1-42.

Early findings of esophagitis caused by *Candida* with plaques not yet becoming confluent. As the infection worsens, there is associated hyperemia. (*Courtesy of* Dr. A. Tsuchida, Madigan Army Medical Center.)

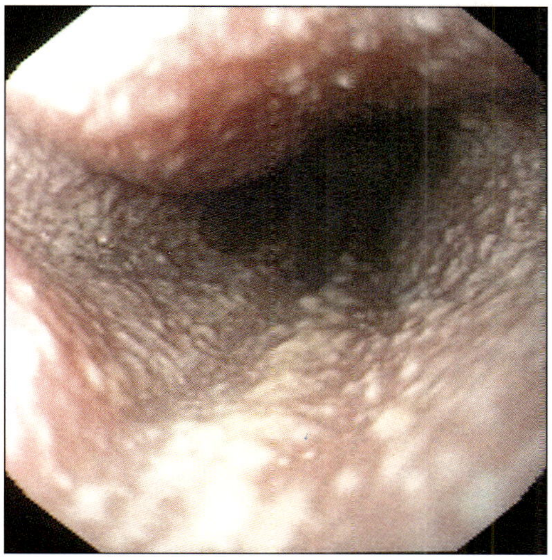

FIGURES 1-43.

Progression of esophageal disease caused by candidiasis. (*Courtesy of* Dr. M. Lyons, Madigan Army Medical Center.)

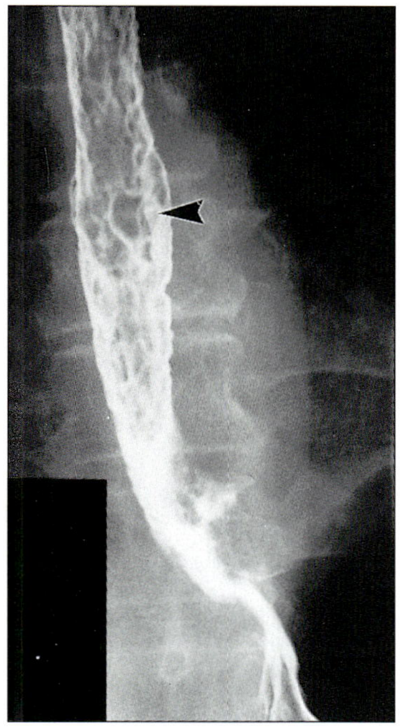

FIGURE 1-44.

Classic findings in acute esophagitis caused by *Candida*. Discrete plaque-like lesions, oriented longitudinally, producing linear or irregular filling defects with distinct margins (*arrowhead*).

TREATMENT OF *CANDIDA*-INDUCED ESOPHAGITIS

Drug formulation	No or minimal lymphocyte defects and normal granulocytes	Decreased lymphocyte function but normal granulocytes	Decreased granulocyte function
Oral, nonabsorbable drugs			
Nystatin suspension (1,000,000 units/mL)	1–3 MU orally, 4 times daily	Not applicable	Not applicable
Amphotericin B lozenge (10 mg) or suspension (100 mg/mL)*	1–2 lozenges or 1 mL suspension, 4 times daily	Not applicable	Not applicable
Miconazole oral gel (25 mg/mL)	10 mL orally, 4 times daily	Not applicable	Not applicable
Clotrimazole troches (10 mg)	**10 mg troche, dissolved in mouth 5 times daily**	Not applicable	Not applicable
Clotrimazole vaginal tablets (100 mg)	100 mg tablet, dissolved in mouth 3 times daily	100 mg tablet, dissolved in mouth 3–5 times daily	Not applicable
Oral, absorbable drugs			
Ketoconazole tablets (200 mg)	200 mg orally, once daily	400–800 mg orally, once daily	400–800 mg orally, once daily
Fluconazole capsules (50 or 100 mg)	50 mg orally, once daily	**100 mg orally, once daily**	100–200 mg orally, once daily
Flucytosine capsules (250 or 500 mg)†	Not applicable	Not applicable	50–150 mg kg^{-1} day^{-1}, at 6 hr intervals
Intravenous drugs			
Amphotericin B for IV use (5 mg/mL)	Not applicable	0.3 mg kg^{-1} day^{-1}, intravenously	**0.5 mg kg^{-1} day^{-1}, intravenously**
Fluconazole for IV use (2 mg/mL)‡	100 mg intravenously, once daily	100 mg intravenously, once daily	100–200 mg intravenously, once daily

*Not available in the USA.
†Not for use as a single agent. See text for discussion of the use of this drug.
‡When oral route is not available.
The therapy of choice under each column is given in bold.

FIGURE 1-45.

Treatment of esophagitis caused by *Candida*. (*Adapted from* Baehr and McDonald [25].)

Herpes simplex

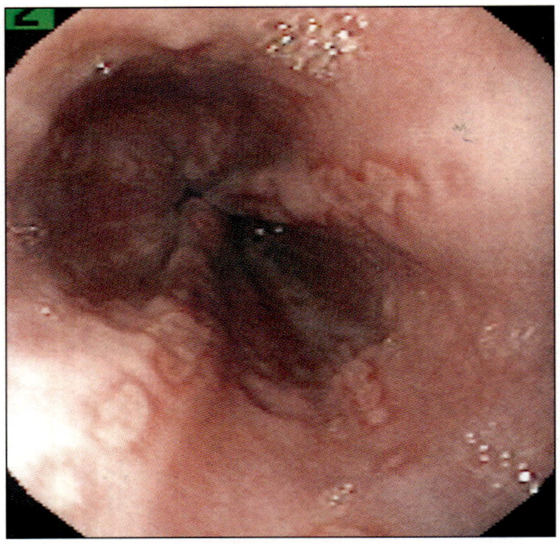

FIGURE 1-46.

Endoscopic findings in esophagitis caused by herpes simplex virus (HSV). In the necrotic phase of the disease process, diffuse esophagitis is noted with confluent esophageal ulcers. (*Courtesy of* Dr. K. Yamamoto, Madigan Army Medical Center.)

PREVENTION AND TREATMENT OF ESOPHAGITIS CAUSED BY HERPES SIMPLEX VIRUS (HSV)

DRUG FORMULATION	PREVENTION OF HSV INFECTION*	TREATMENT OF ESTABLISHED HSV INFECTION
Acyclovir, capsules (200 mg)	200–400 mg orally 4–5 times daily, or 800 mg orally twice daily	200–400 mg orally 5 times daily for 2 weeks
Acyclovir, for IV use (500 mg/10 mL vial, admixed to final concentration <7 mg/mL)	250 mg/m^2 every 12 hours IV	250 mg/m^2 every 8 hours IV for 2 weeks†
Foscarnet, for intravenous use (12 g/500 mL)‡	Not applicable	60 mg/kg every 8 hours (or 90 mg/kg every 12 hours) IV for 2 weeks, then 90–120 mg/kg daily for maintenance (if indicated)§

**For patients at risk.*
†Intravenous acyclovir therapy can be converted to oral route for completetion of induction therapy in responders.
‡For treatment of HSV resistant to acyclovir.
§Induction therapy should be extended if the patient has not completely responded and other etiologies are excluded.

FIGURE 1-47.

Current therapeutic strategies are based on the severity of disease and immune status of the patient. Clinical decisions must be made to determine if a patient is at significant risk to merit the use of prophylaxis. Options include supportive care, acyclovir or foscarnet. (*Adapted from* Baehr and McDonald [25].)

Cytomegalovirus

PREVENTION AND TREATMENT OF ESOPHAGITIS CAUSED BY CYTOMEGALOVIRUS

Drug formulation	Prevention of CMV infection*	Treatment of established CMV disease
Acyclovir, for IV use (500 mg/10 mL vial, admixed to final concentration <7 mg/mL)†	For seropositive patients‡ or recipients of organs from seropositive donors: 500 mg/m^2 BSA IV every 8 hours	Not applicable
Ganciclovir, for IV use (500 mg/10 mL vial, admixed to final concentration < 10 mg/mL)§	For seropositive patients‡ or recipients of organs from seropositive donors: 5 mg/kg every 12 hours IV for 5 days, then once daily as maintenance therapy	5 mg/kg every 12 hours IV for 2 weeks,¶ then once daily for maintenance (if indicated)
Foscarnet, for IV use (12 g/500 mL)	Not applicable	60 mg/kg every 8 hours (or 90 mg/kg every 12 hours) IV for 2 weeks,¶ then 90–120 mg/kg daily for maintenance (if indicated)
Epidemiologic methods	For seronegative patients: Transfusion of CMV seronegative blood products; Organ transplants from CMV seronegative donors; Leukofiltration of CMV seropositive blood products	

*For patients at risk.
†Adjust dose for renal function.
‡Marrow transplantation patients; trials of prophylactic ganciclovir for patients infected with HIV have not been completed.
§Use of oral ganciclovir formulations are under current study.
¶Induction therapy should be extended if the patient has not completely responded and other etiologies are excluded.

FIGURE 1-48.

Therapy for cytomegalovirus (CMV) can be given as prevention of disease in patients known to be immunocompromised or a therapy against established disease proven by tissue biopsy. Current therapy includes ganciclovir and acyclovir for prophylaxis and ganciclovir and foscarnet for treatment of established disease. In AIDS patients with biopsy-proven CMV esophageal ulceration, both ganciclovir and foscarnet therapy have been associated with endoscopically documented ulcer healing in some patients in 2 weeks or less. (*Adapted from* Baehr and McDonald [25].)

HIV

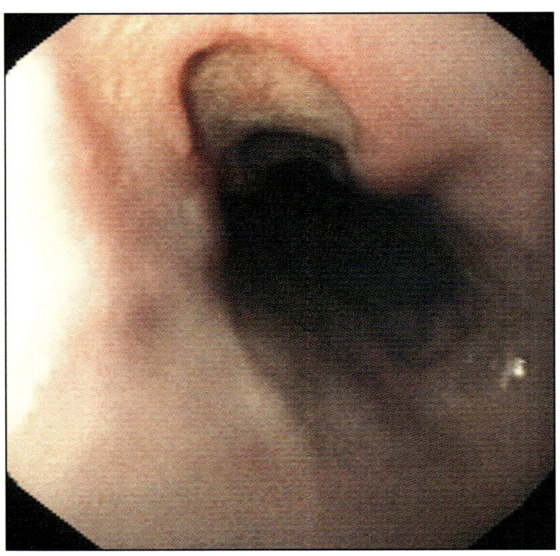

FIGURE 1-49.

The endoscopic characteristics of an esophageal ulcer caused by HIV are variable, ranging from small, superficial shallow aphthous ulcers (0.5 to 1.0 cm) to large, deep ulcers with undermining borders (1 to 5 cm). To be considered as an ulcer caused by HIV other causes of esophageal ulceration must be excluded. This endoscopic photograph demonstrates a large 6-cm chronic ulcer with deep undermining edges and nodularity within the ulcer base. Idiopathic HIV-associated ulcers have been treated with intravenous corticosteroid therapy. In one study, 23 of 24 patients (95.8%) improved. Relapses were common after discontinuation of therapy. To maintain remission, long-term therapy was required. Trials of sucralfate four times daily mixed with dexamethasone (0.5) mg given as a slurry have been promising. These results must be tempered by the risk of additional long-term immunosuppressive therapy.

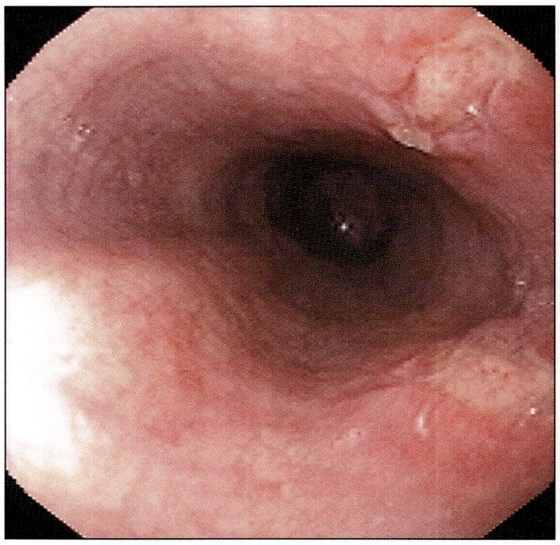

FIGURE 1-50.
Pill ulcer. A 25-year-old female was prescribed doxycycline for treatment of acne. After she developed dysphagia and odynophagia acutely, she remembered that she had taken a dose of doxycycline just before she went to bed the night before. Endoscopy showed two ulcers in the midesophagus. The history and endoscopic appearance are perfectly compatible with the diagnosis of esophagitis caused by medication in pill form.

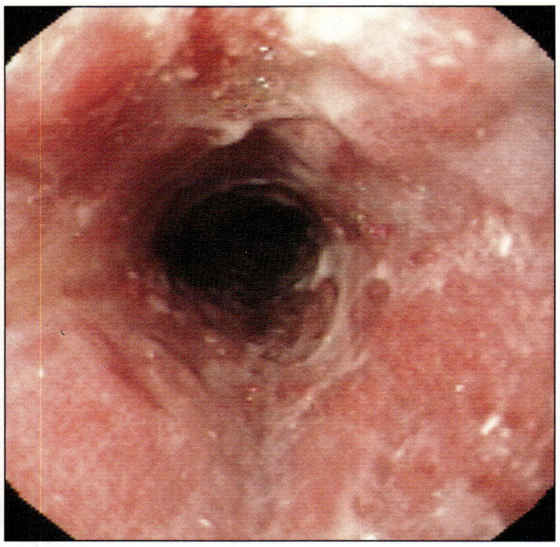

FIGURE 1-51.
Caustic injury. This endoscopic photograph demonstrates a desquamated esophageal epithelium from the middle to the distal esophagus. The likelihood of stricture formation in this patient with circumferential injury is high.

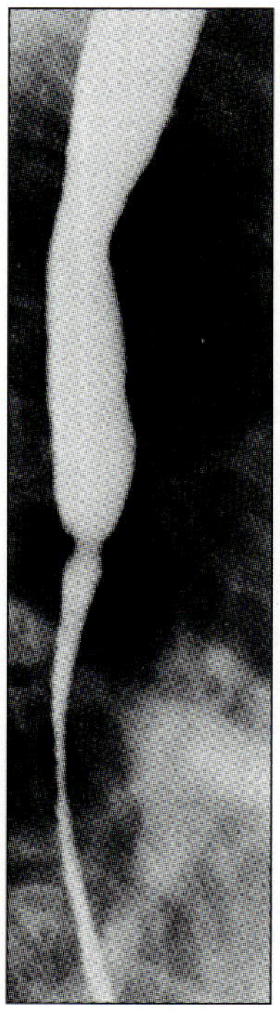

FIGURE 1-52.
Radiation esophagitis. Esophagitis induced by combined radiation and chemotherapy (doxorubicin). Patients often present during the third to fifth week of radiation therapy, although the natural history of the radiation injury may be altered with the coadministration of chemotherapeutic agents. Retrosternal burning, dysphagia, or odynophagia are typical symptoms that may be persistent and require supportive care to maintain hydration and nutrition. Additionally, patients must be considered for the possibility of superinfection with organisms such as *Candida*. High-grade stenosis involving about 9 cm of the distal esophagus with significant obstruction was found on examination 2 months after the onset of symptoms. The lumen of the stricture is irregular. The transition from the proximal esophagus, although abrupt, appears benign and is characterized by concentric narrowing. (*From* Boal *et al.* [26]; with permission.)

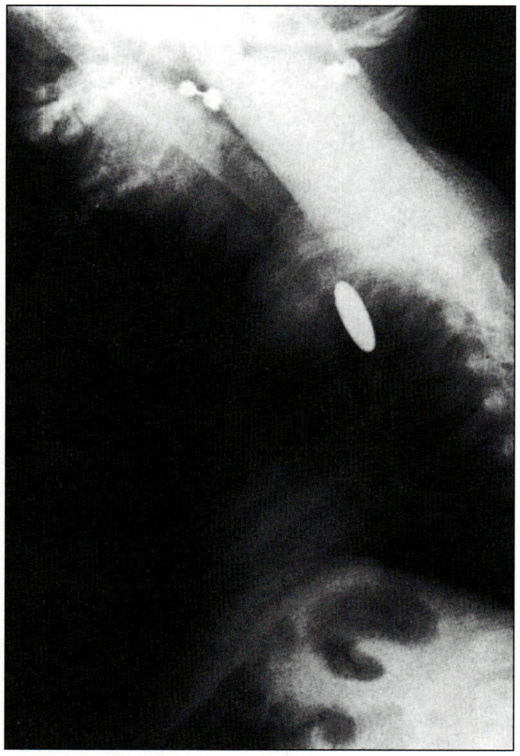

FIGURE 1-53.
Foreign body. Taking plain radiographic films of the neck when evaluating foreign body impaction is important. Note coin in the child's esophagus. (*From* Yoshida and Peura [27]; with permission.)

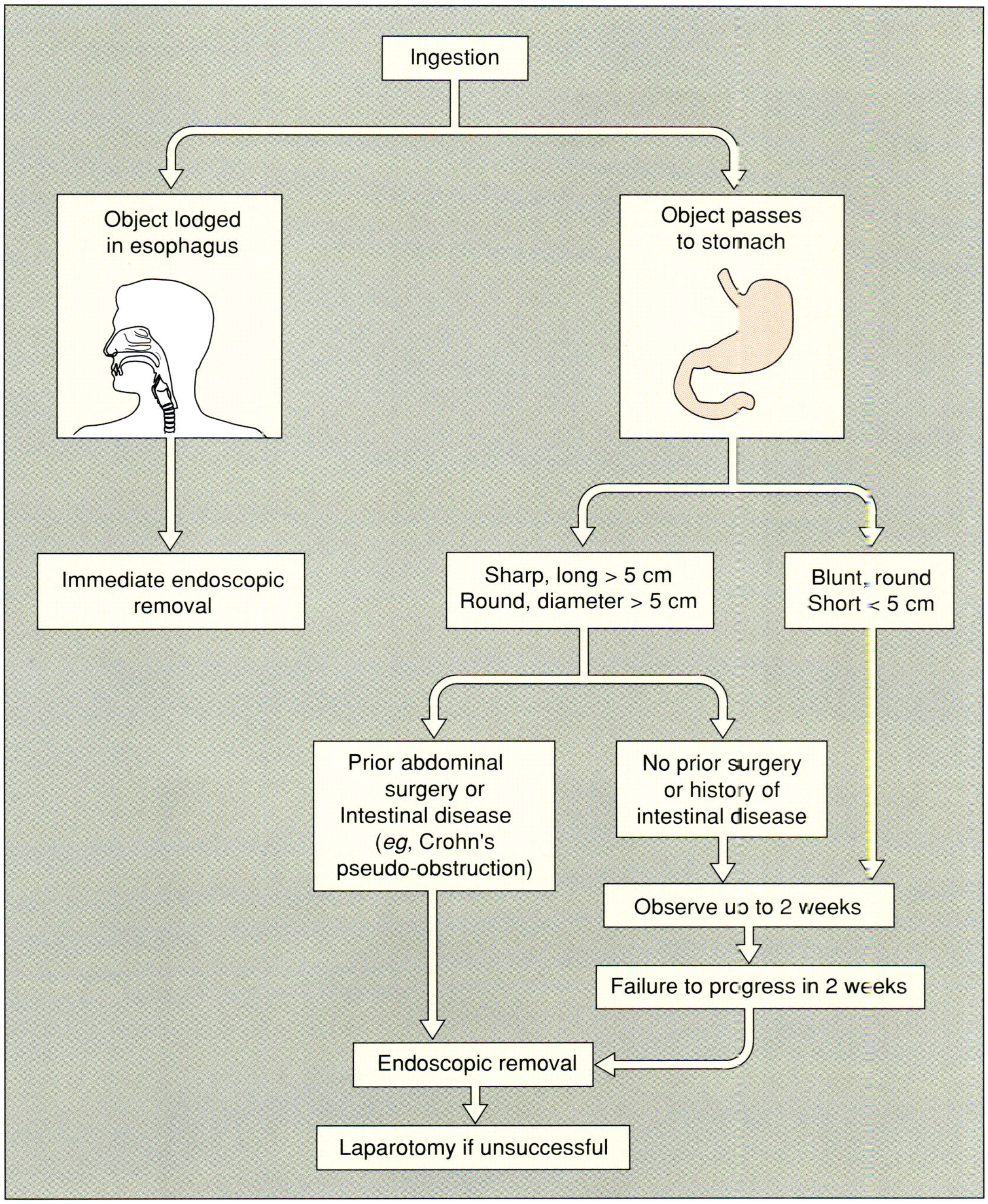

FIGURE 1-54.

Foreign body. This figure shows an algorithmic approach to a patient with foreign body ingestion.

Diagnostic evaluation should precede with a complete history and physical examination. The patient is usually able to give specifics concerning the size, consistency, and time of foreign body ingestion. A past history of gastroesophageal reflux disease, dysphagia, loss of teeth, or change in dentures are clues concerning the etiology. Posteroanterior and lateral chest radiographs, as well as neck radiographs with radiographic technique to emphasize soft tissues, are important to assess impaction in the hypopharynx and cervical esophagus as well as airway compromise. Barium swallow is generally not indicated in suspected foreign body impaction because aspiration may occur and the barium may prevent endoscopic visualization. Additionally, other objects should not be swallowed to try to "drive" the impacted object into the stomach.

The first consideration when approaching the patient would be the nature of the ingested object. Sharp objects should be considered for removal. Toxic or caustic objects should also be considered for early removal. Location, as determined by radiology studies, is also important. All objects stuck in the esophagus should be considered for removal if adequate resources are available. (*Adapted from* Cotton *et al.* [28].)

MUCOSAL RING (B RING, SCHATZKI'S RING)

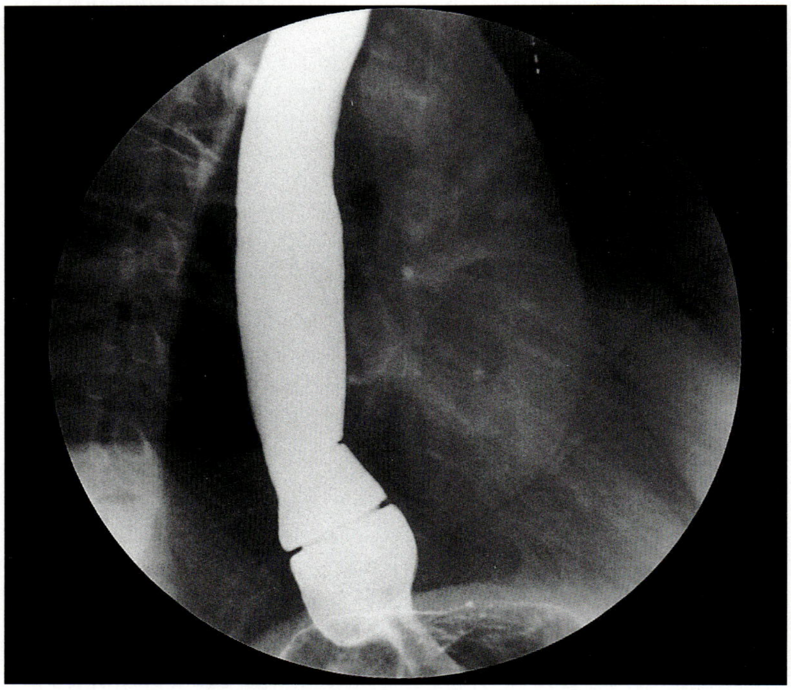

FIGURE 1-55.

Schatzki's ring on barium esophagram. Esophageal webs and rings are thin esophageal stenoses typically composed of only mucosa. Rings formed at the gastroesophageal junction, as described by Schatzki, are usually silent but become symptomatic when the internal diameter is less than 13 mm. (*From* McBride and Ergun [29]; with permission.)

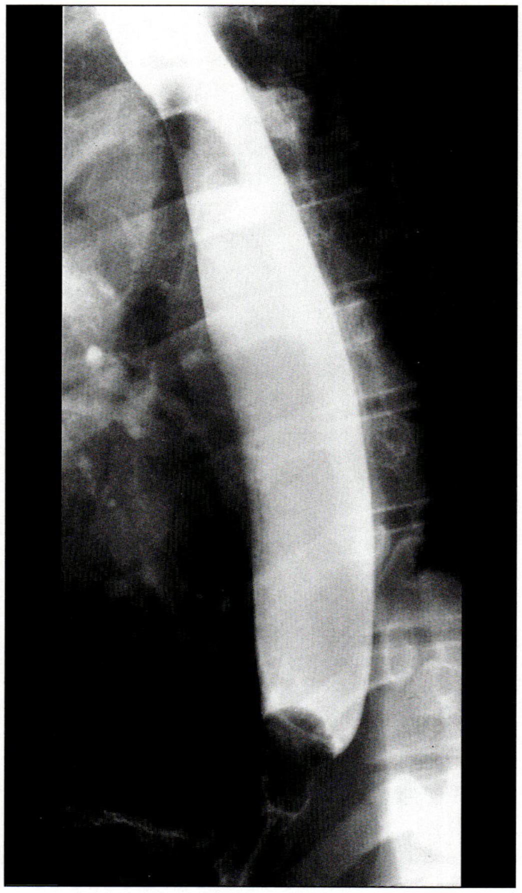

FIGURE 1-56.

Adequate examination of the lower esophagus by both radiology and endoscopy is impossible without adequate distension. For this reason a common lesion, such as lower esophageal mucosal ring, can be missed by both techniques. The radiologist may also challenge the esophagus with a solid bolus such as a marshmallow or a barium tablet. This patient had intermittent solid food dysphagia for many years. Previous evaluation using esophagography, manometry, and endoscopy were normal. The marshmallow distended the lower esophagus and brought out the lower esophageal mucosal ring. In addition, impaction of the marshmallow reproduced the patient's symptom. Esophageal dilatation rendered this patient asymptomatic.

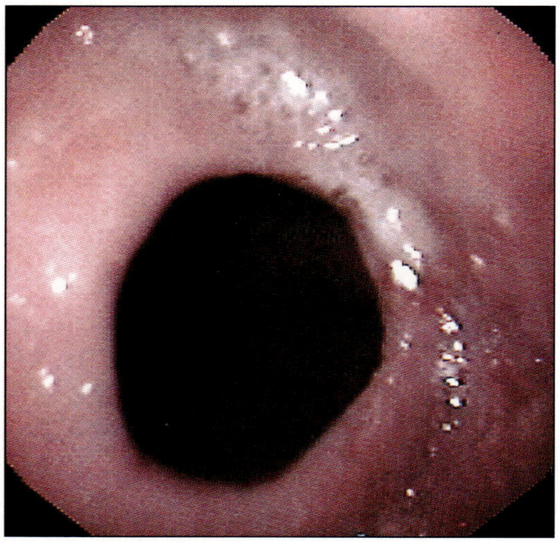

FIGURE 1-57.

Endoscopic appearance of a lower esophageal mucosal ring. Its pathogenesis is unknown. Its upper surface is always covered by esophageal (squamous) epithelium, its lower surface by gastric (columnar) epithelium. In general, rings smaller than 13 mm in diameter are always symptomatic and those over 20 mm never produce any symptoms. Intermittent solid food dysphagia is the main presenting symptom. Treatment consists of passing a single large-caliber dilator (*ie*, 15 mm or larger) through the esophagus to disrupt the ring, although the ring may recur.

VASCULAR LESIONS

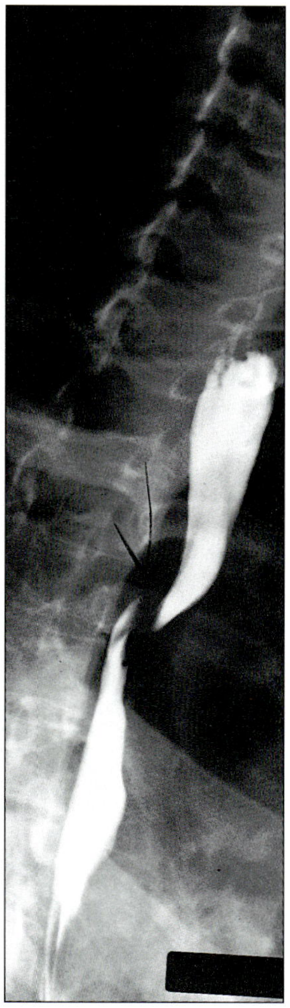

FIGURE 1-58.

Arteria lusoria. Dysphagia lusoria is caused by extrinsic esophageal compression caused by an aberrant right subclavian artery arising from the descending aorta and passing behind the esophagus. (*From* McBride and Ergun [29]; with permission.)

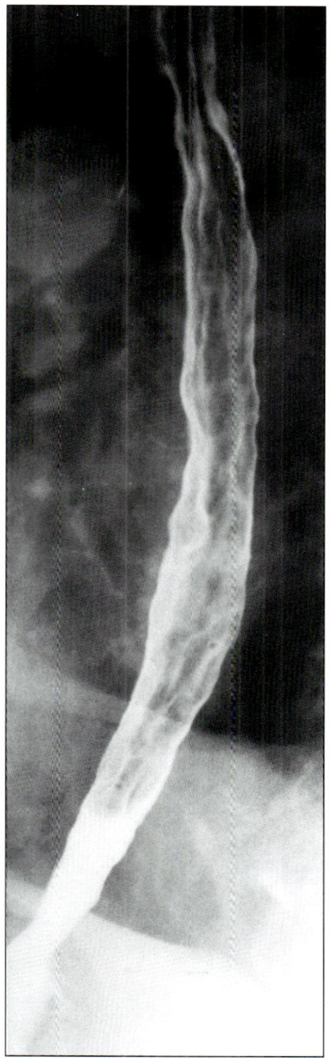

FIGURE 1-59.

Esophageal varices as seen on barium swallow. Portal hypertension results in congestion and dilation with the deep intrinsic veins becoming grossly enlarged, thus displacing the more superficial venous systems. The deep veins eventually occupy a superficial subepithelial location and are identified radiographically and endoscopically as esophageal varices. (*Courtesy of* Dr. Frank Miller, Northwestern University Medical School.)

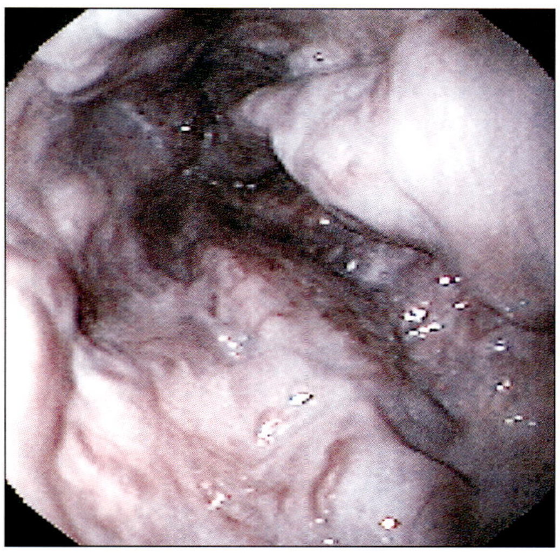

FIGURE 1-60.

Endoscopy showing large esophageal varices. Liver biopsy showed cirrhosis. Varices were treated with sclerotherapy.

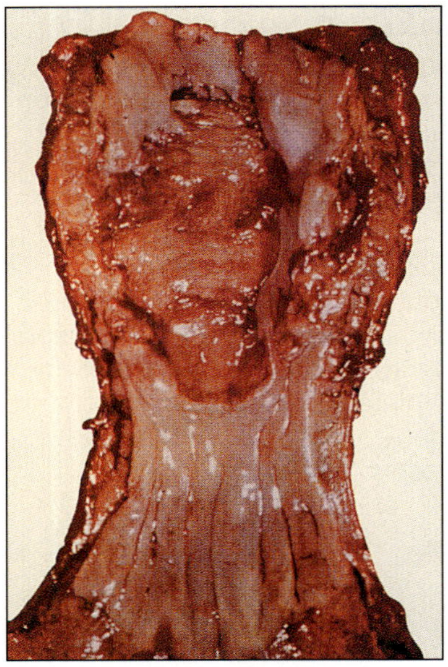

FIGURE 1-61.

Squamous cell carcinoma is the most common malignant neoplasm of the esophagus and constitutes 90% to 95% of all esophageal carcinomas. It commonly affects males, with the peak age of onset between 50 and 70 years. Smoking tobacco and excessive alcohol consumption are the two most important risk factors. Human papillomavirus infection and a variety of dietary triggers have also been suggested as risk factors. Among the predisposing conditions and attendant associations are celiac sprue, prior irradiation, tylosis palmaris et plantaris, Plummer-Vinson syndrome, achalasia, and stricture resulting from the ingestion of lye. Squamous cell carcinoma may occur anywhere in the esophagus but is most commonly found in the middle, and secondly, in the lower third portions. Macroscopic appearance of advanced esophageal carcinomas vary from exophytic mass to ulcerated, infiltrating lesion, to a combination of all these. Squamous cell carcinoma may present as a large excavating esophageal ulcer, as seen in this figure. The carcinoma had infiltrated into the periesophageal soft tissue. Note the tumor nodules in the surrounding periesophageal soft tissue. The esophagus has a rich lymphatic supply, which accounts for the frequent lymphatic spread to surrounding lymph nodes. Metastasis to distant organs is also common, especially to the liver, lungs, pleura, and adrenals. Occasionally the tumor extends directly into the mediastinum. (*From* Ming [30].)

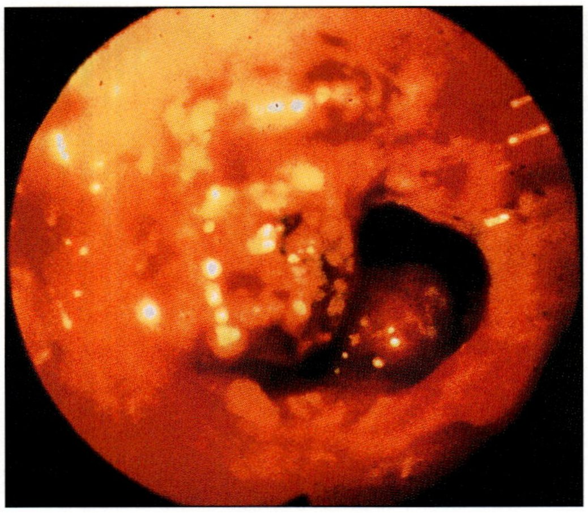

FIGURE 1-62.

Endoscopic appearance of an exophytic tumor obstructing the esophagus.

MALIGNANT TUMORS OF THE ESOPHAGUS
Squamous cell carcinoma >90%
Special types
Verrucous carcinoma
Basaloid carcinoma
Spindle cell variant
Small cell carcinoma
Adenosquamous carcinoma
Adenocarcinoma 6%
Mucoepidermoid carcinoma
Choriocarcinoma
Adenocystic carcinoma
Leiomyosarcoma (rare)
Malignant melanoma
Malignant lymphoma and plasmacytoma
Metastatic tumors
Rare sarcomas

FIGURE 1-63.

Malignant tumors of the esophagus. The great majority of malignant tumors of the esophagus are carcinomas. Among these, squamous cell carcinoma is the most common primary neoplasm, followed by adenocarcinoma. Other malignant tumors are uncommon. Primary lymphoma is very rare in the esophagus but several cases have been reported in the AIDS setting. Kaposi's sarcoma has also been reported in patients with AIDS. Tumor metastatic to the esophagus is infrequent. More commonly, the esophagus is involved by direct spread from tumors arising in contiguous organs, such as lung, stomach, thyroid, and larynx.

ESOPHAGEAL TNM PATHOLOGIC STAGING

Classification	
Primary tumor (T) class	
Tis	Carcinoma in situ
T1	Invades lamina propria or submucosa
T2	Invades muscularis propria
T3	Invades adventitia
T4	Invades adjacent structures
Nodal (N) class	
N0	No regional node metastases
N1	Regional node metastases
Distant metastases (M) class	
M0	No distant metastases
M1	Distant metastases
Stage grouping	
0	Tis N0 M0
I	T1 N0 M0
IIA	T2–T3, N0 M0
IIB	T1–T2, N1 M0
III	T3 or T4 N1 M0
IV	AnyT AnyN M1

FIGURE 1-64.

Accurate staging of esophageal cancer is important for therapeutic management and evaluation of treatment. This table illustrates the staging scheme developed by the American Joint Committee on Cancer in Cooperation with the TNM Committee of the International Union Against Cancer. The classification given here applies to all esophageal carcinomas. The pathologic stage is based on examination of the resected esophagectomy specimen. The clinical staging is based on clinical examination before treatment is given and includes physical examination, endoscopy, imaging, and endoscopic ultrasonography. Computed tomography and endoscopic ultrasound scanning are particularly useful in the evaluation of the depth of invasion and of the status of the lymph nodes. (*Adapted from* American Joint Committee on Cancer [31].)

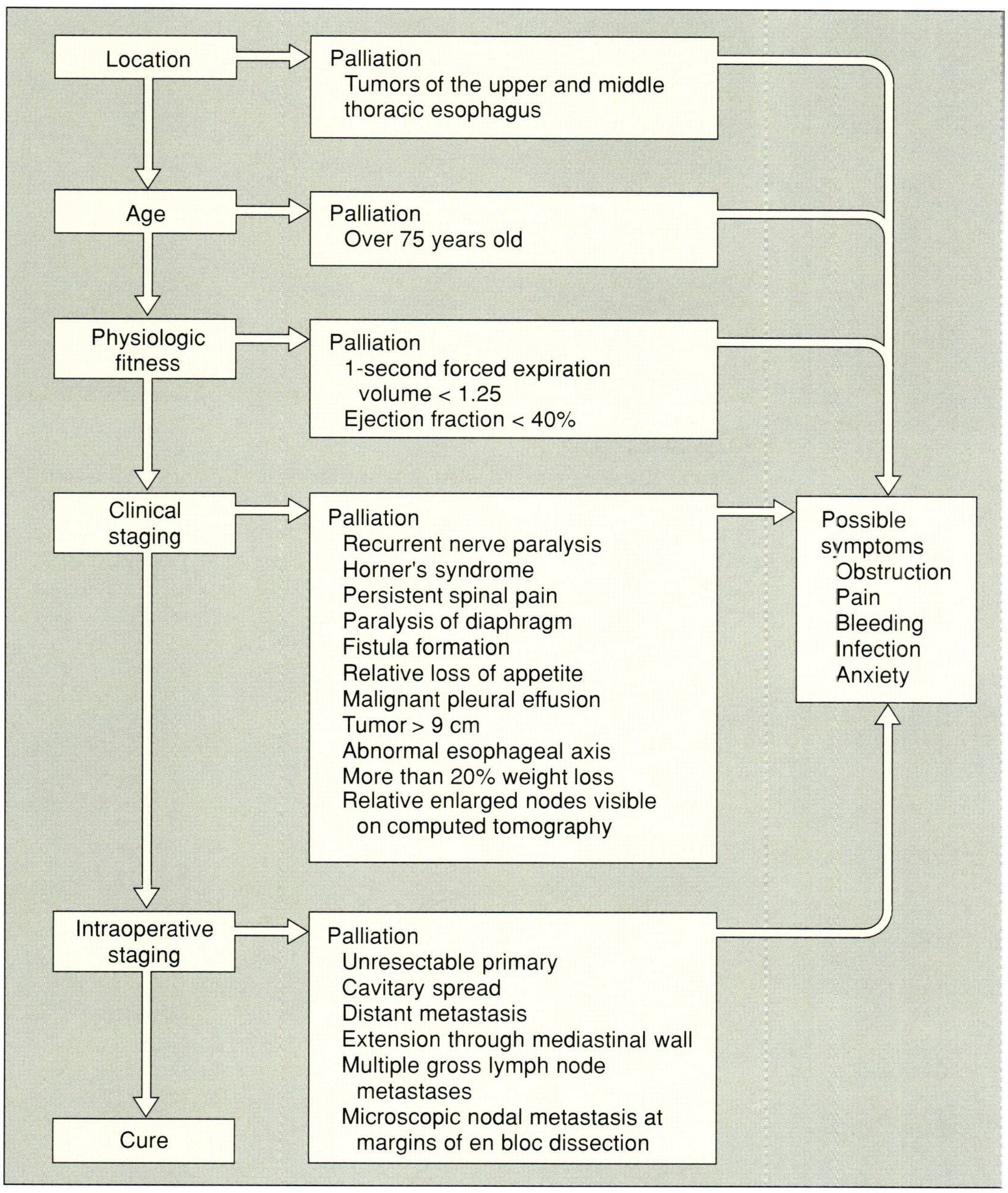

FIGURE 1-65.

Algorithm for therapeutic decisions in esophageal carcinoma. This algorithm is quite pessimistic because of the aggressiveness of esophageal carcinoma. Overall, rates of survival are poor, even with surgical resection. Palliation and a good quality of life plays a vital role in the treatment of this disease. (*Adapted from* Peters and DeMeester [32].)

CUTANEOUS MANIFESTATIONS OF ESOPHAGEAL DISEASE

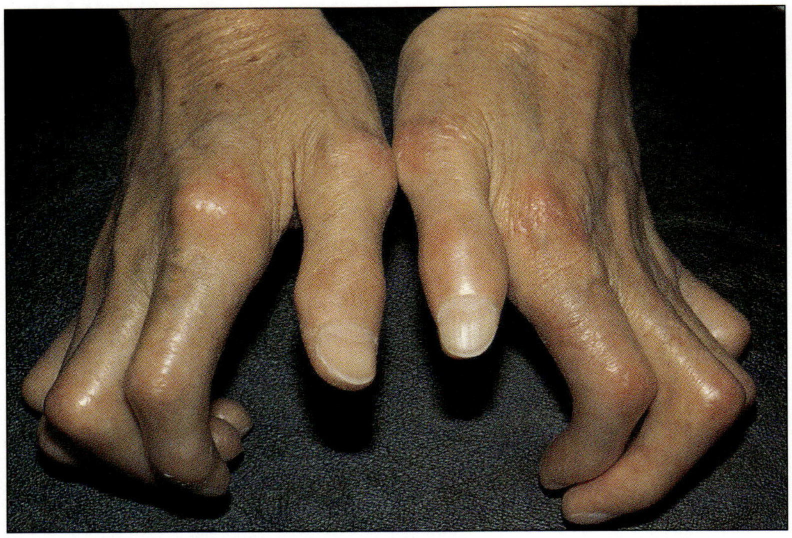

FIGURE 1-66.

Scleroderma, or progressive systemic sclerosis, is characterized by sclerodactyly as seen in this patient. The skin is shiny, thickened, firm, and bound down on the hands, arms, face, and shoulders. Gastroesophageal reflux diseases resulting from loss of lower esophageal sphincter function and reduced or absent peristalsis leads to esophagitis and stricture formation. Dysphagia may result from stricture or from esophageal dysmotility.

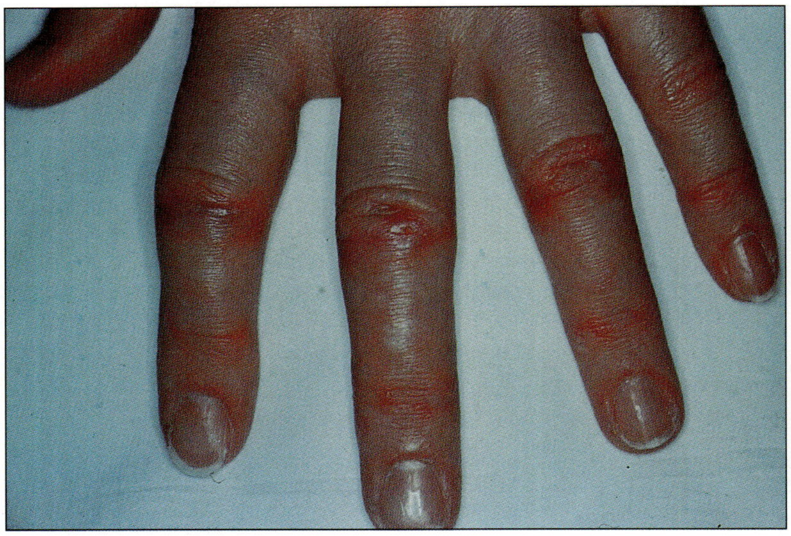

FIGURE 1-67.

The musculature of the oropharynx and upper esophagus may be involved in dermatomyositis, leading to dysphagia. Characteristic cutaneous signs include Gottron's sign, in which a violaceous, scaly erythema appears on the skin over the tendons of the hands, particularly over the knuckles, as seen in this patient. Papules occurring in this location are referred to as *Gottron's papules*. Pruritic, erythematous plaques may be present over the elbows, knees, posterior neck, buttocks, and other extensor surfaces. Edema and erythema of the eyelids may occur, producing the characteristic "heliotrope rash."

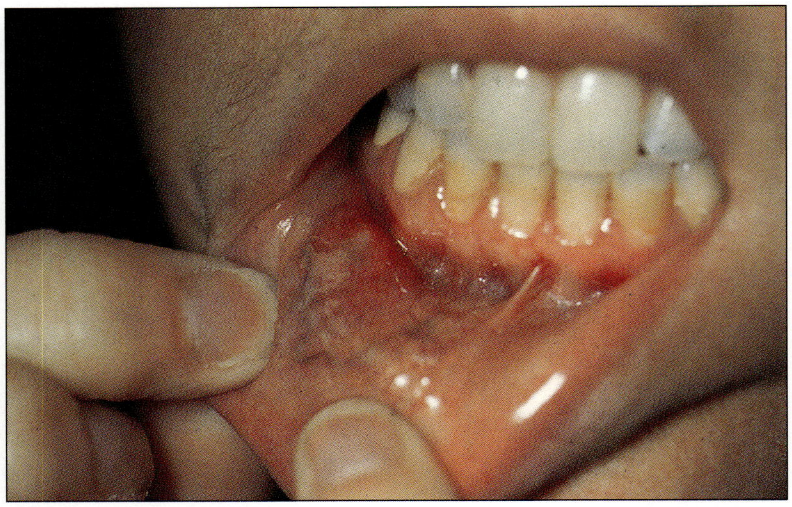

FIGURE 1-68.

Behçet's disease presents with oral and genital ulcers, as well as with eye disease. Esophageal lesions may cause dysphagia. Oral lesions usually appear as punched-out ulcers, similar to those seen with aphthous stomatitis. Colitis may also be present. (*Courtesy of* P. Eichhorn, Dallas, TX)

REFERENCES

1. Kahrilas PJ: The anatomy and physiology of dysphagia. In *Dysphagia, Diagnosis, and Treatment*. Edited by Gelfand DW, Richter JE. New York: Igaku-Shoin; 1989:11–28.
2. Goyal RK, Rattan S: Neurohumoral, hormonal, and drug receptors for the lower esophageal sphincter. *Gastroenterology* 1978, 74:598.
3. Mittal RK, Rochester DF, McCallum RW: Sphincteric action of the diaphragm during a relaxed lower esophageal sphincter. *Am J Physiol* 1989, 256:G139–G144.
4. Boyle JT, Altschuler SM, Nixon TE, *et al.*: Role of the diaphragm in the genesis of lower esophageal sphincter pressure in the cat. *Gastroenterology* 1985, 88:723–730.
5. Mittal RK, Rochester DF, McCallum RW: Electrical and mechanical activity in the human lower esophageal sphincter during diaphragmatic contraction. *J Clin Invest* 1988, 81:1182–1189.
6. Mittal RK, Rochester DF, McCallum RW: Sphincteric action of the diaphragm during a relaxed lower esophageal sphincter in humans. *Am J Physiol* 1989, 256:G139–G144.
7. Miller LS, Liu JB, Klenn PJ, *et al.*: Endoluminal ultrasonography of

the distal esophagus in systemic sclerosis. *Gastroenterology* 1993, 105:31–39.

8. Alban-Davies H, *et al.*: Angina-like pain: differentiation for cardiac pain by history. *J Clin Gastroenterol* 1985, 7:477–481.
9. Alban-Davies H: Anginal pain of esophageal origin: Clinical presentation, prevalence and prognosis. *Am J Med* 1992, 92:5s–10s.
10. Hewson EG, *et al.*: Twenty-four-hour esophageal pH monitoring: the most useful test for evaluating noncardaice chest pain. *Am J Med* 1991, 90:576–583.
11. Schofield PM, *et al.*: Exertional gastroesophageal reflux: a mechanism for symptoms in patients with angina pectoris and normal coronary angiograms. *Br Med J* 1987, 294:1459–1461.
12. Squillace SJ, Young MF, Sanowski RA: Single dose omeprazole as a test for noncardiac chest pain [Abstract]. *Gastroenterology* 1993, 104:A197.
13. Stahl WG, *et al.*: Diagnosis and treatment of patients with gastroesophageal reflux and noncardiac chest pain. *South Med J* 1994, 87:739–742.
14. Achem SR, *et al.*: Chest pain associated with nutcracker esophagus: a preliminary study of the role of gastroesophageal reflux. *Am J Gastroenterology* 1993, 88:187–192.
15. Orlando RC: Reflux esophagitis. In *Textbook of Gastroenterology*. Edited by Yamada T, Alpers DH, Owyang C, *et al.* Philadelphia: JB Lippincott; 1991:1123–1147.
16. A Gallup Organization National Survey: *Heartburn Across America*. Princeton: The Gallop Organization; 1988.
17. Nebel OT, Fornes MF, Castell DO: Symptomatic gastroesophageal reflux: incidence and precipitating factors. *Am J Dig Dis* 1976, 21:953.
18. Rasmussen CW: A new endoscopic classification of chronic esophagitis. *Am J Gastroenterol* 1976, 65:409.
19. Spechler SJ: Epidemiology and natural history of gastro-oesophageal reflux disease. *Digestion* 1992, 51(suppl 1):24–29.
20. Tytgat GNJ: Upper gastrointestinal endoscopy. In *Textbook of Gastroenterology*. Edited by Yamada T, Alpers DH, Owyang C, *et al.* Philadelphia: JB Lippincott; 1991:435–436.
21. Weinstein WM, Goboch ER, Bowes KL: The normal human esophageal mucosa: a histologic reappraisal. *Gastroenterology* 1975, 68:40.
22. Orlando RC: Gastroesophageal reflux. In *Current Therapy in Gastroenterology and Liver Disease*, ed 3. Edited by Bayless TM. Philadelphia: BC Decker, 1990:7.
23. Pope CE II: Gastroesophageal reflux disease (reflux esophagitis). In *Gastrointestinal Disease: Pathophysiology, Diagnosis, Management*. Edited by Sleisenger MH, Fordtran JS. Philadelphia: WB Saunders; 1983:449.
24. Negre JB, Markkula HT, Keyrilainen O, *et al.*: Nissen fundoplication: results at 10-year follow-up. *Am J Surg* 1983, 146:635.
25. Baehr PM, McDonald GB: Esophageal infections: risk factors, presentation, diagnosis and treatment. *Gastroenterology* 1994, 106:509–532.
26. Boal DKB, Newburger PE, Teele RL: Esophagitis induced by combined radiation and adriamycin. *Am J Roentgenol* 1979, 132:567–570.
27. Yoshida CM, Peura DA: Foreign bodies. In *The Esophagus*, ed 2. Edited by Castell DO. Boston: Little, Brown and Company; 1995:379.
28. Cotton PB, Tytgat GNJ, Williams CB: *Annual of Gastrointestinal Endoscopy*. 1988:13.
29. McBride MA, Ergun GA: Role of upper endoscopy in the management of esophageal strictures. *Gastrointest Endosc Clin North Am* 1994, 4:595–621.
30. Ming S-C: *Atlas of Tumor Pathology, series 2–Fascicle: Tumors of the Esophagus and Stomach*. Bethesda, MD: Armed Forces Institute of Pathology; 1973
31. American Joint Committee on Cancer: *Manual for Staging of Cancer*, ed 4. Philadelphia: JB Lippincott Company; 1992.
32. Peters JH, DeMeester TR: Esophagus and diaphragmatic hernia. In *Principles of Surgery*, ed 6. Edited by Schwartz SL, Shires GT, Spencer FC. New York: McGraw-Hill; 1994:1092.

Chapter 2

Disorders of the Stomach and Duodenum

EDITOR

Mark Feldman

CONTRIBUTORS

Byron Cryer
Daniel C. DeMarco
Karl Fukunaga
Robert T. Jensen
Douglas Kliewer
Juan Lechago
Edward L. Lee
Felix W. Leung
Amit G. Pandya
Neal E. Seymour
Vasundhara Tolia
C. Mel Wilcox
Russell David Yang

GENERAL CLASSIFICATION OF GASTRITIS

Category	Nomenclature	Diagnostic modality	Etiology
Endoscopic	Gastropathy	Endoscopy	NSAIDs, physiologic stress, alchohol, chemical agents, and idiopathic
Histologic			
Acute	Acute erosive hemorrhagic gastritis	Endoscopic biopsy and histologic evaluation	NSAIDs, physiologic stress, alchohol, chemical agents, and idiopathic
Chronic			
Nonspecific	Chronic active superficial gastritis Chronic superficial gastritis Chronic atrophic gastritis	Endoscopic biopsy and histologic evaluation	*Helicobacter pylori*, autoimmune, and bile reflux
Specific	Depends on etiology	Endoscopic biopsy and histologic evaluation	Bacterial, viral, fungal parasitic, granulomatous, eosinophilic, and hypertrophic

FIGURE 2-1.

General classification of gastritis. Gastritis may be determined endoscopically or histologically. Endoscopic gastritis is defined by gross findings of mucosal erosions or focal hemorrhagic lesions. On mucosal biopsy of these endoscopic abnormalities, epithelial and vascular changes predominate and, about half the time, no increased inflammatory cell infiltrate is present.

Classifications of histologic gastritis vary because there is no general agreement on its classification. Histologic gastritis, by definition, is associated with increased mucosal inflammation on microscopic examination and, in our classification, is separated into acute and chronic forms. Acute erosive hemorrhagic gastritis is the histologic correlate of acute mucosal injury detected endoscopically. Chronic gastritis is divided into nonspecific and specific categories.

Before the discovery of the involvement of *Helicobacter pylori*, few of the nonspecific forms of gastritis could be linked to a single etiologic agent or disease process. Most of the nonspecific forms now, however, appear to be related to the effects of *H. pylori*. Morphologically, nonspecific gastritis is characterized by variable microscopic patterns, and, depending on the pattern, can be further classified as chronic active superficial gastritis, chronic superficial gastritis, or chronic atrophic gastritis. Specific histologic gastritis is associated with a specific etiologic agent or disease process and most forms have a distinctive morphology. NSAIDs—nonsteroidal anti-inflammatory drugs.

CHRONIC GASTRITIS: SPECIFIC (DISTINCTIVE) GASTRITIS

Infections	Gastrointestinal tract disease
Bacterial	Crohn's disease
Tuberculosis	Eosinophilic gastroenteritis
Syphilis	Systemic disease
Phlegmonous and emphysematous gastritis	Sarcoid
Viral	Graft-vs-host disease
Cytomegalovirus	Chronic granulomatous disease
Herpesviruses	Miscellaneous (unknown association)
Fungal	Ménétrier's disease
Candidiasis	Focal lymphoid hyperplasia
Histoplasmosis	Granulomatous gastritis
Mucormycosis	
Cryptococcosis	
Aspergillosis	
Parasites and Nematodes	
Cryptosporidiosis	
Strongyloidiasis	
Amebiasis	
Toxoplasmosis	
Pneumocystis carinii infection	

FIGURE 2-2.

Chronic gastritis: specific or distinctive gastritis. The designation specific or distinctive gastritis refers to histologic features that are suggestive of a specific diagnosis. Viewed endoscopically, these disorders may or may not have mucosal abnormalities. Listed in this table are some of the various etiologies that have been associated with a specific form of gastritis. Compared with the nonspecific forms of gastritis, the specific forms are rarer. (*Adapted from* Weinstein [1].)

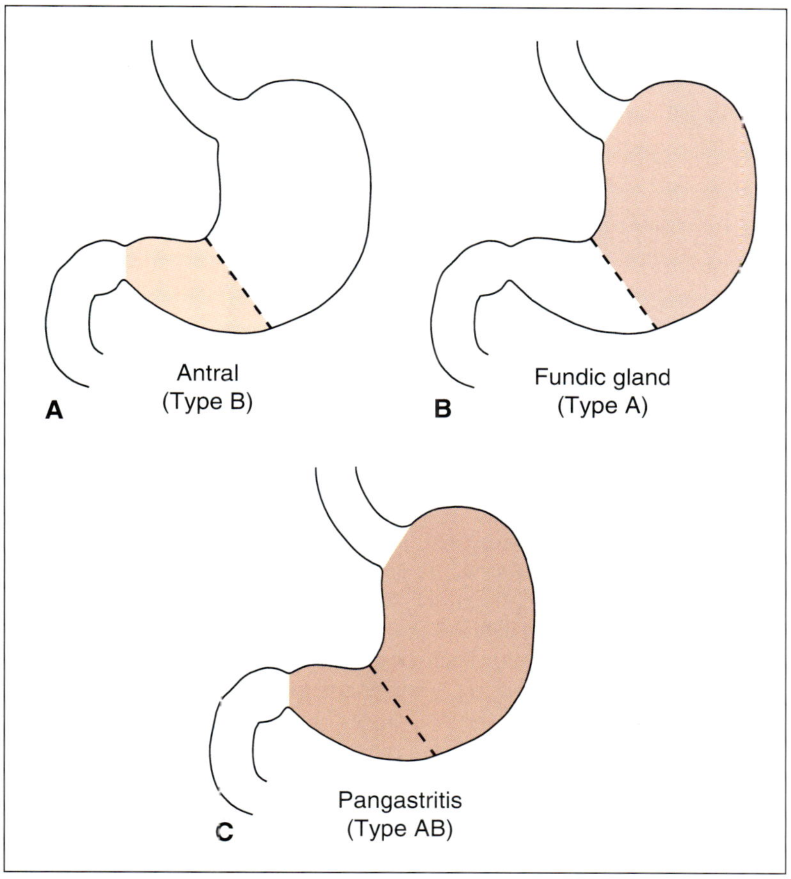

FIGURE 2-3.

Topographic distributions of nonerosive, nonspecific gastritis. The three panels of this figure demonstrate the three major gastric topographic distributions for nonspecific gastritis.

A, Antral gastritis, also referred to as *type B*, is almost always associated with *Helicobacter pylori*. In duodenal ulcer patients, more than 90% have antral gastritis, and 50% to 80% of gastric ulcer patients have this type of gastritis. Type B gastritis is most intense in the antrum. It commonly coexists, however, with a less severe inflammation in the fundic mucosa.

B, Fundic gastritis, also referred to as *type A*, is most intense in the body of the stomach. This pattern of gastritis is seen in pernicious anemia. Although type A gastritis is most intense in body of the stomach and has been described to "spare the antrum", it is frequently associated with a less severe antral gastritis. Thus, type B and A gastritis are actually pangastritides with the predominance of inflammation confined to either the gastric antrum or body.

C, A third type of gastritis, a pangastritis (*Type AB*), has been described and is represented by gastritis in the antrum and body. Type AB gastritis most likely represents proximal extension of Type B gastritis and is also highly associated with *H. pylori* colonization.

There is a fourth topographic pattern of gastritis (not shown) called *multifocal atrophic gastritis*, which begins in the region of the incisura and extends out both proximally and distally and is commonly associated with intestinal metaplasia. (*Adapted from* Weinstein [1]).

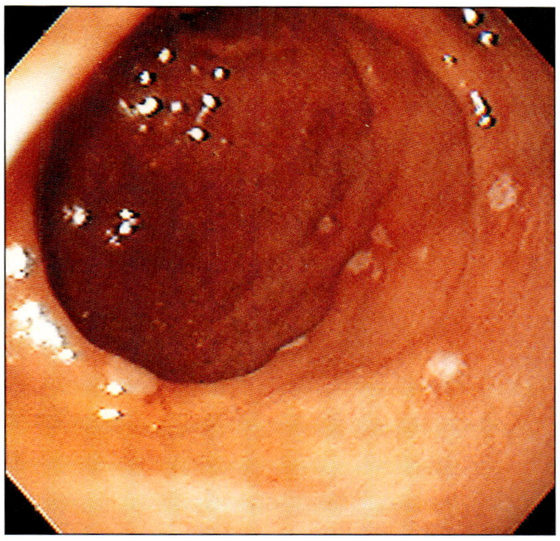

FIGURE 2-4.

Endoscopic erosive gastritis. The observations of multiple erosive and hemorrhagic lesions may be defined endoscopically as gastritis. This figure is an example of endoscopic erosive gastritis. Common settings that may lead to endoscopic gastritis include use of nonsteroidal anti-inflammatory drugs, alcohol abuse, and the physiologic stress associated with serious illnesses (stress gastritis). Other less common causes include ingestion of corrosives, chemotherapeutic agents, or irradiation. There may also be no known demonstrable associated factor present (idiopathic). (*Courtesy of* W. Harford, Dallas, TX.)

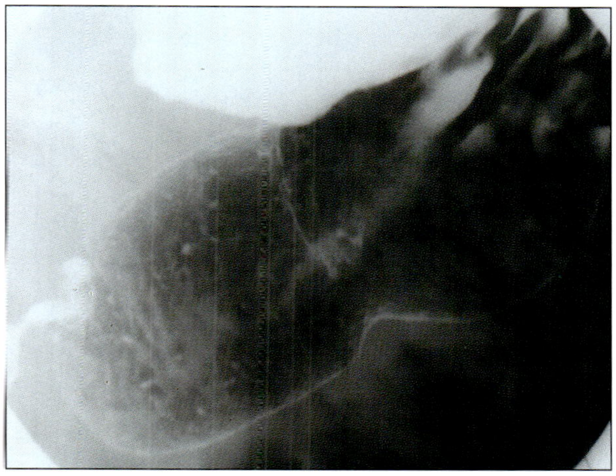

FIGURE 2-5.

Erosive gastritis on upper gastrointestinal barium examination. Superficial gastric erosions appear radiographically as multiple tiny flecks of barium, which represent the erosions, surrounded by radiolucent halos, which represent surrounding mounds of edematous mucosa. Superficial gastric erosions can also appear as flat defects that coat with barium without surrounding reaction and are represented by reproducible linear streaks or dots of contrast. This barium study is an example of the radiographic appearance of erosive gastritis showing multiple tiny flecks, some surrounded by halos. It also shows areas of coalescence of lesions into linear streaks. (*Courtesy of* W. L. Peterson, Dallas, TX.)

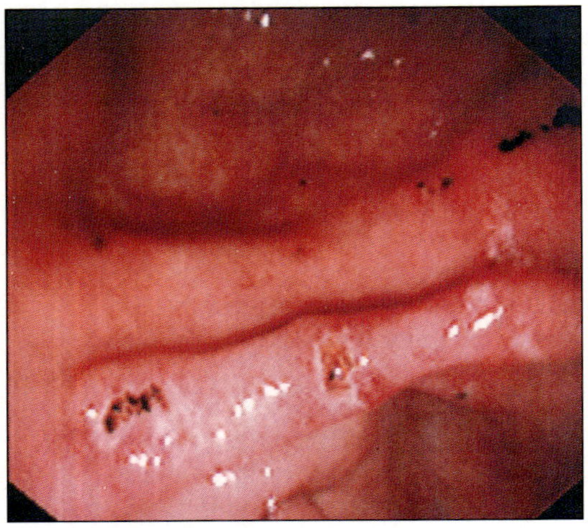

FIGURE 2-6.

Aspirin and other nonsteroidal anti-inflammatory drugs (NSAIDs). As shown in this figure, ingestion of aspirin and other NSAIDs can produce acute gastric mucosal erosions and subepithelial hemorrhages. Although found in all gastric locations, these NSAID–associated lesions have a predilection for the fundus and body. The constellation of multiple small erosions and multiple small submucosal hemorrhages throughout the stomach is very suggestive of NSAID use. On microscopic evaluation, the occurrence of a mucosal inflammatory infiltrate is not greater than that expected for age-matched controls who are not taking NSAIDs. Thus, NSAIDs do not actually cause a histologic gastritis. A more appropriate term for this condition is *NSAID gastropathy*.

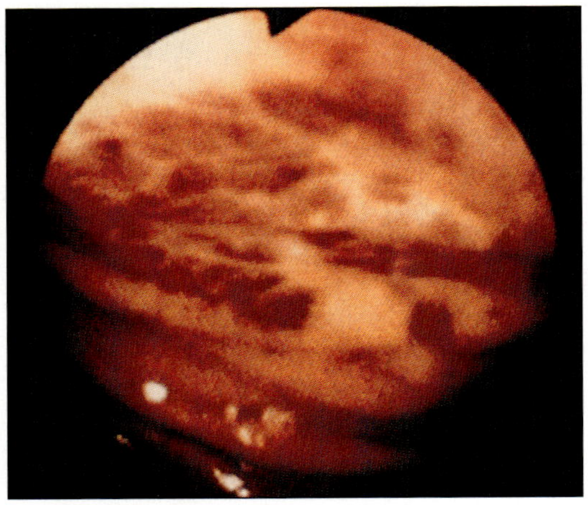

FIGURE 2-7.

Alcohol consumption can result in endoscopic mucosal abnormalities termed *alcoholic hemorrhagic gastritis*. As shown in this figure, endoscopically such patients will have multiple subepithelial hemorrhages without any visible breaks in the mucosa. The appearance has been described as that of "blood under plastic wrap." These lesions are mainly confined to the body and fundus of the stomach and are infrequently seen in the antrum. (*From* Laine and Weinstein [2]; with permission.)

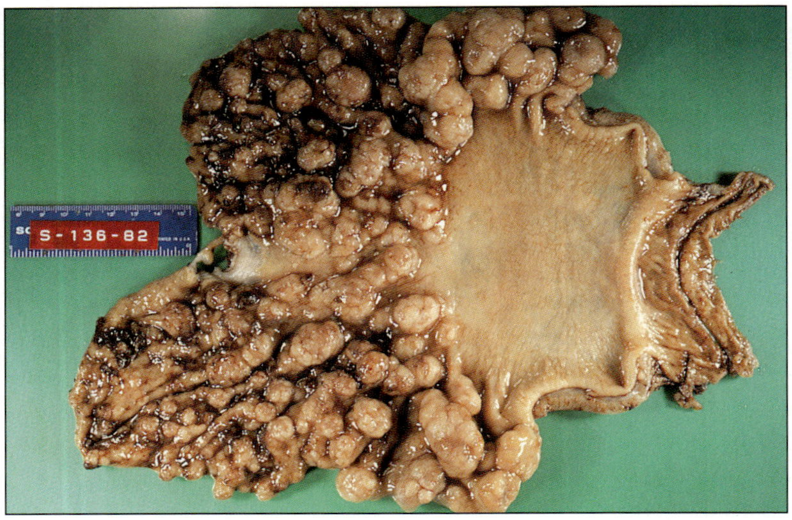

FIGURE 2-8.

Ménétrier's disease. The clinical features diagnostic of Ménétrier's disease are giant folds, especially in the fundus and body of the stomach, protein-losing enteropathy with hypoalbuminemia, hypochlorhydria in advanced stages, and a marked increase in mucosal thickness overall. As shown in this figure, its gross pathological characteristics are enlarged gastric folds in the gastric body that typically spare the antrum. These folds have a nodular or polypoid configuration and may have associated erosions or ulcerations. This condition is rare today.

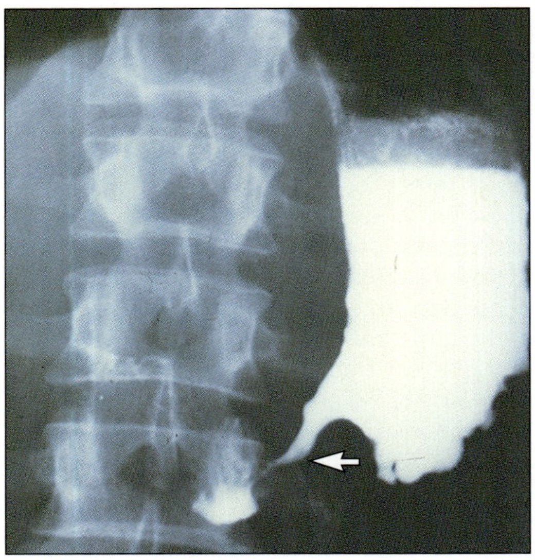

FIGURE 2-9.

Caustic-induced gastritis. Ingestion of caustic agents (typically, they are strongly acidic, but similar effects with strong alkaline substances may also be seen) can cause gastric injury, especially in the antrum. Pathologically, caustic injuries to the gastric mucosa are classified as a continuum starting with superficial injury associated with inflammation, edema, and erythema which generally does not result in scar or stricture formation (first degree).

The next levels of injury are characterized by inflammation, granulation tissue, and ulceration extending down to the muscularis (second degree) or penetration which extends through the gastric wall (third degree). From 2 to 3 weeks following second- and third-degree gastric injuries, a fibroblastic reaction develops most prominently in the antrum, which can result in antral stricturing.

The upper gastrointestinal system barium study shown here is from a patient who had ingested a caustic agent. Note the long tapering antral stricture (*open arrow*) resulting from luminal compression from extensive mucosal scarring noted radiographically as a nodular mass effect. The same nodularity resulting from scarring is also noted in the gastric body along the greater curvature. (*Courtesy of* M. Feldman, Dallas, TX.)

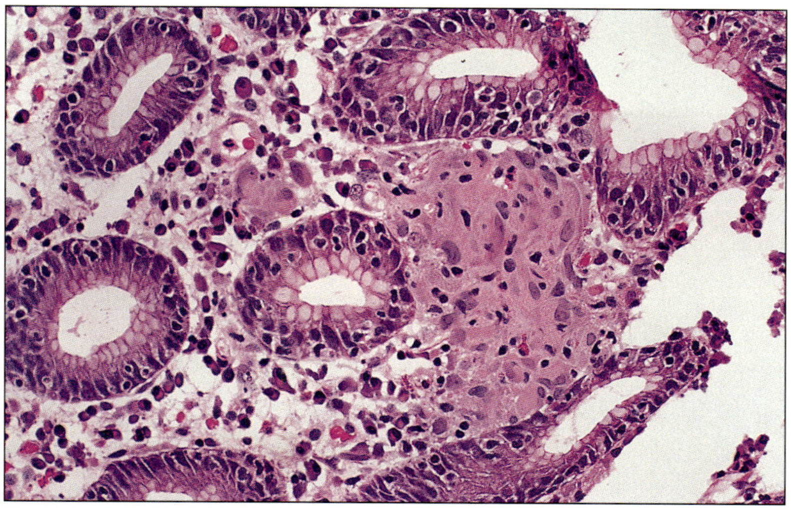

FIGURE 2-10.

Crohn's gastritis. Histologically, gastric Crohn's disease appears as a granulomatous gastritis. Thus, in the absence of other clinical manifestations to suggest Crohn's disease, the diagnosis is difficult to make solely on the basis of histologic evidence. This figure shows two (one large and one small) granulomas (nodular collections of histiocytes) within the lamina propria. Acute and chronic inflammatory infiltrates involving the lamina propria are also present.

GASTRIC AND DUODENAL INFECTIONS IN AIDS

INFECTIOUS AGENTS ASSOCIATED WITH GASTRITIS AND DUODENITIS IN AIDS

- Bacteria
  - *Salmonella*
    - *Mycobacterium avium-intracellulare*
    - *Mycobacterium tuberculosis*
- Viruses
  - Cytomegalovirus
    - Herpes simplex virus
- Protozoa
  - *Cryptosporidium*
  - *Isospora belli*
    - *Microsporidia*
    - *Giardia lamblia*
- Fungal
  - Histoplasmosis
    - Coccidiomycosis

FIGURE 2-11.

A wide range of bacterial, viral, protozoal, and fungal organisms may cause gastritis and duodenitis in patients with AIDS.

HELICOBACTER PYLORI GASTRITIS

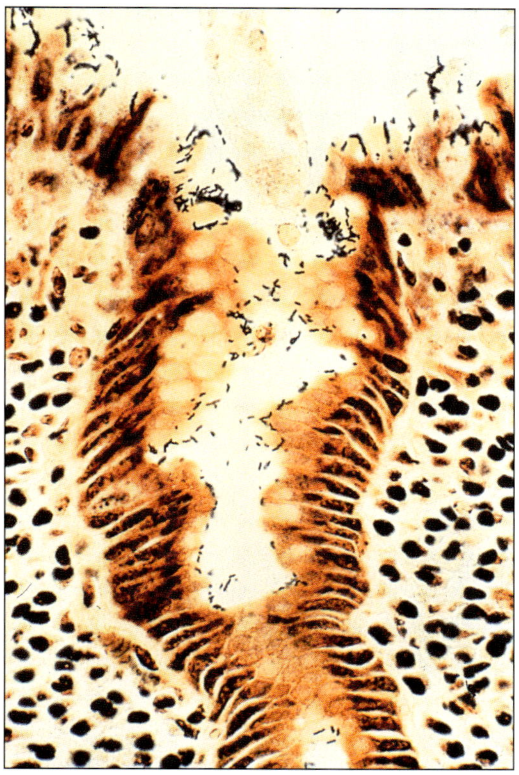

FIGURE 2-12.

Helicobacter pylori in gastric mucosa. As shown, at high-power magnification, *H. pylori* can be easily identified (Warthin-Starry silver stain). *H. pylori* can be almost as easily identified using the routine hematoxylin and eosin stain. Acute and chronic inflammation is present as well. (From Peterson *et al* [3] with permission.)

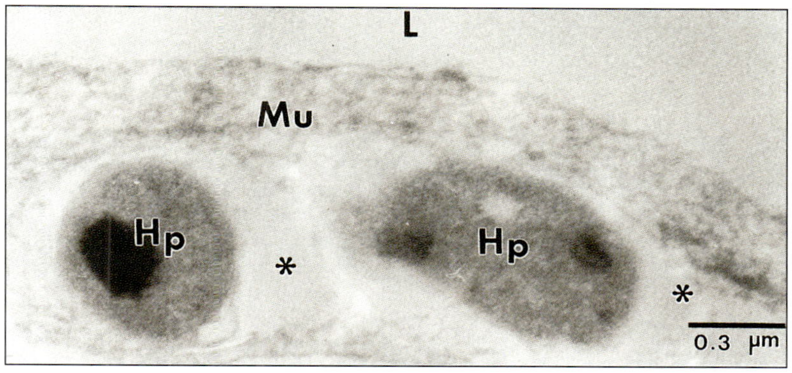

FIGURE 2-13.

Electron micrograph showing *Helicobacter pylori* (Hp) in the mucous layer (Mu). In the vicinity of the bacteria, there is a dramatic reduction in mucus (*asterisks*). L—lumen. (*From* Mauch *et al.* [4]; with permission.)

ASSOCIATION OF *HELICOBACTER PYLORI* WITH GASTROINTESTINAL DISEASE

Group	Seroprevalence of *H. pylori* infection, %
Healthy subjects	20*
Chronic active gastritis	100
Duodenal ulcer	>90
Gastric ulcer	50–80
Gastric adenocarcinoma	90
Gastric lymphoma	85

Will vary with age and ethnic group.

FIGURE 2-14.

Association of *Helicobacter pylori* with gastrointestinal disease. *H. pylori* may be found in healthy asymptomatic individuals, and rates of infection vary depending on age, country of origin, and ethnic group (*see* Figs 2-18 and 2-19). In this table, however, individuals with certain gastrointestinal diseases have higher rates of *H. pylori* infection than nondiseased, healthy subjects.

TESTS FOR *HELICOBACTER PYLORI* INFECTION

Noninvasive

Test	Sensitivity, %	Specificity, %	Comments
Serology	88–96	86–95	Antibody titers do not return to negative after eradication of *H. pylori*; thus, serology is not a suitable test to document effectiveness of eradication
Urea breath tests	90–100	89–100	Because this test has high sensitivity and specificity and is noninvasive, when commercially available, it will be useful for documentation of *H. Pylori* eradiction

Invasive

Test	Sensitivity, %	Specificity, %	Comments
Histology	93–99	95–99	Requires histologic evaluation of mucosal biopsy; thus, it is expensive
Rapid urease test (CLOtest™, Delta West Limited, Bentley, Western Australia)	89–98	93–98	Inexpensive, it can provide relatively rapid diagnosis
Culture	77–92	100	Technically difficult and accuracy varies with laboratory; also expensive

FIGURE 2-15.

The tests for diagnosis of *Helicobacter pylori* can be categorized noninvasive (*ie*, do not require endoscopy) or invasive (*ie*, require endoscopy). The advantages and disadvantages of each diagnostic method are listed. The urea breath test is a good test for *H. pylori* screening and for follow-up of efficacy of *H. pylori* eradication because it is noninvasive and has good sensitivity and acceptable specificity.

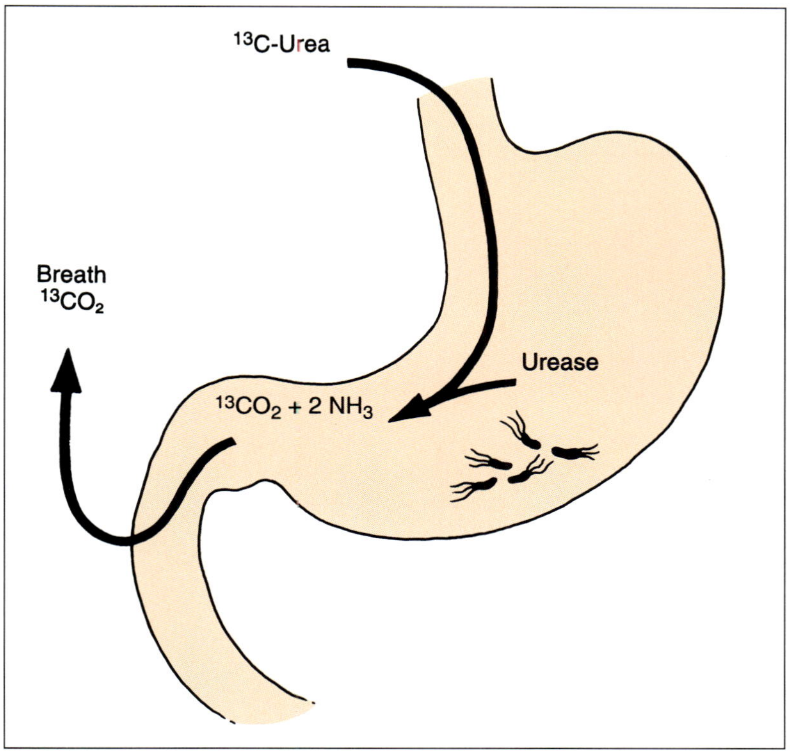

FIGURE 2-16.

Urea breath tests (^{13}C and ^{14}C). Diagnosis of *Helicobacter pylori* by the urea breath test is based on urease metabolism of ingested urea. Either ^{14}C– or ^{13}C–labeled urea is ingested. (The C^{13}–labeled urea is a nonradioactive carbon isotope). If *H. pylori* is present, urea is metabolized to ammonia and carbon-labeled carbon dioxide. The labeled carbon dioxide is then excreted in breath as labeled carbon dioxide, which is then collected and quantified. Although this illustration demonstrates the breath test using ^{13}C, the urea breath test can be similarly performed using ^{14}C.

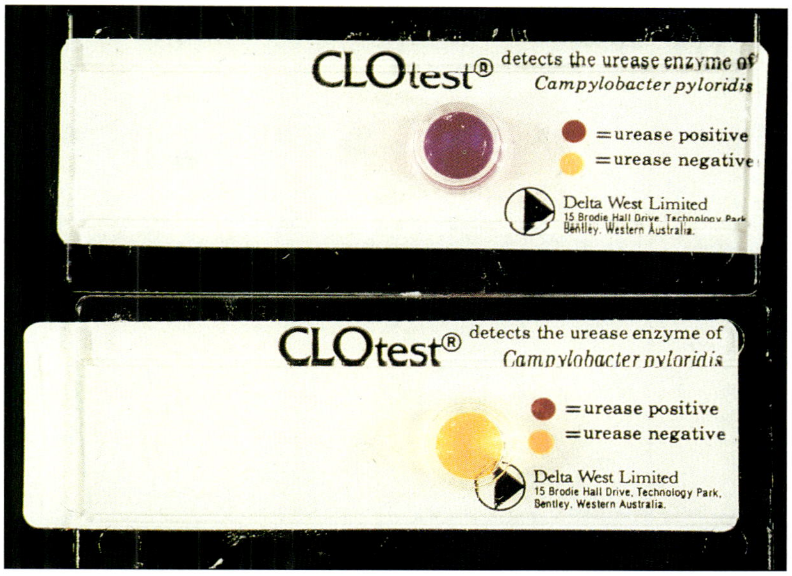

FIGURE 2-17.

The rapid urease test. The rapid urease test involves inoculation of the biopsy specimens into a liquid or gel medium containing urea and phenol red, which turns pink if the pH rises above 6.0. Such a change occurs when urea in the gel is metabolized to ammonia by the urease of the organism. One such test, called CLOtest™ (Delta West Limited, Bentley, Western Australia), is shown in this figure. Its low cost and dependability make it the most quick and desirable endoscopic method of diagnosis [5]. The rapid urease test is 89% to 98% sensitive and 93% to 98% specific.

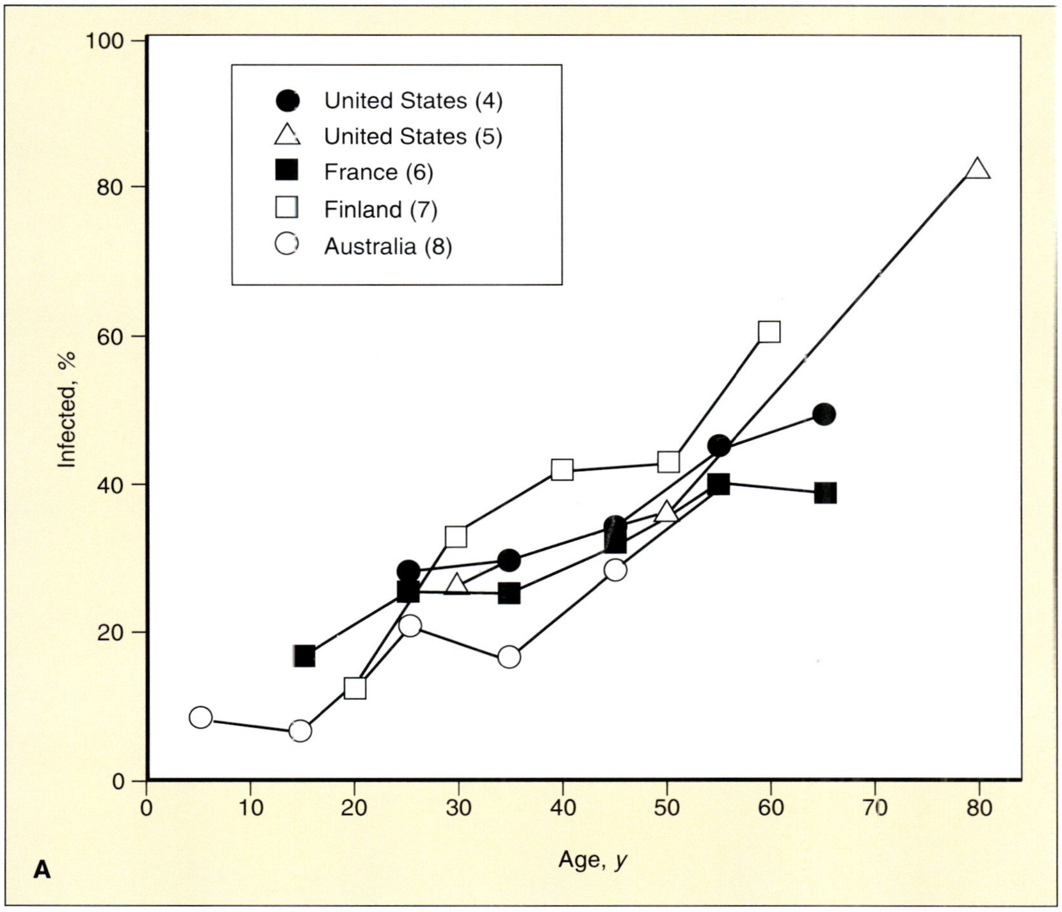

FIGURE 2-18.

Serologic prevalence by age and country of origin. The prevalence of *Helicobacter pylori* colonization in healthy individuals varies greatly with age and country of origin. **A**, In developed countries, it is uncommon for children to be infected with *H. pylori*, whereas up to 50% of adults older than 60 years of age are infected.

(*continued on next page*)

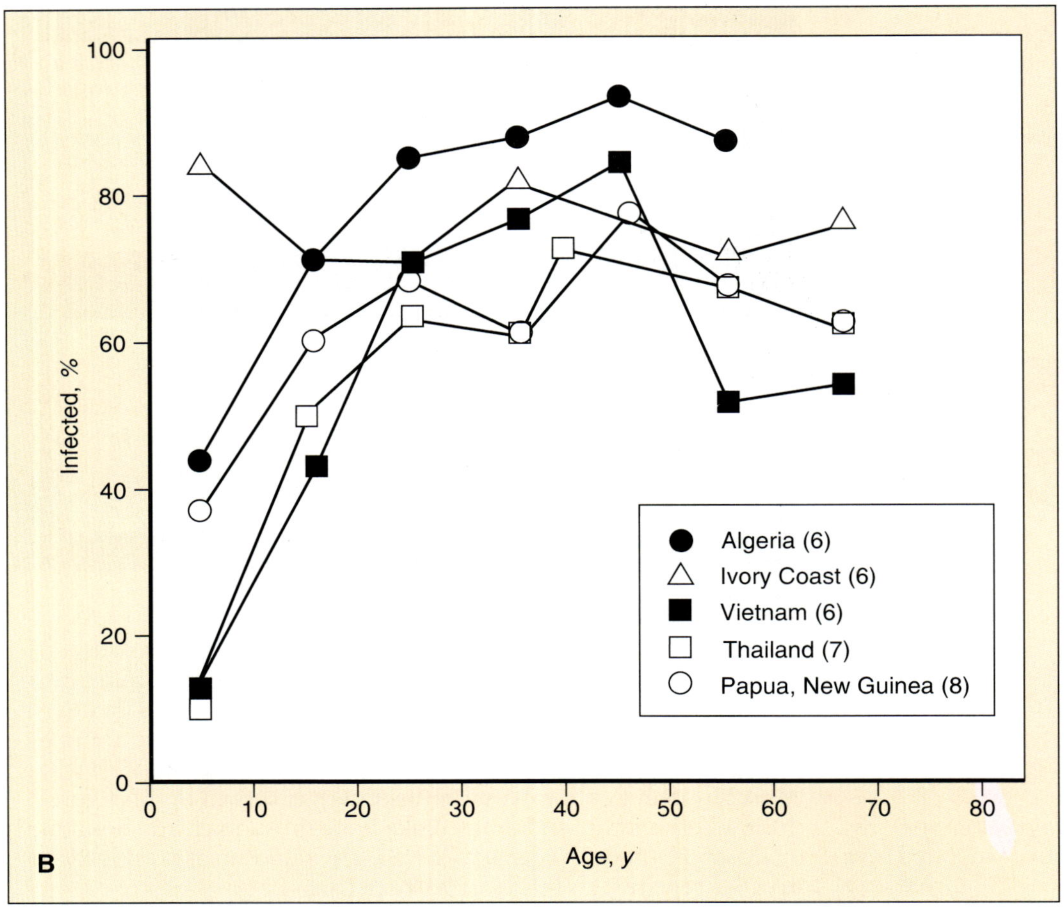

FIGURE 2-18. *CONTINUED*

B, These rates of infection compare with underdeveloped countries where approximately 40% of children younger than 10 are infected with *H. pylori* and, depending on the country, this percentage may increase to greater than 80% by 50 years of age. The mode of transmission of *H. pylori* is thought to be person-to-person through fecal-oral or oral-oral routes. In underdeveloped countries, where many people live in close quarters or where sanitation systems are less advanced or nonexistent, greater opportunities for transmission of *H. pylori* may exist. (*Adapted from* Taylor and Blaser [6]; with permission.)

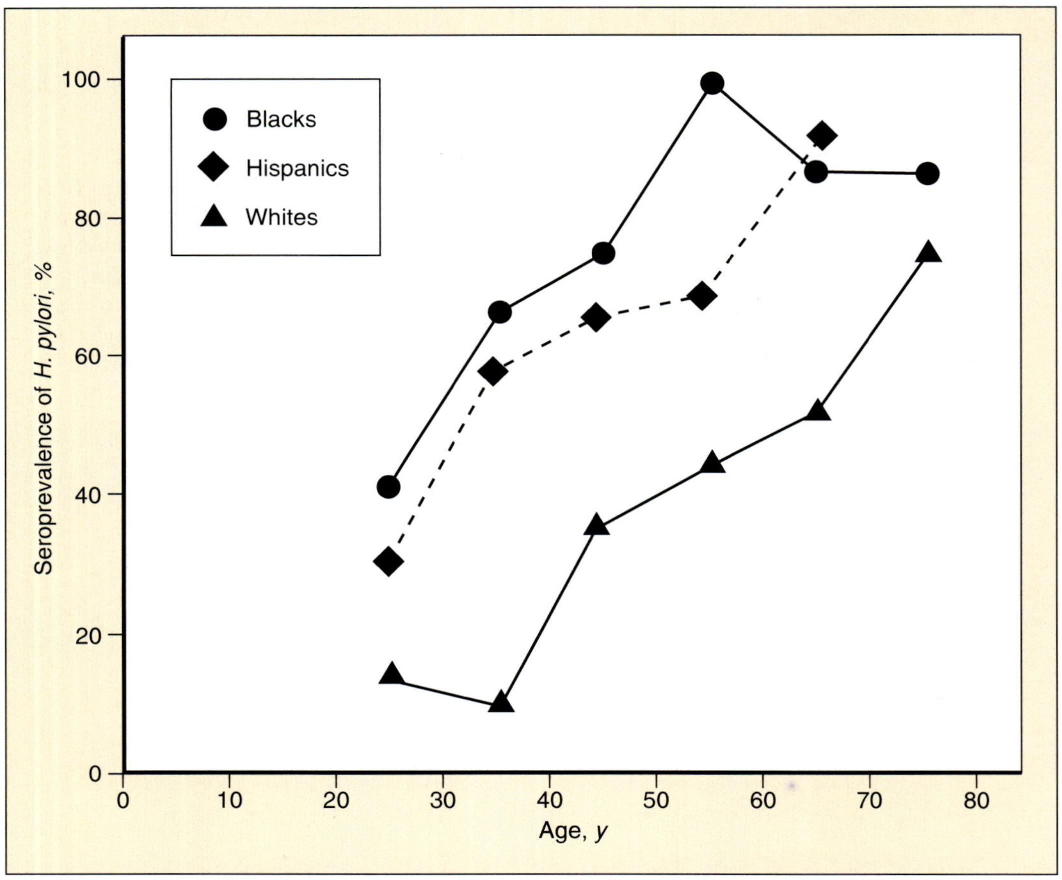

FIGURE 2-19.

Prevalence by ethnic group. In developed countries such as the United States, prevalence of *Helicobacter pylori* varies among different ethnic groups matched for socioeconomic status. (*Data from* Malaty *et al.* [7].)

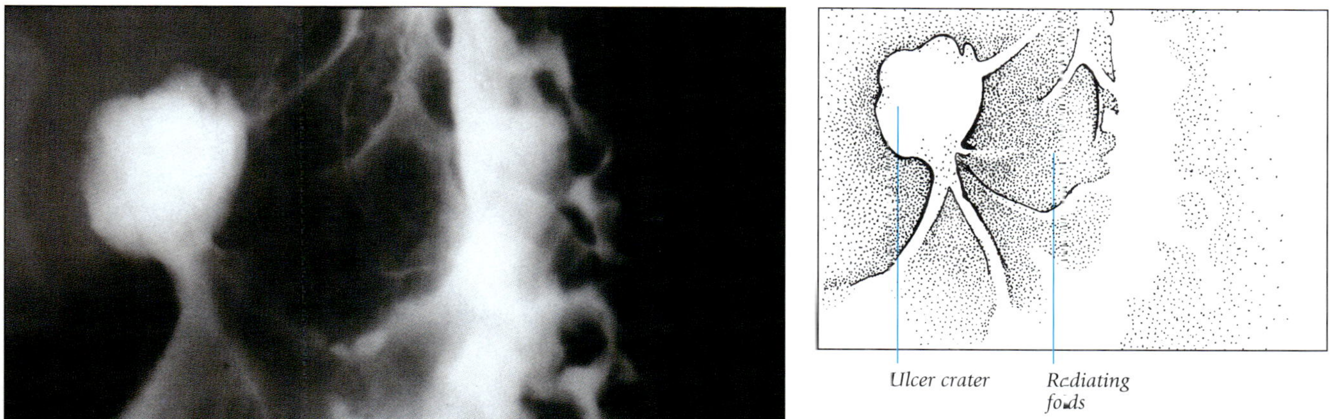

FIGURE 2-20.

Typical radiographic features of a benign gastric ulcer. A large well-circumscribed ulcer is seen on the angularis. Rugal folds can be seen radiating to the crater.

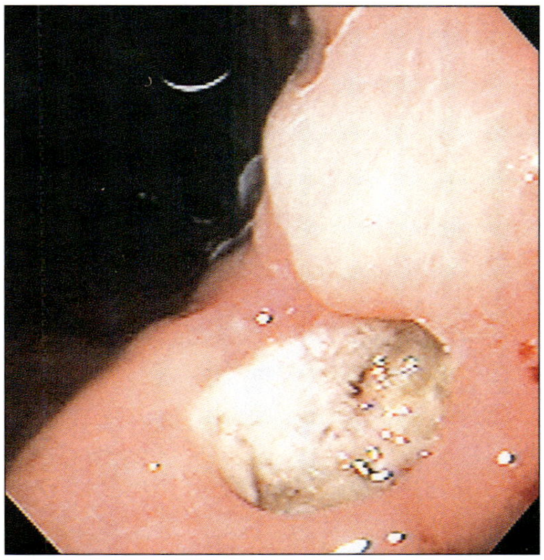

FIGURE 2-21.

The ulcer crater at endoscopy. The lesion is large and well circumscribed with a symmetrical appearance. Multiple biopsies did not demonstrate carcinoma and the ulcer was demonstated to heal on follow-up endoscopy. Radiographic features suggestive of a benign ulcer include projection of the ulcer away from the lumen, abscence of mass effect or mucosal nodularity, and rugal folds of normal appearance, which extend to the ulcer crater. The sensitivity of barium radiography for the diagnosis of gastric ulcer is approximately 65% to 90%; the sensitivity increases with the size of the lesion.

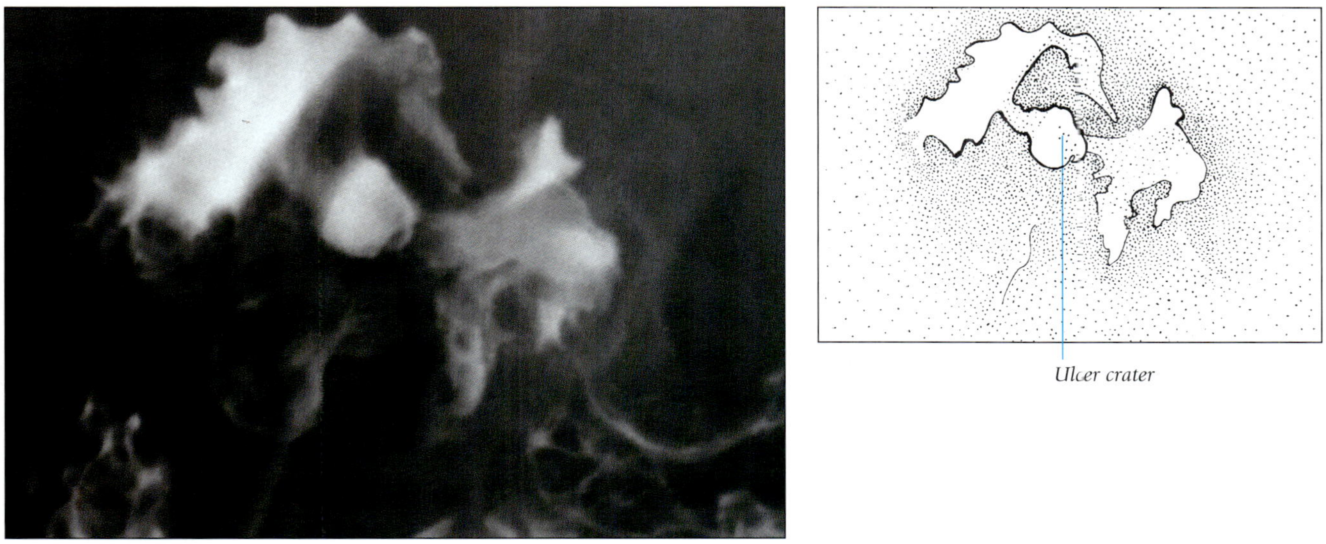

FIGURE 2-22.

Typical radiographic features of duodenal ulcer. This duodenal bulb ulcer is associated with marked edema, resulting in the appearance of radiating folds to the ulcer crater. The bulb is also distored secondary to previously existing ulceration.

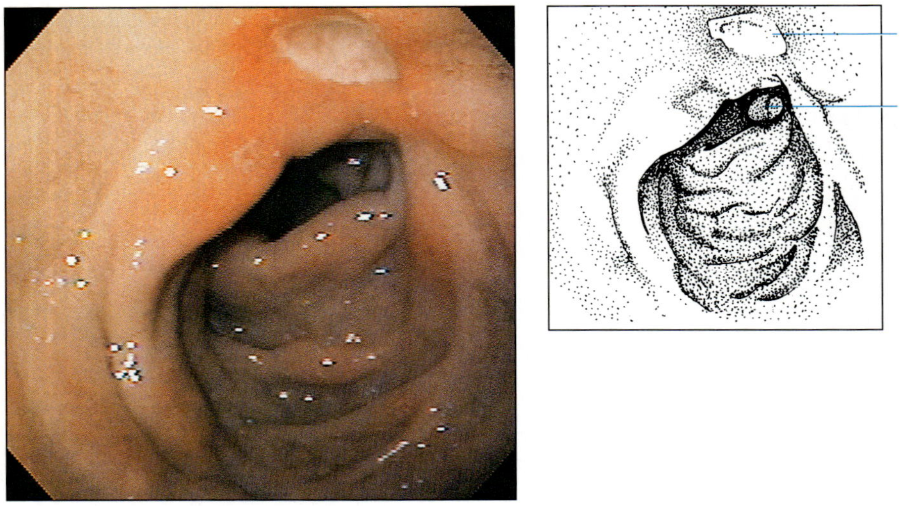

FIGURE 2-23.

Duodenal ulcer endoscopy. A well-circumscribed lesion as seen in a superior view. The remaining portion of the bulb is mildly edematous but without any associated subepithelial hemorrhage or erosions.

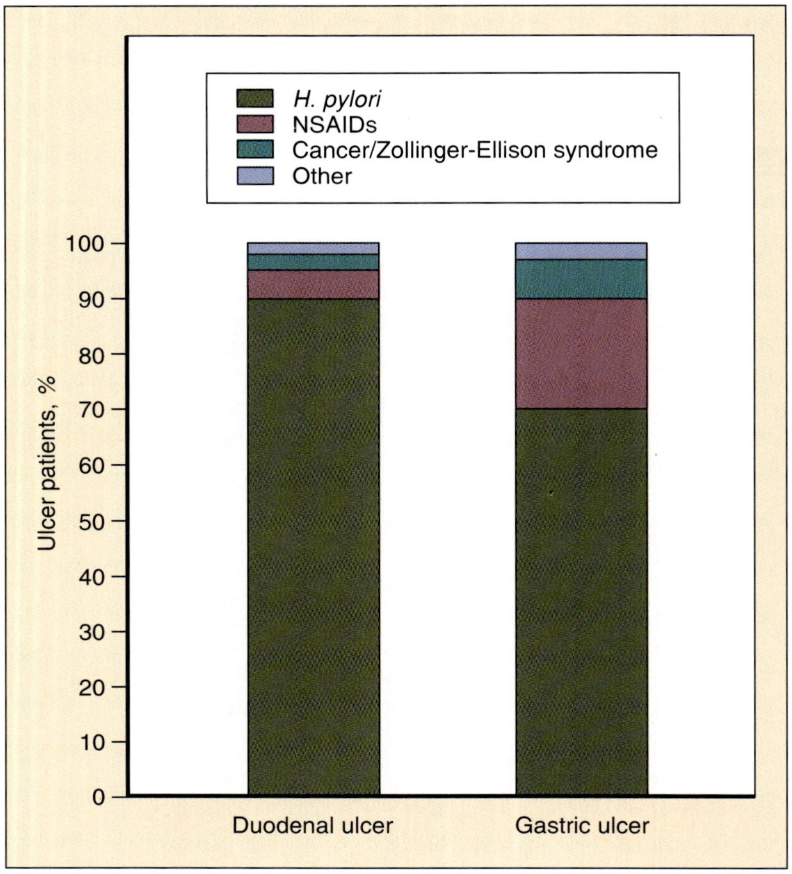

FIGURE 2-24.

Helicobacter pylori and peptic ulcer disease. *H. pylori* has a higher prevalence in gastric and duodenal ulcer patients than in noninfected, healthy controls (*see* Fig. 2-14). Although *H. pylori* has a stronger association with duodenal ulcers than with gastric ulcers, *H. pylori* is the most common cause of gastric ulcers. Depending on the series, *H. pylori* has been associated from 50% to 80% of all gastric ulcers. NSAIDs—nonsteroidal anti-inflammatory drugs.

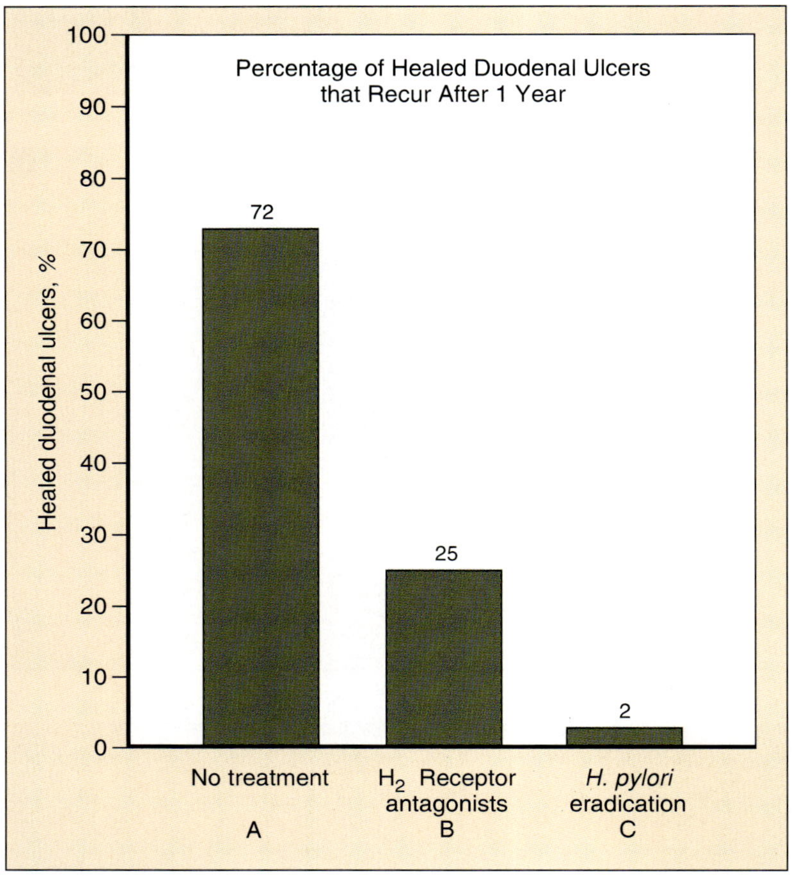

FIGURE 2-25.

Helicobacter pylori and peptic ulcer disease. When duodenal ulcers are healed by eradication of *H. pylori* (**C**), rates of recurrent ulcers are much lower than when ulcers are healed but *H. pylori* is not eradicated (**A** and **B**). (*Data from* Freston [8] and Tytgat and Rauws [9].)

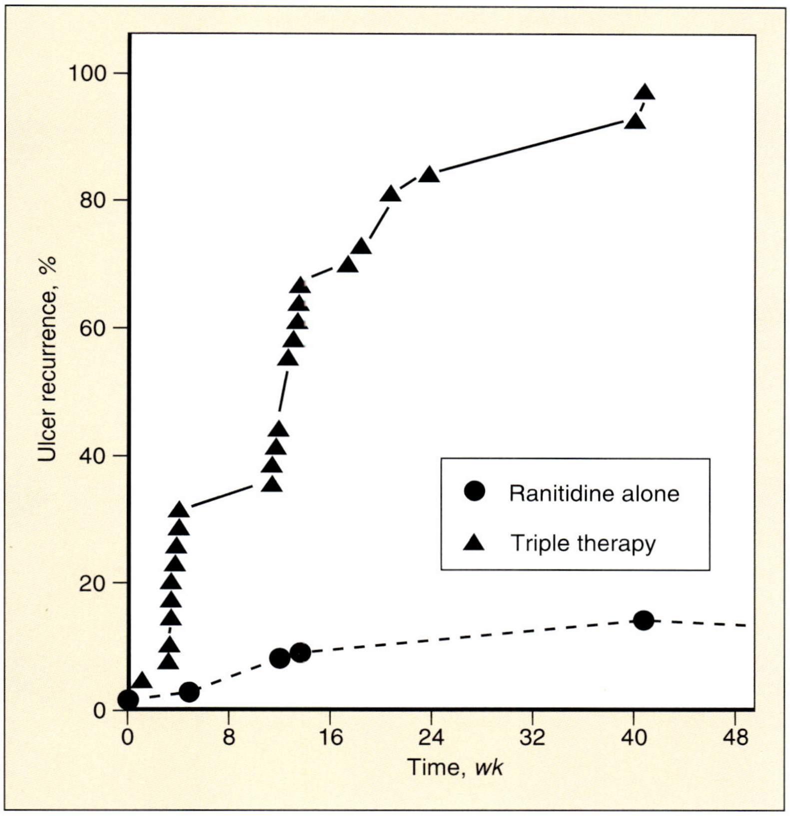

FIGURE 2-26.

Effect of *Helicobacter pylori* eradication on duodenal ulcer recurrence. In the results of the study, when triple therapy (bismuth, metronizadole, and either amoxicillin or tetracycline) is given for *H. pylori* eradication and is added to ranitidine for duodenal ulcer healing, duodenal ulcer recurrence rates at 1 year are much lower than when initial healing is accomplished with ranitidine alone. After the treatment period of ulcer healing, no ulcer maintenance therapy was given. Other popular regimens now include omeprazole plus clarithyromycin; ranitidine-bismuth (Tritec; Glaxo-Wellcome Research, Triangle Park, NC) plus clarithyromycin; and omeprazole, clarithyromycin, and either amoxicillin or metronidazole. (*From* Graham *et al.* [10]; with permission.)

ULCER COMPLICATIONS

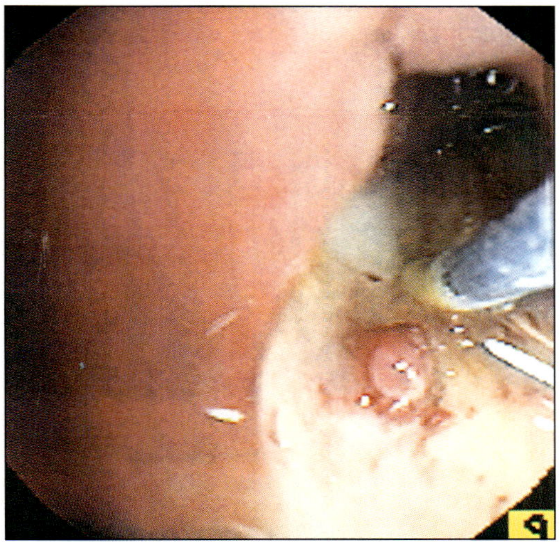

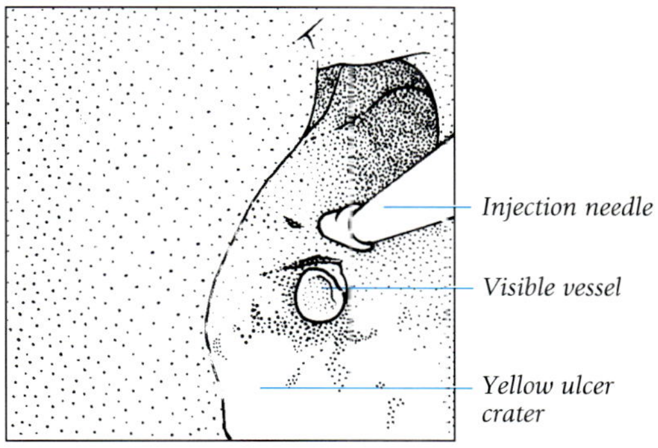

FIGURE 2-27.

Bleeding. Approximately 50% of patients with upper gastrointestinal hemorrhage have experienced bleeding from a peptic ulcer. Bleeding duodenal ulcers are twice as common as gastric ulcers. Endoscopic appearance of an ulcer, that is, the presence or absence of stigmata predicting recurrent bleeding, is of value in assessing prognosis. This visible vessel was seen in an edematous duodenal bulb (hence the close-up view). It is actively oozing. A bipolar electrocoagulation probe is poised in the lower left corner before therapy.

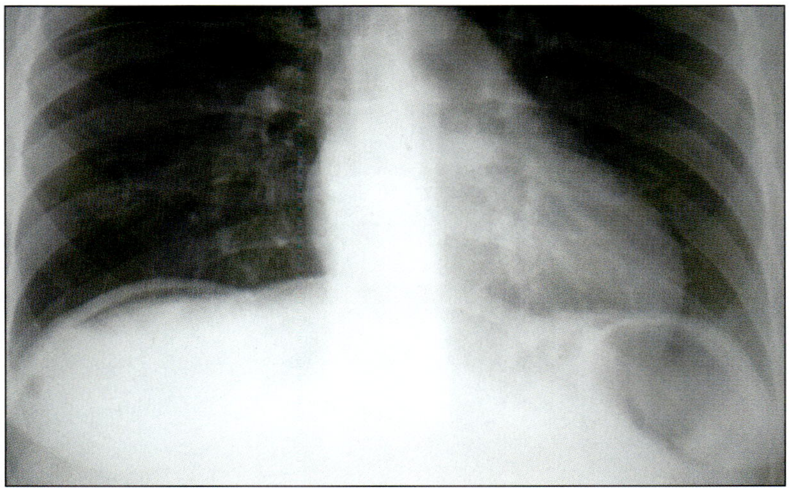

FIGURE 2-28.

Perforated peptic ulcer. Air is present under the right hemidiaphragm in a patient with acute severe abdominal pain. This patient had a perforated anterior duodenal bulbar ulcer. Recently, perforated ulcer has also been associated with cocaine use.

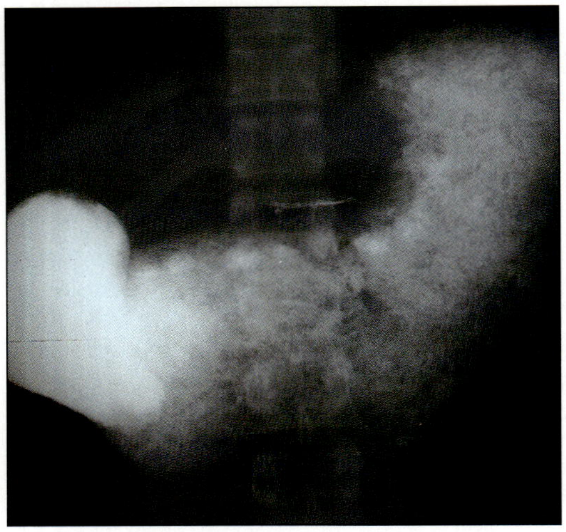

FIGURE 2-29.

Pyloric outlet obstruction related to peripyloric ulcer disease is uncommon. Acutely, obstruction may result from edema. In some patients, however, chronic disease results in fixed fibrosis and outlet obstruction. Barium upper gastrointestinal study demonstrates the size of the stomach.

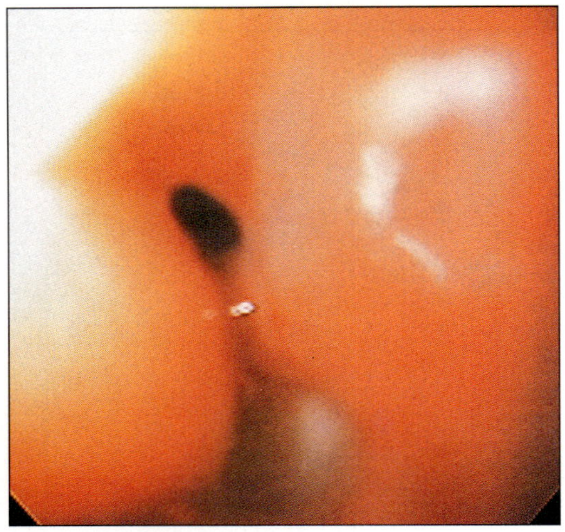

FIGURE 2-30.

Endoscopy demonstrates pyloric obstruction with an active ulcer crater seen in the pyloric channel. Nasogastric suction and intravenous H_2-receptor antagonists resulted in a clinical cure. In some patients, surgery may be required. Endoscopic balloon dilation has been useful in some patients with fixed obstruction without active ulcer disease.

SURGERY FOR ULCER DISEASE

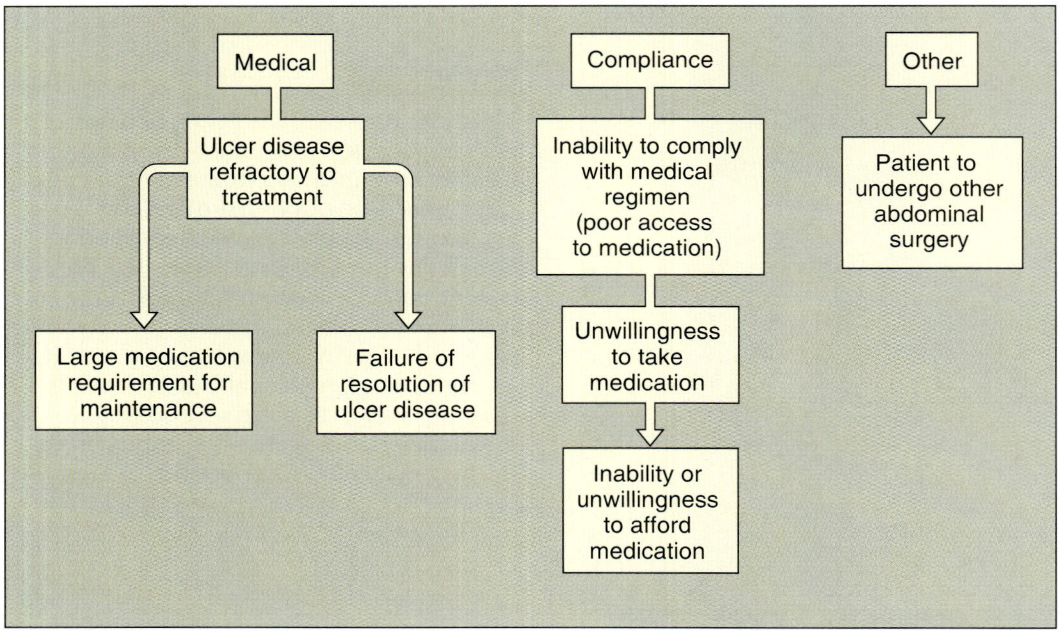

FIGURE 2-31.

Indications for elective operative treatment of peptic ulcer disease (PUD). Until the 1970s, treatment of benign ulcers of the stomach and duodenum comprised an enormous bulk of general surgical practice. Since the advent of effective antisecretory medications and now the recognition and eradication of *Helicobacter pylori*, surgery for PUD has been relegated to a secondary role, most often in a more complicated disease state. Indications for elective surgery remain but are far more circumscribed than they were in the past. Refractoriness to treatment occurs very rarely in the case of duodenal ulcers, but large maintenance medication requirements or intolerance of treatment are occasional indications for surgery. The possibility of carcinoma in gastric ulcers that fail to heal necessitates surgery even if endoscopic biopsies are negative. Patients undergoing other abdominal surgery can be considered for highly selective vagotomy depending on the magnitude of the primary procedure. With the advent of laparoscopic antiulcer surgery, straightforward procedures, such as cholecystectomy, have been combined with laparoscopic vagotomy in selected patients with concurrent symptomatic gallstone and PUD [11]. Data examining such combined operations should be available in the near future.

ULCER RECURRENCE RATES FOLLOWING SURGICAL PROCEDURES

Operation	Recurrence rate, %	Remarks
Gastric resection	2–5	Varies according to amount resected 75% Optimal
Vagotomy and drainage	10–15	Pyloroplasty most frequent drainage procedure
Vagotomy and antrectomy	0–2	Lowest recurrence rates
Parietal cell vagotomy [12,13]	10–17	Operator dependent

Figure 2-32.

Ulcer recurrence rates following surgical procedures. Ulcer recurrence rates after operations for peptic ulcer disease (PUD) vary according to the nature of the procedure, the pathophysiology of the underlying disease, as well as operator skill. Gastric resection alone, although cited for historical purposes, is rarely undertaken for peptic ulcer management. The standard surgical criterion for PUD is vagotomy and antrectomy if protection from recurrent ulcers is taken as the major goal of treatment. Technical pitfalls associated with this procedure include incomplete vagotomy and retained antrum or residual antral mucosa left on the duodenal stump, which can produce hypergastrinemia and recurrent ulcer after restoring foregut continuity by gastrojejunostomy. Although unsuspected gastrinoma must be considered in any patient with marginal ulcer after vagotomy and antrectomy, routine serum gastrin testing before elective surgery has made this situation rare. Most surgeons and patients are willing to accept the slightly higher risk of recurrent ulcers with highly selective vagotomy to avoid postgastrectomy and postvagatomy complications. (*Adapted from* McFadden and Zinner [14]; with permission.)

GASTRINOMA (ZOLLINGER-ELLISON SYNDROME)

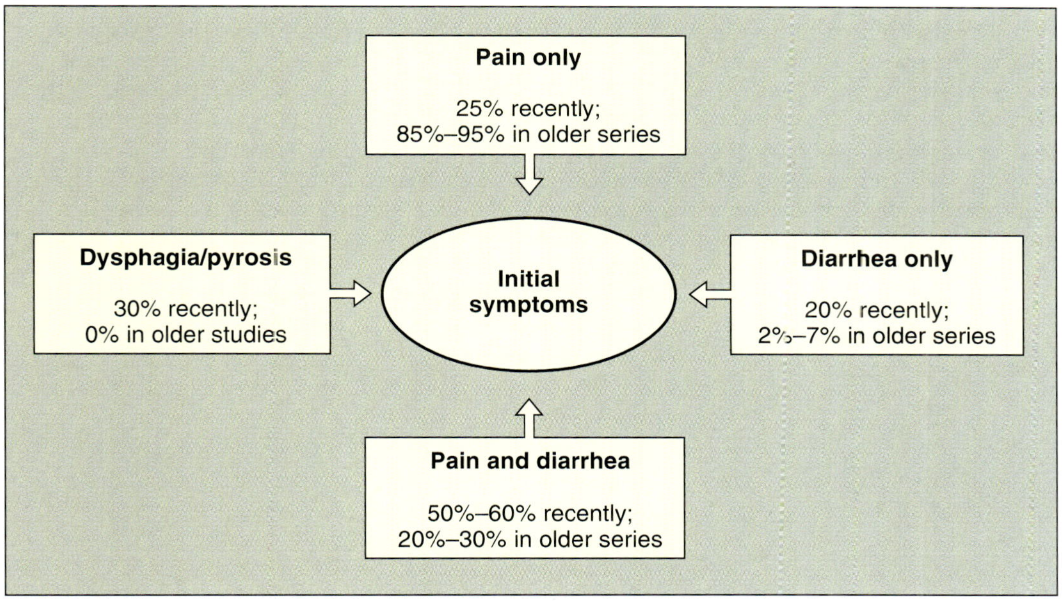

Figure 2-33.

Clinical features of Zollinger-Ellison syndrome (ZES). The results in this figure are based on data from two recently published large series of patients with ZES involving 165 [15] and 144 [16] patients analyzed in a recent review [17], and from other earlier studies involving 34 [18], 40 [19], 26 [20], and 260 [21] patients with ZES. The percentages given in the figure refer to the percentages of all patients with the indicated symptom as the initial presenting symptom. Abdominal pain remains the most common initial feature of the disease, either alone or with diarrhea. Increasingly, however, diarrhea and esophageal reflux disease symptoms are being recognized. In the past, patients frequently presented with complications of severe peptic disease, however, at present, a typical patient first has symptoms indistinguishable from those seen in a patient with routine peptic ulcer disease, resulting in an average delay of 6 years in making the diagnosis of ZES [17]. At present, bleeding, severe nausea and vomiting, or perforation occur in 10%, 30%, and 7% of patients with ZES [17,22,23].

CLINICAL FEATURES OR LABORATORY TESTS THAT SHOULD LEAD TO A SUSPICION OF ZES

I. Clinical features
- A. In a patient with duodenal ulcers
  - 1. No *Helicobacter pylori* present
  - 2. Presence of diarrhea
  - 3. Failure of the duodenal ulcer to heal with *H. pylori* eradication or with standard doses of histamine H_2 blockers
- B. Multiple duodenal ulcers or ulcers in unusual locations
- C. Severe peptic ulcer disease leading to a complication (*eg*, bleeding perforation, intractability)
- D. Severe or resistant peptic esophageal disease
- E. History of nephrolithiasis or endocrinopathies
- F. Family history of nephrolithiasis, endocrinopathies, or peptic ulcer disease

II. Laboratory features in a patient with peptic ulcer that should suggest ZES
- A. Hypergastrinemia
- B. Hypercalcemia
- C. Endocrinopathy
- D. Prominent gastric folds on upper gastrointestinal tract radiograph or at upper gastrointestinal endoscopy

FIGURE 2-34.

Clinical features or laboratory results that should lead to a suspicion of Zollinger-Ellison syndrome (ZES). Because most patients with ZES present with pain that is indistinguishable from pain observed in patients with routine peptic ulcer disease, resulting in a mean delay in diagnosis of 6 years [17,24], it is important to have a high index of suspicion for this disease. Diarrhea particularly should suggest the diagnosis, because even in patients with routine peptic ulcer disease who are gastric acid hypersecreters, diarrhea is rare [25]. *Helicobacter pylori* is found in 90% to 98% of patients with duodenal ulcers with routine peptic ulcer disease [17,24,26] but is found in less than 50% of patients with ZES [27–29]. *H. pylori* eradication results in healing in 90% of patients with routine peptic ulcer disease, but it will not result in ulcer healing in ZES. Any feature suggesting multiple endocrine neoplasia type 1 syndrome (associated endocrinopathy) or a family history of peptic ulcer disease should raise the suspicion of ZES in a patient with peptic ulcer disease.

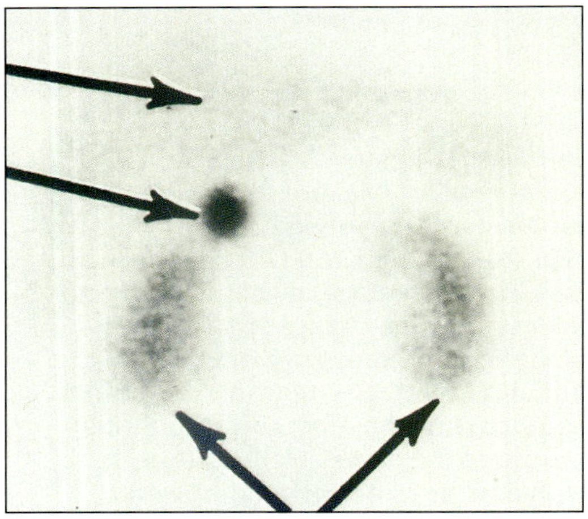

FIGURE 2-35.

Somatostatin receptor scintigraphy (SRS) localization of a gastrinoma in the pancreatic head area in a patient with Zollinger-Ellison syndrome (ZES). This figure shows the localization of a gastrinoma (*lower arrow at left*) in a patient with ZES using SRS with [^{111}In-DTPA-DPhe^{1}]-octreotide. As this figure shows [^{111}In-DTPA-DPhe^{1}]-octreotide is primarily excreted in the urine (kidneys [*arrows at bottom*]), however, a small amount also is taken up by the liver (*upper arrow at left*). Recent data suggest SRS will be particularly helpful in diagnosis of gastrinomas [30–33]. Nearly 100% of gastrinomas are reported to possess increased numbers of somatostatin receptors [34]. Another advantage of SRS is its ability of also frequently detecting previously unrecognized distal metastases [32]. The false-positive rate, whether SRS will detect small duodenal gastrinomas, and whether it is more sensitive than angiography remain unclear [30,35].

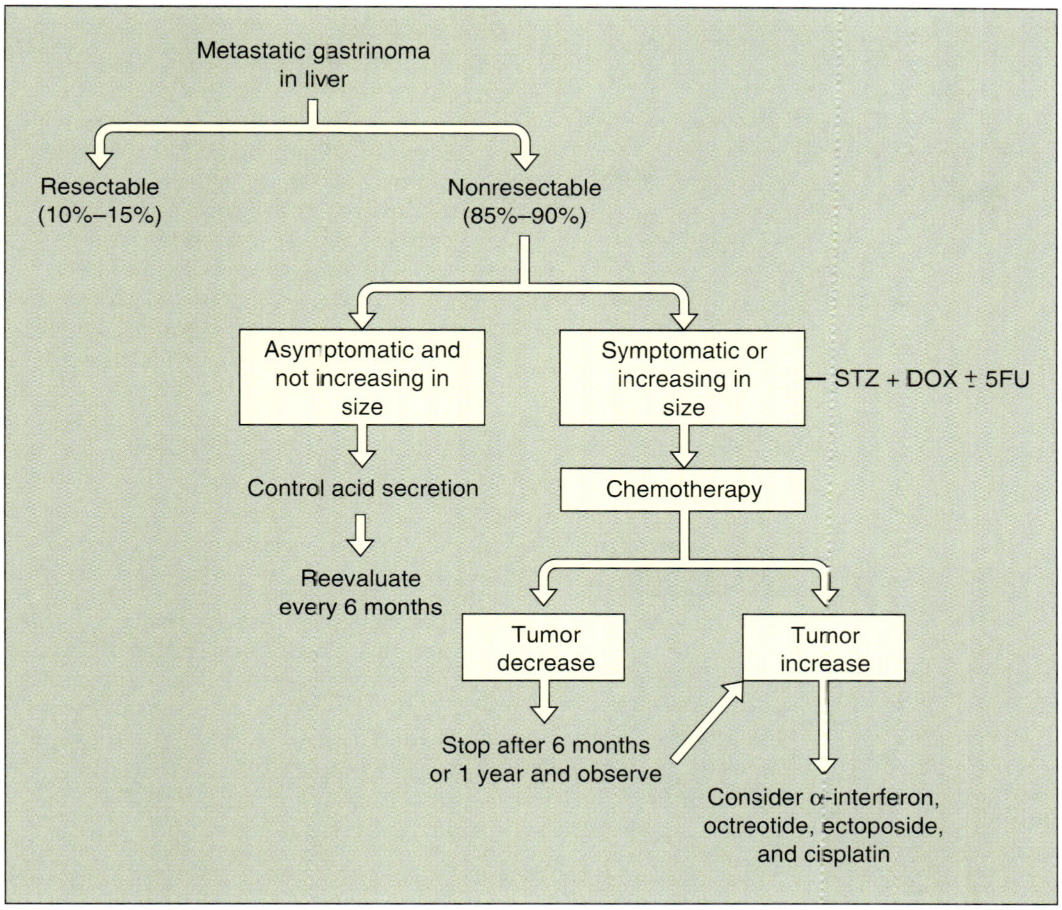

FIGURE 2-36.

Treatment of metastatic gastrinoma. Up to 15% of metastatic gastrinomas found in the liver may be resectable [36]. Most patients have diffuse metastases involving both hepatic lobes, however, the decision needs to be made whether chemotherapy or some other treatment should be instituted because of the patients poor prognosis. A small percentage of patients do not demonstrate progressive disease and after acid secretion is controlled, are asymptomatic, and thus no further treatment is required [37]. If the tumor progresses in size or becomes symptomatic, chemotherapy with streptozotocin (STZ) and doxorubicin (DOX) with or without 5-fluorouracil (5FU) is recommended. Approximately 50% will respond with a decrease in tumor size, but with time the tumor usually begins to grow again [38–40]. Subsequent treatment with interferon, octreotide, or possibly ectoposide and cisplatin might be considered [38,41–44].

OTHER COMMON BLEEDING GASTRODUODENAL LESIONS

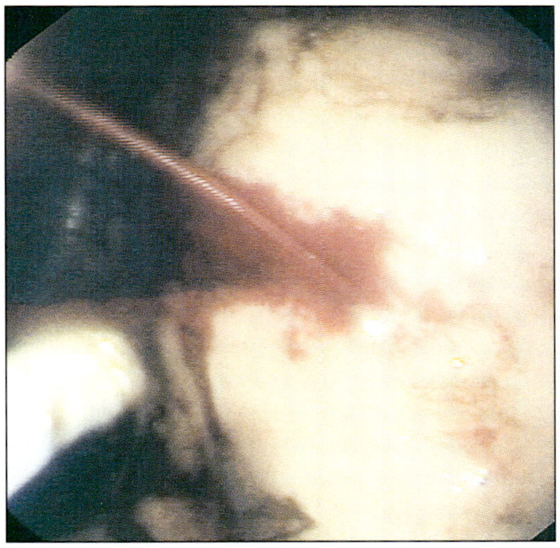

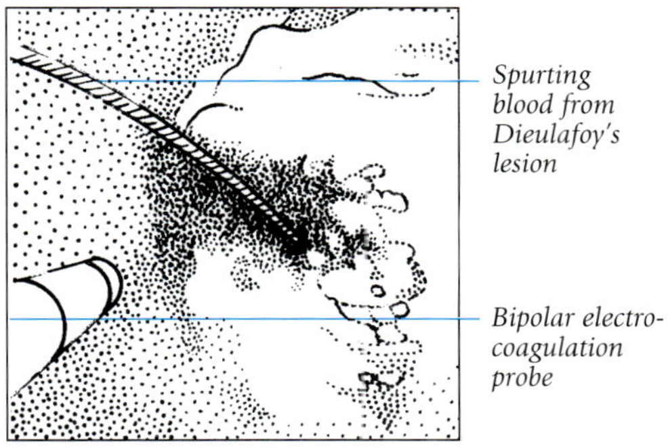

FIGURE 2-37.

Dieulafoy's lesion. Dieulafoy's lesion is a rare cause of massive and recurrent upper gastrointestinal hemorrhage. The lesion is an extramural caliber artery present in the submucosa. Bleeding probably results from pressure exerted by such a blood vessel on the overlying mucosa so that it is ultimately exposed to the lumen. Dieulafoy's lesion is most common in the gastric cardia, 6 cm from the gastroesophageal junction. Mortality is high because the bleeding site is often difficult to identify. When exposed to the lumen, the vessel's wall may actually break down and lead to dramatic bleeding.

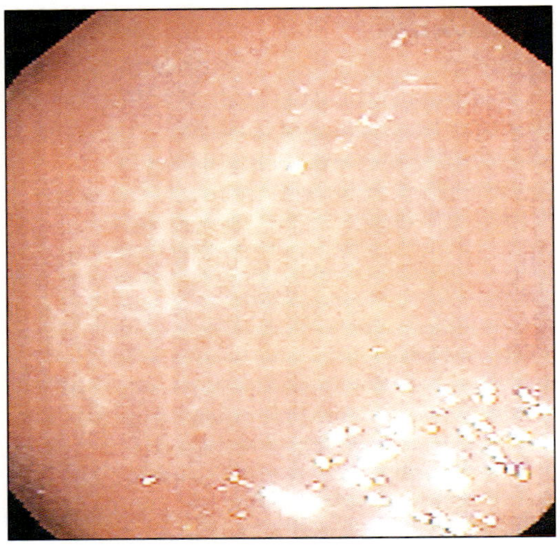

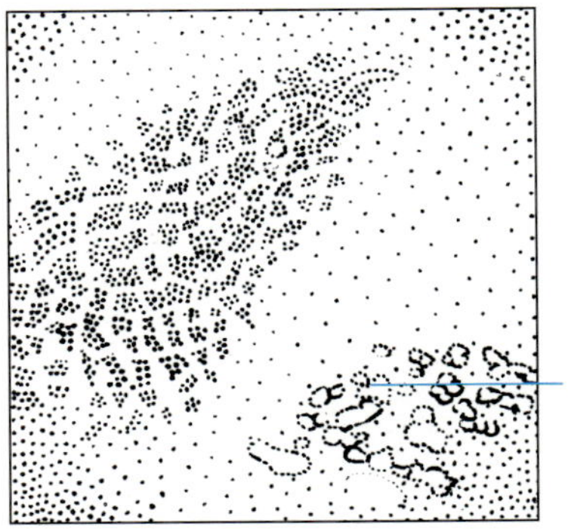

FIGURE 2-38.

Portal hypertensive gastropathy. Typically portal hypertensive gastropathy has the appearance of a mucosal mosaic pattern with a speckling of subepithelial hemorrhages superimposed upon it. Histologically, it consists of vascular dilation and ectasia. Despite being very common in patients with portal hypertension, it has not been proven that portal hypertensive gastropathy by itself is responsible for significant upper gastrointestinal hemorrhaging; although this is likely.

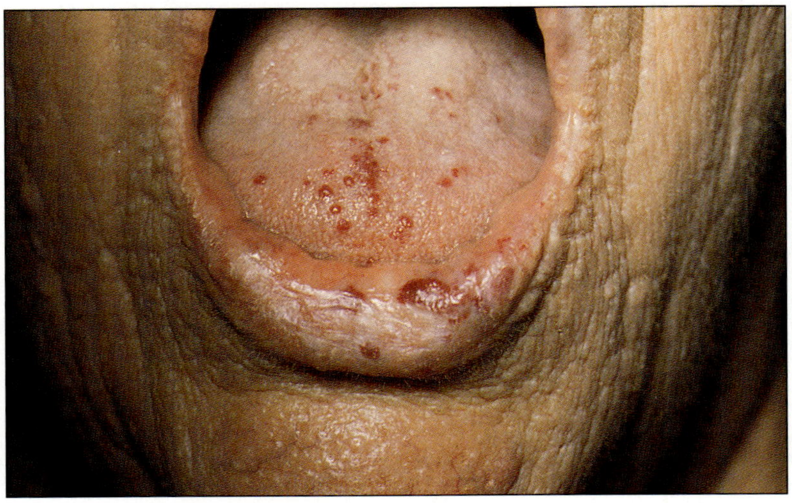

FIGURE 2-39.

A patient with Rendu-Osler-Weber syndrome, demonstrating multiple telangiectasias on the tongue and lips. The lesions usually begin as flat macules, then slowly enlarge to form papules. They commonly occur on the face, lips, tongue, palate, ears, hands, chest, and feet. Arteriovenous malformations and aneurysms may develop throughout the body, causing epistaxis and gastrointestinal tract bleeding. Although the syndrome is autosomal dominant, up to 46% of patients develop the syndrome without a positive family history.

MALIGNANT GASTRIC NEOPLASMS

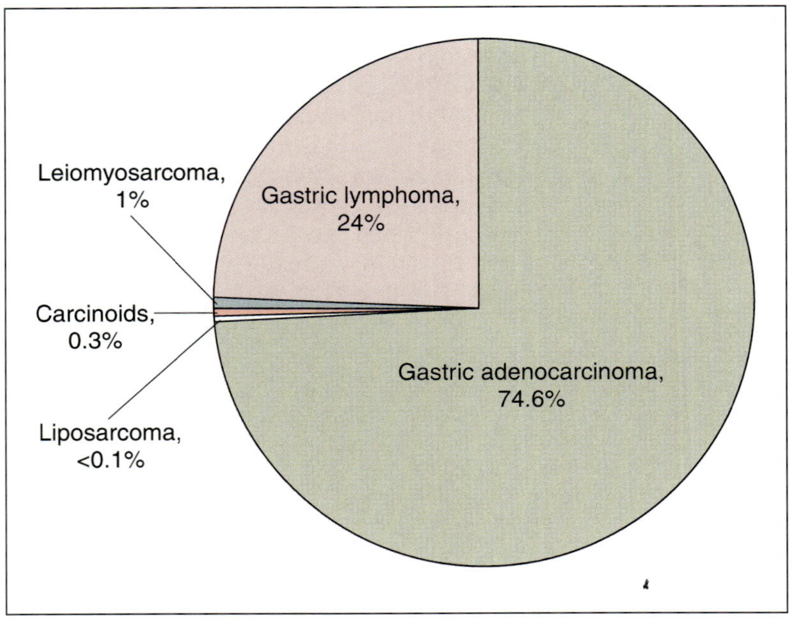

FIGURE 2-40.

Malignant gastric neoplasms. Pie chart demonstrating the relative incidence of malignant tumors of the stomach. The vast majority of these malignancies and neoplasms are gastric adenocarcinomas [45].

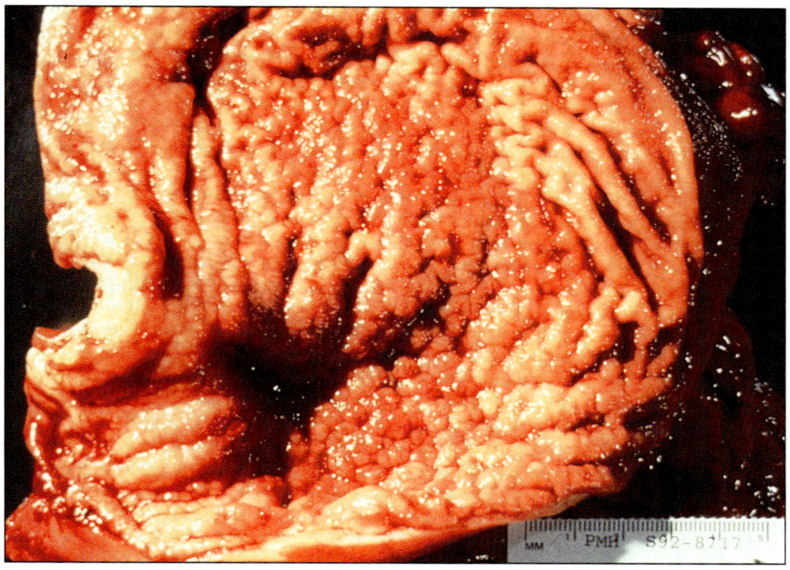

FIGURE 2-41.

Gastric adenocarcinoma. *Helicobacter pylori* is epidemiologically associated with adenocarcinoma of the gastric body and antrum. This association of *H. pylori* is not, however, seen with adenocarcinomas of the gastric cardia. Shown is a resected stomach with diffuse gastric adenocarcinoma of the "linitis plastica" type. A very large, deep ulcer is seen at the junction of the gastric body and antrum. Diffuse thickening of the entire stomach is seen as producing multiple, nodular folds. On microscopic sections, *H. pylori* and adenocarcinoma were both visualized. (*Courtesy of* C. Vardaman, Dallas, TX)

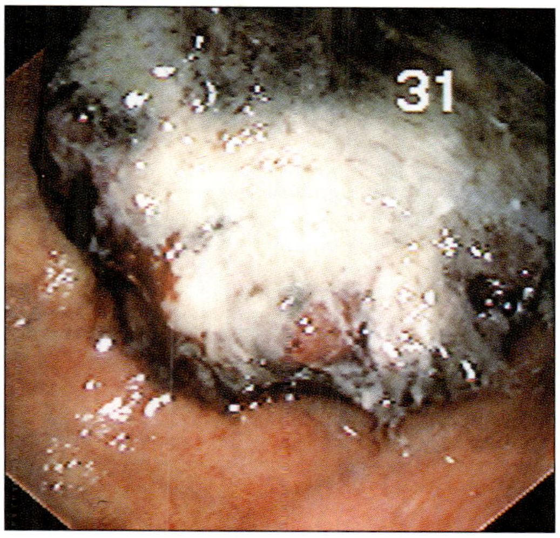

FIGURE 2-42.

This endoscopic view reveals the presence of an obviously ulcerated mass. Biopsy is one type of modality frequently used to reveal the presence of adenocarcinoma.

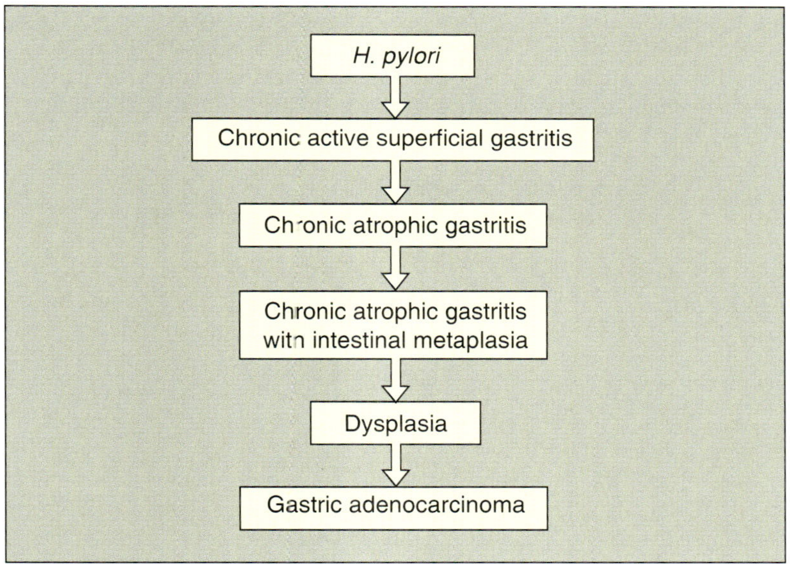

FIGURE 2-43.

Relationship of *Helicobacter pylori* to gastric cancer. Sequence of gastric mucosal histologic events through which chronic gastric inflammation may predispose to gastric adenocarcinoma is shown. *H. pylori* is the major cause of chronic active superficial gastritis which, in some patients, may progress to chronic atrophic gastritis. As important as *H. pylori* appears to be in gastric cancer, however, other cofactors must also play a role. Only a small proportion of patients progress to atrophic gastritis, much less dysplasia and adenocarcinoma. At this time it is uncertain whether eradication of *H. pylori* in infected, but otherwise healthy, subjects will prevent gastric cancer or reduce its incidence.

EARLY VERSUS ADVANCED GASTRIC CANCER

Depth of invasion	Lymph node involvement, %	5-year survival, %
Early gastric cancer	7	91
Advanced gastric cancer	66	4

FIGURE 2-44.

Neoplasms of the stomach. Early gastric cancer involves the mucosa, with or without involvement of the submucosa, but does not involve the muscularis propria. It has an excellent prognosis with surgical resection compared to advanced gastric cancer. (*From* Davis [45]; with permission.)

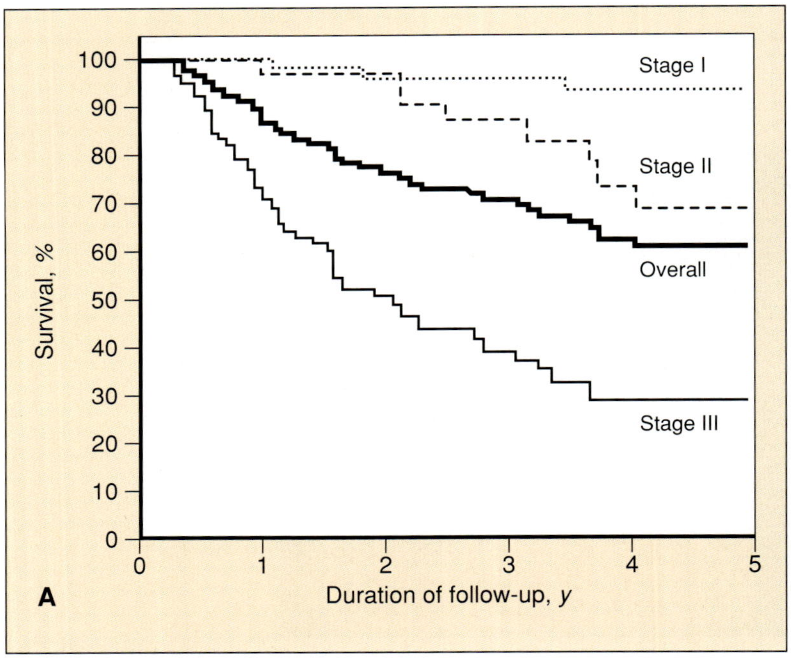

B. 1987 UNIFIED INTERNATIONAL TUMOR, NODE, METASTASES STAGING OF GASTRIC CANCER

Stage of disease	TNM		
I	T1N0M0	T1N1M0	T2N0M0
II	T1N2M0	T2N1M0	T3N0M0
IIIa	T2N2M0	T3N1M0	T4N0M0
IIIb	T3N2M0	T4N1M0	

T1=confined to mucosa/submucosa
T2=invading muscularis propria to subserosa
T3=through serosa
T4=through serosa with involvement of contiguous structures
N0=no nodal involvement
N1=affected nodes < 3 cm from tumor
N2=affected nodes > 3 cm from tumor
M0=no distant metastases

FIGURE 2-45.

Survival after operation for gastric cancer by tumor stage. In a recent study of gastric cancer in England, 42% (207 of 493) of treated patients were able to undergo potentially curative resection. Survival results after potentially curative treatment are shown here by stage of disease (*panel A*) along with the Unified International Tumor, Node, Metastasis (UICC TNM) staging system for gastric cancer (*panel B*) [46]. UICC TNM stage I and II patients had generally good results, and although they were the smallest group of patients overall (24%), they constituted 58% of potentially curative treatments. Stage III disease, as in other studies, fared considerably worse than patients staged earlier and were the single largest group receiving potentially curative treatment (42%). This experience was felt to reflect an increase in the incidence of curable cases being detected. (*Adapted from* Sue-Ling *et al.* [47]; with permission.)

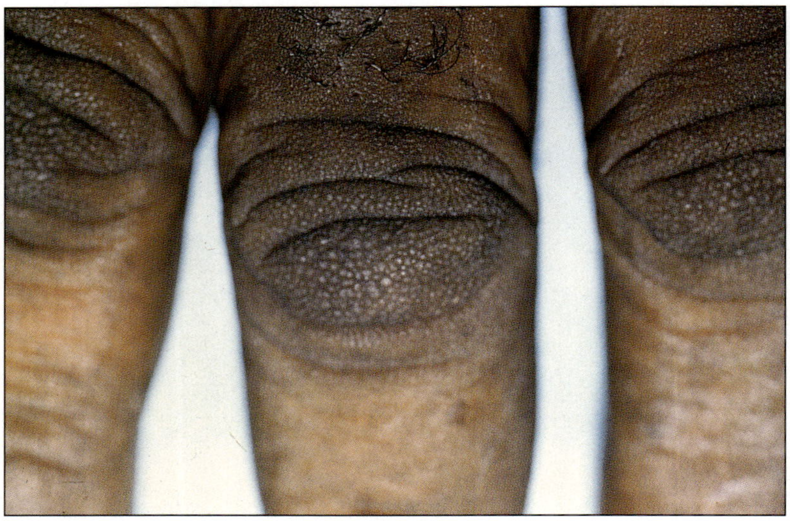

FIGURE 2-46.

Malignant acanthosis nigricans is a disorder of sudden onset that appears in unusual locations, such as the hands in addition to other more common locations. This disorder is frequently caused by a tumor, with gastric carcinoma as the associated malignancy in two-thirds of patients.

Gastric lymphoma

HELICOBACTER PYLORI AND GASTRIC NON-HODGKIN'S LYMPHOMAS

	Cases, *n*	Infected, %	Matched controls infected, %	Odds ratio	95% Confidence interval
Gastric non-Hodgkin's lymphoma	33	85	55	6.3*	2.0 to 19.9
Nongastric non-Hodgkin's lymphoma	31	65	59	1.2	0.5 to 3.0

*P=0.02

Figure 2-47.

Non-Hodgkin's lymphoma of the stomach is a rare disorder that accounts for only 3% of gastric malignancies, but is the most common type of extranodal lymphoma. Epidemiologic data have suggested an association between *H. pylori* infection and gastric lymphomas. Similar to the nested case control studies previously described, in this study, stored sera from patients with non-Hodgkin's gastric lymphomas and control subjects without cancer were analyzed for *H. pylori*. The sera were collected years before the diagnosis of gastric lymphoma. Patients with non-Hodgkin's gastric lymphoma were six times more likely to have been previously infected with *H. pylori* than were control subjects without lymphoma.

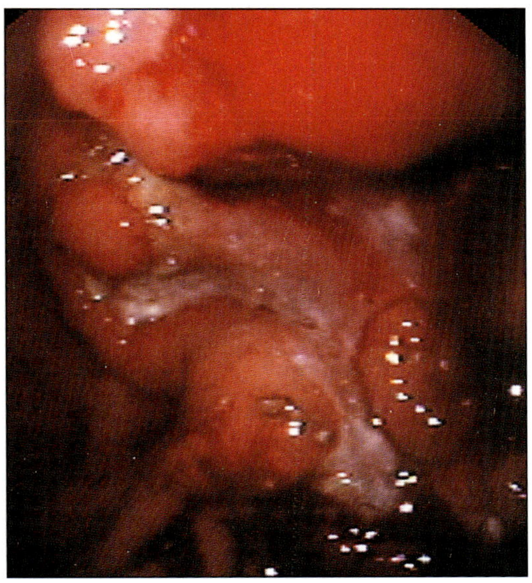

Figure 2-48.

Gastric lymphoma. Gastric lymphoma represents less than 5% of the gastric malignant neoplasms seen. The stomach remains the most common site of involvement for extranodal non-Hodgkin's lymphoma. Using only endoscopy and radiographic barium studies, lymphoma may be difficult to differentiate from gastric adenocarcinoma. Biopsies also are not particularly helpful in making the diagnosis. The 5-year survival rate for patients who have gastric lymphoma is approximately 50% when all combinations of patients and therapeutic modalities are considered. This endoscopic view reveals thickened folds. The differential diagnosis of thickened gastric folds includes many entities such as Zollinger-Ellison syndrome, Ménétrier's disease, varices lues, idiopathic hypertrophic gastrophy, eosinophilic gastritis, pseudolymphoma, and lymphoma.

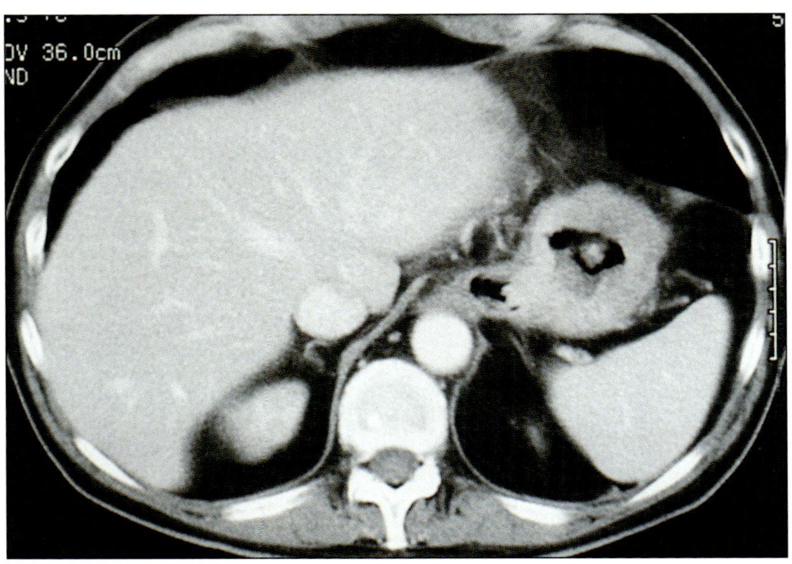

Figure 2-49.

Image from a computed tomographic scan demonstrating gastric involvement with lymphoma. The duodenum, pancreas, liver, spleen, and retroperitoneum remain uninvolved.

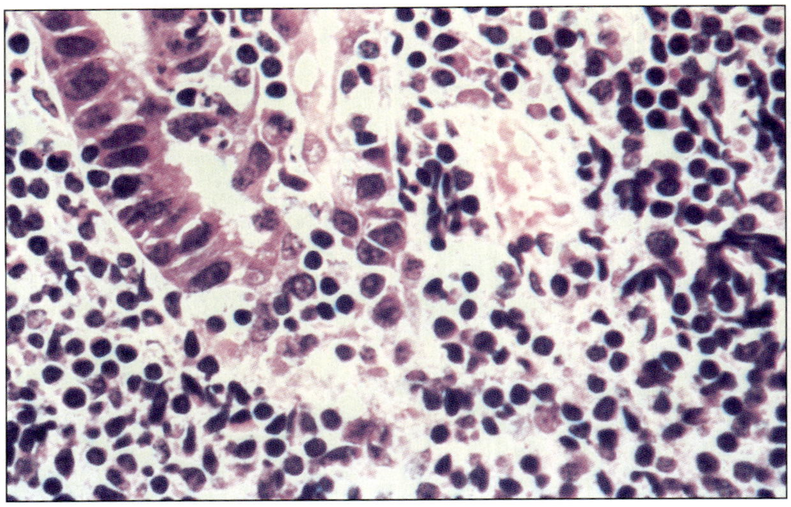

FIGURE 2-50.

Lymphoepithelial lesion. The transition from a *Helicobacter pylori*–related dense lymphoid infiltrate to a true mucosa-associated lymphoid tissue (MALT) lymphoma is felt to be represented histologically by the appearance of numerous lymphoepithelial lesions (LEL). Although LELs on histology are strongly suggestive of a MALT lymphoma, the diagnosis is confirmed through demonstration of monoclonality using gene rearrangement studies. As shown, a dense lymphoid infiltrate and glandular dropout are both present. The LEL is characterized by gland infiltration and destruction by lymphocytes.

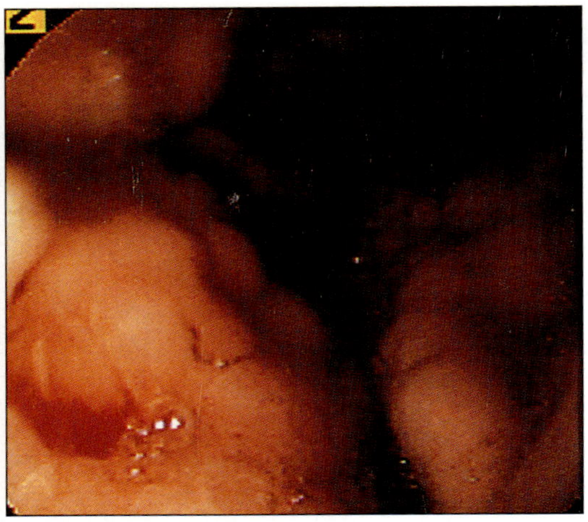

FIGURE 2-51.

Maltoma. Endoscopic view of an edematous gastric mucosa with marked erythema and friability.

REGRESSION OF GASTRIC MUCOSA-ASSOCIATED LYMPHOID TISSUE (MALT) LYMPHOMA WITH *HELICOBACTER PYLORI* ERADICATION

RESPONSE TO *H. PYLORI* ERADICATION	PATIENTS, *n**
Regression of MALT lymphoma	6
Reduction of MALT lymphoma	19
Persistence of MALT lymphoma	4
Status uncertain	3

**Total equals 32*

FIGURE 2-52.

Regression of gastric mucosa-associated lymphoid tissue (MALT) lymphoma with *Helicobacter pylori* eradication. Further evidence for a etiologic role of *H. pylori* in gastric MALT lymphomas comes from studies in which MALT lymphomas have been observed to regress after *H. pylori* eradication. In results of this study, 32 patients with MALT lymphoma and *H. pylori* were treated with antibiotics to eradicate *H. pylori*. Six patients showed regression and 19 patients showed a reduction in their MALT lymphomas with *H. pylori* eradication.

Gastric carcinoid tumors

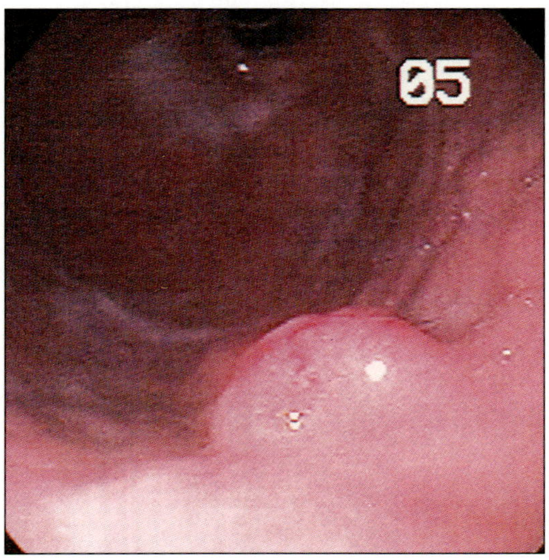

FIGURE 2-53.

Carcinoid tumor. Gastric carcinoids are rare tumors arising from enterochromaffin cells and are thought to be promoted by achlorhydria alone or combined with hypergastrinemia. They are rarely seen, even in persons on potent acid-inhibiting medication. This image shows gastric carcinoids in a patient with chronic pernicious anemia.

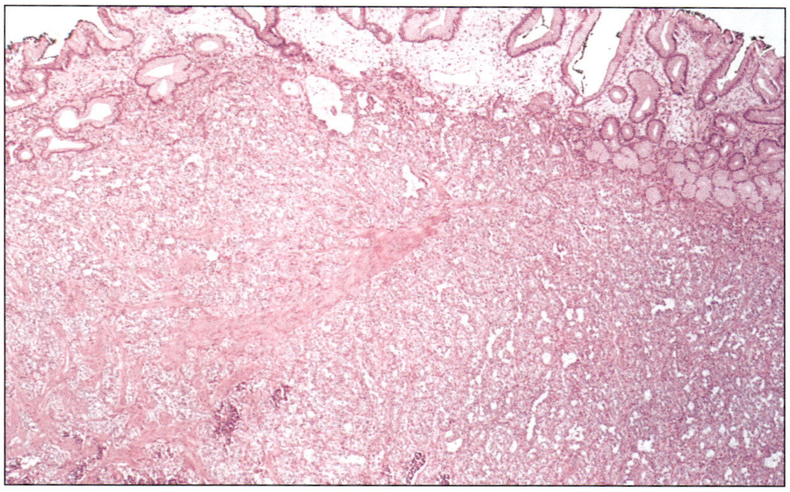

FIGURE 2-54.

Gastric carcinoid: morphologic aspects. Low-power view of a gastric carcinoid arising in the corpus of the stomach in a patient with pernicious anemia. The neoplasm replaces the lower mucosa and extends into the submucosa (hematoxylin and eosin stain).

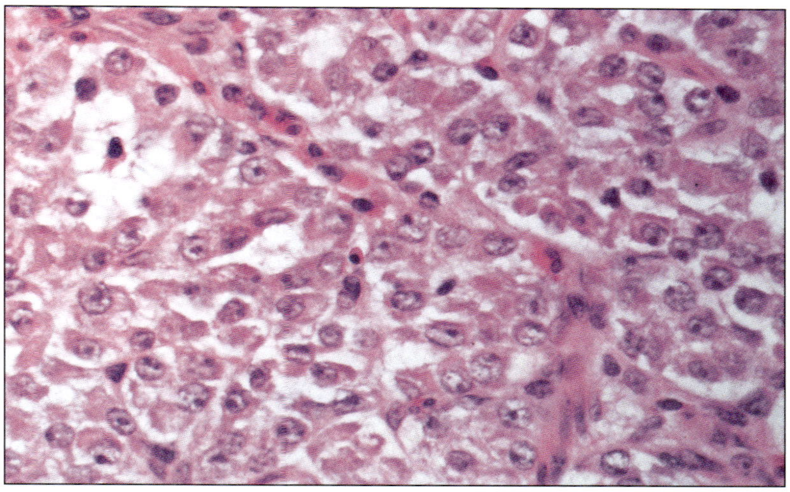

FIGURE 2-55.

High-power view of the carcinoid tumor depicted in Figure 2-54. The tumor cells, arranged in large clusters and sheets, show little atypia and negligible mitotic activity (hematoxylin and eosin stain).

GASTRIC CARCINOIDS: TREATMENT

Hypergastrinemia-associated	Sporadic
Observation only	Resection
Antrectomy	? Endoscopic
Resection of tumor(s)	Surgical
? Endoscopic	
Surgical	

FIGURE 2-56.

Gastric carcinoid tumors (more appropriately called *neuroendocrine tumors* or *ECLomas* in the stomach) usually follow an indolent course and were at one time felt to be entirely benign. Histologically and cytologically, they appear indolent with a low mitotic rate and little atypia. Despite this, 20% of carcinoids will have metastasized when surgery is performed. In general, carcinoids greater than 2 cm in size follow a malignant course, whereas those smaller than 1 cm in size rarely metastasize. Multiple approaches for treatment have been proposed including observation, antrectomy, or endoscopic removal for small tumors smaller than 1 cm, and wide excision including regional node metastasizes for those greater than 2 cm. Chemotherapy has been used for those with metastasis who are deemed unsuitable for surgery with mild success [48].

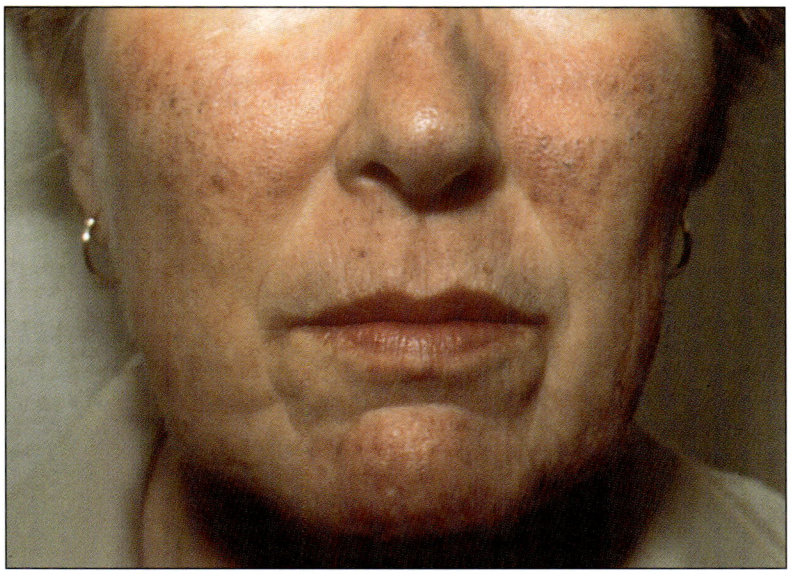

FIGURE 2-57.

A patient with carcinoid syndrome demonstrating facial telangiectasias and flushing. Other skin manifestations include pruritus, rhinophyma, xerosis, and angular cheilitis. Gastrointestinal changes, such as diarrheal malabsorption, abdominal pain, and small bowel obstruction, may precede or coexist with the syndrome. (*Courtesy of* D. Whiting, Dallas, TX.)

Kaposi's sarcoma

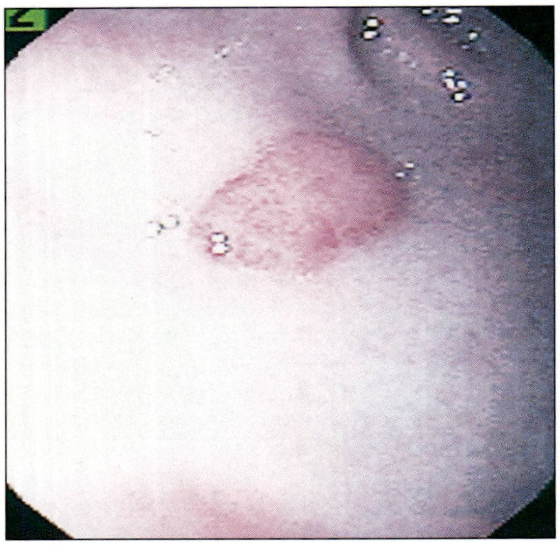

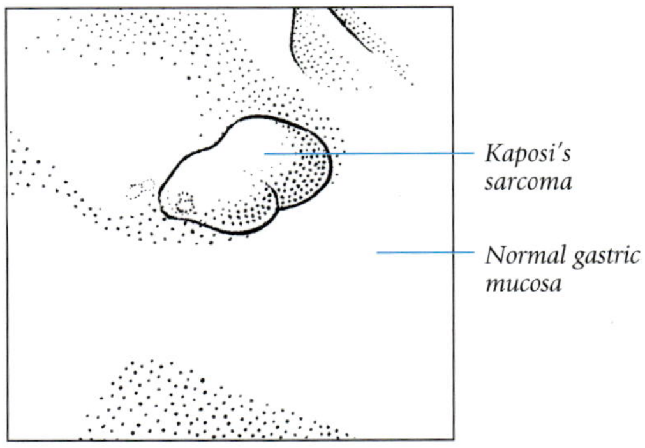

FIGURE 2-58.

Gastric Kaposi's sarcoma. In the area of AIDS, a variety of bleeding gastrointestinal lesions have been noted. Kaposi's sarcoma is a spindle cell tumor that often has a submucosal location histologically; hence the yield of biopsy is low, 23%, despite a typical endoscopic appearance [49]. Although gastrointestinal Kaposi's sarcoma can occur in the absence of cutaneous lesions, increasing numbers of skin lesions predict a higher incidence of gastrointestinal lesions. The lesion is typically a well-circumscribed, submucosal, erythematous or violaceous mass lesion. Bleeding gastrointestinal Kaposi's sarcoma lesions are a reflection of advanced immunosuppression and poor long-term survival. Some authors have, however, reported good acute control of active bleeding with endoscopic sclerotherapy [50].

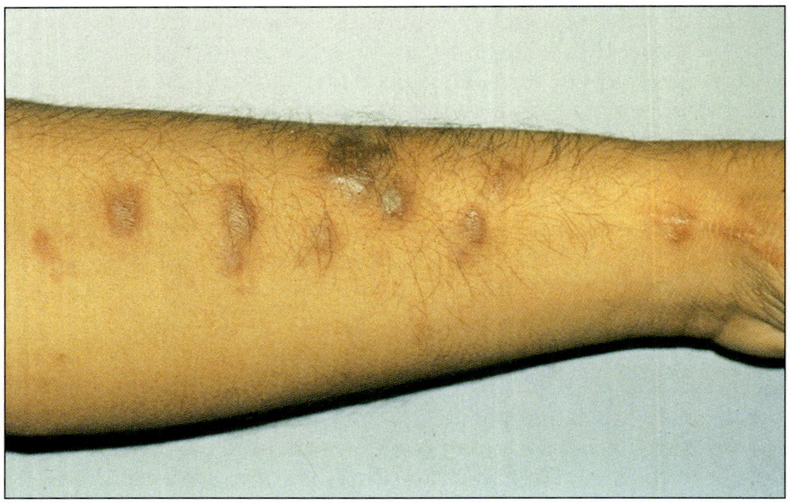

FIGURE 2-59.

Multiple firm, purple nodules on the arm resulting from Kaposi's sarcoma in a patient with AIDS. Most patients with Kaposi's sarcoma lesions, especially those of the mucous membranes, will have gastrointestinal tract lesions. The cutaneous lesions begin as brown or purple macules, which enlarge to form firm papules and nodules. Multiple lesions are common, and they may occur anywhere on the skin. Treatment includes local and systemic chemotherapy, radiation, cryotherapy, and interferon.

REFERENCES

1. Weinstein WM: Gastritis and gastropathies. In *Gastrointestinal Disease*, ed. 5. Edited by Sleisenger MH, Fordtran JS. Philadelphia: WB Saunders; 1993:549.
2. Laine L, Weinstein WM: Histology of hemorrhagic "gastritis": a prospective evaluation. *Gastroenterology* 1989, 94:1254–1262.
3. Peterson WL, Lee E, Feldman M: Relationship between *Campylobacter pylori* and gastritis in healthy humans after administration of placebo or indomethacin. *Gastroenterology* 1988, 95:1185–1197.
4. Mauch F, Bode G, Ditschuneit H, Malfertheiner P: Demonstration of a phospholipid-rich zone in the human gastric epithelium damaged by *Helicobacter pylori*. *Gastroenterology* 1993, 105:1698–1704.
5. Marshall BJ, Warren JR, Francis GI, *et al.*: Rapid urease test in the management of *Campylobacter pylori* disease-associated gastritis. *Am J Gastroenterol* 1987, 182:200–210.
6. Taylor DH, Blaser MJ: The epidemiology of *Helicobacter pylori* infection. In *Helicobacter pylori in Peptic Ulceration and Gastritis.* Edited by Marshall BJ, McCallum RW, Guerrant RL. Boston: Blackwell Scientific; 1991:46–54.
7. Malaty HM, Evans DG, Evans DJ Jr, Graham DY: *Helicobacter pylori* in Hispanics: Comparison with blacks and whites of similar age and socioeconomic class. *Gastroenterology* 1992, 103:813–816.
8. Freston JW: H_2-receptor antagonists and duodenal ulcer recurrence: analysis of efficacy and commentary on safety, costs, and patients selection. *Am J Gastroenterol* 1987, 82:1242–1249.
9. Tytgat GNJ, Rauws EAJ: *Campylobacter pylori* and its role in peptic ulcer disease. *Gastroenterol Clin North Am* 1990, 19:183–196.
10. Graham DY, Lew GM, Klein PD, *et al.*: Effect of treatment of *Helicobacter pylori* infection on the long-term recurrence of gastric or duodenal ulcer: a randomized, controlled study. *Ann Intern Med* 1992, 116:705–708.

11. Bailey RW, Flowers JL, Graham SM: Combined laparoscopic cholecystectomy and selective vagotomy. *Surg Laparosc Endosc* 1991, 1:45–49.
12. Byrne DJ, Brock BM, Morgan AC, *et al.*: Highly selective vagotomy: A 14-year experience. Br J Surg 1988, 75:869–872.
13. Jordan PH: Indications for parietal cell vagotomy without drainage in gastrointestinal surgery. *Ann Surg* 1989, 210:29–41..
14. McFadden DW, Zinner MJ: Reoperation for recurrent peptic ulcer disease. *Surg Clin North Am* 1991, 71:77–92.
15. Jensen RT, Gardner JD: Zollinger-Ellison syndrome: clinical presentation, pathology, diagnosis and treatment. In *Peptic Ulcer and Other Acid-Related Diseases*. Edited by Dannenberg A, Zakim D. Armonk: Academic Research Associates; 1991:117–212.
16. Bonfils S, Landor JH, Mignon M, Hervoir P: Results of surgical management in 92 consecutive patients with Zollinger-Ellison syndrome. *Ann Surg* 1981, 194:692–697.
17. Jensen RT, Gardner JD: Gastrinoma. In *The Pancreas: Biology, Pathobiology and Disease*, ed 2. Edited by Go VLW, DiMagno EP, Gardner JD, *et al.*: New York: Raven Press, 1993:931–978.
18. Stage JG, Stadil F: The clinical diagnosis of the Zollinger-Ellison syndrome. *Scand J Gastroenterol* 1979, 53(suppl):79–91.
19. Regan PT, Malagelada JR: A reappraisal of clinical, roentgenographic, and endoscopic features of the Zollinger-Ellison syndrome. *Mayo Clin Proc* 1978, 53:19–23.
20. Cameron AJ, Hoffman HN: Zollinger-Ellison syndrome: clinical features and long-term follow-up. *Mayo Clin Proc* 1974, 49:44–51.
21. Ellison EH, Wilson SD: The Zollinger-Ellison syndrome: re-appraisal and evaluation of 260 registered cases. *Ann Surg* 1964, 160:512–530.
22. Jensen RT, Maton PN: Zollinger-Ellison syndrome. In *The Stomach*. Edited by Gustavsson S, Kumar D, Graham DY. London: Churchill Livingstone; 1992:341–374.
23. Waxman I, Gardner JD, Jensen RT, Maton PN: Peptic ulcer perforation as the presentation of Zollinger-Ellison syndrome. *Dig Dis Sci* 1991, 16:19–24.
24. Isenberg JI, Walsh JH, Grossman MI: Zollinger-Ellison syndrome. *Gastroenterology* 1973, 65:140–165.
25. Collen MJ, Jensen RT: Idiopathic gastric acid hypersecretion: comparison with Zollinger-Ellison syndrome. *Dig Dis sci* 1994, 39:1434–1440.
26. Tytgat GNJ, Noach LA, Rauws EAJ: *Helicobacter pylori* infection and duodenal ulcer disease. *Gastroenterol Clin North Am* 1993, 22:127–139.
27. Saeed ZA, Evans DJ Jr, Evans DG, *et al.*: *Helicobacter pylori* and the Zollinger-Ellison syndrome. *Dig Dis Sci* 1991, 36:15–18.
28. Fich A, Talley NJ, Shorter RG, Philips SF: Zollinger-Ellison syndrome: relation to *Helicobacter pylori*-associated chronic gastritis and gastric acid secretion. *Dig Dis Sci* 1991, 36:10–14.
29. Weber HC, Orbuch M, Jensen RT: Diagnosis and treatment of the gastric and hypersecretion in patients with Zollinger-Ellison syndrome. In *Pancreatic Endocrine Tumors: Seminars in Gastrointestinal Diseases*. Edited by Jensen RT. Duluth: WB Saunders; 1995:79–89.
30. Orbuch M, Doppman JL, Strader DB, *et al.*: Imaging for pancreatic endocrine tumor localization: recent advances. In *Endocrine Tumors of the Pancreas: Recent Advances in Research and Management*. Edited by Mignon M, Jensen RT. Basel: Karger; 1995:268–281.
31. Kwekkeboom DJ, Krenning EP, Oei HY, *et al.*: Use of radiolabeled somatostatin to localize islet cell tumors. In *Endocrine Tumors of the Pancreas: Recent Advances in Research and Management*. Edited by Mignon M, Jensen RT. Basel: Karger; 1995:298–308.
32. Lamberts SW, Bakker WH, Reubi JC, Krenning EP: Somatostatin-receptor imaging in the localization of endocrine tumours. *N Engl J Med* 1990, 323:1246–1249.
33. Lamberts SWJ, Chayvialle JA, Krenning EP: The visualization of gastro-enteropancreatic endocrine tumors. *Digestion* 1993, 54(suppl 1):92–97.
34. Krenning EP, Kwekkeboom DJ, Bakker WH, *et al.*: Somatostatin receptor scintigraphy with [^{111}In-DTPA-D-Phe^{1}]- [^{123}I-Tyr^{3}]-octreotide: the Rotterdam experience with more than 1000 patients. *Eur J Nucl Med* 1993, 20:716–731.
35. Nakamura Y, Larsson C, Julier C, *et al.*: Localization of the genetic defect in multiple endocrine neoplasia type I within a small region of chromosome 11. *Am J Hum Genet* 1989, 44:751–755.
36. Norton JA, Sugarbaker PH, Doppman JL, *et al.*: Aggressive resection of metastatic disease in selected patients with malignant gastrinoma. *Ann Surg* 1986, 203:352–359.
37. Arnold R, Neuhaus C, Benning R, *et al.*: Somatostatin analog sandostatin and inhibition of tumor growth in patients with metastatic endocrine gastroenteropancreatic tumours. *World J Surg* 1993, 17:511–519.
38. Gibril F, Doppman JL, Jensen RT: Treatment of metastatic pancreatic endocrine tumors. In *Pancreatic Endocrine Tumors: Seminars in Gastrointestinal Disease*. Edited by Jensen RT. Duluth: WB Saunders; 1995:114–121.
39. von Schrenck T, Howard JM, Doppman JL, *et al.*: Prospective study of chemotherapy in patients with metastatic gastrinoma. *Gastroenterology* 1988, 94:1326–1334.
40. Moertel CG, Lefkopoulo M, Lipsitz S, *et al.*: Streptozotocin-doxorubicin, streptozotocin-fluorouracil or chlorozotocin in the treatment of advanced islet cell carcinoma. *N Engl J Med* 1992, 326:519–523.
41. Norton JA, Levin B, Jensen RT: Cancer of the endocrine system. In *Cancer: Principles and Practice of Oncology*, ed 4. Edited by DeVita VT Jr, Hellman S, Rosenberg SA. Philadelphia: JB Lippincott; 1993:1333–1435.
42. Moertel CG, Kvols LK, O'Connell MJ, Rubin J: Treatment of neuroendocrine carcinomas with combined etoposide and cisplatin: evidence of major therapeutic activity in the anaplastic variants of these neoplasms. *Cancer* 1991, 68:227–232.
43. Pisegna JR, Slimak GG Doppman JL, *et al.*: An evaluation of human recombinant alpha interferon in patients with metastatic gastrinoma. *Gastroenterology* 1993, 105:1179–1183.
44. Arnold R, Frank M: Systemic chemotherapy for endocrine tumors of the pancreas: recent advances. In *Endocrine Tumors of the Pancreas: Recent Advances in Research and Management*. Edited by Mignon M, Jensen RT. Basel: Karger; 1995:431–438.
45. Davis GR: Neoplasms of the stomach. In *Gastrointestinal Disease*. Edited by Sleisenger MH, Fordtran JS. Philadelphia: WB Saunders; 1993:763–789.
46. Jeyasingham K: Oesophageal and gastric carcinoma. In *Operative Surgery and Management*, ed 2. Edited by Keen G. New York: Macmillan; 1987:71.
47. Sue-Ling HM, Johnston D, Martin IG, *et al.*: Gastric cancer: a curable disease in Britain. *BMJ* 1993, 307:591–596.
48. Lechago J: Neuroendocrine cells of the gut and their disorders. In *Gastrointestinal Pathology*. Edited by Goldman H, Appelman HR. Baltimore, MD: Williams & Wilkins, 1990:181–219.
49. Friedman S, Wright T, Altman D: Gastrointestinal Kaposi's sarcoma in patients with acquired immunodeficiency syndrome: endoscopic and autopsy findings. *Gastroenterology* 1985, 89:102–108.
50. Lew E, Dieterich D: Severe hemorrhage caused by gastrointestinal Kaposi's syndrome in patients with the acquired immunodeficiency syndrome. *Am J Gastroenterol* 1992, 87:1471–1474.

Chapter

3

Disorders of the Small Intestine

EDITOR

Lawrence R. Schiller

CONTRIBUTORS

Ralph A. Giannella
Samuel Klein
Edward L. Lee
Gordon D. Luk
Amit G. Pandya
Eamonn M.M. Quigley
Francisco C. Ramirez
Arvey I. Rogers
Charles M. Rosen
David B. Sachar
Ellen J. Scherl
Herbert J. Smith
Robert W. Summers

ANATOMY OF THE SMALL INTESTINE

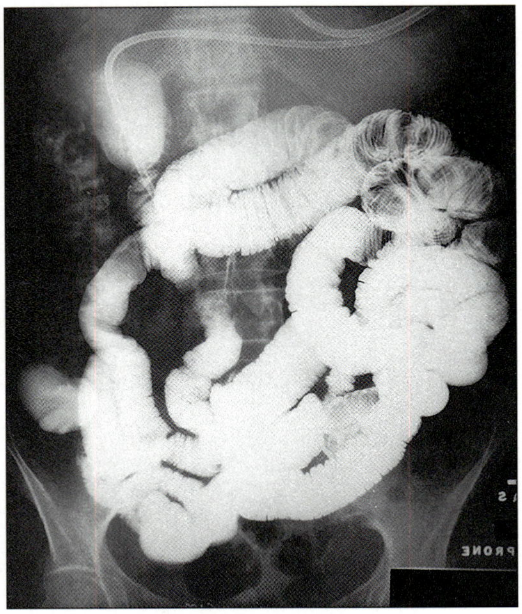

FIGURE 3-1.

The small intestine is approximately 5 m in length, depending on the degree of contraction or relaxation. It is clearly defined on this small bowel enteroclysis study. The duodenum extends about 25 cm from the pylorus to the ligament of Treitz. It has the largest diameter and the thickest wall, but the shortest length of all of the three intestinal regions. The jejunum is about 2 m long, with a proximal diameter about twice that of the distal ileum. The ileum is about 3 m long; its wall is thinner than that of the jejunum. Although the jejunum differs structurally from the ileum, no sharp anatomic distinction exists between the two. In the duodenum and jejunum, the mucosa is redundant and arranged so that it produces circular folds (valvulae conniventes). These folds probably act as baffles to disrupt laminar flow and contribute to more turbulence, enhancing mixing of intestinal contents with digestive secretions and exposure to the absorbing surface. Valvulae do not exist in the ileum, giving it a smoother contour. (*Courtesy of* Dr. Charles Lu, University of Iowa.)

ACUTE (INFECTIOUS) DIARRHEA

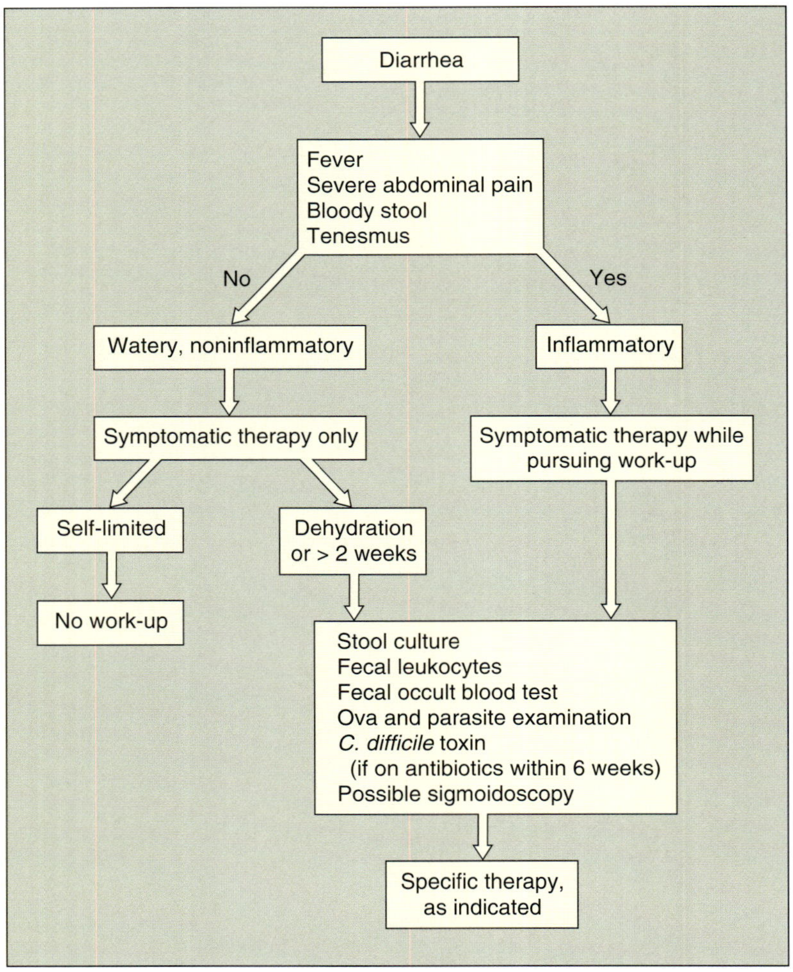

FIGURE 3-2.

Approach to the patient with acute diarrhea. Most cases of acute diarrhea are self-limited and require neither specific diagnosis nor therapy. In the absence of fever, severe abdominal pain, bloody stools, or tenesmus, watchful waiting and symptomatic therapy should be given. If either fever, severe abdominal pain, bloody stools, or tenesmus is present, this finding suggests inflammatory diarrhea and increases the likelihood of a specific, treatable enteropathogen. In such cases, symptomatic therapy can be applied while a diagnostic evaluation is pursued. (*Adapted from* Saxe and Giannella [1]; with permission.)

INFLAMMATORY VERSUS NONINFLAMMATORY DIARRHEA: COLON VERSUS SMALL INTESTINE

Characteristic	Inflammatory diarrhea	Noninflammatory diarrhea
Fecal leukocytes	Positive	Negative
Clinical presentation	Bloody, small-volume diarrhea; lower left quadrant abdominal cramps; may be febrile and toxic	Large-volume, watery diarrhea; may have nausea, vomiting, cramps
Causes	*Shigella*, *Salmonella*, amebic colitis, *Campylobacter*, *Yersinia*, invasive *Escherichia coli*, *Yersinia*, *Clostridium difficile*	Viruses, *Vibrio*, *Giardia*, Enterotoxigenic *E. coli*, enterotoxin-producing bacteria, food-borne gastroenteritis
Site of involvement	Colon	Small intestine
Diagnostic evaluation	Indicated	If severely volume-depleted or toxic

FIGURE 3-3.

Features of inflammatory and noninflammatory diarrhea. Acute diarrhea can be divided into inflammatory or noninflammatory types. Inflammatory diarrhea is characterized by the presence of fecal leukocytes, by bloody or small-volume bowel movements, by tenesmus, and frequently by fever. Invasive or cytotoxin-producing bacteria characteristically cause this syndrome. The primary target organ is the colon. Noninflammatory diarrhea, however, is characterized by the absence of fecal leukocytes, large-volume, watery diarrhea, and lack of fever. Organisms causing noninflammatory diarrhea are enterotoxin-elaborating bacteria and certain minimally destructive viruses. The primary target organ is the small intestine [2,3]. (*Adapted from* Park and Giannella [3]; with permission.)

DIFFERENTIAL DIAGNOSIS OF FOOD POISONING SYNDROMES

Symptoms	Incubation Period, *hr*	Possible Agents
Acute upper gastrointestinal symptoms, nausea, vomiting	6	Preformed heat-stable toxins of *Staphylococcus aureus*, *Bacillus cereus*; also *D. latum*, anisakis, heavy metals
Upper small-bowel symptoms; watery noninflammatory diarrhea	6–72	*Clostridium perfringens* type A, *B. cereus*, enterotoxigenic *E. coli*, *Vibrio cholerae*, *Giardia lamblia*
Inflammatory ileocolitis	16–72	Salmonella, shigella, *Campylobacter jejuni*, *V. parahaemolyticus*, enteroinvasive *E. coli*, Yersinia, Aeromonas
Sensory or motor neurologic symptoms with or without gastrointestinal symptoms, suggesting botulism, fish, shellfish, or chemical poisoning	—	Histamine-like scombrotoxin, dinoflagellate neurotoxins, monosodium glutamate, mushrooms, solanine, pesticides

FIGURE 3-4.

Differential diagnosis of food poisoning syndromes. Food poisoning syndromes can present in various ways. An acute syndrome characterized by upper gastrointestinal symptoms, nausea, and vomiting is one of the more common. Nausea and vomiting accompanied by watery diarrheal syndrome or inflammatory diarrhea also occurs. The least common is a syndrome characterized by sensory and motor neurologic symptoms with or without accompanying gastrointestinal symptoms. The organisms causing each of these syndromes are shown in this table. (*Adapted from* Guerrant and Bobak [4]; with permission.)

CAMPYLOBACTER DIARRHEA SUMMARY

Characteristics

Prodrome (fever, malaise, myalgias)

Colicky pain, watery diarrhea, and ± dysentery

Mimics salmonellosis, shigellosis, yersinosis, and antibiotic-associated diarrhea

Enteritis with or without colitis

Causes 5%–10% of cases of acute diarrhea

Positive stool culture for 2–5 weeks

Diagnosis

Fecal leukocytes, positive stool culture (on selective media grown at 42°C, in a CO_2-enriched environment)

Treatment

Erythromycin, tetracycline, chloramphenicol, gentamicin

Complications

Acute abdomen

Chronic diarrhea

Septicemia

Mimics idiopathic inflammatory bowel disease

FIGURE 3-5.

Campylobacter diarrhea. The usual clinical manifestations and course are described. The clinical syndrome mimics those of shigellosis, salmonellosis, and other enteric infections, and therefore cannot be reliably distinguished on clinical grounds alone. *Campylobacter* infection is extremely widespread and, in many surveys, is the most common definable cause of acute intestinal infection.

Most cases of *Campylobacter* infection are self-limited, resolve before a specific diagnosis is made, and do not require specific treatment. In severe cases, however, and in cases with prolonged diarrhea, antibiotic administration is required. Erythromycin is the preferred therapeutic agent. Various complications of *Campylobacter* diarrhea should be noted; they include abdominal pain so severe as to mimic an acute abdomen, occasional septicemia, and a chronic illness that mimics idiopathic inflammatory bowel disease.

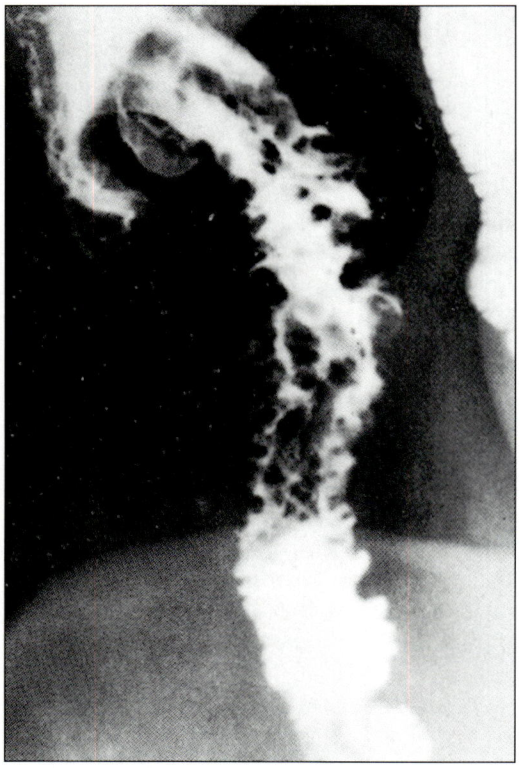

FIGURE 3-6.

Yersinia enterocolitica. *Yersinia enterocolitica* can cause both acute and chronic diarrheal syndromes. These organisms can infect both the small bowel and colon. The typical location is the distal ileum. Two clinical syndromes are possible: a watery diarrheal syndrome or a typical dysenteric syndrome. Although the typical case lasts only 2 to 3 weeks, illness *can* be prolonged for many weeks, and thus the illness can mimic Crohn's disease. This radiograph illustrates the appearance of *Yersinia enterocolitica* ileitis. Films of the terminal ileum reveal markedly thickened folds with a nodular pattern. This can mimic Crohn's disease, lymphoma, or lymphoid hyperplasia. (*From* Vantrappen *et al.* [5]; with permission.)

CRYPTOSPORIDIOSIS: SUMMARY

Features

Diarrhea, cramps, nausea, vomiting, weight loss

An enteritis or enterocolitis

Common in normal host (self-limited)

Occurs in clusters (*ie*, families and day-care centers)

Common among AIDS patients (chronic and devastating)

One third of cases have an associated second pathogen, especially giardia

Diagnosis

Acid-fast stain—oocysts in stool

Small-intestinal biopsy

Colonic biopsy

Therapy

Not required in normal host

Only partially successful in immunocompromised patients

FIGURE 3-7.

Cryptosporidiosis. Cryptosporidiosis is an illness characterized by diarrhea, abdominal cramps, nausea, vomiting, and weight loss. It can cause either an enteritis or an enterocolitis. It is common both in the normal immunocompetent host and especially in the immunodeficient host, such as patients with AIDS. In such patients, the diarrhea is frequently chronic and devastating, and may be associated with nutrient malabsorption.

Diagnosis of cryptosporidiosis is made by demonstration of oocysts in stool, which are most easily appreciated when stool is stained with an acid-fast stain. Small intestinal biopsy and colonic biopsy are other methods of making this diagnosis. Treatment usually is not required in the normal host and is only partially effective in the immunosuppressed host [6–8].

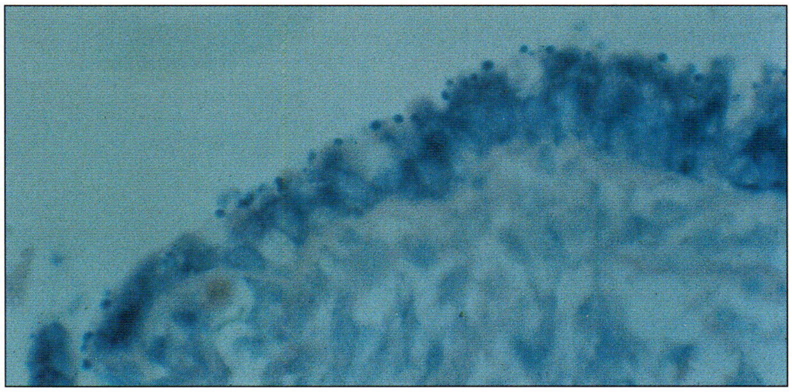

FIGURE 3-8.

Photomicrograph of intestinal biopsy—cryptosporidiosis. A small intestinal biopsy reveals cryptosporidia adherent to the surface of the enterocytes. The organism does not invade and is confined to the surface of the epithelial cell [9]. A similar appearance can be seen in the colon. (*From* Banwell and Lake [9]; *courtesy of* R.L. Owen, MD, Cell Biology Section, VA Hospital, San Francisco, CA.)

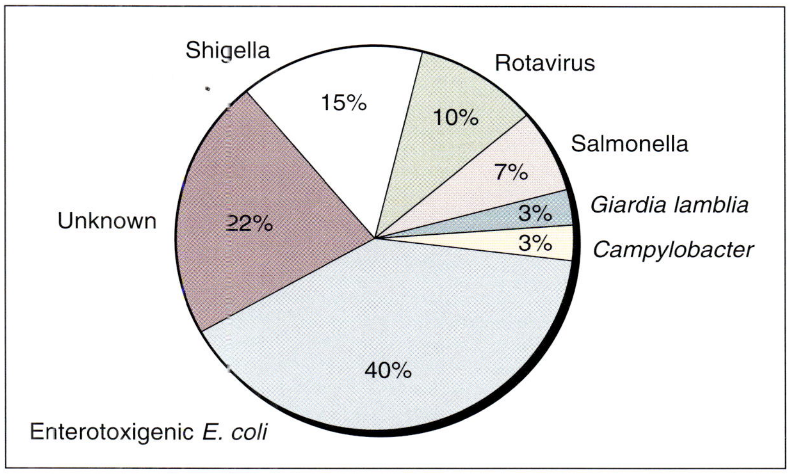

FIGURE 3-9.

Causes of traveler's diarrhea. Traveler's diarrhea is a syndrome occurring during or shortly after travel. A large array of enteropathogenic agents can cause the syndrome; however, the most common single cause is enterotoxigenic *Escherichia coli*. Other organisms causing this syndrome are shown. In all studies, 20% to 35% of patients elude specific diagnosis, thus suggesting the existence of other undefined infectious agents [9]. ETEC—Enterotoxigenic *Escherichia coli*. (*Adapted from* Banwell and Lake [9].)

PROPHYLAXIS FOR TRAVELER'S DIARRHEA AND TARGET GROUPS

Effective Prophylaxis	Groups Recommended for Prophylaxis
Antibiotics (ciprofloxacin, TMP-Sulfa)	Patients with gastrectomy
Bismuth subsalicylate	Patients with inflammatory bowel disease
	Those susceptible to dehydration (*ie*, patients with ileostomy or short-bowel syndrome)
	Those with severe systemic illnesses
	Immunosuppressed patients

FIGURE 3-10.

Effective prophylaxis of traveler's diarrhea and specific groups recommended. Two means are effective in preventing traveler's diarrhea: antibiotics and bismuth subsalicylate; they appear to be equally effective. The preferred antibiotics in adults are ciprofloxacin or trimethoprim-sulfa.

Most authorities do not recommend routine prophylaxis for all Americans traveling to other countries. However, certain high-risk groups, as shown, should receive prophylaxis.

CHRONIC DIARRHEA

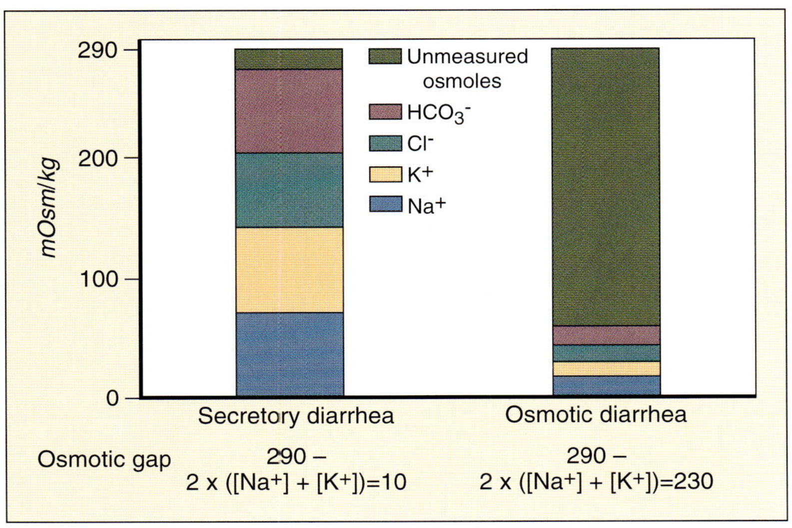

FIGURE 3-11.

Calculation of stool osmotic gap. Because colonic luminal contents are in osmotic equilibrium with body fluids, the sum of the concentrations of ions and small molecules contributing to osmolality must equal plasma osmolality, usually 290 mOsm/kg. In secretory diarrhea, electrolyte absorption is compromised so that sodium, potassium, and their counterions account for most of the osmoles in stool water. In osmotic diarrhea, electrolyte absorption is normal so that measured cations and their corresponding anions account for only a fraction of the osmoles in stool water. Unmeasured osmoles (*eg*, carbohydrate or magnesium ion) comprise most of the "osmotic space." Osmotic gaps more than 50 mOsm/kg are associated with ingestion of a poorly absorbed substance [10].

MECHANISMS AND CAUSES OF SECRETORY DIARRHEA

Reduction in mucosal surface area
- Postresection diarrhea
- Short-bowel syndrome

Extensive mucosal disease and inflammation
- Viral gastroenteritis
- Celiac disease
- Whipple's disease
- Crohn's disease
- Lymphoma

Absence of ion transport mechanism
- Congenital chloridorrhea

Bacterial toxins
- Cholera
- Enterotoxigenic *Escherichia coli*
- Shigella
- Staphylococcus
- *Clostridium perfringens*

Luminal secretagogues
- Bile acids
- Fatty acids, hydroxy-fatty acids
- Phenolphthalein, ricinoleic acid, bisacodyl

Circulating secretagogues
- Gastrin (Zollinger-Ellison syndrome)
- Vasoactive intestinal polypeptide (VIPoma, ganglioneuroma, neuroblastoma, pheochromocytoma)
- Calcitonin, prostaglandins (medullary carcinoma of the thyroid)
- Somatostatin (somatostatinoma)
- Glucagon (glucagonoma)
- Serotonin, kinins (carcinoid tumor)
- Thyroxine (hyperthyroidism)
- Histamine (mastocytosis)

Drugs and poisons
- Misoprostol
- Olsalazine
- Colchicine
- Propranolol
- Quinidine
- Heavy metals

Abnormal circulation
- Radiation enteritis
- Mesenteric ischemia
- Mesenteric venous thrombosis
- Lymphangiectasia

Disordered regulation
- Postvagotomy diarrhea
- Postsympathectomy
- Diabetic autonomic neuropathy
- Addison's disease

Undetermined or complex mechanism
- Collagen-vascular diseases
- Giardiasis
- Tuberculosis
- Niacin deficiency
- "Idiopathic" secretory diarrhea

Secretory diarrheas of exclusively colonic origin
- Ulcerative colitis, Crohn's disease of colon
- Microscopic ("lymphocytic") colitis
- Collagenous colitis
- Secreting villous adenoma

FIGURE 3-12. Mechanisms and causes of secretory diarrhea.

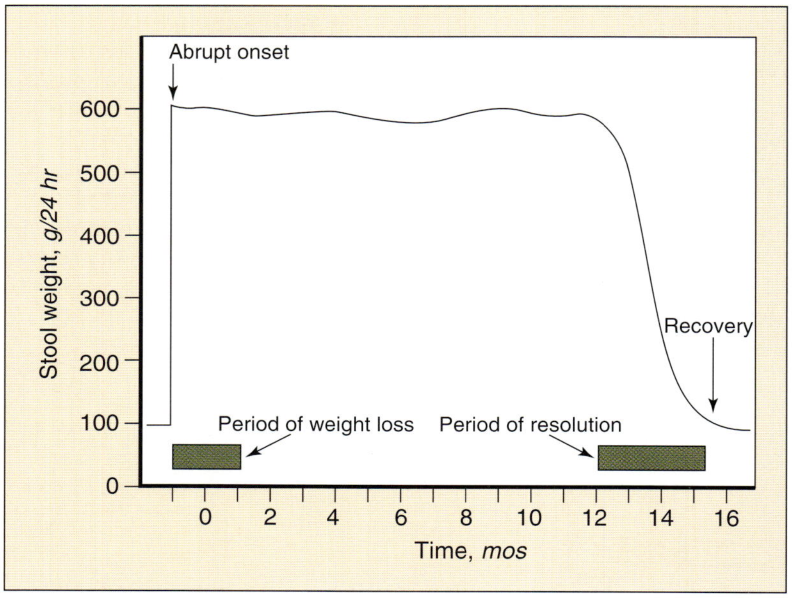

FIGURE 3-13. Idiopathic secretory diarrhea. Patients who have been extensively evaluated for chronic watery diarrhea without finding a cause are a remarkably homogeneous group [11]. They typically give a history of good health until the acute onset of diarrhea, often after domestic travel. This is followed by continuous diarrhea and a limited period of weight loss. Diarrhea persists at a constant intensity for 1 to 3 years and then subsides spontaneously over a few months. No causative organism has been identified, but the sudden onset and spontaneous disappearance suggest an infectious etiology. Outbreaks of a similar syndrome have been reported to be associated with consumption of milk or water, but sporadic idiopathic secretory diarrhea usually occurs in isolated individuals, even though others may have had identical food or water exposures. Nonspecific antidiarrheal therapy with opiates is helpful in most such patients.

DRUGS ASSOCIATED WITH DIARRHEA

- Antibiotics
- Antineoplastic drugs
- Antiarrhythmics
  - Quinidine
  - Procainamide
- Antihypertensives
  - Beta-blockers
  - Angiotensin-converting enzyme inhibitors
  - Hydralazine
- Antidepressants
  - Lithium
  - Fluoxetine (Prozac)
- Tranquilizers
  - Alprazolam (Xanax)
  - Meprobamate
- Anticonvulsants
  - Ethosuximide
  - Valproic acid
  - L-Dopa
- Hypocholesterolemic drugs
  - Lovastatin
  - Gemfibrozil
  - Clofibrate
  - Probucol
- Gastrointestinal drugs
  - Magnesium-containing antacids
  - H_2-receptor antagonists
  - Prostaglandin analogues (misoprostal)
  - Sulfasalazine
  - Olsalazine
  - Prokinetic drugs (cisapride)
- Miscellaneous agents
  - Methysergide
  - Theophylline
  - Diuretics
  - Oral hypoglycemic drugs
  - Colchicine
  - Thyroid hormone

FIGURE 3-14. Drugs associated with diarrhea [12]. Several different categories of drugs can cause diarrhea as a side effect. Some examples are shown under each category. The mechanisms causing diarrhea are not known for most of these drugs.

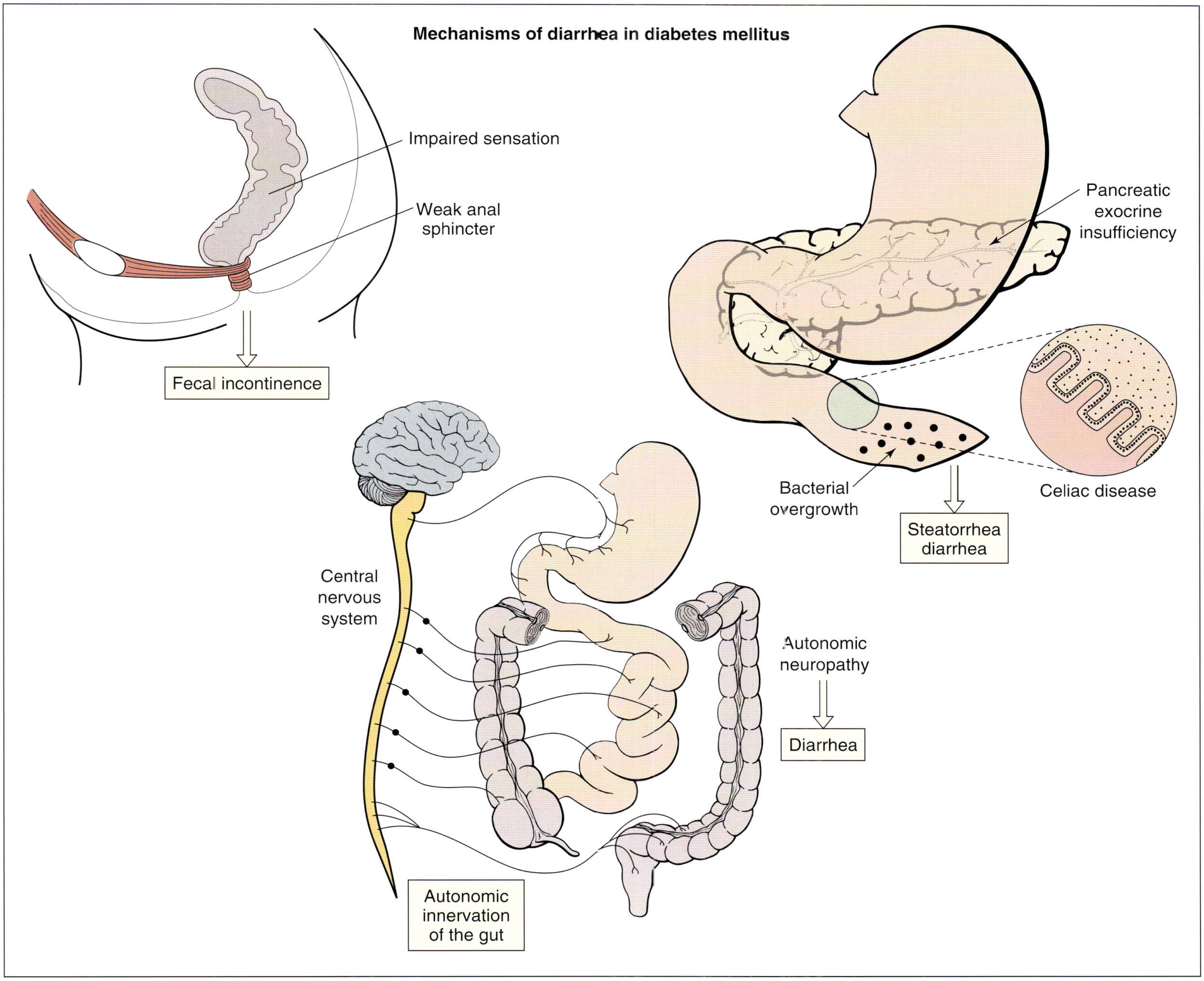

FIGURE 3-15.

Diabetes mellitus. Longstanding diabetes mellitus is complicated by the development of chronic diarrhea in roughly 20% of patients. In some this results from fecal incontinence, misreported as diarrhea, but in others, stool weight may be abnormally high. Clinically, it is important to distinguish steatorrhea from chronic watery diarrhea in these patients. Steatorrhea may be caused by coexisting small-bowel bacterial overgrowth, celiac disease, or pancreatic exocrine insufficiency. Watery diarrhea has been attributed to dysregulation by the enteric nervous system as a manifestation of diabetic autonomic neuropathy. Studies in animals suggest the possibility of adrenergic dysfunction in diabetes, but attempts to treat diabetic diarrhea in people with clonidine, an α_2-adrenergic agonist agent, have been only variably successful [13].

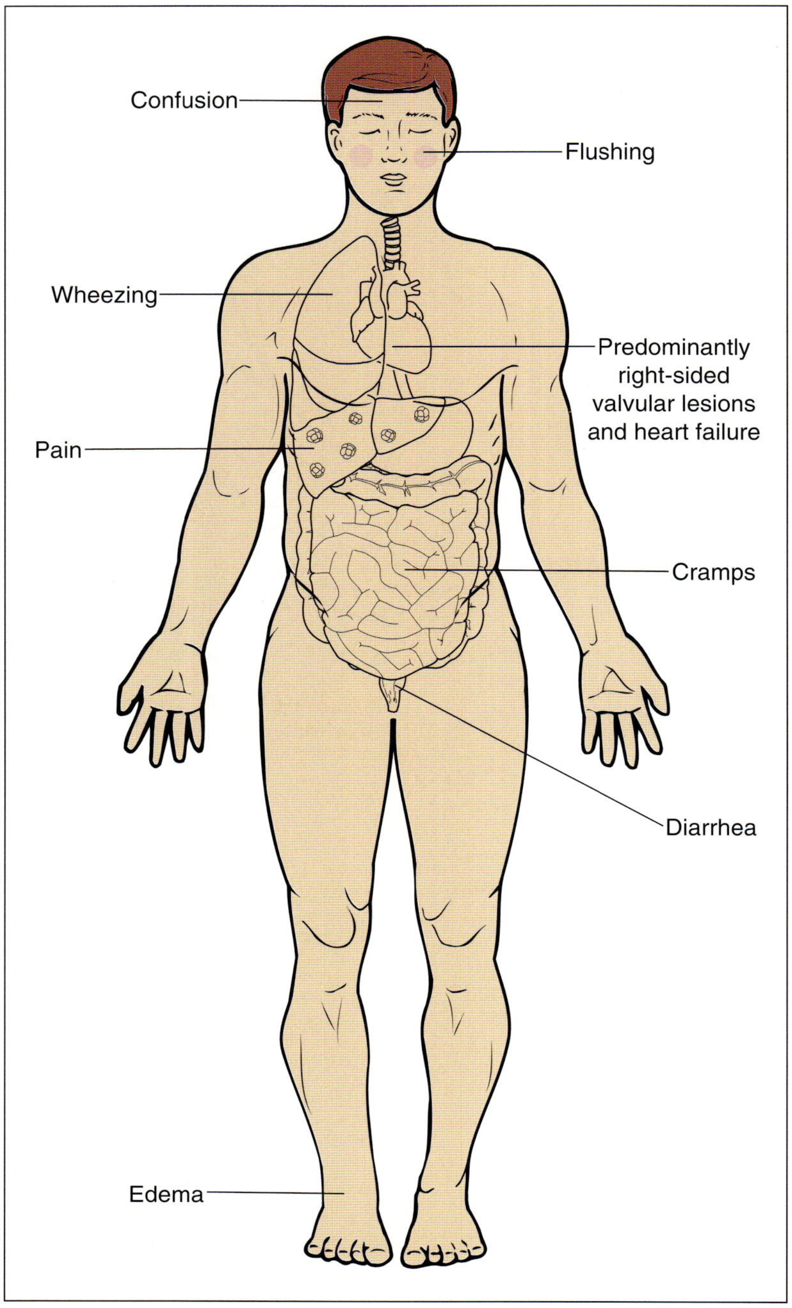

Figure 3-16.

Carcinoid tumors of the gastrointestinal tract are fairly common tumors, but carcinoid syndrome is less common [14]. To produce carcinoid syndrome, a carcinoid tumor must secrete mediators capable of producing symptoms and must be either metastatic to the liver or lung or primary at a site where direct access to the systemic venous circulation (bronchus, ovary) exists. The liver is capable of inactivating many of the mediators that may be produced by tumors in the intestine. After access to the systemic circulation has been achieved, the intensity of symptoms tends to be related to the tumor burden and the circulating levels of mediators. Progression of tumor is slower than that of carcinomas arising in the intestine; a course of up to 10 years from the onset of symptoms until death is not unusual. Diarrhea may be caused largely by hurried intestinal transit rather than by development of a secretory state, and usually is of only moderate volume.

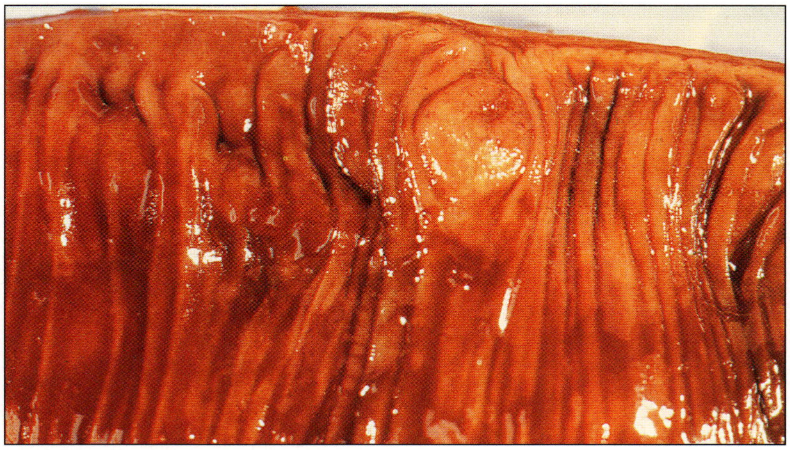

Figure 3-17.

Carcinoid. This surgical resection specimen shows a well-circumscribed intraluminal mass with apparently normal overlying mucosa and a central umbilication. On cut section, the tumor showed a pale-yellow meaty appearance, suggestive of a carcinoid; the muscular layer and setosa has undergone retractile changes that resulted in the formation of a knuckle of bowel, also suggestive of a carcinoid.

Figure 3-18.

Clinical diagnostic algorithm for the approach to patients with chronic diarrhea (> 4 weeks' duration to exclude most acute infectious causes). A careful history can largely define the potential causes of chronic diarrhea. The key diagnoses that can be evaluated by history include iatrogenic diarrhea (*ie,* caused by drugs, radiation, or surgery) and systemic diseases producing diarrhea (such as hyperthyroidism, diabetes, or vasculitis). The history also provides evidence of risk factors for AIDS and the need to test for HIV infection. Physical examination and routine laboratory tests provide information on the effects of diarrhea (fluid status, electrolyte depletion) and the need for rehydration or nutritional support. Serum chemistries can disclose evidence of malabsorption, hypogammaglobulinemia, or dysgammaglobulinemia. A quantitative stool collection provides information about the severity of diarrhea, the presence of steatorrhea, the presence of an osmotic gap in stool water, indicating an osmotic component, and the presence of laxatives. If secretory diarrhea is confirmed, chronic infectious processes should be excluded by examining the stool for bacterial pathogens, parasites, and protozoa. The next step is to exclude structural and inflammatory disease with carefully conducted small-bowel radiography and colonoscopy with biopsies, even if the mucosa appears normal, to exclude microscopic and collagenous colitis. If the diagnosis remains uncertain, computerized tomography (CT) and a small-bowel biopsy with aspirate for quantitative culture are appropriate. Selective evaluation for circulating secretagogues might include serum gastrin, calcitonin, vasoactive intestinal polypeptide (VIP), and thyroid-stimulating hormone (TSH) levels, and measurement of urinary excretion of 5-hydroxyindole-acetic acid (5-HIAA), metanephrines, and histamine.

(*figure on opposite page*)

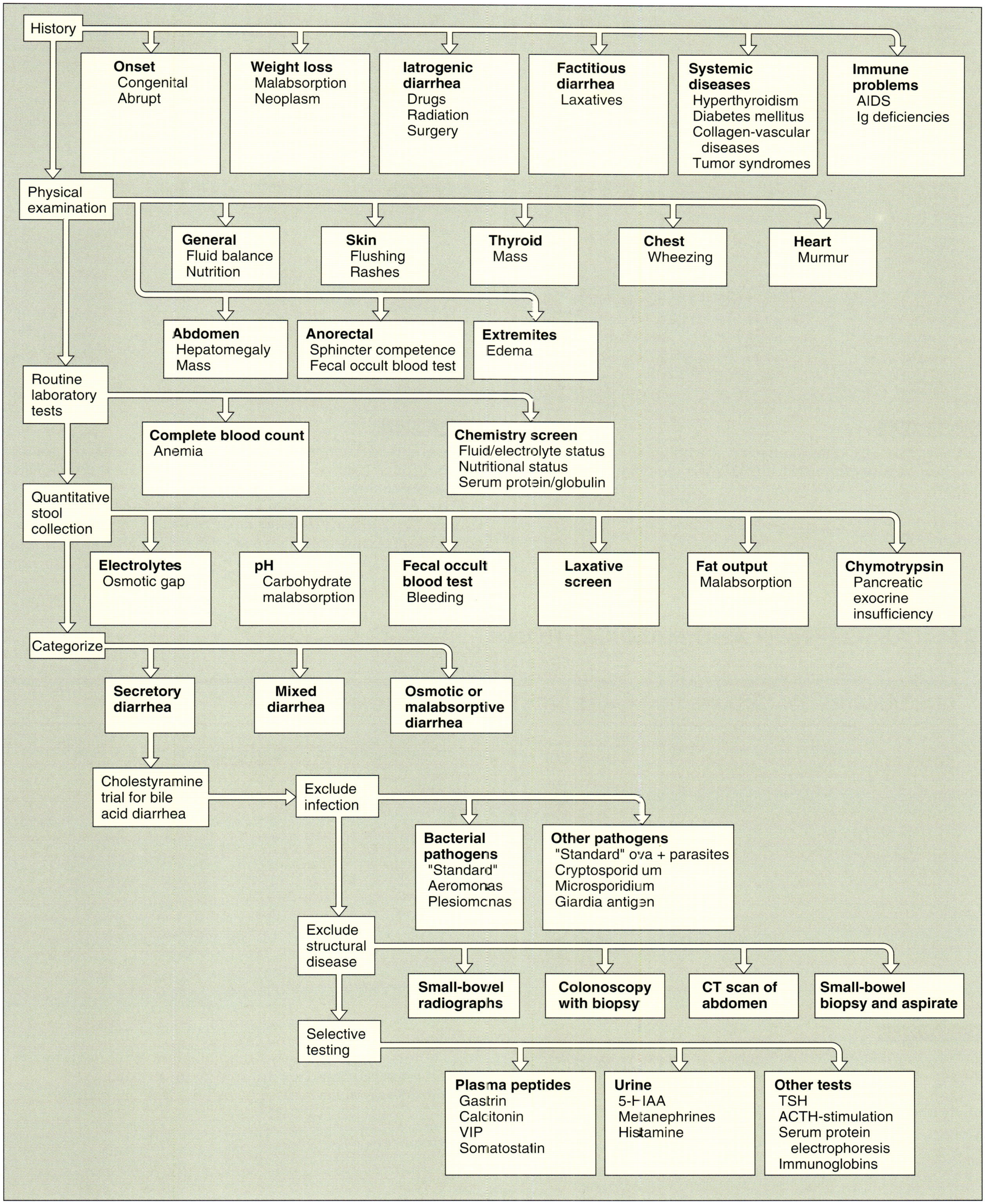
History
Onset
Congenital
Abrupt
Weight loss
Malabsorption
Neoplasm
Iatrogenic diarrhea
Drugs
Radiation
Surgery
Factitious diarrhea
Laxatives
Systemic diseases
Hyperthyroidism
Diabetes mellitus
Collagen-vascular diseases
Tumor syndromes
Immune problems
AIDS
Ig deficiencies
Physical examination
General
Fluid balance
Nutrition
Skin
Flushing
Rashes
Thyroid
Mass
Chest
Wheezing
Heart
Murmur
Abdomen
Hepatomegaly
Mass
Anorectal
Sphincter competence
Fecal occult blood test
Extremites
Edema
Routine laboratory tests
Complete blood count
Anemia
Chemistry screen
Fluid/electrolyte status
Nutritional status
Serum protein/globulin
Quantitative stool collection
Electrolytes
Osmotic gap
pH
Carbohydrate malabsorption
Fecal occult blood test
Bleeding
Laxative screen
Fat output
Malabsorption
Chymotrypsin
Pancreatic exocrine insufficiency
Categorize
Secretory diarrhea
Mixed diarrhea
Osmotic or malabsorptive diarrhea
Cholestyramine trial for bile acid diarrhea
Exclude infection
Bacterial pathogens
"Standard"
Aeromonas
Plesiomonas
Other pathogens
"Standard" ova + parasites
Cryptosporidium
Microsporidium
Giardia antigen
Exclude structural disease
Small-bowel radiographs
Colonoscopy with biopsy
CT scan of abdomen
Small-bowel biopsy and aspirate
Selective testing
Plasma peptides
Gastrin
Calcitonin
VIP
Somatostatin
Urine
5-HIAA
Metanephrines
Histamine
Other tests
TSH
ACTH-stimulation
Serum protein electrophoresis
Immunoglobins

PATIENTS SUSPECTED OF LAXATIVE ABUSE

Type	Characteristics
Patients with bulimia	Usually adolescent to young adult women; concerned about weight or manifesting an eating disorder
Secondary gain	May have disability claim pending; illness may induce concern or caring behavior in others
Münchausen's syndrome	Typically, a peripatetic patient who "enjoys" being a challenge to doctors; may undergo extensive testing repeatedly
Polle syndrome (Münchausen by proxy)	Dependent child poisoned by parent with laxatives to show how effective parent can be as a caregiver; may have history of sibling who died with chronic diarrhea

FIGURE 3-19.

Laxative abuse suspects. Some patients who present with chronic diarrhea are surreptitiously using laxatives. Some of the causes are listed here.

LAXATIVES AND DETECTION METHODS

Laxative	Detection Method
Phenolphthalein	Alkalinization of stool produces pink color; spectrophotometry
Bisacodyl	Thin-layer chromatography
Ipecac	Thin-layer chromatography
Senna	Urinary assay for anthraquinone
Magnesium	Osmotic gap in stool water; increased concentration of magnesium in stool water
Phosphate	Increased concentration in stool water
Sulfate	Increased concentration in stool water
Water	Creation of factitious diarrhea by addition of water to stool specimen can be detected by measurement of low-stool osmolality (<< 290 mosm/kg)

FIGURE 3-20.

Laxatives and detection methods. Phenolphthalein, bisacodyl, senna, and some other laxatives reduce water and electrolyte absorption in the intestine and cause a secretory diarrhea, usually for therapeutic laxation. Some patients surreptitiously induce diarrhea using these laxatives [15,16]. Such patients can be difficult to detect unless the possibility of laxative abuse is considered and appropriate diagnostic tests are done. (*Adapted from* Schiller [15].)

MALABSORPTION AND MALDIGESTION

CLASSIFICATION OF DISEASES THAT CAUSE INTESTINAL MALABSORPTION

Premucosal	Mucosal	Postmucosal
Pancreatic insufficiency	Celiac sprue	Congenital lymphangiectasia
Hepatobiliary disease	Tropical sprue	Secondary lymphangiectasia
Bacterial overgrowth	Whipple's disease	
Rapid intestinal transit	Eosinophilic enteritis	
Gastrectomy	Brush border enzyme deficiency	
	Lymphoma	
	Short-bowel syndrome	
	Prolonged malnutrition	
	Radiation enteritis	
	Parasitic infection	
	Mesenteric ischemia	

FIGURE 3-21.

The diseases that impair nutrient absorption can be classified by the site of their primary pathophysiologic abnormality. Premucosal diseases are those that affect the digestion of nutrients in the lumen of the intestine. Mucosal diseases are those that affect the mucosal brush border digestion with or without uptake of nutrients by the small intestine. Postmucosal diseases are those that affect the systemic delivery of nutrients absorbed by the small intestine.

SELECTED SYMPTOMS AND SIGNS OF NUTRIENT DEFICIENCIES

	Symptoms or sign	Possible nutrient deficiency
General	Weakness, weight loss, muscle wasting	Protein, calorie
Skin	Pallor	Folate, iron, vitamin B_{12}
	Follicular hyperkeratosis	Vitamin A, vitamin C
	Perifollicular petechiae	Vitamin C
	Dermatitis	Protein, calorie, niacin, riboflavin, zinc, vitamin A, essential fatty acids
	Bruising, purpura	Vitamin C, vitamin K
Hair	Easily plucked, alopecia	Protein, zinc, biotin
	Corkscrew hairs, coiled hair	Vitamin C, vitamin A
Eyes	Night blindness, keratomalacia, photophobia	Vitamin A
	Conjunctival inflammation	Vitamin A, riboflavin
Mouth	Glossitis	Riboflavin, niacin, folate, vitamin B_{12}, protein
	Bleeding or receding gums, mouth ulcers	Vitamin A, vitamin C, vitamin K, folate
	Decreased taste	Zinc, vitamin A
	Burning or sore mouth and tongue	Vitamin B_{12}, vitamin C, niacin, folate, iron
	Angular stomatitis or cheilosis	Riboflavin, niacin, pyridoxine, iron
Neurologic	Tetany	Calcium, magnesium
	Paresthesias	Thiamine, pyridoxine
	Loss of reflexes, wrist drop, foot drop, loss of vibratory and position sense	Vitamin B_{12}, vitamin E
	Dementia, disorientation	Niacin, vitamin B_{12}
	Ophthalmoplegia	Vitamin E, thiamine
	Depression	Biotin, folate, vitamin B_{12}

FIGURE 3-22. Selected symptoms and signs of nutrient deficiencies. The history and physical examination of the patient with suspected malabsorption should involve an evaluation for specific nutrient deficiencies. In general, rapidly proliferating tissues, such as hair, skin, oral and intestinal mucosa, and bone marrow, are often most affected by nutrient deficiencies.

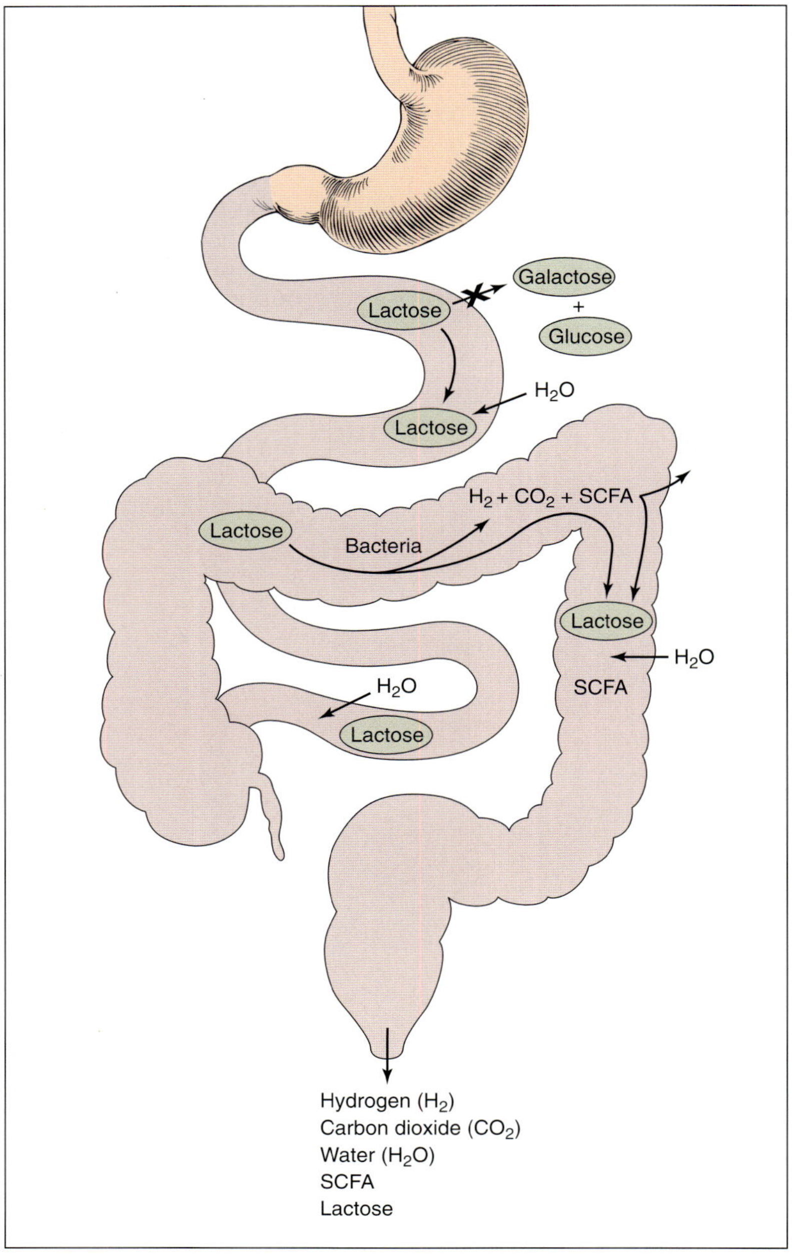

FIGURE 3-23.

Pathophysiology of lactase deficiency. Lactase deficiency is the most common mucosal brush border enzyme deficiency. Clinical symptoms of lactase deficiency include abdominal pain, bloating, flatulence, and diarrhea. These symptoms are caused by osmotic effects of unabsorbed lactose and its metabolic byproducts, increased peristalsis caused by intestinal distension, and gas (H_2, CO_2) produced by bacterial fermentations of lactose. The severity of symptoms after lactose ingestion depends on the load (amount × rate) of lactose delivered to the gastrointestinal tract and the capacity of the colon to absorb short-chain fatty acids (SCFA) produced by bacterial fermentation of lactose.

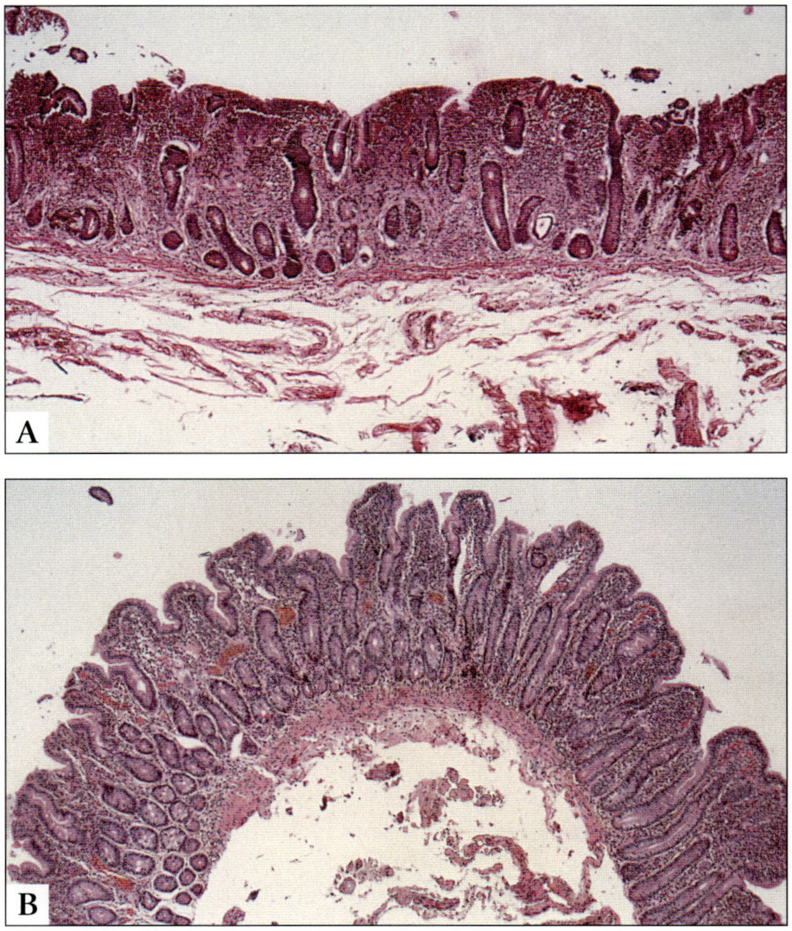

FIGURE 3-24.

Sprue. Jejunal mucosal biopsy from a patient with celiac sprue before (*panel A*) and 3 months after (*panel B*) treatment with a gluten-free diet. Celiac sprue is characterized by small intestinal mucosal damage and nutrient malabsorption in susceptible persons after ingesting gluten, the water-insoluble protein component of certain grains. **Panel A** illustrates the flat mucosal surface, absence of villi, hyperplastic crypts, and increased lamina propria cellularity that are characteristic of the disease. After 3 months of treatment (*panel B*) the mucosa is markedly improved and recognizable villi are present. The villi are short, however, and crypt hyperplasia and lamina propria hypercellularity persist.

The severity of malabsorption and clinical symptoms can vary markedly in patients with celiac sprue, and are directly correlated with the length of the intestinal lesion. Usually, the proximal intestine is most involved and disease severity decreases distally along the length of small bowel. Patients with severe disease have flatulence, progressive weight loss, and multiple nutrient deficiencies. The diarrhea is often voluminous and may float on water because of increased air and fat content. However, some patients have increased fecal mass without loose stools and complain of constipation. Removal of dietary gluten, present in wheat, rye, barely, oats, food additives, emulsifiers, and stabilizers, is essential for successful management. Patients who do not respond to a strict gluten-free diet may have refractory sprue or lymphoma.

PREDICTED NUTRITIONAL OUTCOME IN PATIENTS WHO HAVE HAD MASSIVE INTESTINAL RESECTION

Remaining Jejunal length, cm	Colon	Nutritional outcome
0–50	-	TPN
	+	TPN
51–100	-	IVFM/TPN
	+	Modified oral diet
101–150	-	Regular or modified oral diet
	+	Regular diet
151–200	-	Modified oral diet
	+	Regular diet
>200	- or +	Regular diet

Figure 3-25.

Short-bowel syndrome. Although the gastrointestinal tract has considerable reserve for nutrient absorption, massive small-bowel resection can cause significant malabsorption. The severity of malabsorption depends on the length and functional capacity of the remaining intestine and the site of resection. Jejunal resections are better tolerated than ileal resections because of the specialized functions of the ileum and its adaptive ability to compensate for loss of jejunal function. In addition, the status of the colon is particularly important in patients with little remaining small intestine because the colon can salvage malabsorbed carbohydrates and augment fluid absorption. The need for dietary modifications and intravenous nutritional supplementation can be difficult to predict because of the variability in absorptive capacity of the remaining intestine. This table presents reasonable guidelines that can be used in predicting nutritional outcome based on the length of remaining jejunum and the presence or absence of the colon. IVFM—Intravenous fluids and minerals; modified oral diet—regular diet plus supplemental liquid formula with or without oral rehydration solution; regular diet—table food, including high-caloric diets, frequent feedings, and modification in dietary fat levels; TPN—total parenteral nutrition; (+)—present; (-)—absent. (*Data from* Lennard-Jones [17].)

RECOMMENDATIONS FOR VITAMIN AND TRACE MINERAL SUPPLEMENTATION PATIENTS WITH SHORT-BOWEL SYNDROME

Supplement (representative product)	Dose	Route
Multivitamin with minerals*	1 prenatal vitamin, daily	PO
Vitamin D*	50,000 U 2–3 times per week	PO
Vitamin B_{12}†	1 mg daily	PO
	100–500 µg every 1–2 mo	IM
Vitamin A† (Aquasol)	10,000 to 50,000 U daily	PO
Vitamin K† (Mephyton; AquaMEPHYTON)	5 mg, daily	PO
	5–10 mg/wk	SQ/IM/IV
Vitamin E† (Liqui E)	30 U daily	PO
Zinc gluconate or zinc sulfate†	25 mg elemental zinc daily plus 100 mg/L intestinal output	PO
Ferrous sulfate†	60 mg elemental iron t.i.d.	PO
Iron dextran†	≤ 100 mg elemental iron per day based on formula or table	IV

**Recommended routinely for all patients.*
†Recommended for patients with documented nutrient deficiency or malabsorption.

Figure 3-26.

Most patients with short-bowel syndrome who are maintained on an oral diet should be given vitamin and trace mineral supplements. A daily high-dose vitamin and mineral formula (*eg*, a prenatal multivitamin with minerals), vitamin D, and calcium is recommended. Other micronutrients should be supplemented as needed to prevent or treat specific nutrient deficiencies. IM—intramuscular; IV—intravenous; PO—oral; SQ—subcutaneous.

INITIAL EVALUATION OF PATIENT WITH POSSIBLE MALABSORPTION

History and Physical Examination

Initial blood tests	**Follow-up laboratory tests**
Complete blood count	Serum iron
Prothrombin time	Serum folate
Standard electrolytes	Serum vitamin B_{12}
Calcium	Serum vitamin A
Magnesium	Plasma 25-hydroxy vitamin D
Blood urea nitrogen	Urinary oxalate excretion
Creatinine	Stool for Sudan stain
Alkaline phosphatase	Stool for ova and parasites
Cholesterol	
Total protein and albumin	

FIGURE 3-27.

The approach to the patient with suspected malabsorption requires a careful and appropriate initial evaluation to establish the likelihood of malabsorption and to formulate a list of possible causes. The history and physical examination should assess body weight changes, appetite and food intake, generalized weakness, the presence and volume of diarrhea, stool characteristics suggestive of steatorrhea, signs and symptoms of dehydration, signs and symptoms of specific nutrient deficiencies, abdominal pain and other gastrointestinal symptoms, and extraintestinal manifestations. Follow-up laboratory tests are usually more expensive or more difficult to perform than the initial blood tests, and their use should be reserved for specific indications.

CROHN'S DISEASE

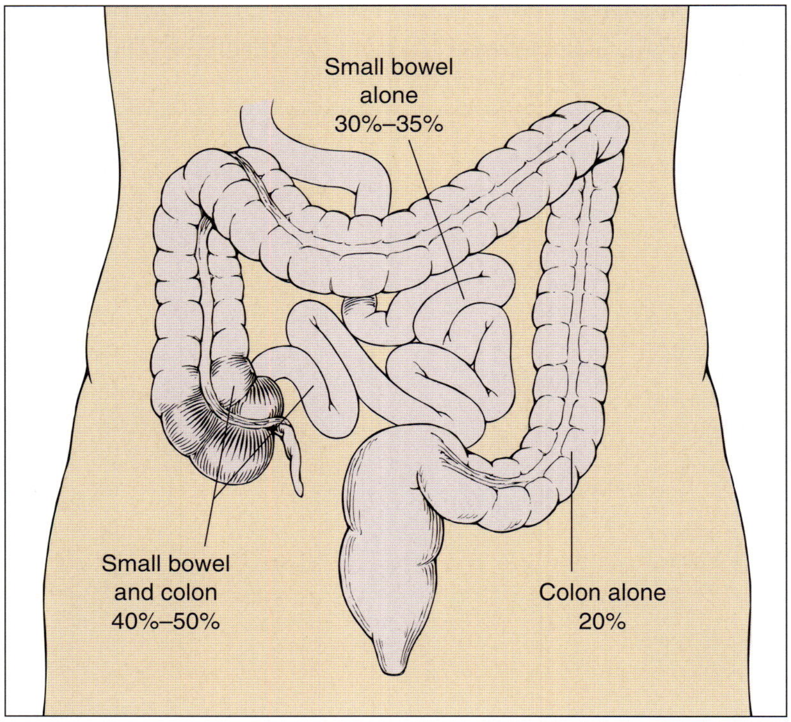

FIGURE 3-28.

Anatomic distribution in Crohn's disease. Crohn's disease affects the small bowel alone in approximately 33% of cases and the colon alone in approximately 20%; nearly 50% of the cases involve both the small and large bowels (ileocolitis). The etiology of Crohn's disease is not known.

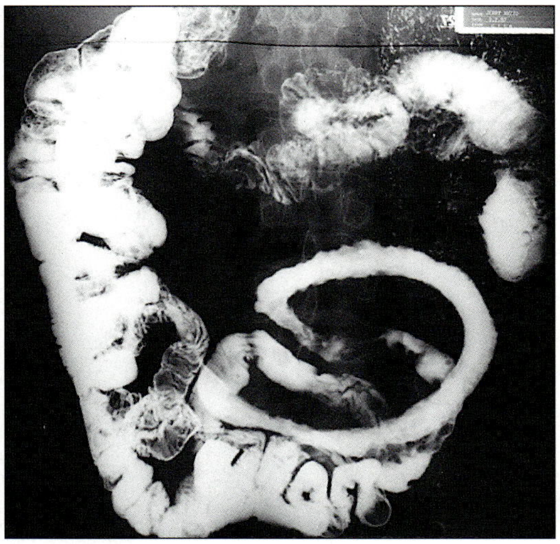

FIGURE 3-29.

Radiographic appearance of Crohn's disease of the terminal ileum. Nodularity, ulceration, narrowing, and irregularity of the lumen, characteristically affecting the terminal ileum, may result from transmural inflammation and lymphoid proliferation. Separation of involved loops of intestine from adjacent segments of bowel reflects luminal narrowing, thickening of bowel wall, and mesenteric hypertrophy.

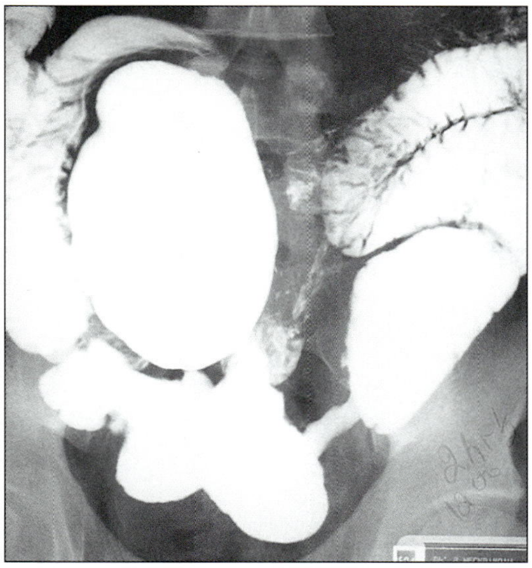

FIGURE 3-30.

When multiple strictures produce multiple areas of massively dilated proximal bowel over periods of many years, huge sacs, or "saddlebags," may develop. This saccular pattern is often accompanied by clinical sequelae of malnutrition due to impaired intake, bacterial overgrowth, and malabsorption.

HISTORY, PHYSICAL EXAMINATION, RADIOGRAPHIC AND LABORATORY FINDINGS IN CROHN'S DISEASE

History
Abdominal pain
Diarrhea
Weight loss or failure of growth
Fever
Family history of inflammatory bowel disease

Physical examination
Right lower quadrant tenderness, with or without mass

Radiography
Abnormal small-bowel follow-through radiographs
Barium enema with ileal reflux showing abnormal terminal ileum

Laboratory
Anemia
Elevated erythrocyte sedimentation rate
Hypoalbuminemia
Hypocholesterolemia

FIGURE 3-31.

The inflammatory pattern of small-bowel Crohn's disease characteristically presents with recurrent episodes of right lower quadrant pain and fever, although a careful history usually uncovers preexisting bowel complaints. Persistent inflammation and scarring may progress to stenosis with repeated bouts of obstruction.

DIFFERENTIAL DIAGNOSIS OF CROHN'S DISEASE

DISEASES OF ADJACENT ORGANS

Appendix and cecum
Appendicitis
Appendiceal abscess
Cecal diverticulitis
Cecal carcinoma

Tuboadnexae
Pelvic inflammatory disease
Ovarian cyst or tumor
Endometriosis

INTRINSIC ILEOCECAL DISEASES

Neoplasms
Carcinoid
Lymphoma
Metastatic tumor

Vascular
Oral contraceptives
Systemic vasculitis

Radiation

Infections
- Acute
  - Anisakiasis
  - *Yersinia enterocolitica*
- Chronic
  - Tuberculosis
  - *Mycobacterium avium-intracellulare*

Miscellaneous diseases
Chronic nongranulomatous ulcerative jejunoileitis
Eosinophilic gastroenteritis
Amyloidosis
Zollinger-Ellison syndrome

FIGURE 3-32.

The clinical and radiologic diagnosis of Crohn's disease of the small bowel is rather straightforward. However, not every ileocecal or right lower quadrant lesion represents Crohn's disease. Two major categories of disease that may be confused with regional enteritis are disorders of the adjacent organs and intrinsic disease of the ileum and cecum that mimic the radiographic picture of Crohn's disease.

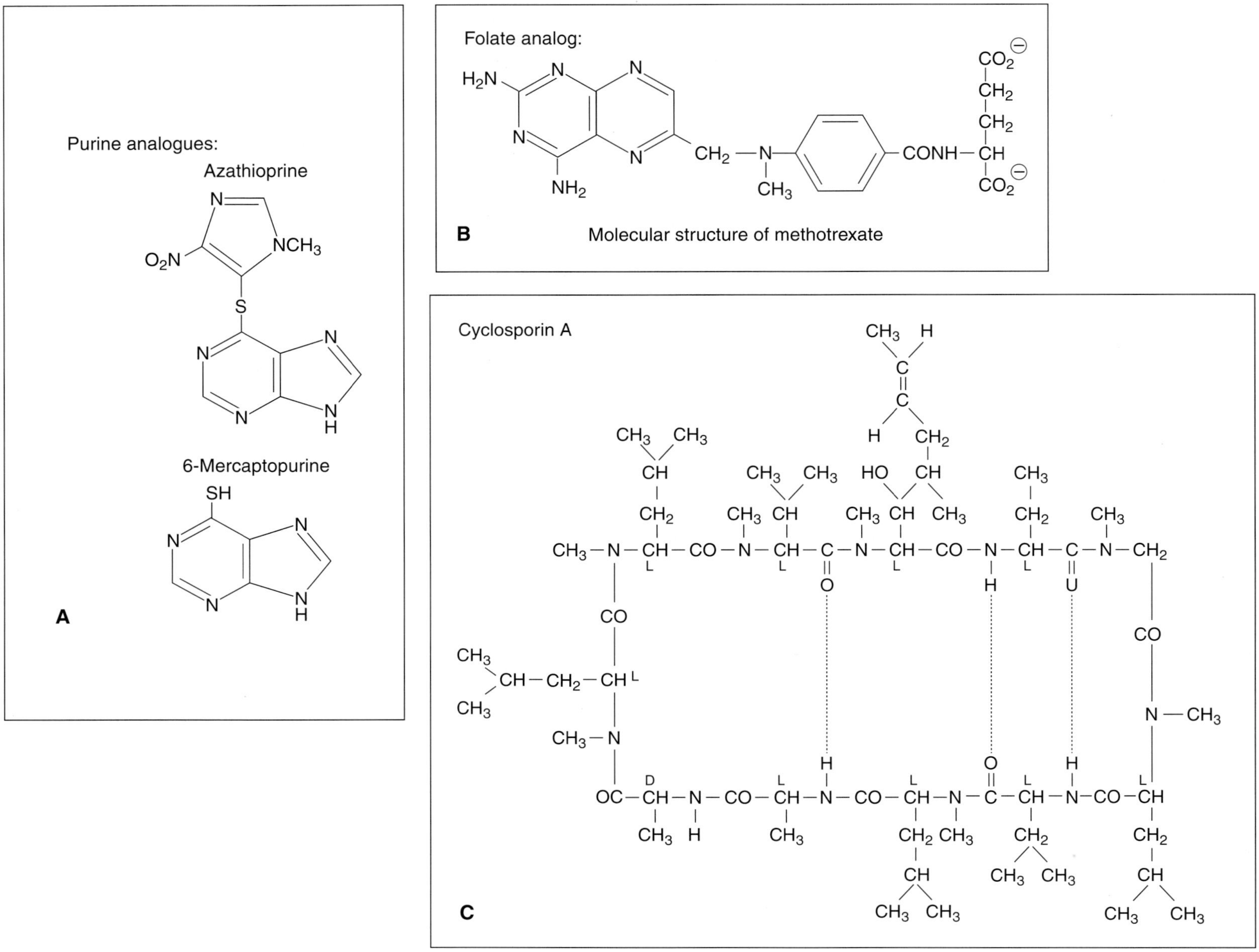

FIGURE 3-33.

Immunomodulators in Crohn's disease. Whereas corticosteroids and 5-aminosalicylates are the standards of therapy in Crohn's disease, immunomodulators are used for refractory, severe cases. **A**, Azathioprine is a prodrug that is quickly converted to 6-mercaptopurine (6-MP) in red blood cells. Azathioprine and 6-MP are purine analogues that inhibit nucleotide biosynthesis. These drugs are effective for inducing and maintaining remission of inflammatory and fistulizing Crohn's disease, and especially for reducing corticosteroid requirements, but they require up to 3 to 6 months before the onset of therapeutic action. 6-MP is administered in doses 1.0 to 1.5 mg/kg/day. Azathioprine is administered 1.0 to 3.0 mg/kg/day. Allergic reactions occur in about 5% of patients, including early fever, rash, arthralgias, and acute, reversible pancreatitis, early in the course, or a drug-induced hepatitis later in the course of therapy. Leukopenia is rare, dose related, and reversible. Neither 6-MP or azathioprine has been associated with increased risk of cancer or adverse outcomes of pregnancy, although two cases of CNS lymphoma have been reported in the world experience.

B, Methotrexate is a folate analogue which, like the purine analogues 6-MP and azathioprine, acts as an antimetabolite that inhibits T-lymphocyte function. Indications for treatment include induction of remission in Crohn's disease and reducing corticosteroid requirements. Methotrexate is most effectively administered at a dose of 15 to 25 mg/week, intramuscularly or subcutaneously, for 12 to 18 weeks. Some experts recommend liver biopsy because of the potential for hepatic fibrosis.

C, Cyclosporin A specifically blocks T-helper cell function and proliferation by inhibiting interleukin-2 gene transcription. Although used primarily for inducing remission in severe steroid refractory ulcerative colitis, cyclosporine has also been useful in promoting rapid fistula closure in Crohn's disease and dramatic healing of pyoderma gangrenosum in both Crohn's disease and ulcerative colitis. The usual IV dose is 4 mg/kg/day to achieve levels of 400 to 600 mcg/L using the monoclonal cyclosporine immunoassay.

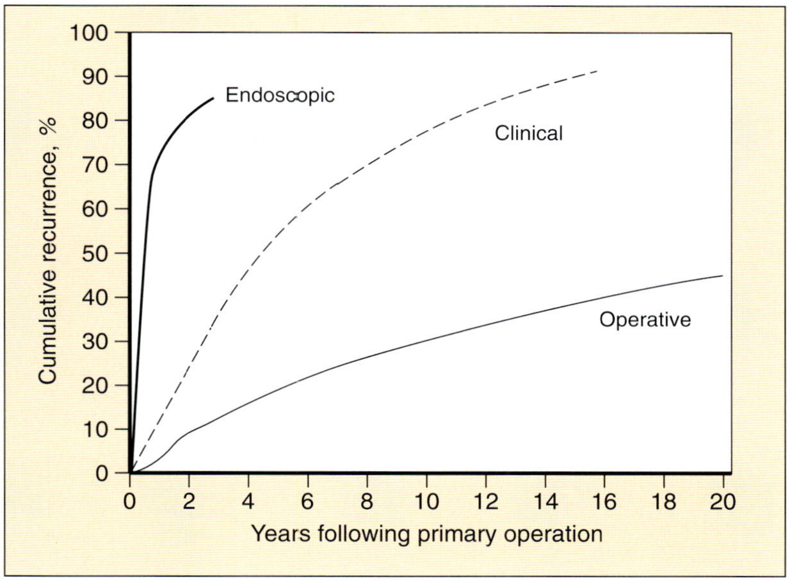

FIGURE 3-34.

Surgery in Crohn's disease is indicated to treat medically refractory cases or complications such as intestinal obstruction. Although surgery is frequently necessary and highly effective in managing complications, achieving rehabilitation, and restoring a healthier quality of life in patients with Crohn's disease, postoperative recurrence is almost inevitable. The magnitude of this problem of postoperative recurrence depends largely on the definition of *recurrence*—whether endoscopic, clinical, or surgical.

SMALL INTESTINAL ISCHEMIA

CAUSES OF MESENTERIC VASCULAR INSUFFICIENCY

Nonocclusive factors (low flow)	*Venous*
Impaired cardiac output	Thrombosis
Reduced systemic arterial flow	Intrinsic
Vasoconstriciton (drugs)	Extrinsic
Occlusive vascular disease	Trauma
Arterial	Neoplasm
Thrombosis	Hypertension (*ie*, Portal)
Embolism	

FIGURE 3-35.

Causes of mesenteric vascular insufficiency. Occlusive or nonocclusive arterial disease leads to insufficiency of blood flow and may result in ischemia or infarction. Decreased cardiac output and systemic blood flow occur in hypotension resulting from hypovolemia, sepsis or hemorrhage, congestive heart failure, aortic stenosis, myocardial infarction, and arrhythmias. Examples of locally vasoconstrictive drugs include norepinephrine, vasopressin, and digitalis.

Arterial occlusion can be caused by a thrombus (usually on or into an atheromatous plaque), embolus, vasculitis, trauma, or neoplasm. Venous occlusion is secondary to thrombus (from a variety of hypercoagulable states), trauma, or neoplasm [18]. (*Adapted from* American Gastroenterological Association [18].)

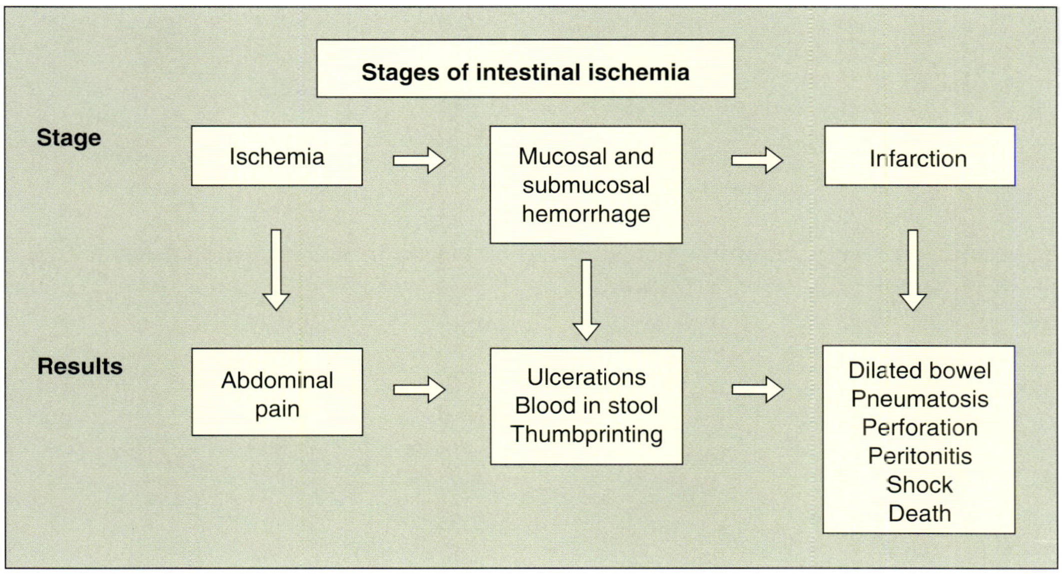

FIGURE 3-36.

Stages of intestinal ischemia. The clinical presentations of intestinal ischemia depend on the completeness and duration of impaired gut blood flow. In mild and potentially reversible ischemia, the only clinical feature is abdominal pain. Blood tests, stool studies, and radiographs are normal. If the ischemia progresses or is more severe initially, necrosis of the surface epithelium occurs with mucosal sloughing and submucosal hemorrhage. Complete infarction, which is irreversible, manifests itself as an "acute abdomen" with features of peritonitis. (*Adapted from* American Gastroenterological Association [18]; with permission.)

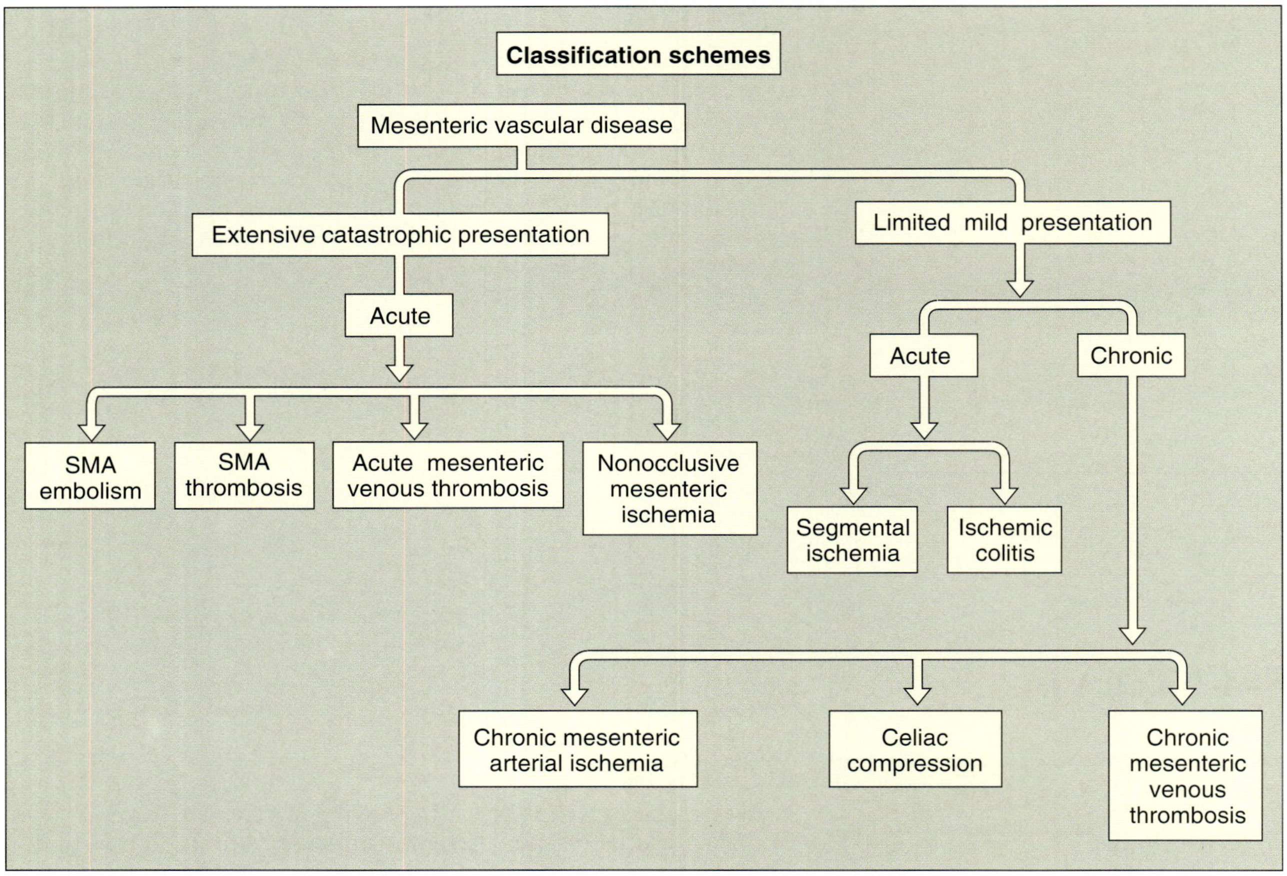

FIGURE 3-37.

Classification of mesenteric vascular disease based on the extent of ischemia. Previous classification schemes have been based on time (acute versus chronic), location (arterial versus venous and mesenteric versus colonic), and the character of the obstruction (occlusive versus nonocclusive). The classification scheme proposed by Williams, which separates disease entities into extensive ischemia and limited ischemia, may facilitate evaluation, diagnosis, and treatment of mesenteric vascular disorders [19]. (*Adapted from* Williams [20].)

CLASSIFICATION OF SMALL INTESTINAL ISCHEMIC DISORDERS

MAJOR PATHOLOGICAL PROCESS	EXAMPLES OF DISEASE ENTITIES
SMA occlusion	SMA thrombosis or embolus
SMA low flow state without occlusion (SMA vasospasm)	Nonocclusive intestinal ischemia as in heart failure, aortic surgery, or circulatory shock
Miscellaneous processes	
Bacterial invasion in susceptible mucosa	Necrotizing enterocolitis
Mesenteric venous occlusion	Extension of a portal thrombus, compression of a mesenteric vein (strangulated hernia, hepatic tumor, ileus, volvulus, adhesions)
Arterial wall connective tissue inflammation	Periarteritis nodosa

FIGURE 3-38.

Classification of small intestinal ischemic disorders according to the pathologic process. This organization is based on the predominant pathogenetic process and emphasizes the most common severe intestinal ischemic states. (*Adapted from* Levine and Jacobson [21]; with permission.)

CONDITIONS THAT MAY CONTRIBUTE TO OR BE ASSOCIATED WITH MESENTERIC VASCULAR OCCLUSION OR INSUFFICIENCY

- Embolic occlusion
  - Cardiac diseases
    - Rhythm
      - Arrhythmia
      - Atrial fibrillation
    - Valvular disease
      - Rheumatic heart disease
      - Prosthetic heart valve
      - Endocarditis
      - Valvular stenosis
    - Heart chamber disease
      - Myocardial infarction
      - Mural thrombus
      - Atrial myxoma
    - Vascular diseases
      - Invasive radiologic procedures, angiographic manipulation
      - Arterial plaques
      - Vascular aneurysms
      - Vascular dissections
      - Trauma
- Thrombotic occlusion
  - Atherosclerosis
  - Hypercoagulable state
    - Sickle-cell disease
    - Polycythemia vera
    - Thrombocytosis
    - Factor V Leiden mutation
    - Antithrombin III deficiency
    - Protein C or S deficiency
    - Neoplasms (especially intra-abdominal)
    - Pregnancy
    - Migratory thrombophlebitis
  - Vascular diseases
    - Invasive radiologic procedures, angiographic manipulation
    - Arterial plaques
    - Vascular aneurysms
    - Vascular dissections
    - Trauma
- Nonocclusive mesenteric ischemia
  - Hypoperfusion
    - Cardiac failure
    - Hypovolemia
    - Sepsis
    - Vasoconstricting drugs
- Mesenteric vein thrombosis
  - Hypercoagulable states
    - Sickle-cell disease
    - Polycythemia vera
    - Thrombocytosis
    - Factor V Leiden mutation
    - Antithrombin III deficiency
    - Protein C or S deficiency
    - Neoplasms (especially intra-abdominal)
    - Pregnancy
    - Migratory thrombophlebitis
  - Local venous stasis
    - Portal hypertension
      - Cirrhosis
      - Congestive splenomegaly
      - After sclerotherapy of esophageal varices
    - Compression of portal venous radicles by tumor
- Portal hypertension
- Intra-abdominal inflammation and sepsis
  - Abscess (pelvic, intra-abdominal)
  - Peritonitis
  - Inflammatory bowel disease
  - Diverticulitis
  - Pancreatitis
- Postoperative states
- Trauma

FIGURE 3-39.

Conditions that may contribute to or be associated with mesenteric vascular occlusion or insufficiency. Whatever the cause, the end result of extensive mesenteric ischemia can be similar and range from mild completely reversible intestinal injury to irreversible, transmural, hemorrhagic necrosis. The degree of ischemia and the length of bowel involved are factors that determine the clinical picture [19]. (*Adapted from* Rogers and David [19].)

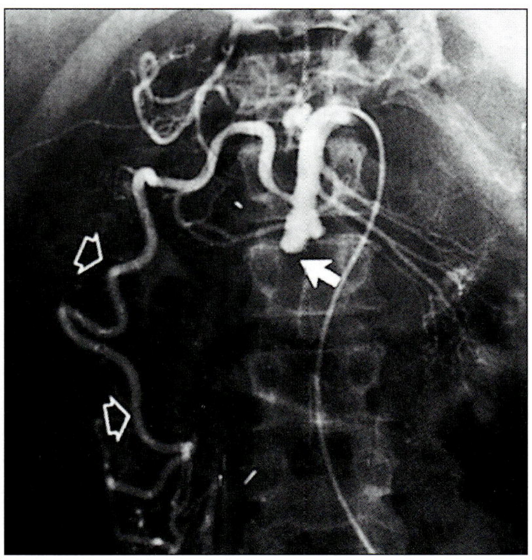

FIGURE 3-40.

Embolic occlusion of the superior mesenteric artery (SMA). The usual origin of a mesenteric arterial embolus is a mural thrombus from the left atrium or ventricle. Predisposing conditions include atrial fibrillation, rheumatic heart disease, prosthetic heart valves, myocardial infarction, ventricular aneurysms, and invasive angiographic procedures. The clinician should be alert to the possibility of embolism to a major mesenteric artery when severe periumbilical abdominal pain, vomiting, diarrhea, and leukocytosis arise acutely in the appropriate clinical setting. Emboli to the SMA most often lodge in the middle colic branch, but can affect any of its four branches. Emboli tend to lodge within 3 to 8 cm of the origin of the SMA, usually where the vessel narrows. This angiogram reveals occlusion of the SMA by a thrombus. The solid arrow points to complete occlusion distal to the origin of the middle colic artery. The open arrows reveal some collateral flow through the middle colic–right colic anastomosis [19]. (*From* Rogers and David [19]; *courtesy of* Stanley Baum, MD, University of Pennsylvania, Philadelphia, PA.)

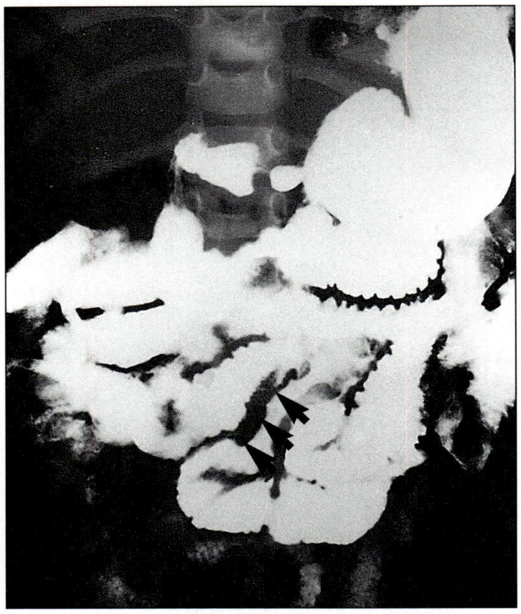

FIGURE 3-41

Henoch-Schönlein purpura. Henoch-Schönlein purpura, a small-vessel vasculitis, frequently involves the gastrointestinal tract. It is characterized by nonthrombocytopenic purpura, renal involvement, and colicky abdominal pain (with or without bloody diarrhea). This disease is most often seen in children between the ages of 4 and 7 years old. Pain may be related to intramural hemorrhage, secondary to the vasculitis. Pain, nausea, and vomiting may also develop if hematoma formation or resultant edema causes intussusception. This upper gastrointestinal series was taken of a 2-year-old child who presented with anemia, abdominal pain, and gastrointestinal bleeding. It reveals narrowing and ulceration of the jejunum and ileum (*arrows*), which are most commonly involved. This appearance can mimic Crohn's disease or lymphoma [22]. (*Courtesy of* Robert Feltman, Miami, FL.) (*See* Figure 3-62 for skin changes in Henoch-Schönlein purpura.)

ROUTINE TESTS FOR PATIENTS WITH SUSPECTED INTESTINAL ISCHEMIA

Tests	Findings with ischemia	Nonvascular causes of finding
Routine Laboratory	Anion gap acidosis	Any abdominal catastrophe
	Leukocytosis/bandemia	Any acute inflammation or sepsis
	Hyperamylasemia	Pancreatitis, bowel perforation, penetrating ulcer
Flat and upright radiographs of the abdomen	Thickened bowel wall	Other inflammatory bowel diseases [IBD] (acute dysentery)
	Free intraperitoneal gas	Perforation (diverticulitis, appendicitis, IBD, ulcer)
	Gas in portal venous system or linear pneumatosis	Any cause of bowel infarction

FIGURE 3-42.

Routine tests for suspected intestinal ischemia. If ischemia is considered likely in a patient with acute abdominal pain, the laboratory and radiologic studies undertaken may offer supporting evidence and assist in establishing a diagnosis far more rapidly. These tests are insensitive, however, and are usually positive only when infarction has already occurred (*eg*, acidosis). In addition, these tests are nonspecific with similar results (*eg*, hyperamylasemia) present in other disease processes. On the contrary, routine abdominal radiographs or computed tomographic scans revealing intraperitoneal free air or gas in the portal venous system in this setting offer compelling evidence of intestinal infarction and should lead to immediate surgical intervention. (*Adapted from* Levine and Jacobson [21]; with permission.)

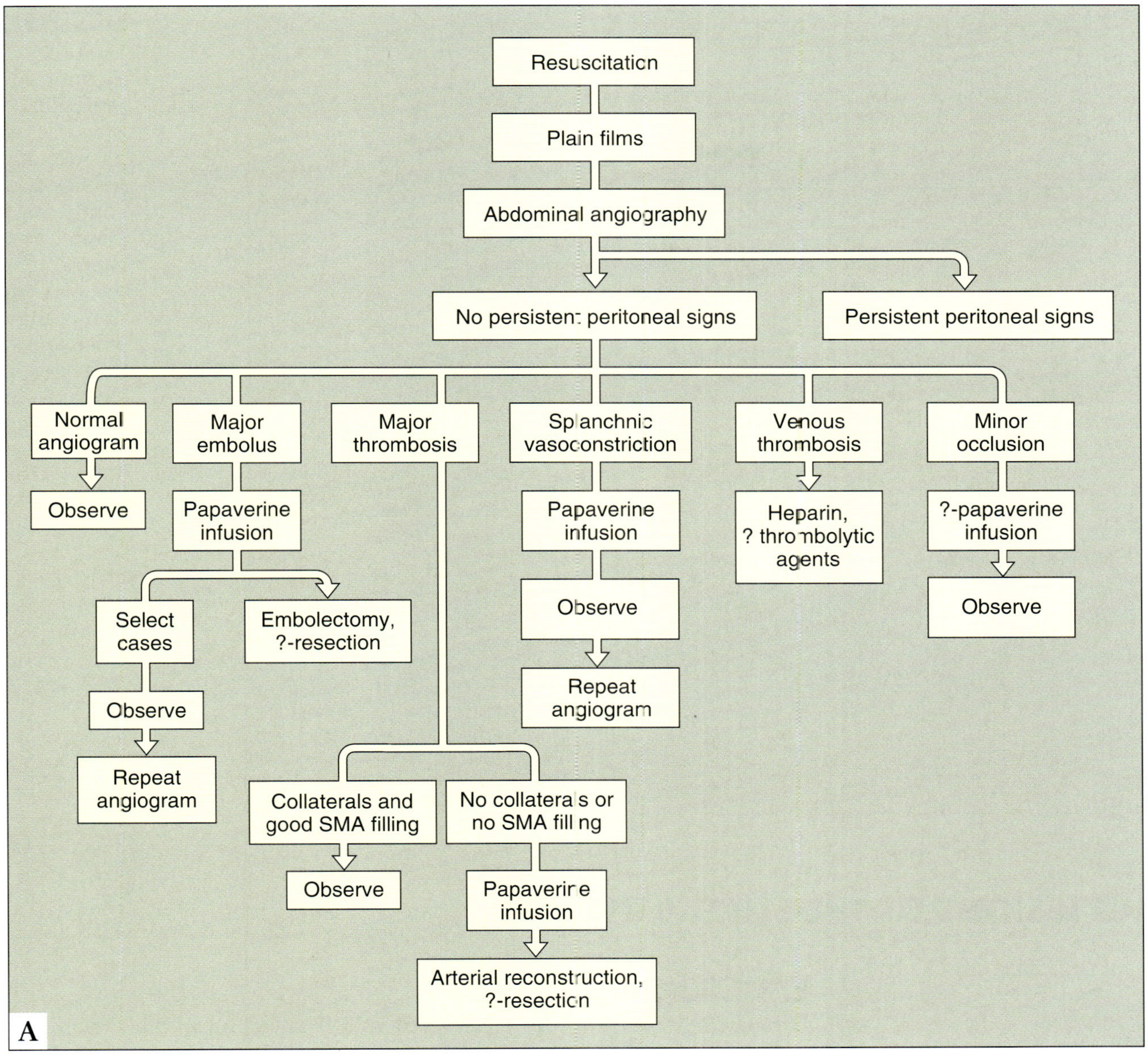

FIGURE 3-43.

Algorithm for the management of extensive mesenteric vascular ischemia in the absence (*panel A*) and presence (*panel B*) of persistent peritoneal signs [19]. Factors that increase the risk of mesenteric ischemia include age greater than 50 years old, previous myocardial infarction or embolic events, cardiac arrhythmia, valvular or rheumatic heart disease, low cardiac output, invasive vascular procedures and the use of oral contraception. As described by Boley *et al* [23,24], if a patient with any of these risk factors presents with acute onset of abdominal pain that persists for more than 2 or 3 hours, the diagnosis of extensive mesenteric ischemia must be suspected, and the above protocol for evaluation and treatment should be initiated.

(continued on next page)

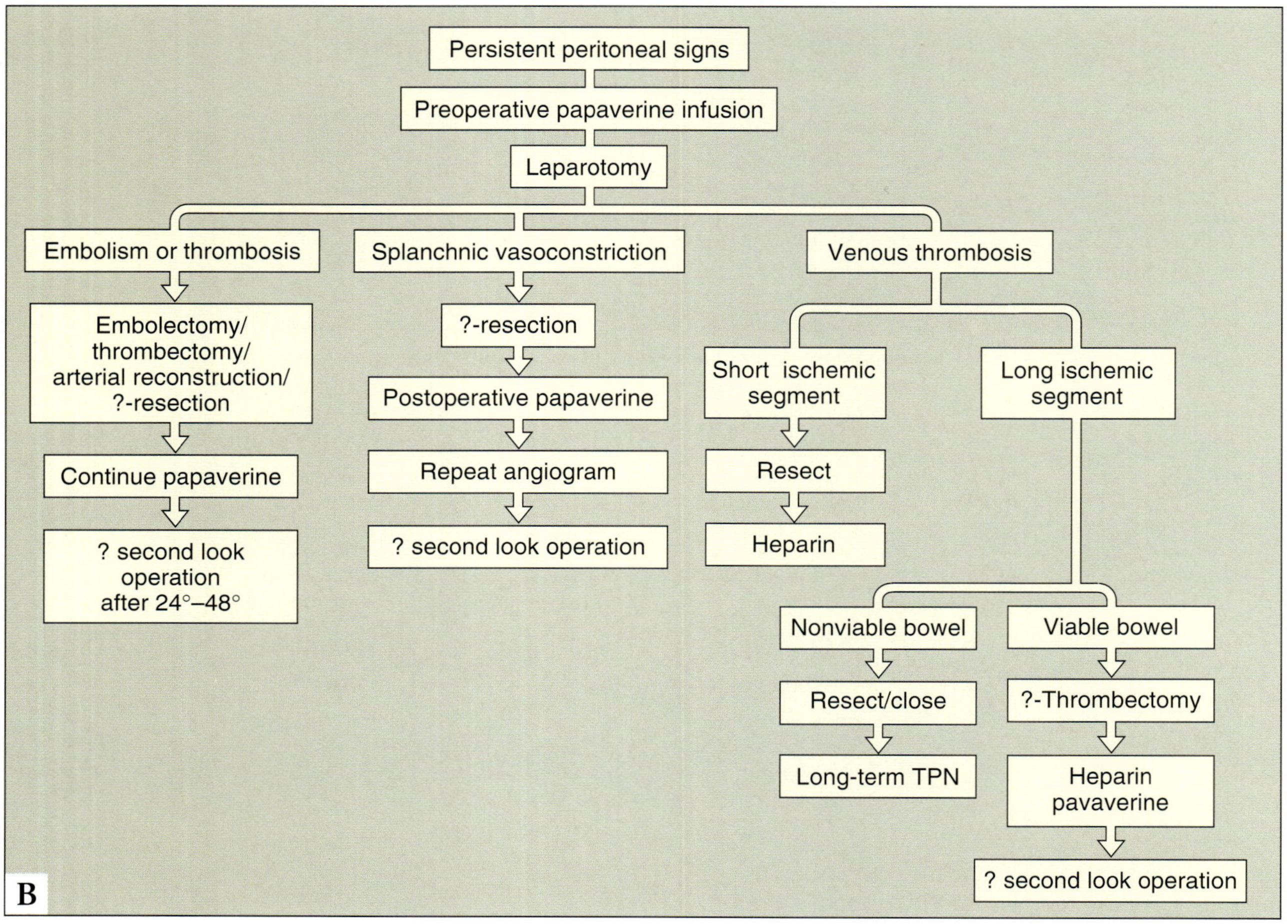

FIGURE 3-43. *CONTINUED*

The only way to decrease the morbidity and mortality of visceral ischemic injury is by having a high index of suspicion and employing early angiographic examination supplemented by selective mesenteric vasodilation or urgent surgery, when appropriate. If the diagnosis is made after intestinal infarction occurs, the mortality rate is between 70% and 90%. (*Adapted from* Rogers and David [19]; with permission.)

BLEEDING LESIONS OF THE SMALL INTESTINE

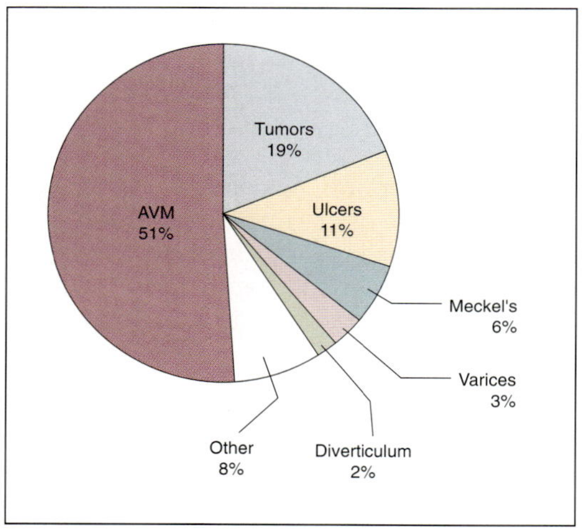

FIGURE 3-44.

Etiology of small-bowel bleeding. Based on 519 patients in whom a lesion thought to be responsible for small-bowel bleeding was identified [25–31], mucosal vascular anomalies (AVMs) were the most frequently found (51%), followed by small-bowel tumors (19%). Of these neoplasms, primary smooth muscle tumors represented 34% (79% benign, 21% malignant). Other malignant solid tumors (primary or metastatic) represented 25% of tumors, lymphoma 15%, nonspecified neoplasms 12%, and others 13% (carcinoid, leukemia, endometrioma, polyps). Small-bowel ulcerations, excluding those induced by nonsteroidal anti-inflammatory drugs (NSAIDs), were responsible for gastrointestinal bleeding in 11% of cases. Meckel's diverticulum was the source of bleeding in 6% of cases, whereas varices and diverticula accounted for 3% and 2%, respectively. Other diagnoses (erosions, aortoenteric fistula, NSAID-associated ulcers, and bleeding without an identified source) were responsible for the remaining 8% of cases.

DIAGNOSTIC TECHNIQUES AVAILABLE FOR EVALUATION OF SMALL-BOWEL BLEEDING

Barium Contrast Radiologic Studies

Small-bowel series

Enteroclysis

Nuclear Medicine Studies

^{99m}Technetium sulfur colloid scintigraphy

^{99m}Technetium-labeled erythrocyte scintigraphy

^{99m}Technetium sodium pertechnetate scan (Meckel's scan)

Enteroscopy

Push enteroscopy (jejunoscopy)

Sonde enteroscopy

Arteriography

Exploratory Laparotomy

Alone

With intraoperative angiography

With intraoperative scintigraphy

With intraoperative enteroscopy

FIGURE 3-45.

A list of the diagnostic techniques available for the work-up of patients with suspected small-bowel bleeding is arranged from the least to the most invasive. Typically, patients with small-bowel bleeding not only have multiple, but also repeated tests during the course of their evaluation. Some of these techniques are also capable of delivering therapy, such as electrocoagulation with jejunoscopy, vasopressin infusion or embolization with arteriography, and resection with exploratory laparotomy. The choice of the diagnostic tool to be used depends on the severity of gastrointestinal bleeding, its mode of presentation, and the patient's overall clinical condition.

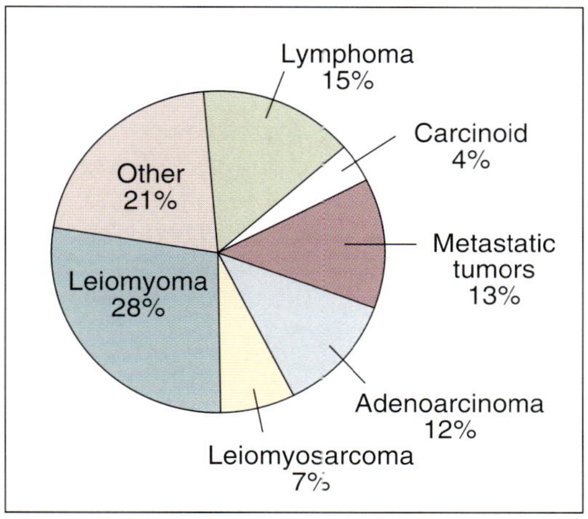

FIGURE 3-46.

Gastrointestinal hemorrhage of obscure origin arising from small-bowel tumors. Small-bowel tumors are found in 19% of patients evaluated for gastrointestinal hemorrhage of obscure origin when standard upper gastrointestinal tract endoscopy and colonoscopy are negative. Among 99 tumors reported as a cause of obscure gastrointestinal hemorrhage [25–35] primary smooth muscle tumors were the most common (35%); 28% were benign (leiomyomas) and 7% were malignant (leiomyosarcomas). Adenocarcinoma was found in 12% and metastatic tumors in 13%. Lymphoma of the small bowel was another common cause of gastrointestinal hemorrhage of obscure origin (15%), but carcinoid tumors represented only 4%. Other tumors, including those reported only as "neoplasms," represented 21% of the total. Small-bowel tumors are the most common cause of bleeding detected through enteroscopy in patients younger than 50 years of age [36].

TREATMENT OPTIONS FOR SMALL-BOWEL BLEEDING LESIONS

Options	Useful in these circumstances	Applications	Limitations
Medical Iron Supplementation Blood Transfusion Estrogen/Progesterone	1. Chronic slow bleeding 2. Patient unfit for invasive diagnostic work-up 3. Patient unfit for surgery 4. After rebleeding despite other therapies	Diffuse arteriovenous malformations (AVMs) Metastatic disease	Temporary Bleeding recurs if therapy stops
Endoscopic Heater Probe Electrocoagulation Laser	1. Active bleeding discovered during endoscopy 2. When multiple lesions are diffuse and therefore not suitable for surgical therapy	AVMs Ulcers	Endoscopic skills needed Persistent/recurrent bleeding
Radiographic Vasopressin Embolization	1. Active bleeding discovered during angiography 2. Patient unfit for surgery 3. Widespread metastasis	Ulcers Tumors AVMs	Temporary Recurrence Invasive
Surgical Excision Local Resection Segmental Resection	1. Bleeding uncontrolled by other modalities 2. Isolated bleeding lesion 3. Suspected malignancy	Tumors Meckel's diverticulum Isolated AVMs	Invasive Persistent/recurrent bleeding

FIGURE 3-47.

Treatment options for small-bowel bleeding lesions. The four major therapeutic options for bleeding small-bowel lesions include medical, which is primarily directed to achieve secondary goals, and include iron supplementation, blood transfusion, or use of estrogen/progesterone preparations (*eg*, diffuse arteriovenous malformations, metastatic disease); endoscopic, directed to achieve primary goals, such as to arrest active bleeding, and remove or ablate the source of bleeding (*eg*, arteriovenous malformations, ulcers); radiographic, which include the use of vasopressin or direct embolization (*eg*, ulcers, tumors, arteriovenous malformations); and surgical, in which excision and local or segmental resection attempts to achieve primary goals (*eg*, tumors, Meckel's diverticulum, isolated arteriovenous malformations). Each option has utility in certain circumstances. Each modality has its own limitations. Thus, recurrent bleeding occurs frequently if medical therapy is stopped, therefore providing only temporary relief of the problem. Some techniques (all surgical and some radiographic) are considered invasive and may not be suitable for the fragile, unfit patient. Recurrent or persistent bleeding may also occur with endoscopic and surgical techniques, especially with multiple diffuse lesions. Special endoscopic skill is needed for performing enteroscopy with or without therapy.

HORMONAL THERAPY OF SMALL-BOWEL ANGIODYSPLASIAS

Author	Study Design	Patients (n)	Drug(s)	Results
Bronner *et al.* [37]	Uncontrolled	7	Mestranol 0.075–0.15 mg + norethisterone 1 mg	Arrested bleeding in all patients
Van Cutsem *et al.* [38]	Placebo-controlled	10	Norethindrone 1 mg + ethinylestradiol 0.05 mg	Significant reduction of bleeding in treated group (P<0.002)
Lewis *et al.* [39]	Cohort	64	Norethynodrel 5–10 mg + mestranol 0.075–0.15 mg or conjugated estrogens 0.625 mg	No difference in transfusion requirements

FIGURE 3-48.

Hormonal therapy of small-bowel angiodysplasias. The mechanism of action of hormonal therapy in the setting of bleeding angiodysplasias (both acquired and inherited) remains unknown. Improvement in the endothelial integrity in patients with Osler-Weber-Rendu disease [40], blood stasis within mesenteric microcirculation in animals [41], shortened bleeding time in dialysis patients [42], and effects on the endothelium such as reduction in prostacyclin production [43] have been some of the phenomena observed in response to estrogen therapy.

TUMORS OF THE SMALL INTESTINE

SMALL-BOWEL TUMORS: SIGNS AND SYMPTOMS

Adenocarcinoma	Carcinoid	Lymphoma	Leiomyosarcoma
Pain	Asymptomatic	Pain	Asymptomatic
Obstruction	Obstruction	Obstruction	Pain
Systemic	Pain	Mass	Gastrointestinal bleeding
(Jaundice with periampullary tumors)		Perforation	Mass
		Gastrointestinal bleeding	Perforation
		Systemic	

FIGURE 3-49.

Small-bowel tumors: signs and symptoms. Although the majority of small-bowel tumors are asymptomatic or present with mild symptoms only, bulkier tumors can lead to abdominal pain, bowel obstruction, and systemic signs and symptoms. Adenocarcinomas tend to grow circumferentially and lead to pain and obstruction. Jaundice is characteristic of periampullary tumors, which are commonly adenocarcinomas. Carcinoids tend to be smaller than 1 to 2 cm, and are typically asymptomatic, although they may result in obstruction and pain becasue of the occasionally intense desmoplastic tissue reaction and contractures. Lymphomas tend to be bulky and commonly lead to pain, obstruction, a palpable mass, perforation, and bleeding. Although occult gastrointestinal (GI) blood loss may be seen with all small-bowel tumors, gross GI bleeding is seen generally only with lymphomas and leiomyosarcomas. Because leiomyosarcomas tend to be slow growing, they are often asymptomatic until reaching a large size of 5 cm or more, when they may present with pain, GI bleeding, or perforation [44–48].

SMALL-BOWEL MALIGNANT TUMORS: RISK FACTORS

Adenocarcinoma
- Familial adenomatous polyposis
- Crohn's disease (involving small bowel)
- Celiac sprue
- Ureteroileostomy
- Neurofibromatosis

Carcinoid
- Multiple endocrine neoplasia syndrome I

Lymphoma
- Celiac sprue
- Immunosuppression and immunodeficiency

FIGURE 3-50.

Small-bowel malignant tumors: risk factors. Although small-bowel malignancies are uncommon in the general population, several risk factors predispose to their development in susceptible individuals. For instance, patients with familial adenomatous polyposis have a greater than 50% chance of developing small-bowel (primarily duodenal) adenomas, which often progress to adenocarcinoma. Generally, these risk factors predispose to a specific histologic tumor type. The exception is celiac sprue, which predisposes affected individuals to adenocarcinomas and lymphomas [44–48].

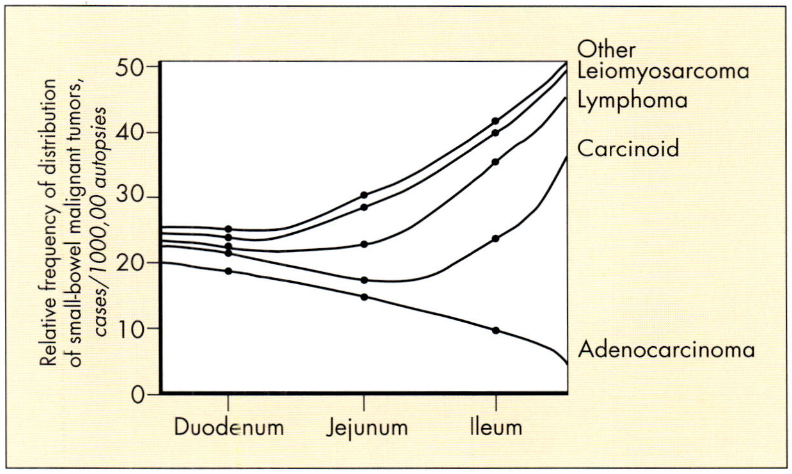

FIGURE 3-51.

Relative frequency of distribution of small-bowel malignant tumors. Adenocarcinomas are the most common among small-bowel malignancies followed by carcinoids, lymphomas, and leiomyosarcomas. Other histologic malignant tumor types are distinctly uncommon. Adenocarcinomas predominate in the duodenum and carcinoids predominate in the distal ileum. Lymphomas and leiomyosarcomas are more common in the distal and mid small bowel, with relatively few being found in the duodenum. A duodenal mass is most likely an adenocarcinoma, and a distal ileal mass is most likely a carcinoid. Jejunal and ileal (except for distal ileal) masses may be of any histologic type [44,48–51]. (*Data from* Lance [44], Donohue [48], Parker *et al.* [49], Weiss and Yang [50], and Zollinger *et al.* [51].)

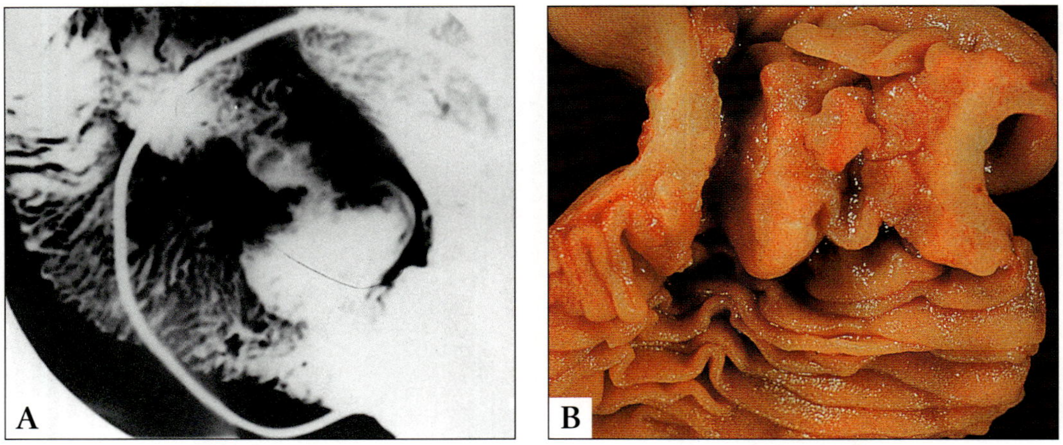

Figure 3-52.

Small bowel adenocarcinoma. Although many duodenal and proximal jejunal tumors may be seen by endoscopy or enteroscopy, most are beyond the reach of even the longest instruments. Such tumors require either conventional small-bowel follow-through radiograms or enteroclysis for their detection. **A**, In this patient, the annular napkin-ringlike lesion was seen to best advantage at enteroclysis. **B**, The marked narrowing of the lumen by the circumferentially growing adenocarcinoma was seen in the resection specimen.

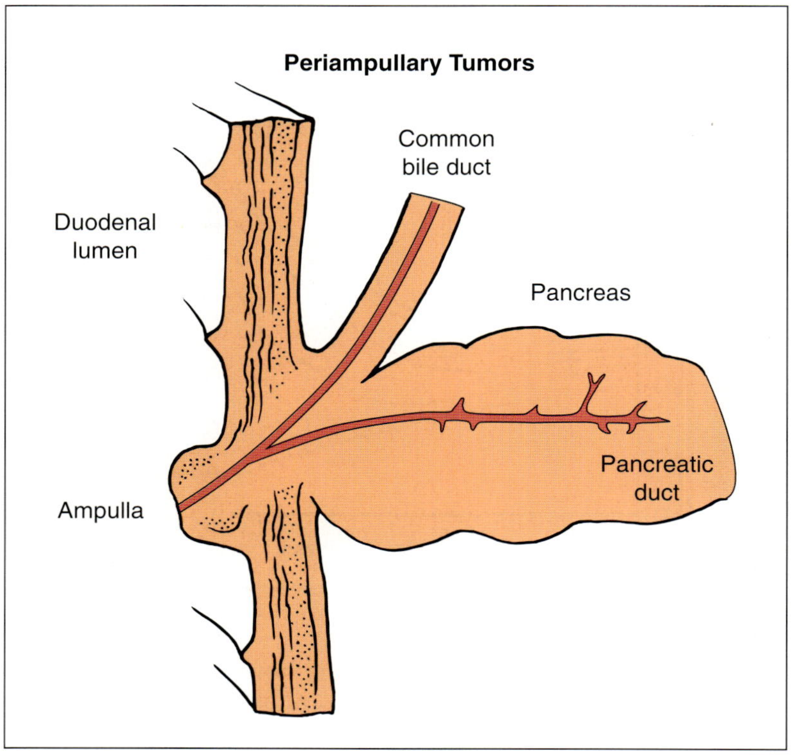

Figure 3-53.

Periampullary tumors. Ampullary and periampullary tumors most commonly arise from the pancreatic duct, but may also arise from the ampulla itself or the periampullary duodenal mucosa (commonly in familial adenomatous polyposis), the common bile duct, and even the gallbladder, liver, and other adjacent organs [44,47,52].

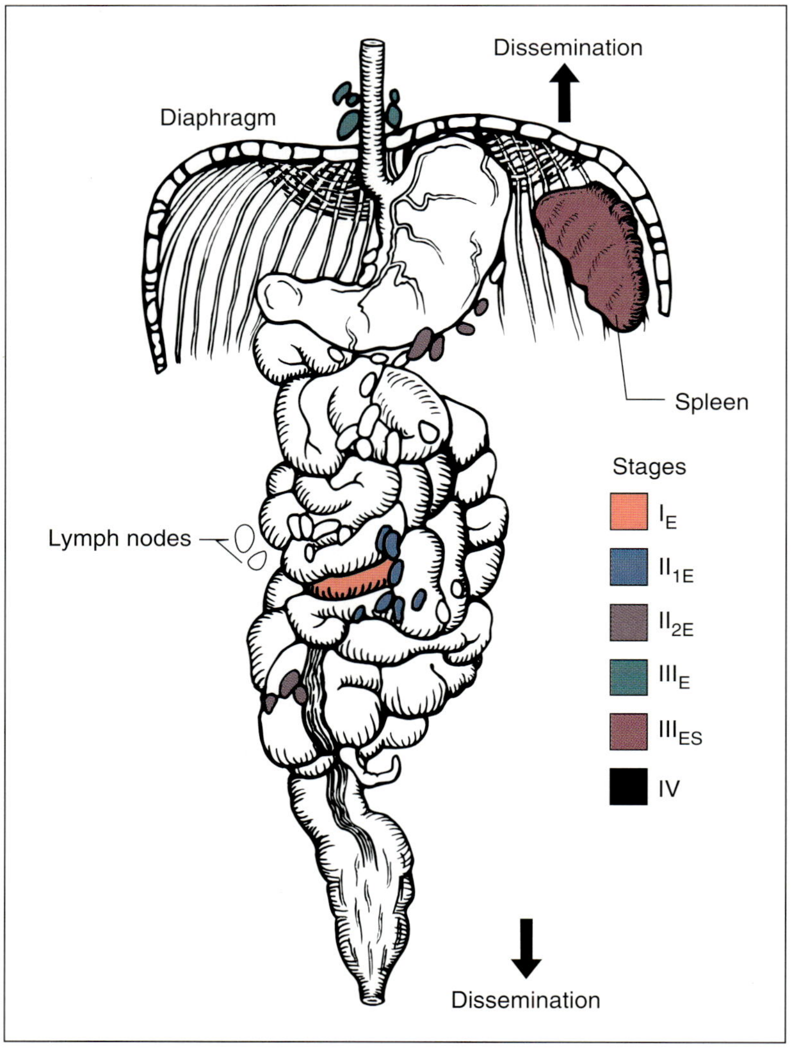

Figure 3-54.

Primary small-bowel lymphoma: clinical staging. Primary small-bowel lymphoma is staged by the extent of disease, analogous to other extranodal lymphomas. Stage I_{1E} is confined to the small bowel, stage II_{IE} involves adjacent nodes, and stage II_{2E} involves nonadjacent regional nodes. Stage III is more extensive and involves nodes on both sides of the diaphragm, with localized extralymphatic or spleen involvement. Stage IV is metastatic disease with involvement of extralymphatic sites.

PRIMARY SMALL-BOWEL LYMPHOMA: PROGNOSIS	
STAGE	5-YR SURVIVAL RATE, %
I_E	80
II_{1E}	50
II_{2E}	35
III_E	15
III_{ES}	10
IV	5

FIGURE 3-55.

Primary small-bowel lymphoma: prognosis. The survival of patients with limited-stage disease (I_E and II_{1E}) who undergo primary excision and radiotherapy or chemotherapy can be very good, with a 5-year survival of 50% to 80% when all gross tumor is resected. With bulky tumors or more advanced-stage disease, management is nonoperative and patients usually receive combination chemotherapy, with the majority of patients dying of their disease within 5 years [44,46,47,53,54]. (*Data from* Lance [44], Jones *et al.* [46], Parker *et al.* [49], Weingrad *et al.* [53], and List *et al.* [54].)

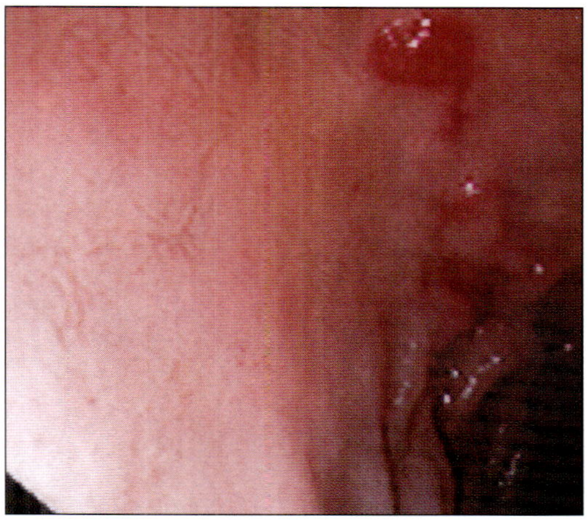

FIGURE 3-56.

Kaposi's sarcoma. Kaposi's sarcoma in patients with AIDS might be considered a systemic disease, and has been found to arise throughout the entire gastrointestinal tract. In this patient there are multiple flat and raised reddish submucosal lesions, with only a thin layer of overlying mucosa in the distal duodenum. Although patients with AIDS are often found to harbor Kaposi's sarcoma on endoscopic examination, it is unclear whether these small lesions cause symptoms. Biopsy will often yield the diagnosis [55].

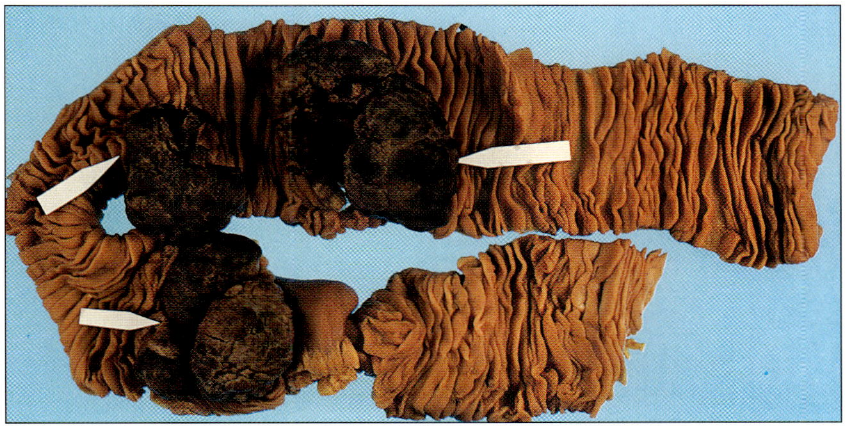

FIGURE 3-57.

Metastatic melanoma. Melanoma is the most common tumor metastatic to the small bowel and is found in about half of patients dying with metastatic melanoma. The metastases may appear as a single mass or multiple masses, as in this case. Most melanoma metastases are pigmented. Because tumors tend to be bulky, patients often develop obstruction or intussusception [56].

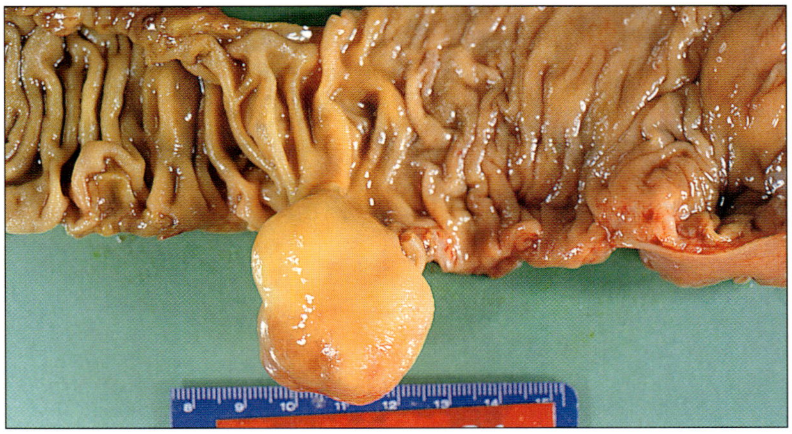

FIGURE 3-58.

Lipoma. This 3-cm polyp was found in the distal ileum of a patient with intermittent intestinal obstruction. The surgical specimen had the characteristic glistening, yellowish appearance of a lipoma. The cut surface revealed the characteristic color and texture of fat.

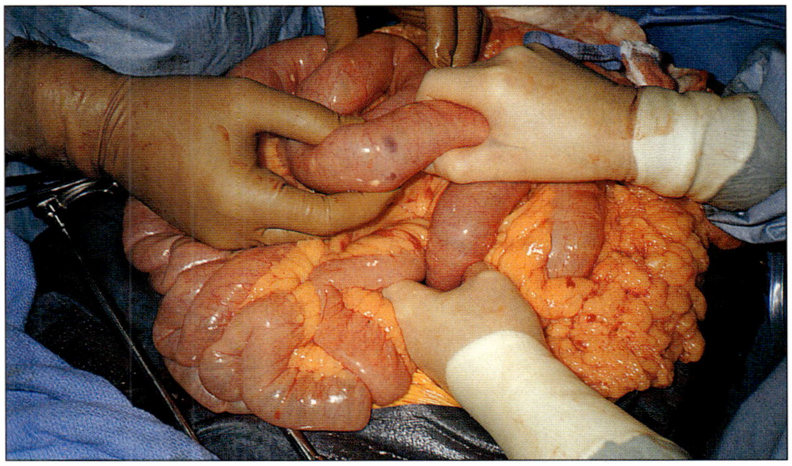

FIGURE 3-59.

Hemangioma. At surgery, this hemangioma was clearly seen through the intact bowel wall, shown here between the surgeon's gloved fingers.

SMALL INTESTINAL PSEUDOOBSTRUCTION

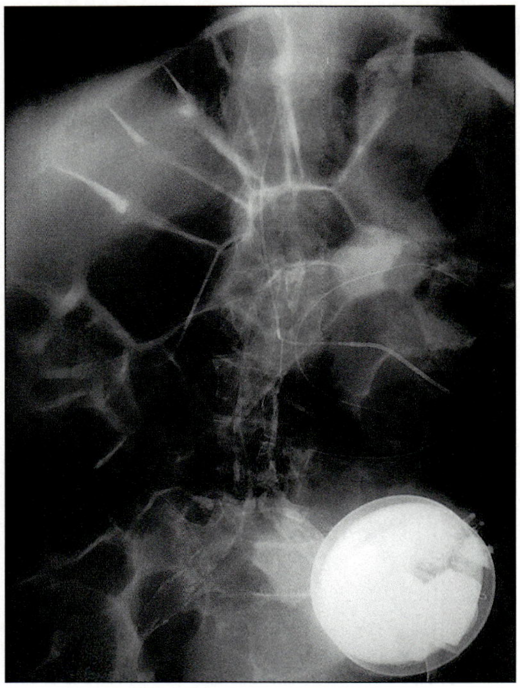

FIGURE 3-60.

Acute intestinal pseudoobstruction or ileus. Although ileus is an expected consequence of abdominal and other surgical procedures, it may also occur in other nonsurgical situations, such as in patients with pneumonia, pancreatitis, cholecystitis, myocardial infarction, and a variety of neurological conditions. Occasionally, ileus may occur without an obvious cause—idiopathic ileus. This figure illustrates marked dilatation of small and large intestine, a finding consistent with ileus, in a patient with multiple sclerosis. Note patient also had an implanted pump to deliver the muscle relaxant baclofen.

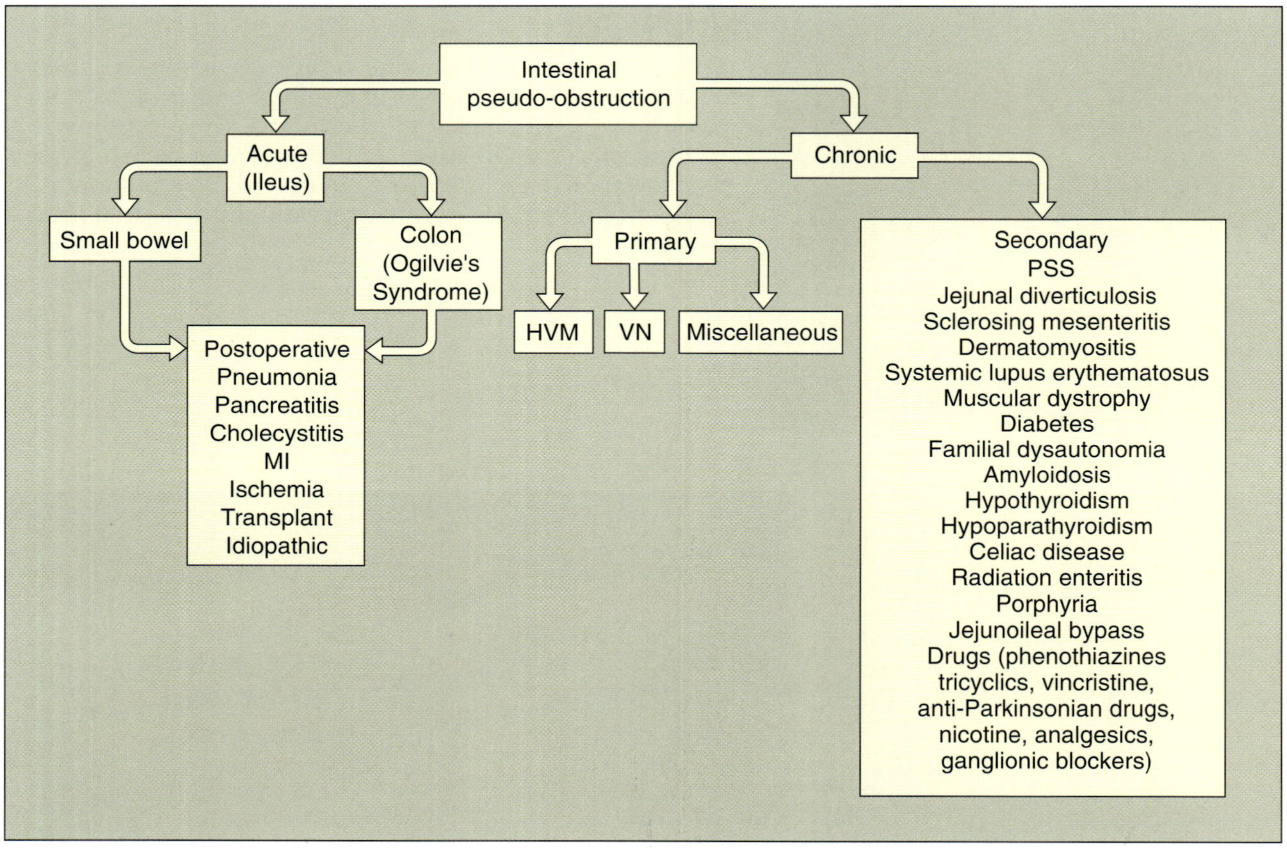

FIGURE 3-61.

Intestinal pseudo-obstruction—etiology and classification. HVM—hollow visceral neuropathy; MI—myocardial infarction; PSS—progressive systemic sclerosis (scleroderma); VN—visceral neuropathy.

DERMATOLOGIC MANIFESTATIONS OF SMALL INTESTINAL DISEASE

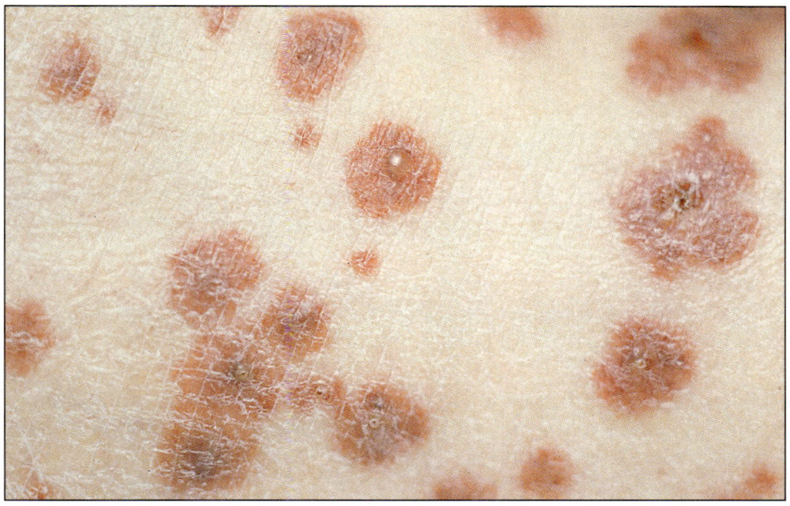

FIGURE 3-62.

Leukocytoclastic vasculitis may produce palpable purpuric lesions on the skin, caused by inflammation and extravasation of erythrocytes from blood vessels. Henoch-Schönlein purpura presents with leukocytoclastic vasculitis, most commonly in children, distributed on the buttocks and legs. Children often have accompanying abdominal pain, musculoskeletal pain, and hematuria. Bowel involvement may be present, resulting in crampy abdominal pain. Gastrointestinal tract bleeding, usually occult, occurs in 40% to 60% of patients, and intussusception and perforation may occur. A skin biopsy of a lesion will often show immunoglobulin A deposited in the vessel walls.

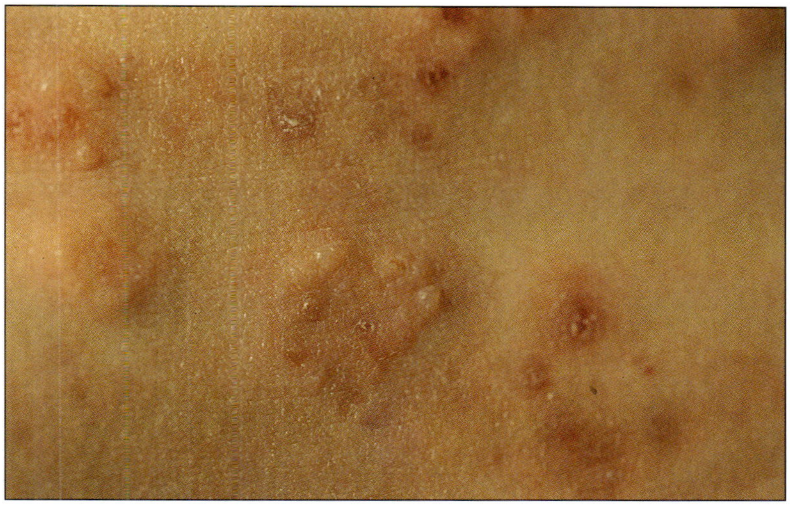

FIGURE 3-63.

Dermatitis herpetiformis presents as grouped papules and vesicles, usually with excoriations, caused by extreme pruritus of the lesions. Clinically evident celiac disease is present in 20% of these patients, whereas 80% have histologic or endoscopic evidence of celiac disease in the jejunum. Weight loss, diarrhea, steatorrhea, and other manifestations of malabsorption are present in patients with symptomatic gastrointestinal disease. Skin lesions usually appear on extensor surfaces as well as on the scalp and lower back. Granular deposition of immunoglobulin A is seen at the dermoepidermal junction. A gluten-free diet can greatly improve skin and gastrointestinal manifestations. Dapsone and sulfapyridine are also effective.

REFERENCES

1. Saxe J, Giannella RA: Bacterial and traveler's diarrhea: diagnosis and management. *Pract Gastroent* 1988, 12:20–28.
2. Giannella RA: Gastrointestinal infections. In *Textbook of Internal Medicine.* Edited by Kelley WN. Philadelphia: JB Lippincott; 1989:554–562.
3. Park SI, Giannella RA: Approach to the adult patient with diarrhea. *Gastroenterol Clin North Am* 1993, 22:483–497.
4. Guerrant RL, Bobak DA: Bacterial and protozoal gastroenteritis. *N Engl J Med* 1991, 325:327–340.
5. Vantrappen G, Gerboes K, Ponette E: *Yersinia enteritis. Med Clin North Am* 1982, 66:639–653.
6. Simth PD, Quinn TC, Strober W, *et al.*: Gastrointestinal infections in AIDS. *Ann Intern Med* 1992, 116:63–77.
7. Smith PD: Infectious diarrheas in patients with AIDS. *Gastroenterol Clin North Am* 1993, 22:549–561.
8. Adal KA, Sterling CR, Guerrant RL: *Cryptosporidium* and related species. In *Infections of the Gastrointestinal Tract*. Edited by Blaser MJ, Smith PD, Ravdin JI, *et al*. New York: Raven Press; 1995:1107–1128.
9. Banwell JG, Lake AM: *Undergraduate Teaching Project. Unit 17. Gut Immunology and Ecology*. Bethesda, MD: American Gastroenterological Association.
10. Eherer AJ, Fordtran JS: Fecal osmotic gap and pH in experimental diarrhea of various causes. *Gastroenterology* 1992, 103:545–551.
11. Afzalpurkar RG, Schiller LR, Fordtran JS: The self-limited nature of chronic idiopathic diarrhea. *N Engl J Med* 1992, 327:1849–1852.
12. Schiller LR: Drug-induced changes in bowel function. *Contemporary Gastroenterology* 1989, 2:29–35.
13. Saslow SB, Camilleri M: Diabetic diarrhea. *Semin Gastrointest Dis* 1995, 6:187–193.
14. Kvols LK: Metastatic carcinoid tumors and the malignant carcinoid syndrome. *Ann NY Acad Sci* 1994, 733:464–470.
15. Schiller LR: Cathartics, laxatives and lavage solutions. In *Gastointestinal Pharmacology and Therapeutics*. Edited by Friedman G, Jacobson ED, McCallum R. Philadelphia: Lippincott-Raven; 1997:159–174.
16. Phillips S, Donaldson L, Geisler K, *et al.*: Stool composition in factitial diarrhea: a 6-year experience with stool analysis. *Ann Intern Med* 1995, 123:97–100.
17. Lennard-Jones JE: Practical management of the short bowel [review article]. *Aliment Pharmacol Ther* 1994, 8:563–577.
18. American Gastroenterological Association: *Undergraduate Teaching Project in Gastroenterology and Liver Disease*. Timonium, Maryland: Milner-Fenwick; 1983.
19. Rogers AI, David S: Intestinal blood flow and diseases of vascular impairment. In Bockus Gastroenterology, vol 2, ed 5. Edited by Haubrich WS, Fenton S. Philadelphia: WB Saunders; 1995:1212–1234.
20. Williams LF Jr.: Mesenteric ischemia. Surg Clin North Am 1988, 68:331–353.
21. Levine JS, Jacobson ED: Intestinal ischemic disorders. Dig Dis 1995, 13:3–24.
22. Harris MT, Lewis BS: Systemic diseases affecting the mesenteric circulation. *Surg Clin North Am* 1992, 72:245–259.
23. Boley SJ, Feinstein FR, Sammartano R, *et al:* New concepts in the management of emboli of the superior mesenteric artery. *Surg Gynecol Obstet* 1981, 153:156–569.
24. Boley SJ, Sprayregan S, Siegelman SS, et al: Initial results from an aggresive roentological and surgical approach to acute mesenteric ischemic. *Surgery* 1977, 82:848–855.

25. Thompson JN, Salem RR, Hemingway AP, *et al.*: Specialist investigation of obscure gastrointestinal bleeding. *Gut* 1987, 28:47–51.

26. Foutch PG, Sawyer R, Sanowski RA: Push enteroscopy for diagnosis of patients with gastrointestinal bleeding of obscure origin. *Gastrointest Endosc* 1990, 36:337–341.

27. Ress AM, Benacci JC, Sarr MG: Efficacy of intraoperative enteroscopy in diagnosis and prevention of recurrent, occult gastrointestinal bleeding. *Am J Surg* 1992, 163:94–99.

28. Lau WY, Yuen WK, Chu KW, *et al.*: Obscure bleeding in the gastrointestinal tract originating in the small intestine. *Surg Gynecol Obstet* 1992, 174:119–124.

29. Berner JS, Mauer K, Lewis BS: Push and sonde enteroscopy for the diagnosis of obscure gastrointestinal bleeding. *Am J Gastroenterol* 1994, 89:2139–2142.

30. Retzlaff JA, Hagedorn AB, Bartholomew LG: Abdominal exploration for gastrointestinal bleeding of obscure origin. *JAMA* 1961, 177:104–107.

31. Briley CA Jr, Jackson DC, Joshrude IS, Mills SR: Acute gastointestinal hemorrhage of small bowel origin. *Radiology* 1980, 136:317–319.

32. Tillotson CL, Geller SC, Kantrowitz L, *et al.*: Small bowel hemorrhage: Angiographic localization and intervention. *Gastrointest Radiol* 1988, 13:207–211.

33. Fiorito JJ, Branch LJ, Kozicky O, *et al.*: The diagnostic yield of superior mesenteric angiography: correlation with the pattern of gastrointestinal bleeding. *Am J Gastoeñterol* 1989, 84:878–881.

34. Rex DK, Lappas JC, Maglinte DDT, *et al.*: Enteroclysis in the evaluation of suspected small intestinal bleeding. *Gastoenterology* 1989, 97:58–60.

35. Chong J, Tagle M, Barkin JS, Reiner DK: Small bowel push-type fiberoptic enteroscopy for patients with occult gastrointestinal bleeding or suspected small bowel pathology. *Am J Gastoenterol* 1994, 89:2143–2146.

36. Lewis BS, Kornbluth A, Wayne JD: Small bowel tumours: yield of enteroscopy. *Gut* 1991, 32:763–765.

37. Bronner MH, Pate MB, Cunningham JT, *et al.*: Estrogen-progesterone therapy for bleeding gastrointestinal telangiectasias in chronic renal failure. *Ann Intern Med* 1986, 105:371–374.

38. Van Cutsem E, Rutgeerts P, Vantrappen G: Treatment of bleeding gastrointestinal vascular malformations with oestrogen-progesterone. *Lancet* 1990, 335:953–955.

39. Lewis BS, Salomon P, Rivera-MacMurray S, *et al.*: Does hormonal therapy have any benefit for bleeding angiodysplasia? *J Clin Gastroenterol* 1992, 15:99–103.

40. Richtmeier W, Weaver G, Stretch W, *et al.*: Estrogen and progesterone therapy receptors in hereditary hemorrhagic telangiectasia. *Otolaryngol Head Neck Surg* 1984, 92:564–570.

41. Nagamine Y, Komatsu S, Suzuki J: New embolization method using estrogen: Effect of estrogen on microcirculation. *Surg Neurol* 1983, 20:269–275.

42. Livio M, Mannucci P, Vigano G: Conjugated estrogens for the management of bleeding associated with renal failure. *N Engl J Med* 1986, 315:731–735.

43. Hull R, Hasbargen J, Fall S, O'Barr T: Conjugated estrogens reduce endothelial prostacyclin production and fail to reduce postbypass blood loss. *Chest* 1991, 99:1116–1119.

44. Lance P: Tumors and other neoplastic diseases of the small bowel. In *Testbook of Gastroenterology*. Edited by Yamada T. Philadelphia: JB Lippincott; 1995:1696.

45. Moertel CG: Gastrointestinal carcinoid tumors and the malignant carcinoid syndrome. In *Gastrointestinal Disease*, ed 5. Edited by Sleisenger MH, Fortran JS. Philadelphia: WB Saunders; 1993:1363.

46. Jones DV, Levin B, Salem PA: Primary small intestinal lymphomas. In *Gastointestinal Disease*, ed 5. Edited by Sleisenger MH, Fordtran JH. Philadelphia: WB Saunders; 1993:1378.

47. Sinar DR: Small bowel neoplasms (other than carcinoid and lymphoma). In *Gastointestinal Disease*, ed 5. Edited by Sleisenger MH, Fordtran JH. Philadelphia: WB Saunders; 1993:1393.

48. Donohue JH: Malignant tumours of the small bowel. *Surg Oncol* 1994, 3:61.

49. Parker SL, Tong T, Bolden S, Wingo PA: Cancer statistics, 1997. *CA Cancer J Clin* 1997, 47:5.

50. Weiss NS, Yang C-P: Incidence of histologic types of the small intestine. *J Natl Cancer Inst* 1987, 78:653.

51. Zollinger RM, Sternfeld WC, Schreiber H: Primary neoplasms of the small intestine. *Am J Surg* 1986, 151:654.

52. Tarazi RY, Hermann RE, Vogt DP, *et al.*: Results of surgical treatment of periampullary tumors: a thirty-five year experience. *Surgery* 1986, 100:716.

53. Weingrad DN, DeCosse JJ, Sherlock P, *et al.*: Primary gastrointestinal lymphoma: a 30-year review. *Cancer* 1982, 49:1258.

54. List AF, Greer JP, Cousar C, *et al.*: Non-Hodgkin's lymphoma of the gastrointestinal tract: an analysis of clinical and pathologic features affecting outcome. *J Clin Oncolc* 1988, 7:1125.

55. Danzig JB, Brandt LJ, Reinus JF, Klein RS: Gastrointestinal malignancy in patients with AIDS. *Am J Gastrenterol* 1991, 86:715.

56. Patel K, Didolkar MS, Pickren JW, Moore RH: Metastatic pattern of malignant melanoma: a study of 216 autopsy cases. *Am J Surg* 1978, 135:807.

Chapter 4

Disorders of the Colon, Rectum, and Anus

EDITOR

C. Richard Boland

CONTRIBUTORS

Jeffrey L. Barnett
Carlos Belmonte-Montes
Robert S. Bresalier
Christopher S. Cutler
Lawrence S. Friedman
Fiona Graeme-Cook
Joel K. Greenson
William L. Hasler
Timothy T. Nostrant
Amit G. Pandya
J. Javier Perez-Ramirez
Douglas K. Rex
David A. Rothenberger
Robert H. Schapiro
Edward T. Stewart
Arnold Wald

ANATOMY OF THE COLON, RECTUM, AND ANUS

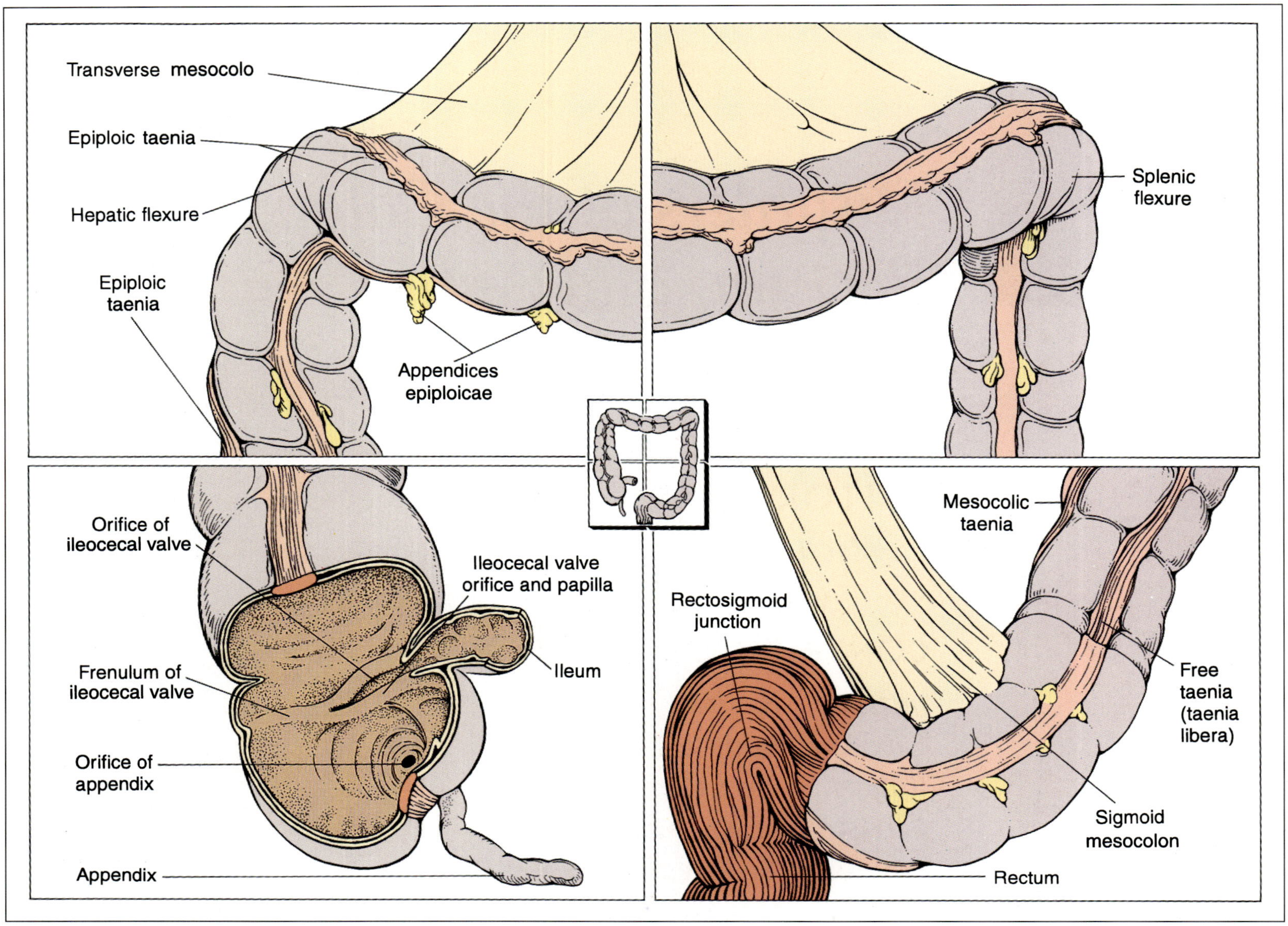

FIGURE 4-1.

The anatomy of the colon is shown. The most proximal region of the colon, the cecum, connects to the distal ileum via the ileocecal valve, a slitlike sphincter that regulates fluid flow from the small intestine into the colon and prevents coloileal reflux. The appendix, an anatomic structure with an unclear physiologic role, joins the cecum via the appendiceal orifice. The ascending, transverse, and descending colonic muscular layers include a circumferential circular layer with three overlying thin strips of longitudinal muscle, the taenia coli (epiploic, libera, and mesocolic), 120° apart. In the rectosigmoid region, the longitudinal muscle merges to envelop the entire circumference of the colon. Overlying the muscle layers of the intraperitoneal portion of the colon is a serosal layer, whereas the retroperitoneal portions of the colon are covered by an adventitial layer. Colonic haustra are defined by the circular muscle folds termed *plicae semilunares coli*. Mesenteric attachment to the intraperitoneal portion of the colon is incomplete, being restricted to the transverse and sigmoid mesocolons. The appendices epiploicae are subserosal fat collections associated with the taenia coli.

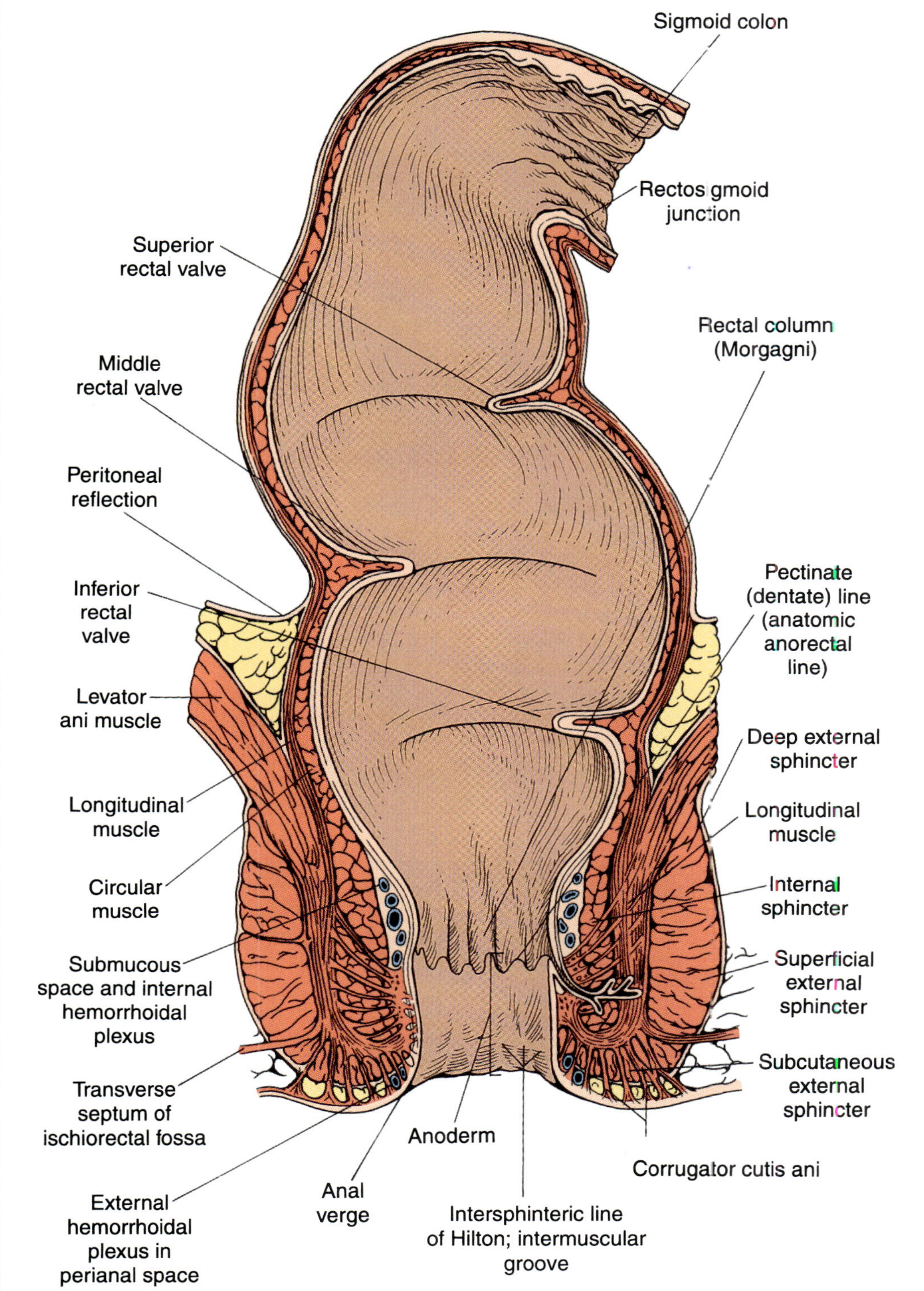

FIGURE 4-2.

The anatomy of the rectum and anus is shown. The most distal 7 to 8 cm of rectum is infraperitoneal and is thereby fixed by surrounding supporting tissues. More orad regions of the rectum and sigmoid colons are intraperitoneal and more mobile. The rectal mucosa is smoother and less corrugated than the more proximal colon, and the rectum is capacious owing to its physiologic function as a storage receptacle for feces before defecation. The rectal mucosa forms three eccentric rectal valves, also known as the *valves of Houston*. The most distal rectum is marked by the rectal columns of Morgagni, which terminate at the pectinate or dentate line delineating the junction of the rectal and anal mucosae. The transition from columnar to squamous mucosa occurs gradually in the distal rectum, usually above the pectinate line. The hemorrhoidal plexuses reside under the mucosa of both the rectum and anus and are believed to serve a cushioning role. The anal musculature is specialized with the circular muscle layer forming a prominent internal anal sphincter. The longitudinal muscle of the rectum projects to the region of the internal anal sphincter but is not as prominent. The external anal sphincter, a skeletal muscle structure, is composed of three muscle groups, the deep external sphincter, the superficial external sphincter, and the subcutaneous external sphincter. The internal sphincter is responsible for much of the resting anal tone. The external sphincter responds to voluntary squeeze commands to maintain continence when feces have moved into the rectum. Finally, the levator ani muscles, three skeletal muscles (puborectalis, pubococcygeus, and iliococcygeus), form the sling musculature surrounding the distal rectum that maintain continence when contracted. When the puborectalis component of the levator ani apparatus relaxes, defecation is permitted.

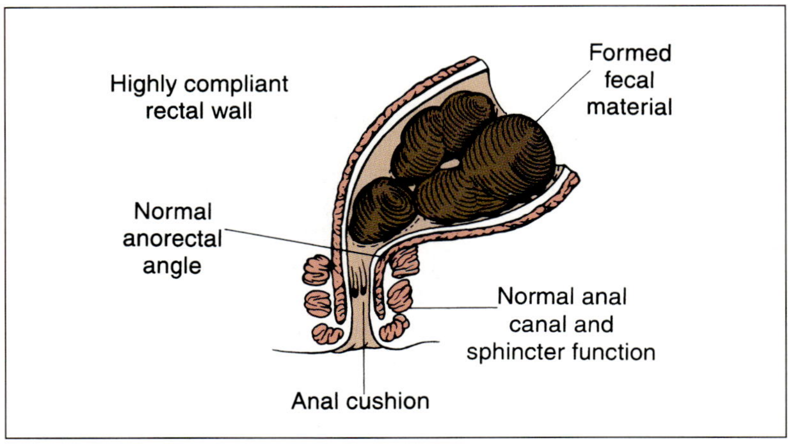

FIGURE 4-3.

The factors necessary for maintenance of fecal continence are shown. During its passage through the colon, fecal material becomes dehydrated and formed such that the stool that reaches the rectum is semisolid to solid. The rectum itself exhibits a highly compliant wall that allows it to serve as a reservoir for the fecal material until it can be conveniently expelled. The internal anal sphincter provides sufficient tone to prevent accidental loss of fecal material, whereas the external sphincter muscles voluntarily contract if unwanted loss of feces is impending. The anal cushions, made up of mucosa, hemorrhoidal plexuses, and the subepithelial-supporting tissue provide a seal that does not permit passage of liquid material under resting conditions. Finally, the anorectal angle created by the puborectalis muscle provides a functional obstruction to accidental loss of stool at rest. (*Adapted from* Irving and Catchpole [1]; with permission.)

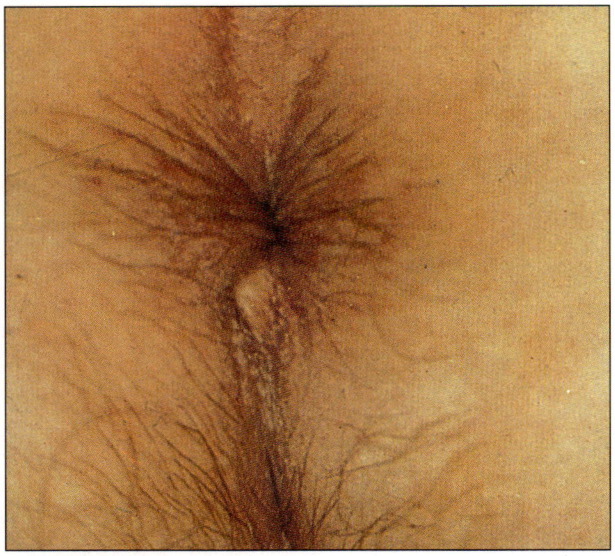

FIGURE 4-4.

A normal perineal examination. Separation of both buttocks with the hands allows full evaluation of the anal and perianal skin. Perianal skin and anal mucosa are normally more granular. No breakdown should be seen. Excoriations may point to pruritus ani, and an evaluation for pin worms would be appropriate. Anal fissures can be seen and are usually observed on the posterior and anterior anal walls. Fistulas can be seen anywhere in the perineal area but are usually concentrated within 3 to 5 cm of the anal verge. Examination of the perineum from the posterior aspect of the anus all the way to the coccyx should be done to exclude pilonidal tracts and cysts.

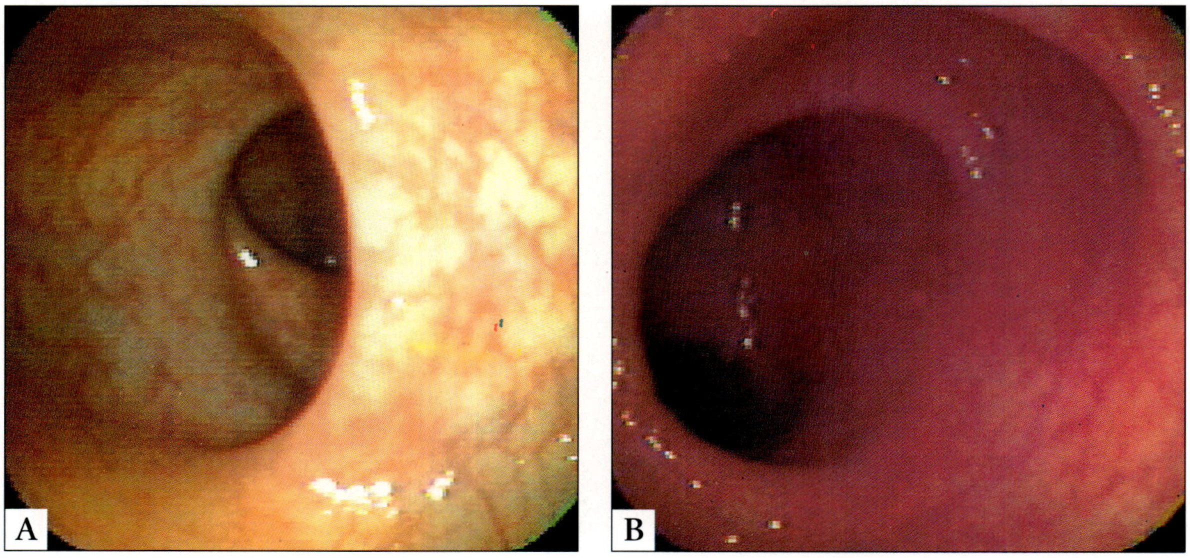

FIGURE 4-5.

Flexible sigmoidoscopy. Approaching the rectosigmoid junction. As the endoscope proceeds up the rectum, mucosal vessels become less prominent, and all three rectal valves can be seen (**A**). Just beyond these three rectal valves is the rectosigmoid junction (**B**).

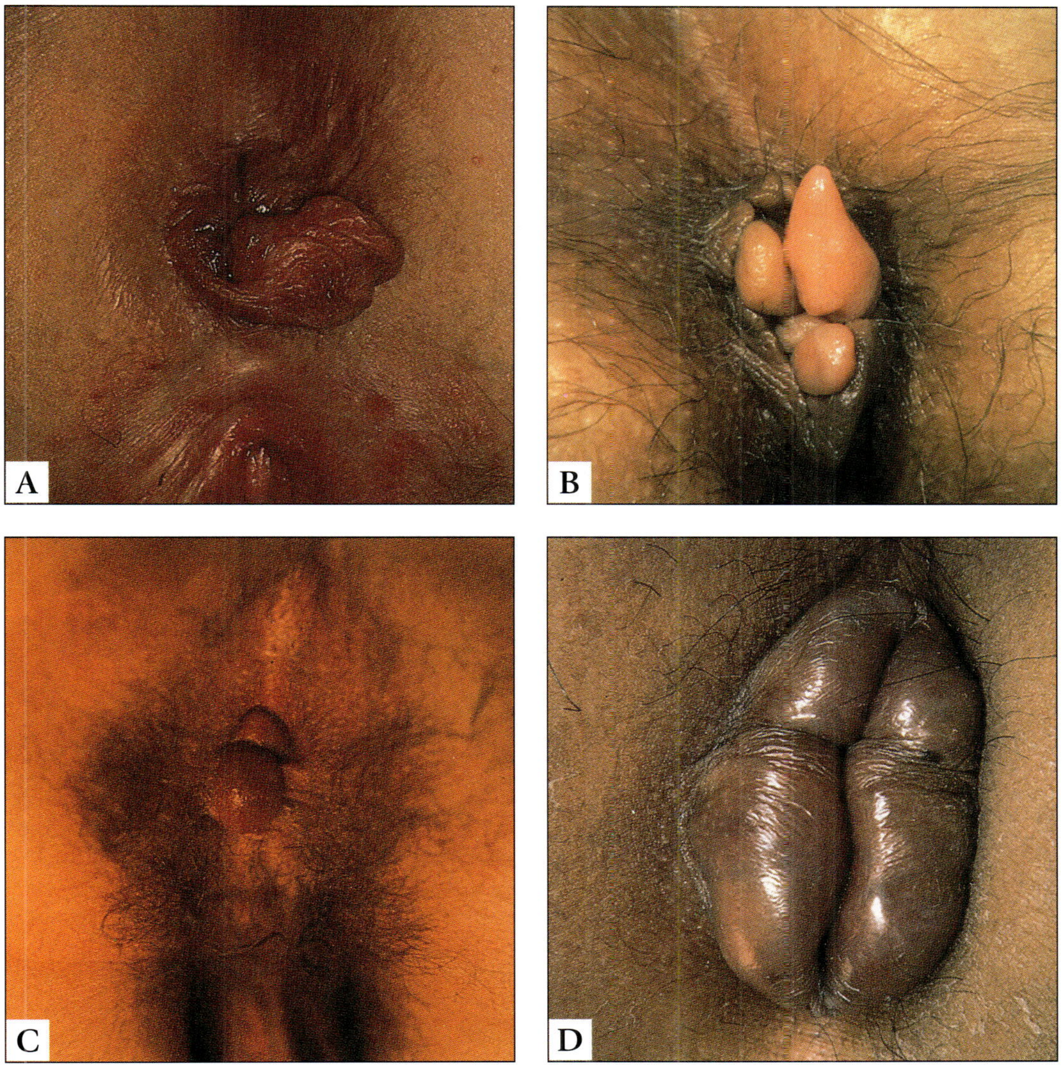

FIGURE 4-6.

External or perianal skin tags are soft, fleshy folds of fibrous connective tissue. They are often the sequelae after the clot from a thrombosed external hemorrhoid has resolved. External hemorrhoids arise from the inferior hemorrhoidal plexus and are located below the dentate line; they are covered by squamous epithelium. External hemorrhoids are usually asymptomatic unless thrombosis occurs. Internal hemorrhoids are submucosal vascular cushions arising from above the dentate line and are covered by rectal mucosa. Internal and external hemorrhoids may coexist as a mixed hemorrhoid. **A**, An external or perianal skin tag. Skin tags may interfere with adequate anal hygiene and may worsen anal irritation or pruritus. Surgical excision is rarely necessary. **B**, Prominent fibroepithelial anal canal tags. **C**, An acutely thrombosed external hemorrhoid. A thrombosed external hemorrhoid may be quite painful, and bleeding may occur if the overlying skin ulcerates and the hematoma is expressed. Most respond to conservative management, but if acute and painful, local incision and clot evacuation afford immediate relief. **D**, Acutely prolapsed large, bilateral external and internal (mixed) hemorrhoids. (*Courtesy of* R. Burney, Ann Arbor, MI)

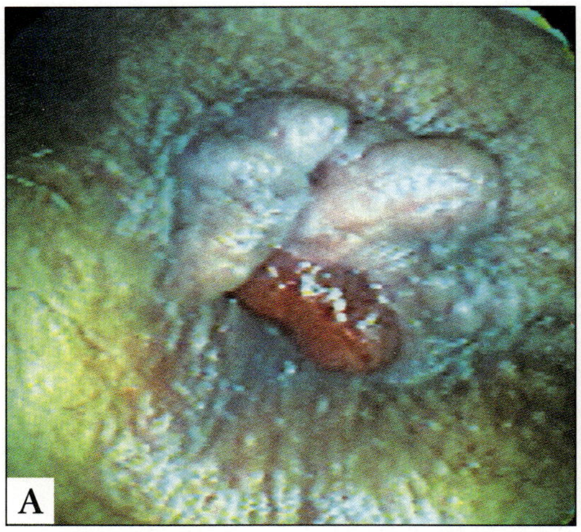

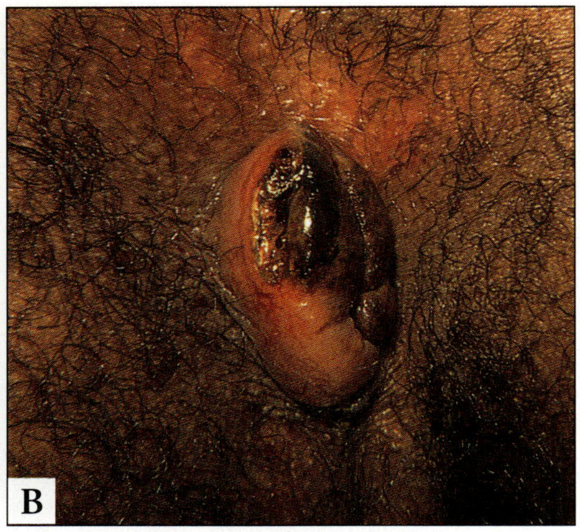

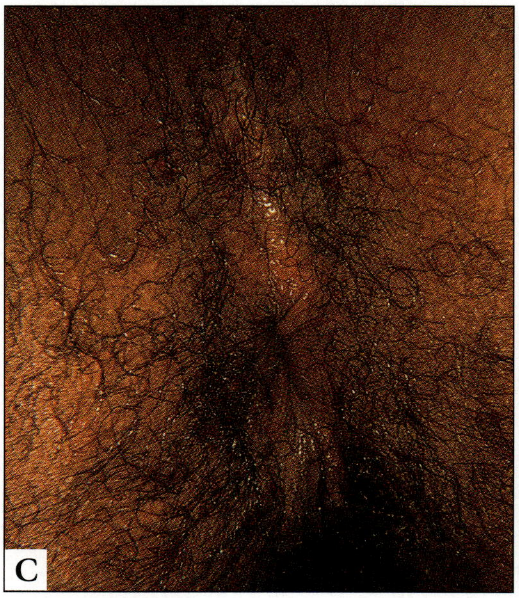

FIGURE 4-7.

Internal hemorrhoids may be associated with pruritus, fecal soiling, discomfort, or no symptoms at all. However, bleeding and prolapse are the most typical complaints and bring the patient to the physician. Internal hemorrhoids may be graded by bleeding and degree of prolapse. With first-degree hemorrhoids, the patient experiences painless, defecatory bleeding without significant prolapse of tissue. The hemorrhoids may be barely visible in the anal canal with straining, and they are best seen through the anoscope. Bleeding and prolapse occur at the time of defecation with second-degree hemorrhoids, but the hemorrhoid reduces spontaneously back into the rectum after straining. Bleeding and prominent prolapse after defecation or straining that require digital reduction characterize third-degree hemorrhoids. Large, usually acute, hemorrhoids that cannot be persistently reduced and are at risk for strangulation are considered fourth-degree hemorrhoids.

A, Prolapsed internal hemorrhoid. This friable internal hemorrhoid was the cause of hematochezia during defecation. External hemorrhoidal skin tags are also shown. Ulcerated, prolapsing internal hemorrhoids before (**B**) and after (**C**) reduction are depicted. (**B** and **C**, *Courtesy of* R. Burney, Ann Arbor, MI)

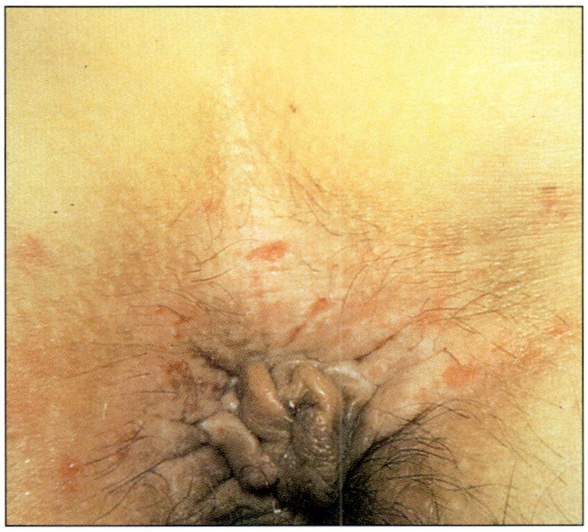

Figure 4-8.

Intense perianal itching and burning discomfort is called *pruritus ani*. Causes include local irritants or sensitivities, benign and malignant dermatoses, infections, and anorectal diseases that lead to fecal contamination or leakage. This excoriated perianal skin was a result of idiopathic pruritus ani. (*Courtesy of* R. Burney, Ann Arbor, MI)

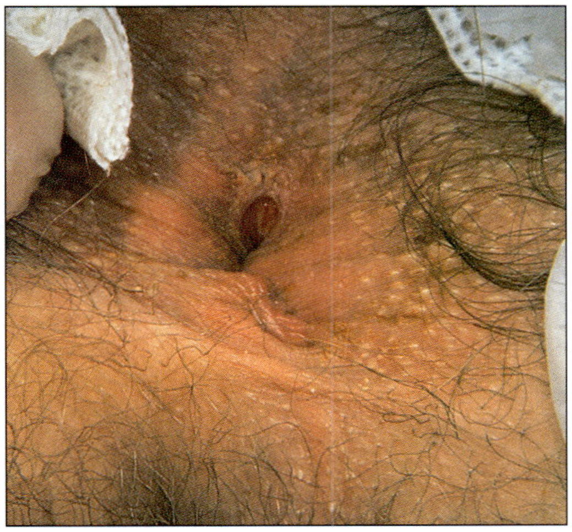

Figure 4-9.

Typical fissure in ano located in the posterior midline. An anal fissure is a painful, linear defect in the anal canal oriented perpendicularly to the dentate line. It is usually caused by a tearing that occurred during passage of a stool. The vast majority are located in the posterior midline; the remainder are anteriorly placed. A fissure located laterally should arouse suspicion of an underlying condition such as inflammatory bowel disease. An anal fissure is best identified by gentle but forceful lateral traction of the buttocks (after topical application of an anesthetic if necessary). Most acute anal fissures will heal with conservative medical management and time. Persistent acute fissures and most chronic fissures require definitive surgery, usually a lateral internal sphincterotomy to reduce resting sphincter tone.

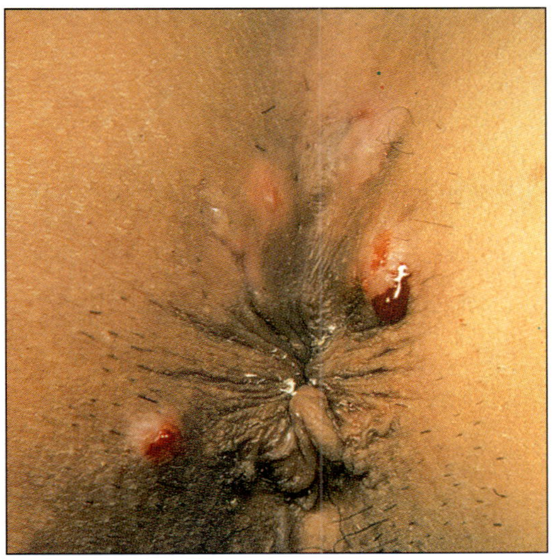

Figure 4-10.

Abscess is the acute manifestation and fistula is the chronic manifestation of suppurative anorectal infection. Fistulous disease and abscess are caused by infection of the anal glands, secondary to ductal obstruction caused by fecal material or anal trauma. The primary fistulous orifice is found at the level of the dentate line and the secondary opening at the anal verge or elsewhere in the perineum. Abscess typically presents as pain and swelling; fistula in ano usually causes discharge with occasional discomfort. Multiple perianal fistula sites from fistula in ano. (*Courtesy of* R. Burney, Ann Arbor, MI)

A. TESTS FOR FECAL OCCULT BLOOD

Test		Reaction		Advantages	Disadvantages
Guaiac-based testing		Hydrogen peroxide (catalyst)		Inexpensive	Low sensitivity
	Phenol (guaiac) Coloress	→	Quinone (blue)	Simple	Low positive predictive value
		Peroxidase activity			
HemoQuant®		Step 1	Step 2		
		Stool heated → in reducing acid to remove heme iron	Purification by extraction to yield free prophyrin solution	Quantitative	Detects upper gastrointestinal bleeding Does not outperform guaiac testing in screening trials
Immunochemical testing HemeSelect®		Direct reaction of antibody with hemoglobin		Highly sensitive for blood Detects only intact hemoglobin	16–24 h Incubation period Not tested in screening trials

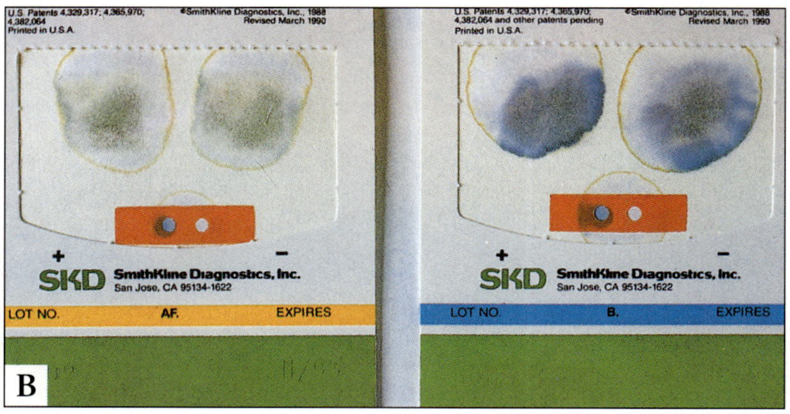

FIGURE 4-11

Fecal occult blood testing has only one purpose in clinical practice, *ie*, the detection of colorectal neoplasia. In clinical practice, fecal occult blood testing is sometimes used in evaluation of patients with upper gastrointestinal tract symptoms such as dyspepsia or to monitor patients ingesting nonsteroidal anti-inflammatory drugs. However, no study has defined the sensitivity, specificity, or clinical implications of fecal occult blood testing in these patients. In fact, fecal occult blood tests performed in these patients are actually still screening tests for colorectal cancer. Any positive fecal occult blood test should lead a patient to colonic imaging for colorectal cancer.

Clinical testing for occult blood can be performed using guaiac-based tests, quantitative tests for porphyrin derivatives such as HemoQuant (University of Minnesota) or immunochemical tests (*panel A*). Only guaiac-based tests are used widely. Several tests employ guaiac-impregnated filter paper on a card. Of these, the best studied is the Hemoccult II Card (SmithKline Diagnostics, San Jose, CA). Hemoccult SENSA (SmithKline Diagnostics) is a newer guaiac-based test which is more sensitive and readable [2] than Hemoccult II (*panel B*). Some guaiac-based tests have been developed that employ guaiac-impregnated paper that is dropped into the toilet bowel. These tests offer the theoretical advantage of improved patient compliance. However, improved compliance has not been proven in large clinical trials. Furthermore, the sensitivity and specificity of such tests has not been thoroughly studied, and it cannot be recommended for clinical practice. Guaiac is a natural occurring phenolic compound. In the presence of an oxidizing agent, guaiac is converted to a quinone, which is a blue color. The product should be unequivocally blue in order to be considered positive. In the guaiac reaction, hemoglobin supplies pseudoperoxidase activity, which permits oxidation. Addition of a developing solution containing hydrogen peroxide is usually necessary. Hydrogen peroxide serves as a catalyst for the oxidative reaction.

The HemoQuant test provides a quantitative measure of stool occult blood. The test measures not only intact heme but also biochemical breakdown derivatives of heme. Therefore, this test is more likely to detect occult bleeding from the upper gastrointestinal tract than other testing methods. In clinical practice, HemoQuant does not perform better than guaiac-based testing as a screening measure for colorectal cancer [3]. Unfortunately, there is a substantial overlap between the amount of bleeding that occurs in normal individuals and the amount that occurs in patients with colorectal cancer. This overlap is an insurmountable obstacle to the effectiveness of occult blood testing for colorectal cancer.

Immunochemical testing, which detects only intact hemoglobin, is probably the most sensitive and specific fecal occult blood test for colorectal cancer [2]. However, it is more expensive than guaiac testing, and major advantages in effectiveness and cost-effectiveness over guaiac testing have not been proven in clinical screening trials. (**B**, *Courtesy of* SmithKline Diagnostics, San Jose, CA)

ADVANTAGES AND LIMITATIONS OF THE GUAIAC-IMPREGNATED SLIDE TEST FOR FECAL OCCULT BLOOD TESTING

- Advantages
  - Readily available
  - Convenient
  - Inexpensive
  - Good patient compliance in motivated groups
- Disadvantages
  - Depends on degree of fecal hydration
  - Affected by storage (hemoglobin degradation)
  - Affected by tumor location
- False-positive tests
  - Exogenous peroxidase activity
    - Red meat (nonhuman hemoglobin)
    - Uncooked fruits and vegetables (vegetable peroxidase)
  - Any source of gastrointestinal blood loss (epistaxis, gingival bleeding, upper gastrointestinal tract pathology, hemorrhoids, etc.)
  - Medications
    - Topical iodine
    - Aspirin, nonsteroidal anti-inflammatory agents (induce upper gastrointestinal bleeding)
- False-negative tests
  - Storage of slides
  - Ascorbic acid (vitamin C)
  - Improper sampling/developing
  - Lesion not bleeding at time of stool collection
  - Degradation of hemoglobin by colonic bacteria

FIGURE 4-12.

Advantages and limitations of the guaiac-based slide tests used for fecal occult blood testing. Although readily available and widely employed clinically, care must be taken to avoid sources of false-positive and false-negative tests. (*From* Bresalier and Kim [4]; with permission.)

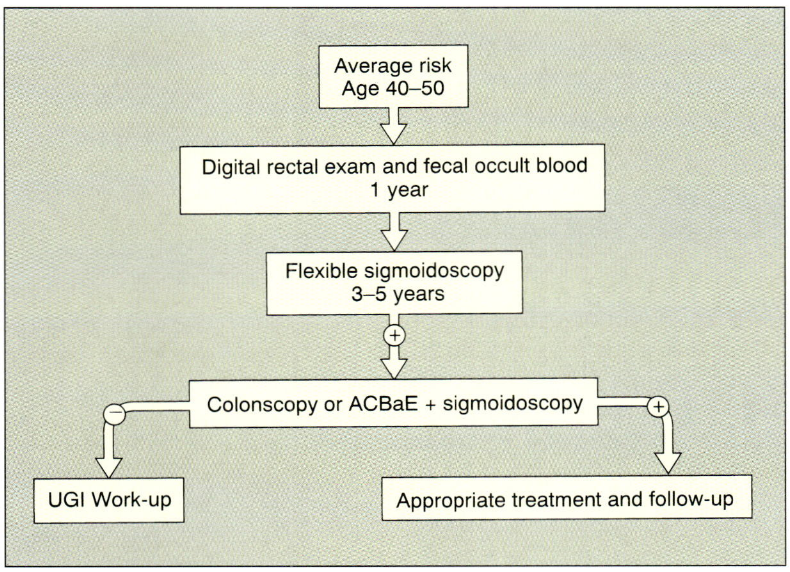

FIGURE 4-13.

Algorithm for colon cancer surveillance of average-risk individuals in the general population. Current data indicate that screening with fecal occult blood testing and sigmoidoscopy can significantly reduce mortality from colorectal cancer. ACBaE—air-contrasted barium enema; UGI—upper gastrointestinal. (*From* Bresalier and Kim [4]; with permission.)

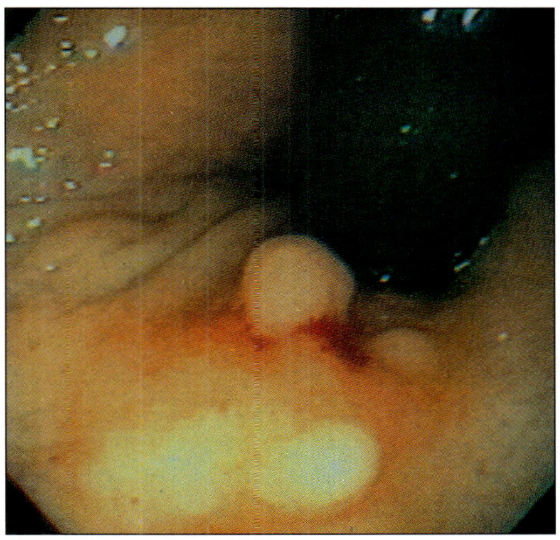

FIGURE 4-14.

Flexible sigmoidoscopic view of the distal rectum upon retroflexion of the sigmoidoscope, which demonstrates several small polyps. Flexible sigmoidoscopy has been shown to detect two- to threefold more neoplasms than rigid sigmoidoscopy. Periodic flexible sigmoidoscopy and polypectomy may reduce cancer incidence and mortality caused by cancer within the reach of the endoscope by approximately 70%.

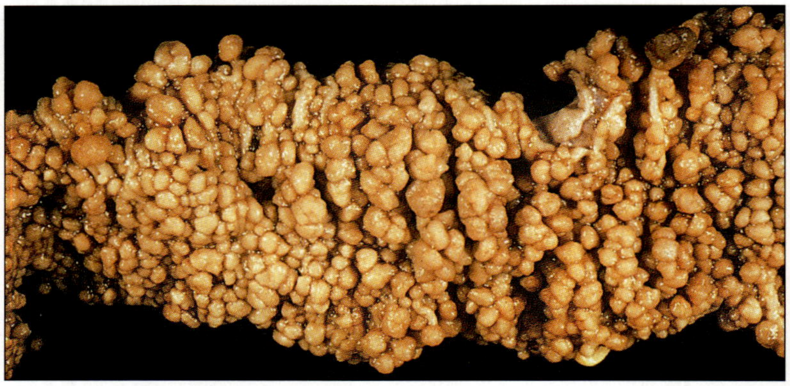

FIGURE 4-15.

Familial adenomatous polyposis. A portion of a colectomy specimen that shows complete carpeting of the mucosal surface by adenomatous polyps. In general, colons containing more than 100 adenomatous polyps are thought to have this autosomal dominant condition. The genetic defect appears to be caused by mutations or deletions in the *APC* gene located on the long arm of chromosome 5.

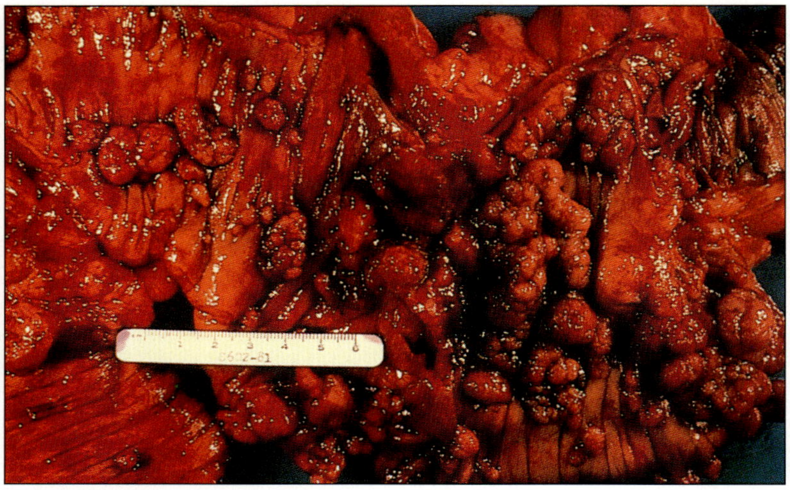

FIGURE 4-16.

Colectomy specimen from a patient with familial adenomatous polyposis coli. In this syndrome, hundreds to thousands of adenomatous polyps arise in the colon. This disease is inherited as an autosomal dominant gene located on chromosome 5q (*APC*). If the colon is not removed in these individuals, the development of colon cancer is inevitable.

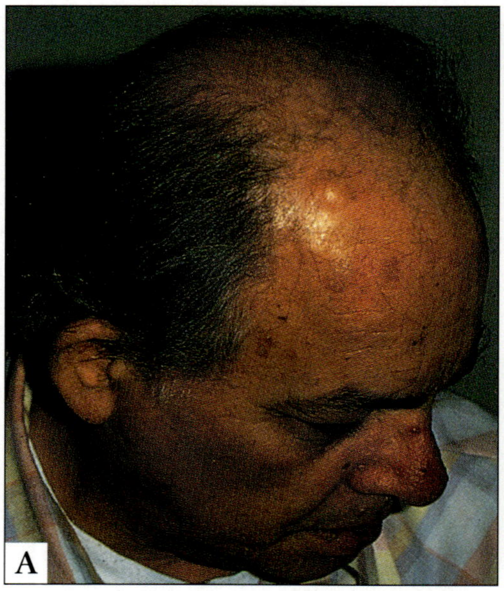

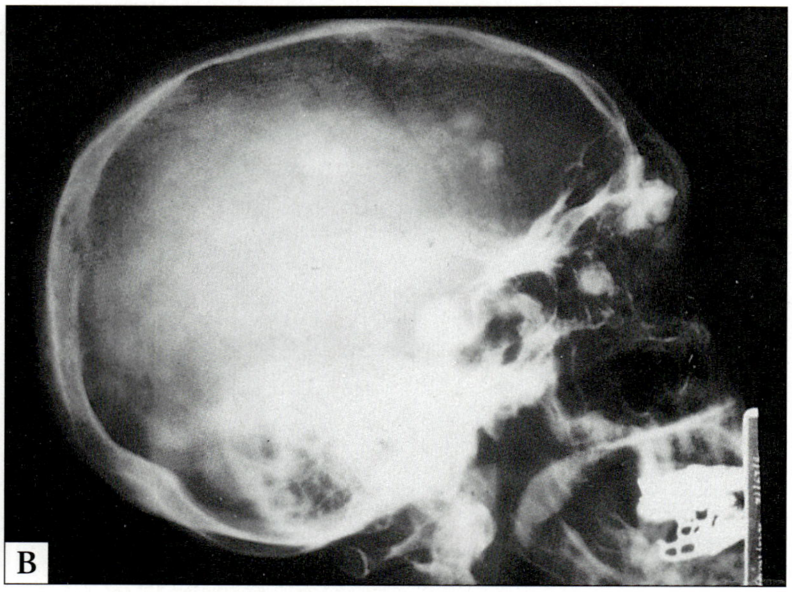

FIGURE 4-17.

Gardner's syndrome is a subset of familial adenomatous polyposis. Familial adenomatous polyposis and Gardner's syndrome are variable manifestations of a disease that may be traced to a single gene locus. The primary features of this syndrome are colonic polyposis, osteomas (particularly in the skull and mandible), and soft-tissue tumors. Periampullary tumors of the duodenum including carcinomas are also common. Soft-tissue tumors include epidermoid cysts, fibromas, lipomas, and desmoid tumors. **A**, Osteoma of the skull in a patient with gross Gardner's syndrome. **B**, Skull radiograph showing multiple osteomas.

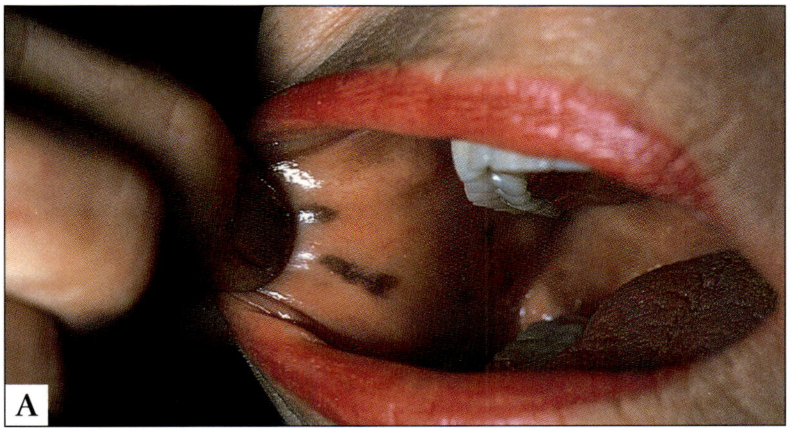

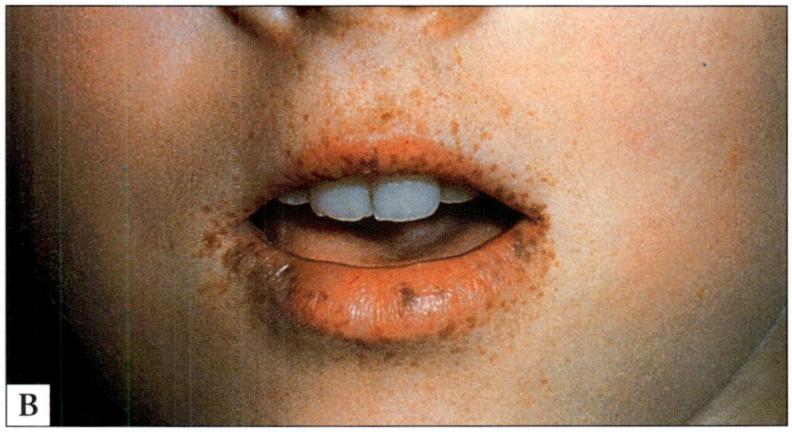

FIGURE 4-18.

A and **B**, Mucocutaneous pigmentation is depicted in a patient with Peutz-Jeghers syndrome. Hamartomas of gastrointestinal tract and mucocutaneous pigmentation define this familial syndrome (autosomal dominant with variable penetrance). Carcinomas of the colon and small intestine may arise in associated adenomatous epithelium.

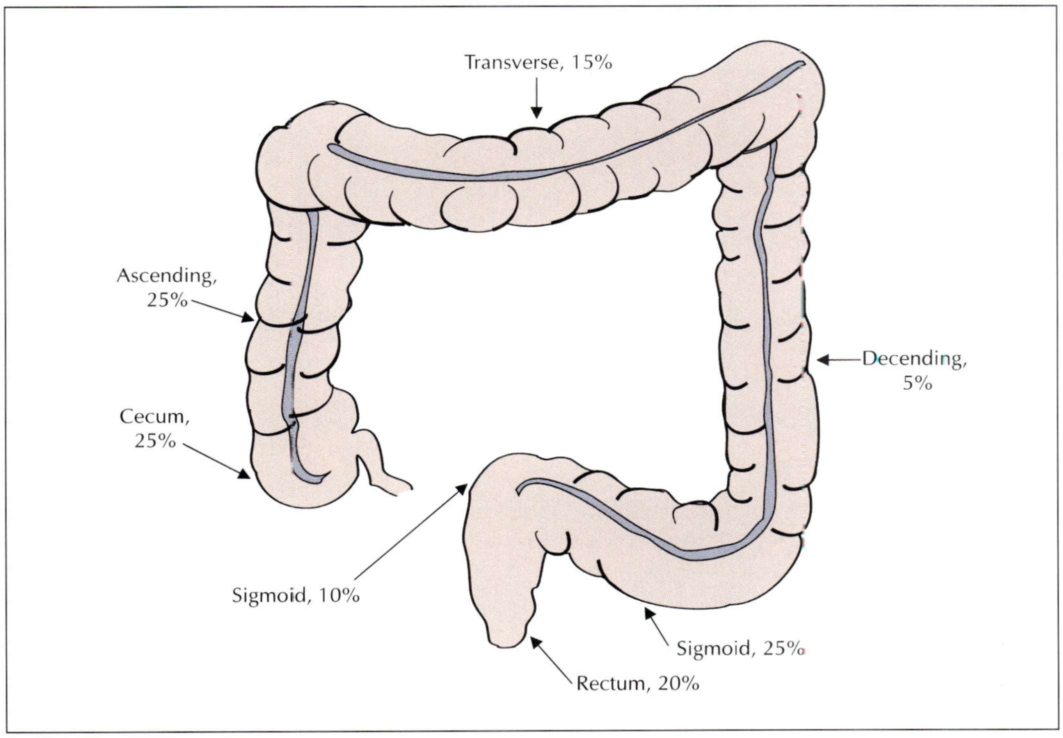

FIGURE 4-19.

Distribution of colorectal cancer in the colon. Although approximately two-thirds of cancers still arise distal to the splenic flexure, an increasing number of cancers are being found in the right colon.

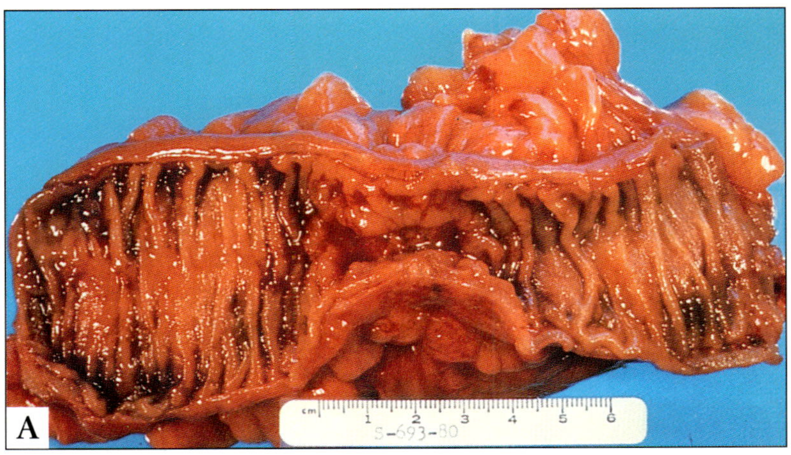

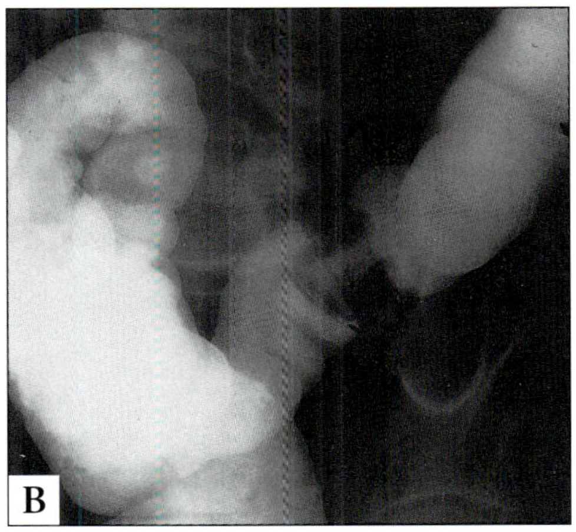

FIGURE 4-20.

A, A gross surgical specimen of annular constricting or napkin-ring carcinoma of the colon. **B**, Full-column barium enema demonstrating the annular constricting lesions.

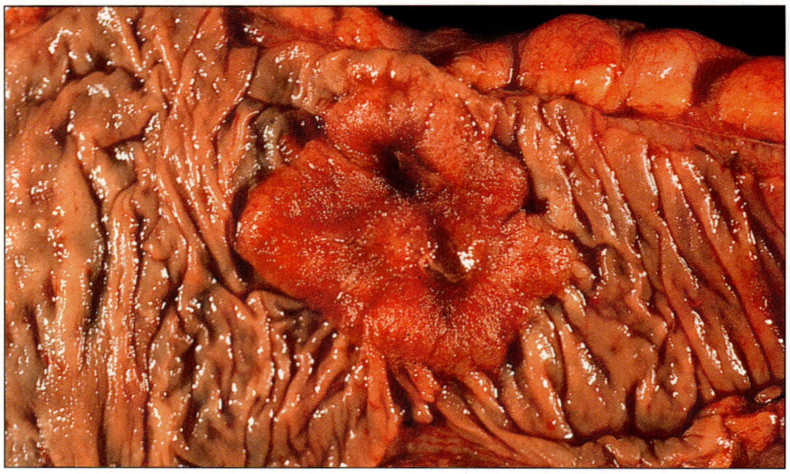

Figure 4-21.

Adenocarcinoma of the colon. This colonic resection specimen shows an erythematous-raised tumor with a central umbilication typical of colon cancer.

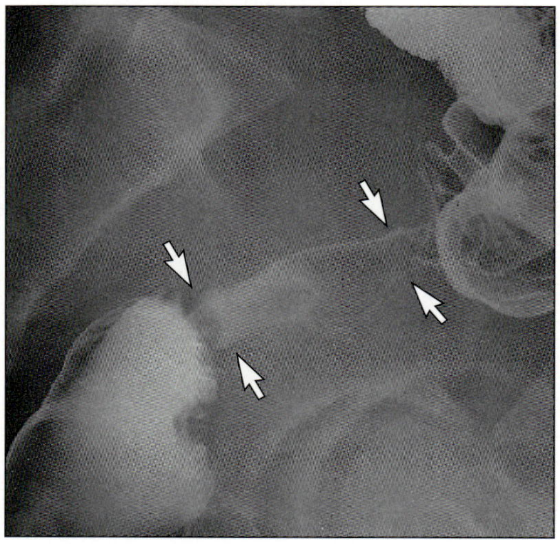

Figure 4-22.

This figure is a lateral view of an air-contrast examination of the colon. There is a long annular infiltrating neoplastic lesion involving the rectosigmoid junction (*arrows*). Although there is very little question as to the nature of this lesion being malignant, neither positive-contrast examination of the colon or endoscopy is sufficient to adequately stage these patients.

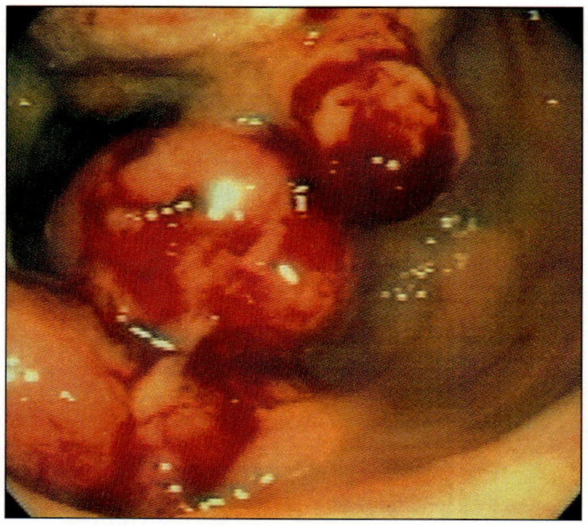

Figure 4-23.

Colonoscopic view of bleeding colon cancer. Colorectal cancers may present with gross bleeding (hematochezia) or result in the presence of occult blood in the stool.

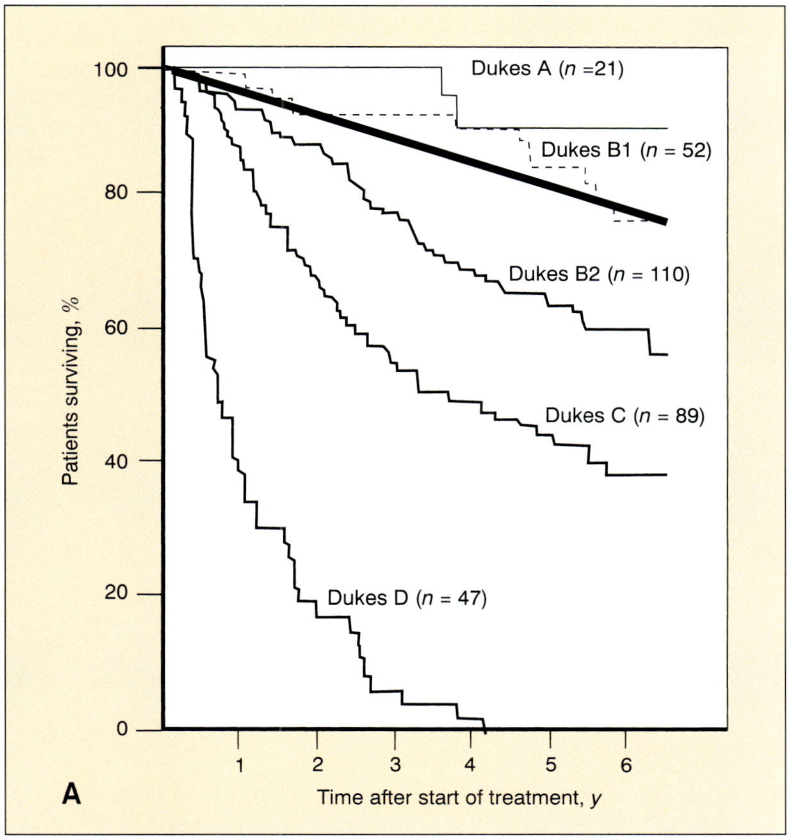

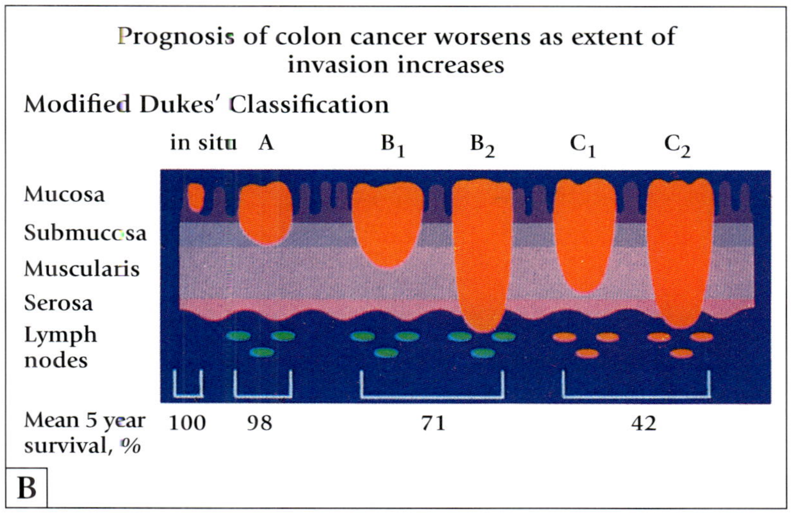

FIGURE 4-24.

A, Survival probabilities according to stage of disease in patients undergoing potentially curative surgery for colorectal cancer. Expected survival among age- and sex-matched general population is indicated by heavy line. **B**, Prognosis worsens as the extent of invasion increases. (**A**, *From* Moertel *et al.* [5]; with permission.) (**B**, *From* Podolsky [6]; with permission.)

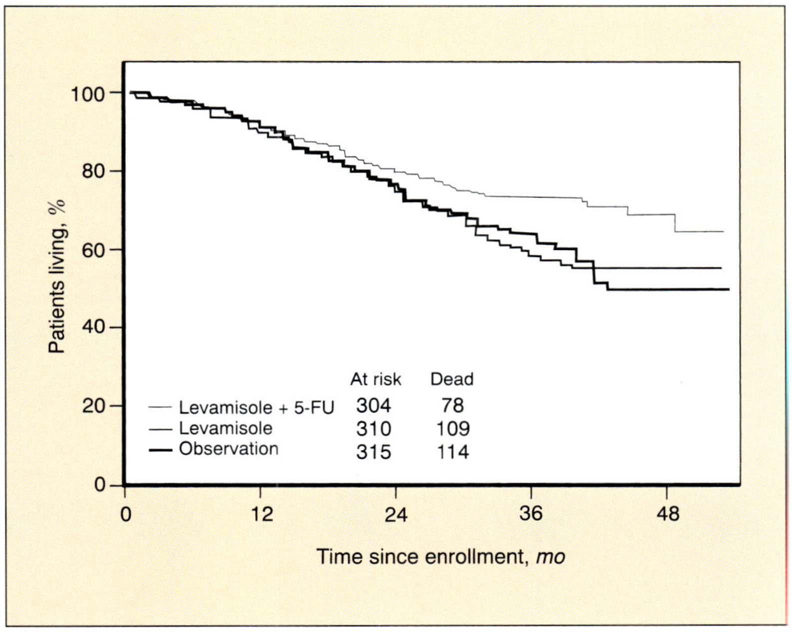

FIGURE 4-25.

Adjuvant chemotherapy of colon cancer in patients with Dukes' C (stage III) disease. Therapy with combined 5-fluorouracil (5-FU; a chemotherapeutic agent) and levamisole (a reported immune system stimulant) results in significantly improved patient survival compared with observation or levamisole alone. (*From* Moertel *et al.* [7]; with permission.)

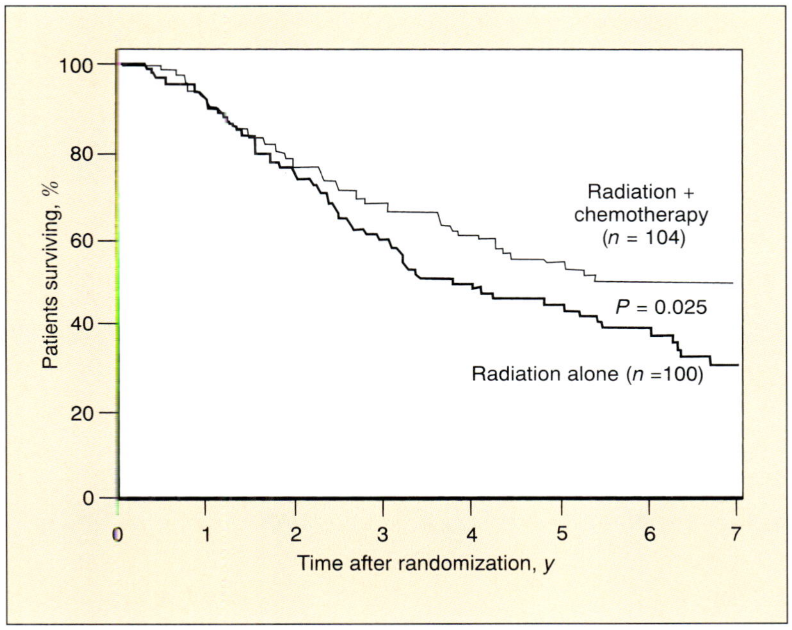

FIGURE 4-26.

Combined modality adjuvant therapy with postoperative radiation (for local disease) and chemotherapy (for microscopic metastatic disease) significantly improves survival in patients with stages II and III rectal cancer. Radiation alone reduces local recurrence but does not prolong survival. (*From* Krook *et al.* [8]; with permission.)

Ulcerative colitis

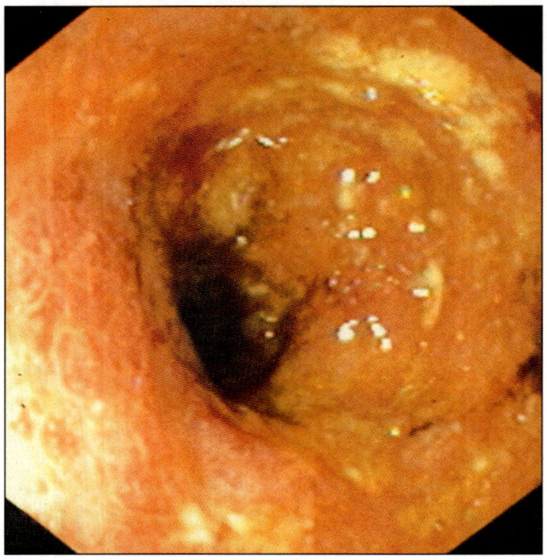

FIGURE 4-27.
Endoscopic features of active ulcerative colitis. Findings include diffusely erythematous, edematous, and granular mucosa with areas of submucosal hemorrhage and, when severe, frank mucopurulent exudate. Inflammation invariably begins in the rectum and extends proximally for varying extents. The chronicity of the process is suggested by the loss of colonic haustrations; otherwise, the endoscopic picture is nonspecific and could be consistent with acute infectious colitis, chronic ulcerative or Crohn's colitis, or any number of other specific causes of colitis. This example shows moderately severe ulcerative colitis with irregular, inflamed, ulcerated mucosa and a patchy exudate.

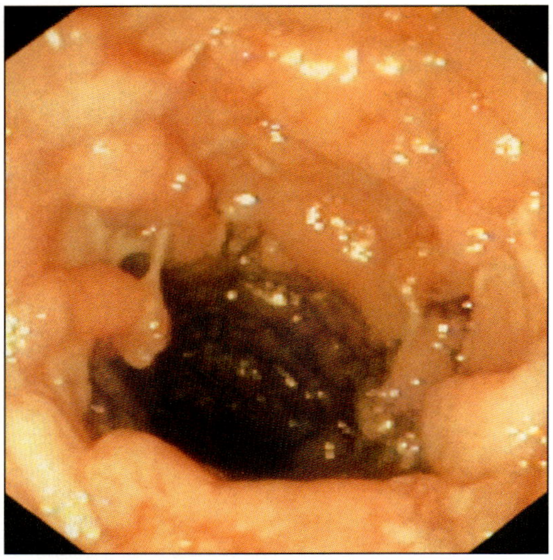

FIGURE 4-28.
Severe ulcerative colitis. The mucosa shows extensive ulceration and diffuse thickening with an inflammatory infiltrate. In contrast to Crohn's colitis, the ulceration lacks depth.

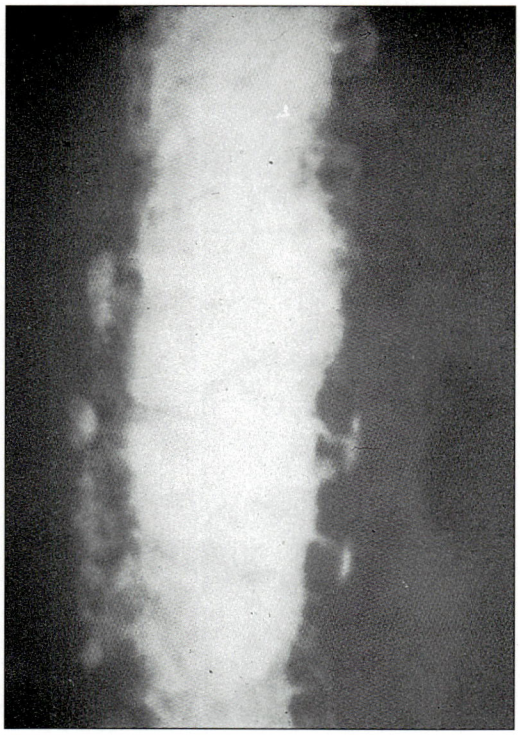

FIGURE 4-29.
Radiographic appearance of severe ulcerative colitis. This single-contrast barium enema demonstrates the typical ragged and ulcerative appearance of the mucosa in active ulcerative colitis. Characteristic collar-button or undermining ulcers are seen. In general, barium enema and colonoscopy should be avoided in fulminant ulcerative colitis because of the possibility of precipitating toxic megacolon.

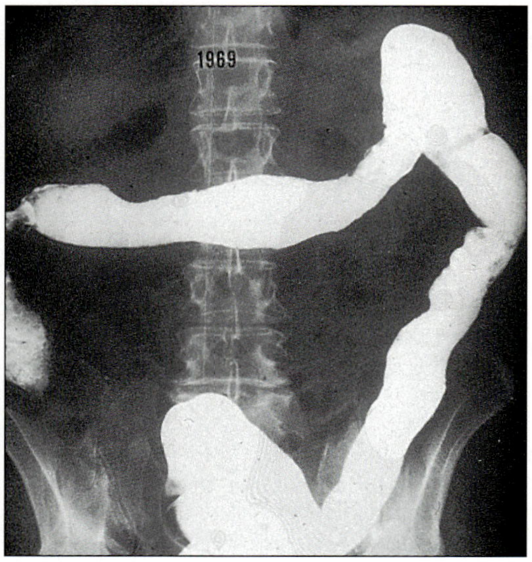

FIGURE 4-30.
Radiographic appearance of chronic ulcerative colitis. Long-standing chronic ulcerative colitis, as shown in this single-contrast barium enema, is characterized by shortening and straightening of the colon with loss of haustrations, resulting in the appearance of a featureless tube. No ulcerations are seen.

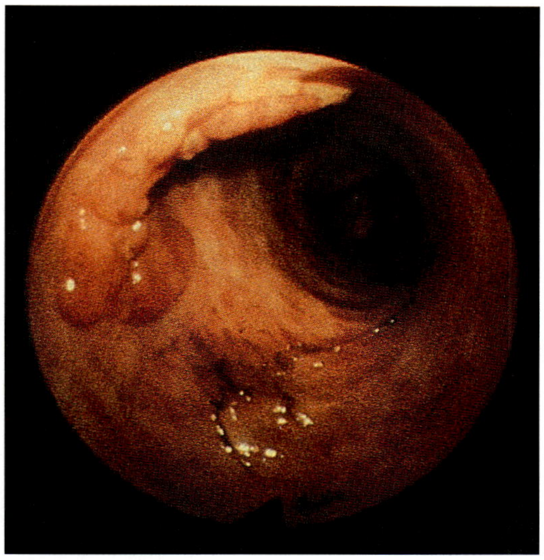

FIGURE 4-31.

Dysplasia-associated mass lesions seen at colonoscopy in a patient with ulcerative colitis. Such lesions may be plaquelike or polypoid and contain dysplastic epithelium. These lesions are highly associated with synchronous carcinoma of the colon.

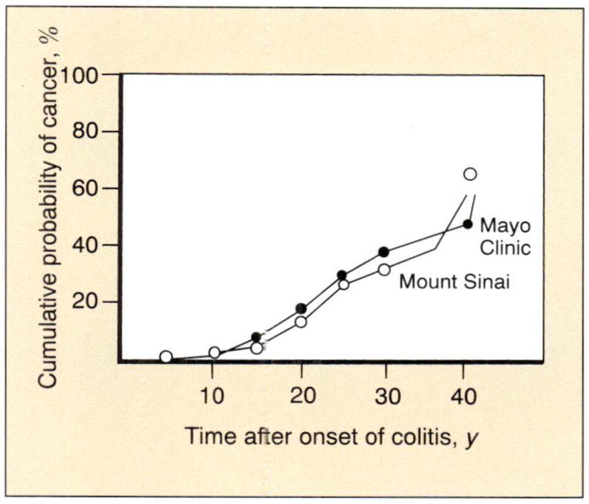

FIGURE 4-32.

Cumulative probability of developing colorectal carcinoma in patients with ulcerative colitis. Data from tertiary referral centers such as the Mayo Clinic and Mount Sinai Medical Center indicate a 1% per year cumulative incidence after 10 years duration of disease. Data from primary care settings suggest an approximately 0.5% per year cumulative incidence. (*From* Bresalier and Kim [4]; with permission.)

Crohn's disease

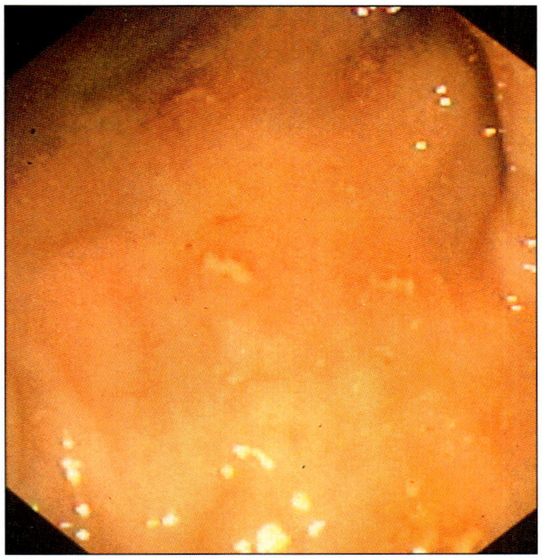

FIGURE 4-33.

Endoscopic features of early Crohn's disease. The earliest lesion of Crohn's disease, shown on colonoscopy, is aphthous ulceration, a focal mucosal defect with surrounding erythema. This finding is nonspecific and may also be seen in herpesvirus infection, cytomegalovirus infection, Yersinia infection, tuberculosis, schistosomiasis, and Behcet's disease.

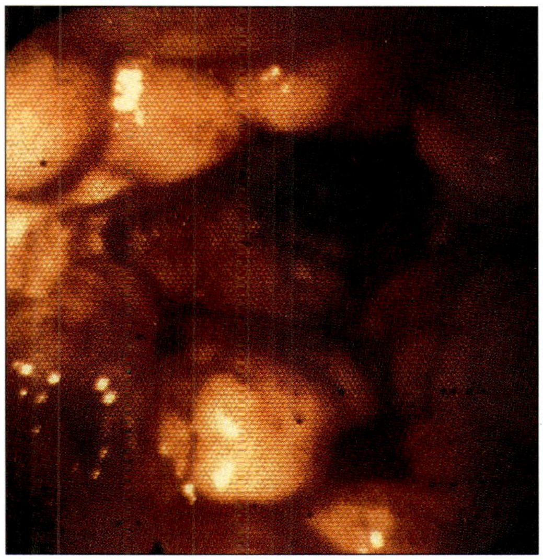

FIGURE 4-34.

Severe Crohn's colitis. A characteristic "cobblestone" appearance is the result of multiple longitudinal ulcers and exuberant inflammation with pseudopolyp formation as well as thickening of the intestinal wall because of transmural inflammation.

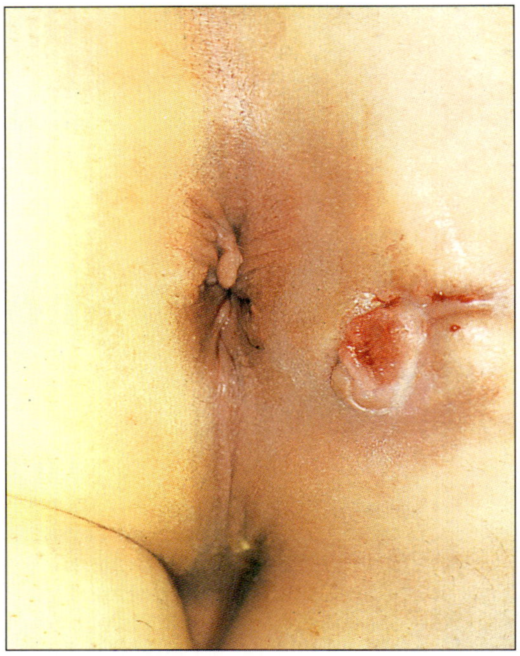

Figure 4-35.

The cutaneous opening of a perirectal fistula is shown. Such fistulas may arise from the crypts of Morgagni in the anus and spread through the internal anal sphincter, resulting in perineal or recto-vaginal fistulas, ischiorectal abscesses, or intersphincteric abscesses.

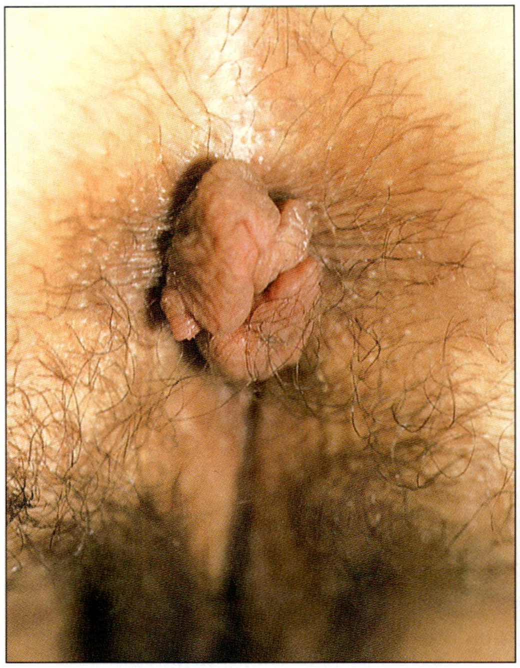

Figure 4-36.

Typical perianal changes of Crohn's disease. The large skin tags of granulation tissue, which are firm and thickened, give an "elephant-ear" appearance.

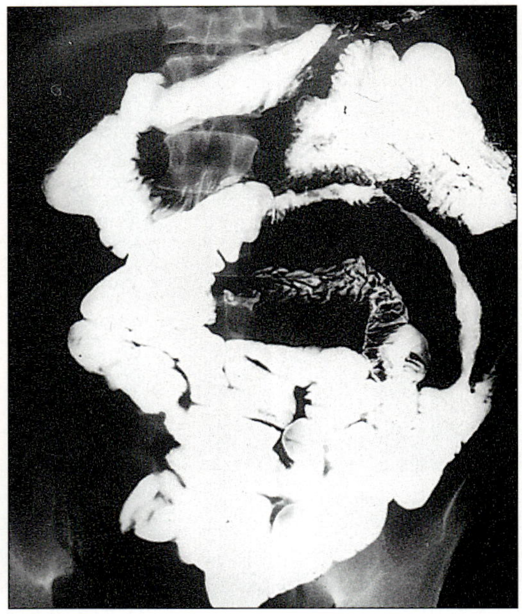

Figure 4-37.

Small bowel follow through showing an isolated segment of Crohn's disease of the jejunum, the so-called "string sign." Lumen of the involved segment is narrowed as a result of either diffuse inflammation of the bowel wall with spasm or a fibrotic stricture from previous inflammation.

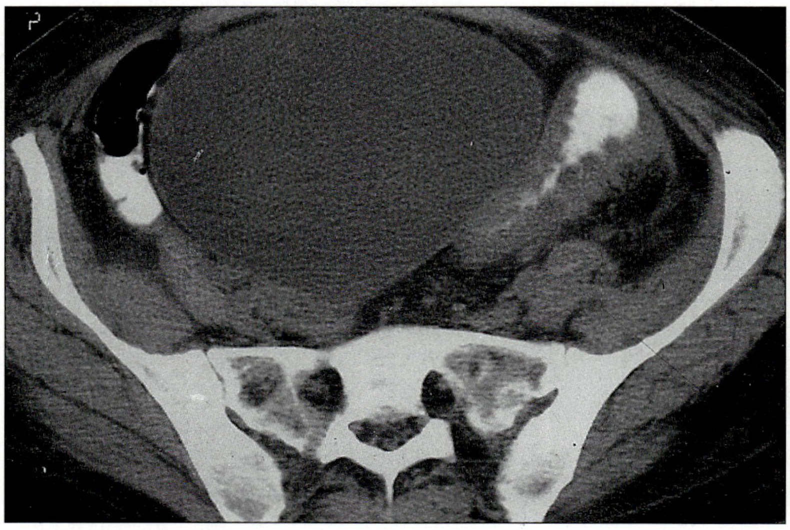

Figure 4-38.

Radiologic findings in Crohn's disease. Computed tomographic scan showing marked thickening of the colonic wall (to the left of the bladder) typical of Crohn's disease. Computed tomographic scanning is also useful for detecting Crohn's abscesses and fistulas. (*Courtesy of* G. J. Whitman, Boston, MA)

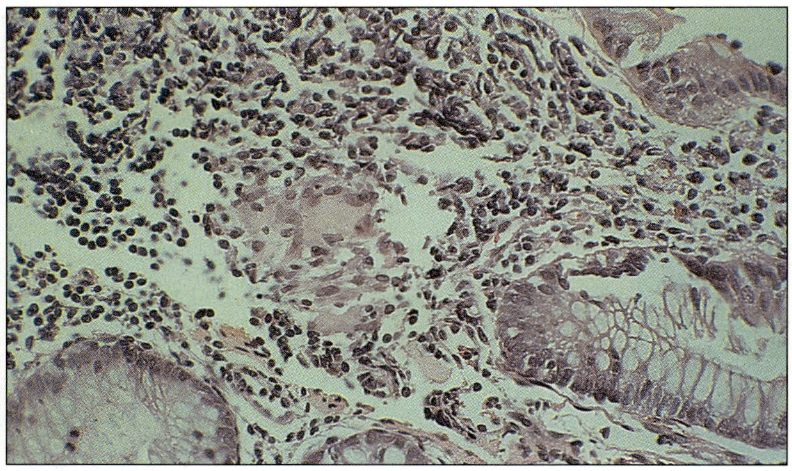

Figure 4-39.

Microscopic specimen from a patient with Crohn's colitis. The specimen has diffuse inflammation of the mucosa and submucosa with a small granuloma in the center.

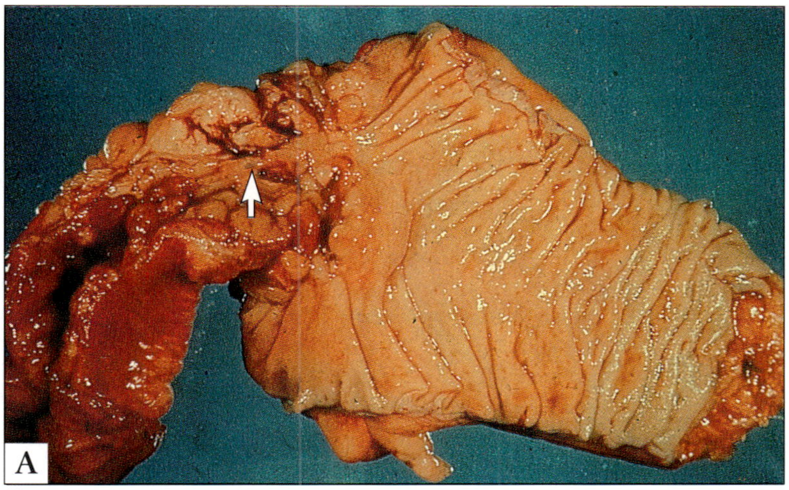

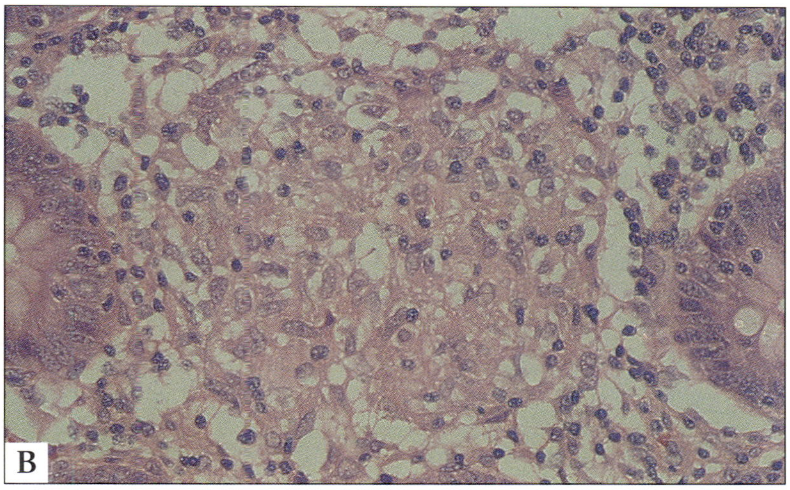

FIGURE 4-40.

Crohn's disease. **A**, This segment of colon shows a stricture in the right colon (*arrow*) with normal appearing mucosa in the distal portion of the specimen. Strictures in the right colon may be seen in both Crohn's disease and ischemic colitis [9]. **B**, An epithelioid granuloma between two colonic crypts is depicted. Although the presence of a granuloma may help establish the diagnosis of Crohn's disease in endoscopic biopsy specimens, serial sections must be examined to be certain that a granuloma is not caused by a ruptured crypt abscess (so-called mucin granuloma). The latter finding may be seen in any active colitis.

ISCHEMIC COLITIS

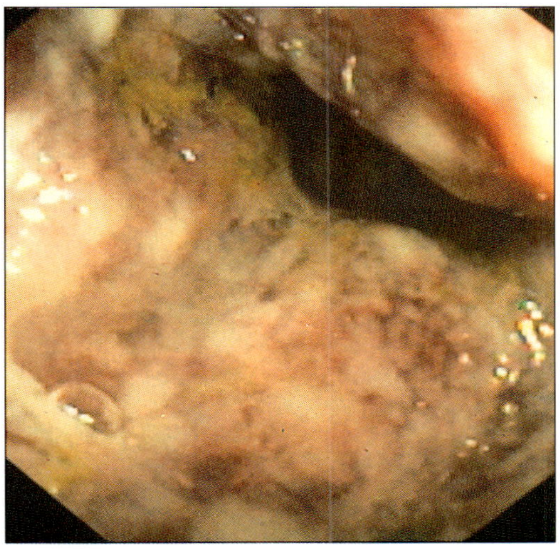

FIGURE 4-41.

Endoscopic appearance of ischemic colitis. In elderly persons, in particular, ischemic colitis enters into the differential diagnosis of inflammatory bowel disease. The etiology is usually nonocclusive ischemic damage to the colon as a result of hypotension or hypoperfusion. Iatrogenic injury to or ligation of the inferior mesenteric artery may also result in ischemic colitis. In contrast with ulcerative colitis, the rectum is typically spared, colonic involvement is segmental, and the symptoms are acute and self-limited. Typical endoscopic features include ulceration, which is patchy and in severe cases, as shown here, associated with necrosis and exudation. In some cases, resolution may be followed by stricture formation.

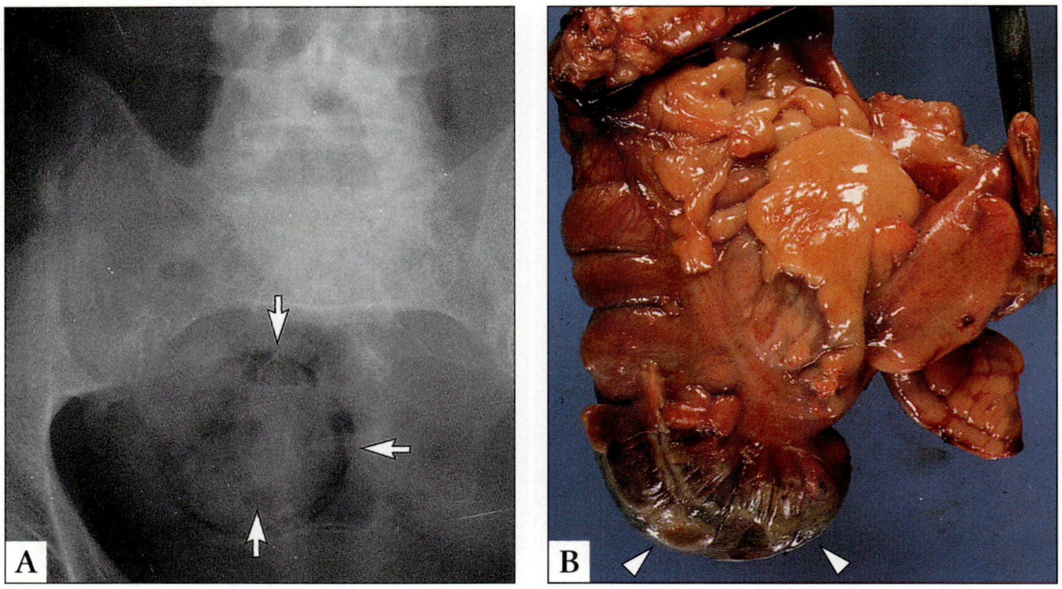

FIGURE 4-42.

Cecal infarction. This 50-year-old man undergoing coronary artery bypass surgery developed right lower quadrant pain 3 days following surgery. A, A persistent gas collection (*arrows*) in the right lower quadrant was thought to represent intramural gas rather than gas surrounding stool; its exact, location, confirmed by positive-contrast study, was in the cecum. **B**, At surgery, the resected cecum demonstrated transmural infarction of the cecal tip (arrowheads). The etiology of the cecal infarction in this patient was thought to be an undetected low flow state sometime during the patients hospital stay. Intramural gas, in this setting, should raise the suspicion of a significant vascular accident with infarction. Although there are benign causes of intramural gas and subserosal gas, in this setting, gas collection of this type is an abnormal finding. Notice how this collection of gas might go undetected if confued with gas in the rectosigmoid area and stool. If in question, computed tomographic scanning through this area would very nicely confirm the location of gas as being in or out of the bowel wall. Gas within the portal venous system is a very poor prognostic sign when bowel infarction is present.

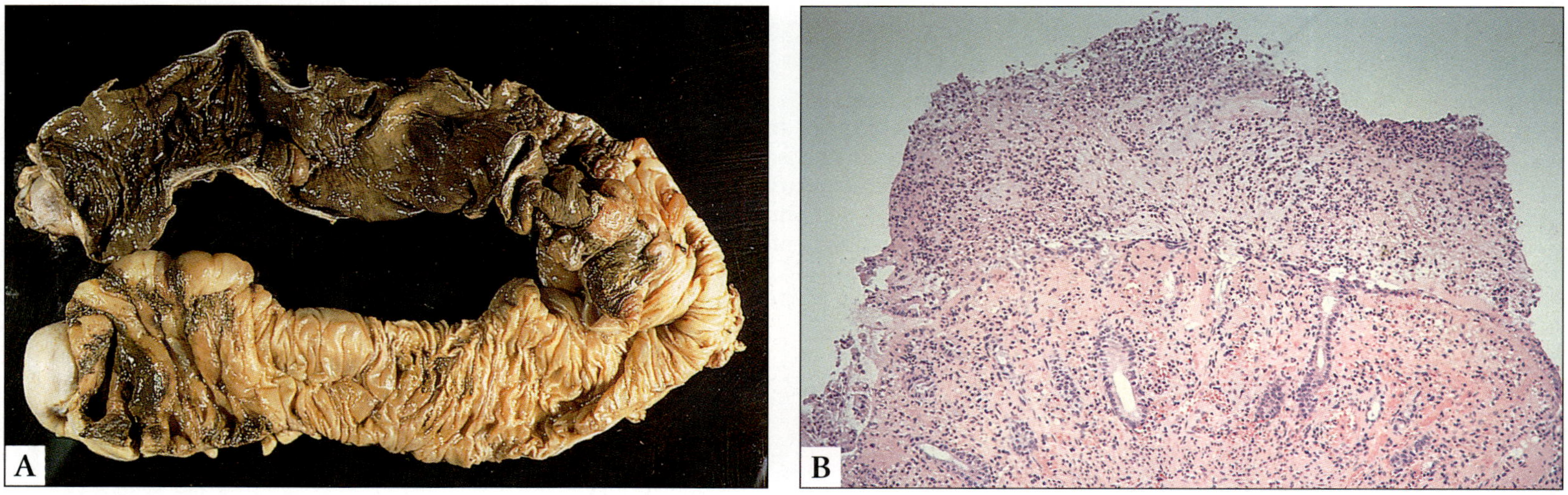

FIGURE 4-43.

Ischemic colitis. **A**, A colectomy specimen that shows a well-demarcated darkened area of hemorrhagic necrosis. The sharp border and diffuse involvement of the affected segment are characteristic of ischemic disease. **B**, This superficial pseudomembrane is identical to that seen in pseudomembranous colitis secondary to *Clostridium difficile* or *Escherichia coli* 0157:H7. The mucosa shows superficial necrosis without much inflammation. The lamina propria often takes on a hyalinized smudgy appearance, and the residual mucosa often shows marked regenerative atypia.

PSEUDOMEMBRANOUS COLITIS

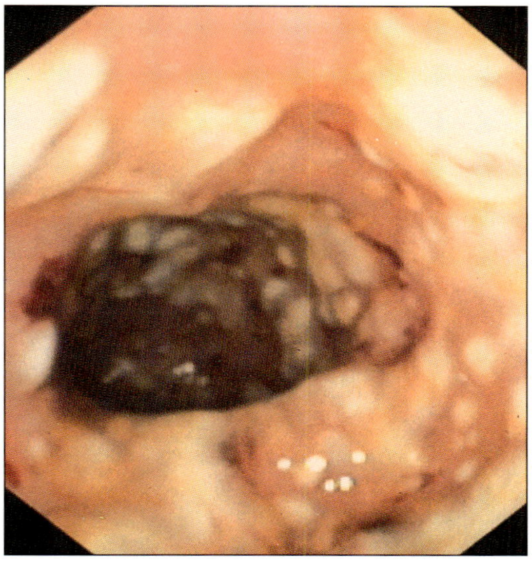

FIGURE 4-44.

Endoscopic appearance of pseudomembranous colitis. Pseudomembranous colitis characteristically results from the use of antibiotics and is caused by the toxin produced by *Clostridium difficile*. The characteristic appearance is yellow-white pseudomembranes on a background of diffuse colonic inflammation. Pseudomembranous colitis also occurs with ischemia and in patients infected with *Escherichia coli* 0157:H7.

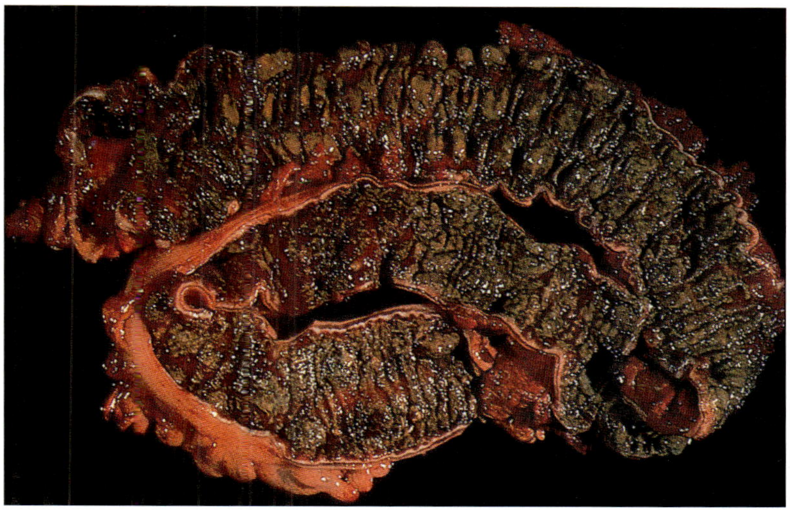

FIGURE 4-45.

Pathologic changes in colitis caused by enterohemorrhagic *Escherichia coli* infection (serotype O157:H7). The endoscopic appearance of infection caused by enterohemorrhagic *E. coli* can mimic that of ischemic colitis or pseudomembranous colitis. On gross pathology, diffuse inflammation of the colonic mucosa is not confined to the distribution of a major mesenteric vessel. There are large areas of pseudomembrane formation and marked edema.

CYTOMEGALOVIRUS COLITIS

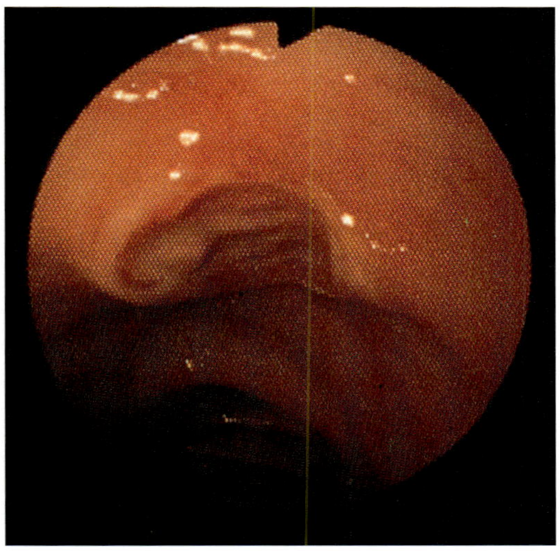

FIGURE 4-46.

Cytomegalovirus colitis. Cytomegalovirus may cause colitis, particularly in immunosuppressed hosts such as patients with AIDS or transplant recipients. Endoscopic findings may include diffuse colitis as well as solitary ulcers of the colon. As shown, the ulcer may be large with raised edges but the surrounding mucosa is normal.

RADIATION COLITIS

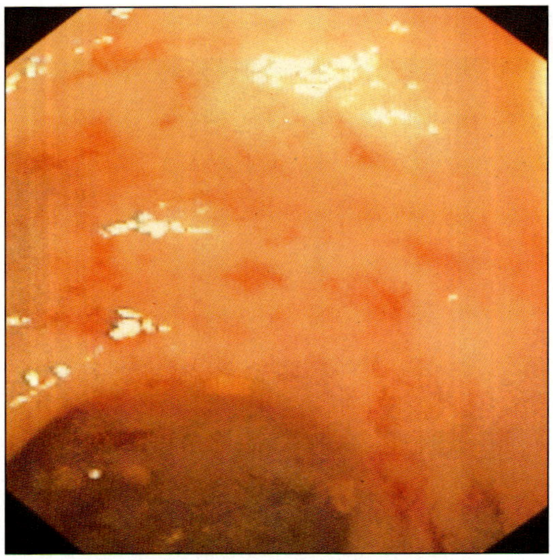

FIGURE 4-47.

Endoscopic features of radiation colitis. Radiation colitis is seen most commonly as a complication of pelvic irradiation for gynecologic malignancy. The endoscopic appearance may be indistinguishable from that of ulcerative colitis, but common characteristic mucosal telangiectatic lesions are seen. Luminal narrowing is frequent and solitary ulcers may occur.

OVERT LOWER GASTROINTESTINAL BLEEDING

CAUSES OF OVERT LOWER GASTROINTESTINAL BLEEDING

Cause	Percent
Upper gastrointestinal tract	10%
Small intestine	5%
Angiodysplasia	
Neoplasms	
Crohn's disease	
Drugs (NSAIDs)	
Aortoenteric fistula	
Meckel's diverticula	
Jejunal diverticula	
Duplication cysts	
Hemangiomas	
Colon	85%
Diverticulosis	
Angiodysplasia	
Neoplasms	
Hemorrhoids	
Inflammatory bowel disease	
Ischemia	
Radiation colitis	
Infectious colitis	
Anal fissures	
Iatrogenic (postpolypectomy)	
Solitary rectal ulcer syndrome	
Herditary hemorrhagic telangiectasia	
Dieulafoy's lesion	
Portal colopathy	
Ecotopic varices	
Drugs (NSAIDs)	
Hemangiomas	
Rectal trauma	
Aortocolonic fistula	
Diversion colitis	
Vasculitis	
Intussusception	
Endometriosis	

FIGURE 4-48.

The causes of lower gastrointestinal bleeding are myriad. Approximately 10% of gastrointestinal bleeds presumed to be lower, based on the history and initial clinical findings, actually originate in the upper gastrointestinal tract, and 5% originate in the small bowel. Five percent to 8% remain undiagnosed despite aggressive diagnostic modalities. The causes of overt lower gastrointestinal bleeding are age specific. In infants and young children, the most common lesions include anal fissures, Meckel's diverticula, and juvenile polyps. This fact holds true for adolescents and young adults, with the addition of hemorrhoids and inflammatory bowel disease. In the elderly, diverticulosis, angiodysplasia, neoplasms, and hemorrhoids constitute the most common etiologies of lower gastrointestinal bleeding [10]. Careful consideration is needed before attributing bleeding to hemorrhoids because 25% of patients who present with rectal bleeding have serious pathology combined with anal disease [11]. NSAIDs—nonsteroidal anti-inflammatory drugs. (*Adapted from* Marshall [12].)

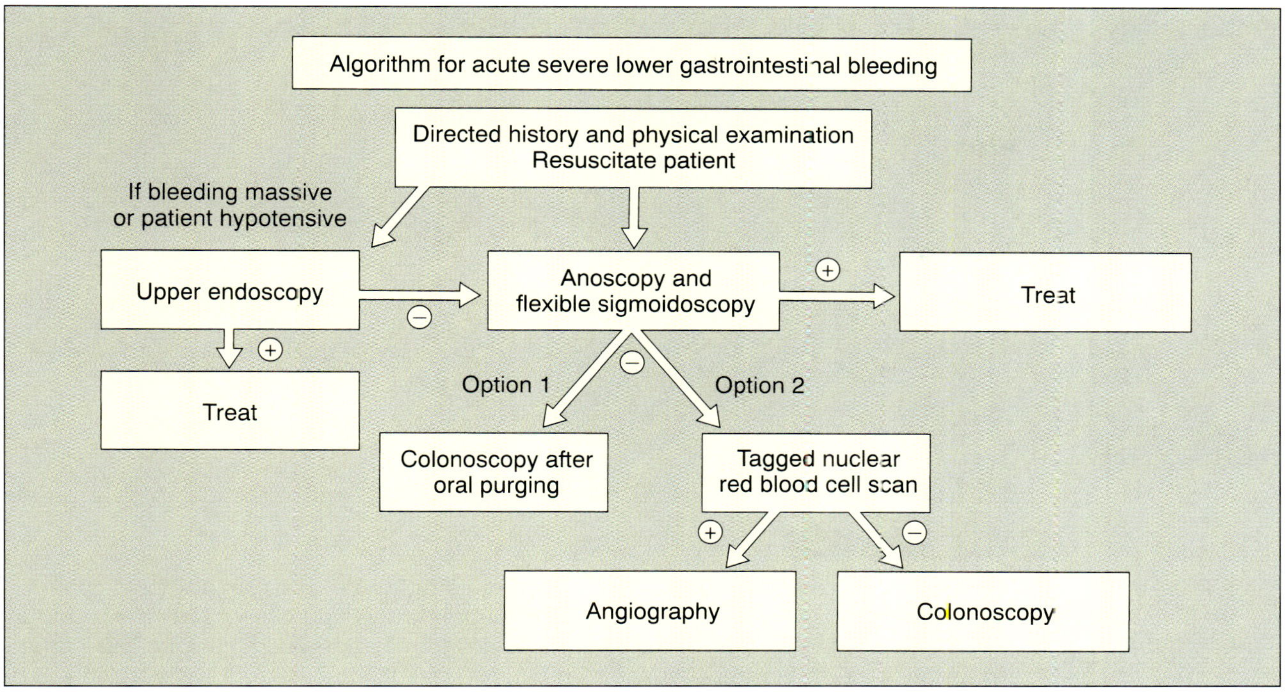

FIGURE 4-49.

The diagnostic approach to the patient with acute lower gastrointestinal bleeding must be individualized. The first steps in the management of these patients is a directed history and physical examination, assessment of the severity of the bleeding, and volume restoration. If bleeding is massive or the patient is hypotensive, an upper endoscopy should be performed to rule out an upper gastrointestinal source of bleeding. If suspicion for an upper gastrointestinal source is low, the patient should undergo anoscopy and flexible sigmoidoscopy to rule out a distal bleeding source. If these studies are not diagnostic, the next appropriate step depends on local preferences and expertise. Some expert endoscopists advocate colonoscopy after oral purging [13]. Another approach uses the radionuclide bleeding scan. A radionuclide-tagged red blood cell scan, prior to an attempt at angiography, can have several benefits. First, if the scan is negative, the bleeding has likely stopped and the patient can be prepared for colonoscopy. If the radionuclide scan is positive, it can direct the angiographer to a particular abdominal vessel, reducing the intravenous contrast load. If the scan is positive but the angiography shows no extravasation or lesion, the scan can direct the angiographer as to which vessel to leave a catheter in for subsequent infusion of vasopressin.

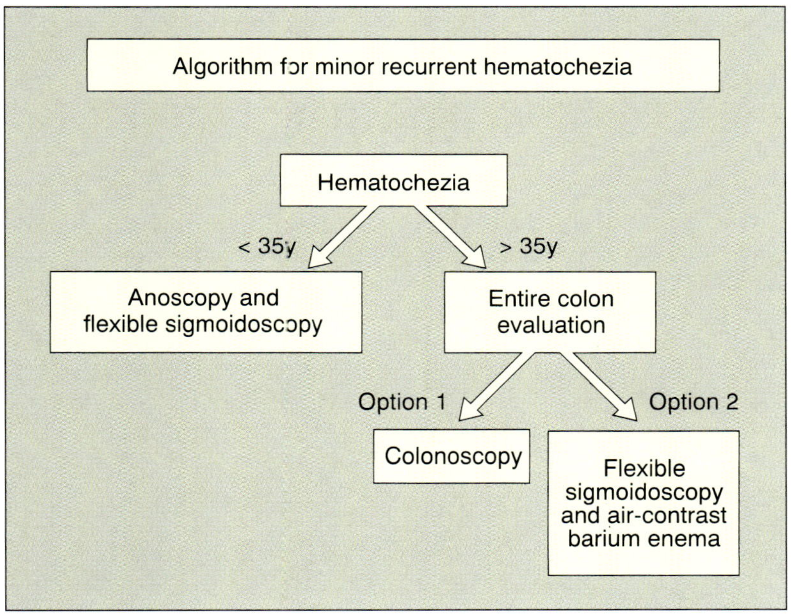

FIGURE 4-50.

Patients frequently present with recurrent minor hematochezia. This presentation may be spotting on the toilet paper, blood dripping into the toilet bowl, or red blood coating or mixed into the stool. The evaluation of these patients is age specific. If the patient is young, anoscopy and sigmoidoscopy may be all that is warranted, because perianal disease and distal colitis are the most common etiologies. If the patient is over 35 years of age, the entire colon should be evaluated because of the increased risk of neoplasm. This evaluation may be accomplished with colonoscopy or flexible sigmoidoscopy plus air-contrast barium enema. In most patients, colonoscopy is preferable and is particularly cost-effective in older patients where there is a high background prevalence of colorectal polyps [14].

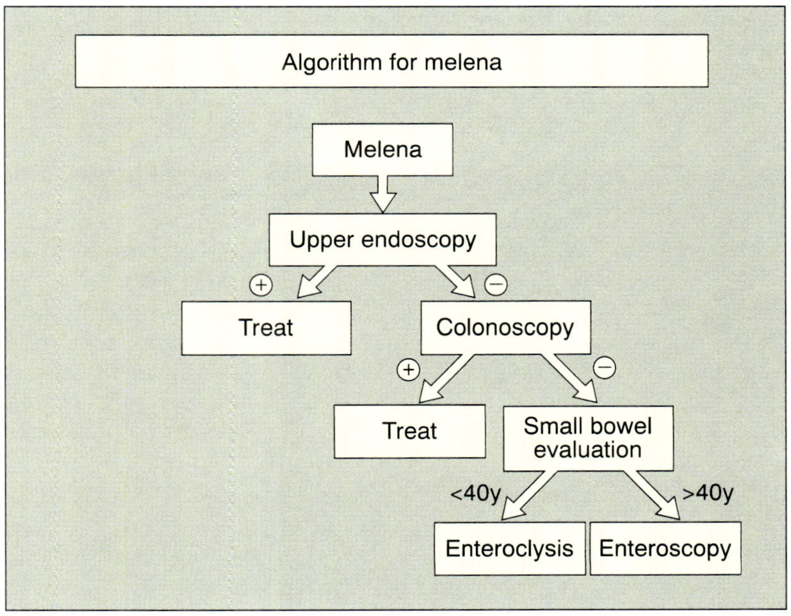

FIGURE 4-51.

The most common cause of melena is bleeding from the upper gastrointestinal tract, and thus the initial diagnostic step should be an upper endoscopy. If this outcome is negative, colonoscopy is performed. If the cause of bleeding is still unclear, the small bowel should be evaluated. If the patient is over 40 years of age, we would favor small bowel push enteroscopy as the first diagnostic test because of a high prevalence of small bowel angiodysplasia. For younger patients, enteroclysis would be an appropriate first option, because of a higher likelihood of small bowel tumors.

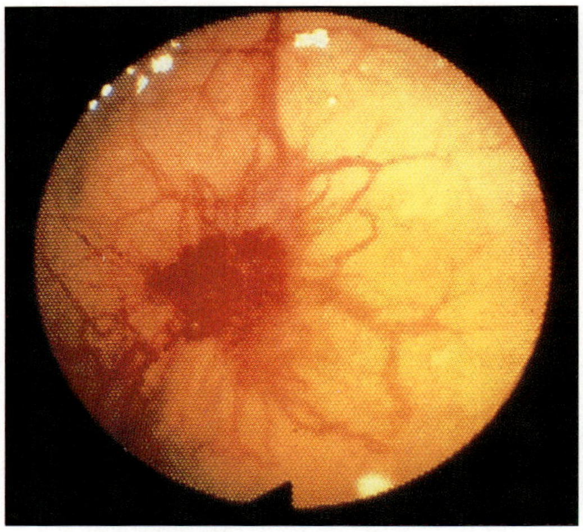

FIGURE 4-52.

Colonoscopy detects approximately 80% of colonic angiodysplasia. Lesions appear flat or slightly raised, red, and 2 to 10 mm in diameter. They may be round, stellate, or fernlike [15]. There may be a prominent feeding vessel or a pale mucosal halo. Many lesions may mimic angiodysplasia, including lesions of hereditary hemorrhagic telangiectasia, ischemia, radiation colitis, and suction artifacts. Lesions may be missed if the patient is anemic or volume depleted. The effect of narcotics on the endoscopic appearance of angiodysplasia is controversial. Narcotics may lead to vasoconstriction and decreased mucosal blood flow, thus obscuring angiodysplasia, whereas naloxone hydrochloride may act to reverse these vasoconstrictive effects [16].

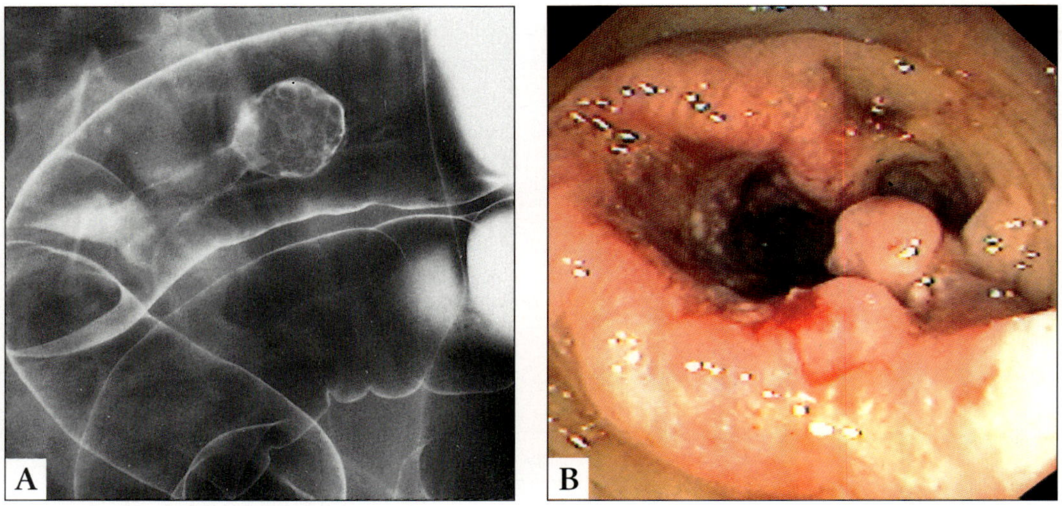

FIGURE 4-53.

Most bleeding from colorectal polyps and cancer is occult or mild and intermittent. Rarely polyps and cancer may cause significant lower gastrointestinal hemorrhage. Left-sided and rectal neoplasms are more likely to cause gross bleeding than right-sided lesions. Diagnosis is made by endoscopy or barium enema. Treatment for bleeding polyps or cancer is usually by colonoscopic removal or surgery. **A,** A pedunculated sigmoid polyp. **B,** An annular rectal adenocarcinoma. (**A**, *Courtesy of* J. Lappas, Indianapolis, IN)

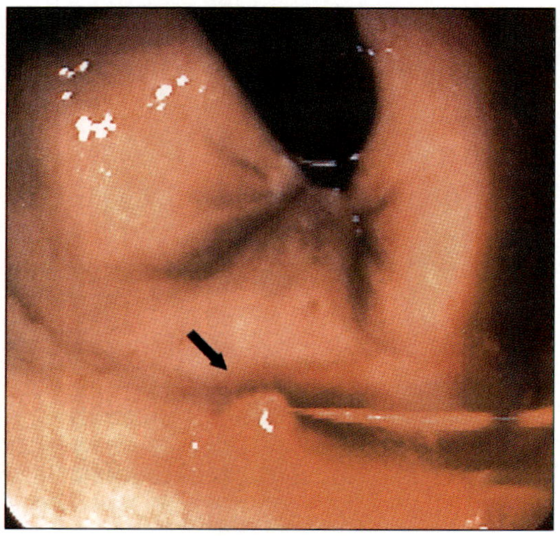

FIGURE 4-54.

Dieulafoy's lesions are usually seen in the proximal stomach, however, they may be found in the colon or small bowel. The pathologic defect is an abnormally large submucosal artery with a small mucosal defect overlying the artery. Bleeding occurs when there is rupture of the artery into the bowel lumen. For small bowel or colonic lesions, the diagnosis is usually made by angiography because bleeding is too massive for endoscopic visualization. Therapeutic options include endoscopic injection or cautery, intra-arterial vasopressin, angiographic embolization, or surgical resection. Pictured is a Dieulafoy's lesion in the rectum with an actively spurting vessel. (*From* Abdulian *et al.* [17]; with permission.)

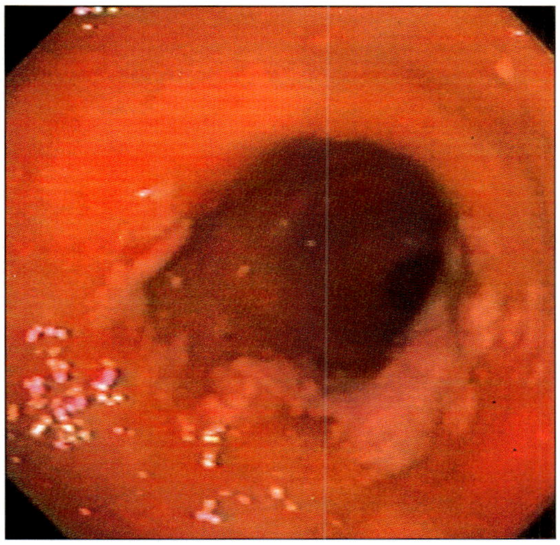

Figure 4-55.

Eighty-five percent to 95% of patients with solitary rectal ulcer syndrome present with hematochezia, usually of low volume and associated with mucus. Symptoms may also include anorectal pain, altered bowel movements, and straining with defecation. It is believed that *solitary rectal ulcer syndrome* is related to prolonged straining during bowel movements and difficulty initiating defecation. Classically, at sigmoidoscopy, there is a shallow, discrete 1-cm ulcer with hyperemic margins 7 to 10 cm from the anal verge on the anterior wall. Lesions, however, may be multiple or vary in size and location. These ulcers follow a benign course, and two thirds of patients improve with conservative measures, including a high-fiber diet, laxatives, and avoidance of straining. Diagnosis is histologic, and the characteristic histologic findings may be seen in patients whose endoscopic findings are only rectal polyps. Pictured is a solitary rectal ulcer seen during flexible sigmoidoscopy.

COLONIC DIVERTICULA

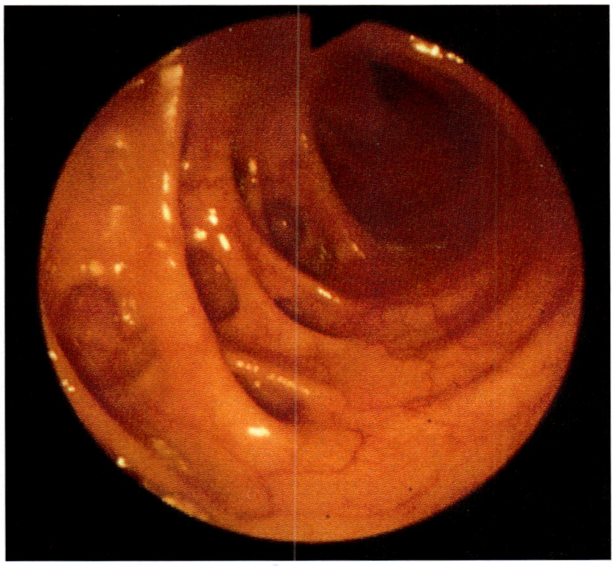

Figure 4-56.

The sigmoid colon. Diverticula with fold thickening should be closely evaluated in the sigmoid colon. Knowledge of the existence of diverticula is important in evaluating patients with left lower quadrant pain and with acute lower GI bleeding.

Diverticulitis

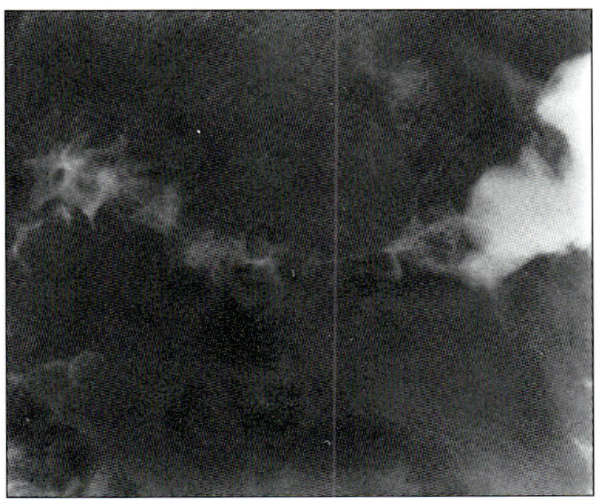

Figure 4-57.

This barium enema demonstrates a classic case of acute sigmoid diverticulitis. Note the long segment of colon involved in the inflammatory process and the luminal narrowing secondary to the inflammation. Endoscopic examination would reveal intense spasm and edema at the rectosigmoid junction.

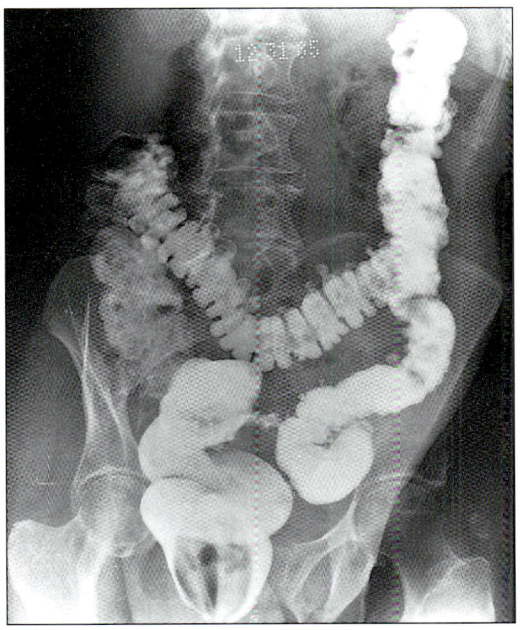

Figure 4-58.

Sigmoid diverticulitis can mimick a carcinoma. Careful endoscopic examination of the sigmoid after resection of the acute phase of the illness may be possible and is necessary to exclude carcinoma. If the stricture and obstructive symptoms resolve as the inflammation subsides and if other pathology can be excluded, nonoperative management is usually indicated, especially after the initial episode of diverticulitis. A high-residue diet supplemented with bulk agents may decrease the luminal pressure and the risk of perforation of diverticula. There is some evidence that a high-fiber diet can decrease recurrences of acute diverticulitis and prevent its complications [18].

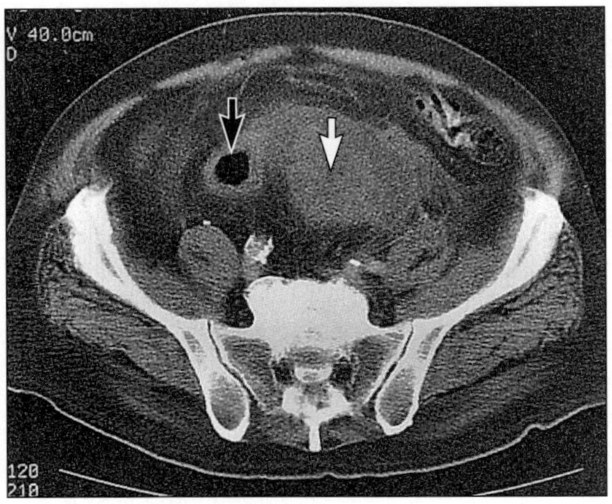

FIGURE 4-59.

A computed tomographic scan of a patient with acute diverticulitis and signs of sepsis demonstrates a large pelvic abscess. The abscess is indicated by the *open arrow* and the distended loop of bowel is indicated by the *closed arrow*. The computed tomographic scan is the most sensitive and specific test to diagnose the inflammatory complications of diverticular disease.

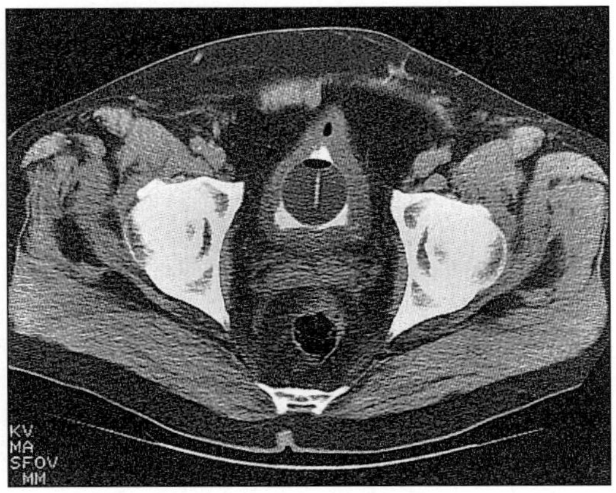

FIGURE 4-60.

Fistulas to other viscera are present in 8% to 42% of patients undergoing surgery for diverticular disease. Colovesical fistulas are the most common type of diverticular disease, accounting for approximately half of all such fistulas. Computed tomographic scanning is the best imaging procedure to establish the diagnosis of colovesical fistula. This computed tomographic scan demonstrates an air-fluid level within the bladder in a patient who presented with sepsis and pneumaturia. Systemic sepsis is usually controlled in such patients as the diverticular abscess drains itself into the bladder. Urosepsis is controlled with antibiotics until an elective colon resection is possible [19].

Diverticular bleeding

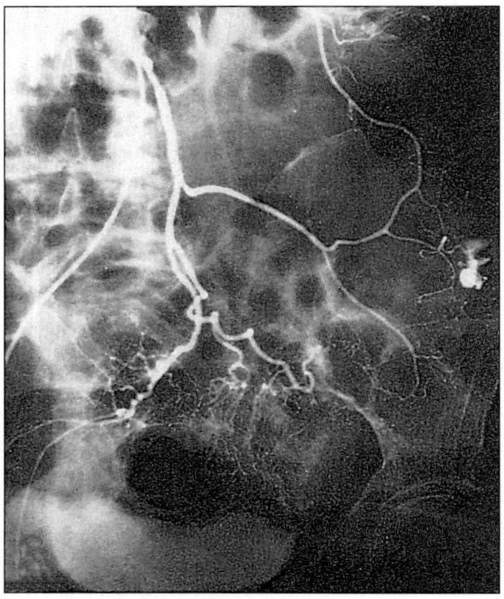

FIGURE 4-61.

Selective mesenteric angiography is effective in the diagnosis of active diverticular bleeding. Extravasation of contrast into a diverticula is the diagnostic radiographic finding. Angiographic infusion of vasopressors may halt diverticular bleeding in 80% to 90% of patients [20]. Typical infusion doses in the superior mesenteric artery range from 0.2 to 0.3 units per minute and in the inferior mesenteric artery from 0.1 to 0.2 units per minute. Fifteen percent to 25% of these patients rebleed and eventually require surgery. Angiographic embolization may also be used, but below the ligament of Treitz, there is a 30% incidence of bowel ischemia or infarction. Radiograph of a patient with an actively bleeding diverticula of the descending colon is shown. (*From* Dietzen and Pemberton [21]; with permission.)

Obstruction from diverticular disease

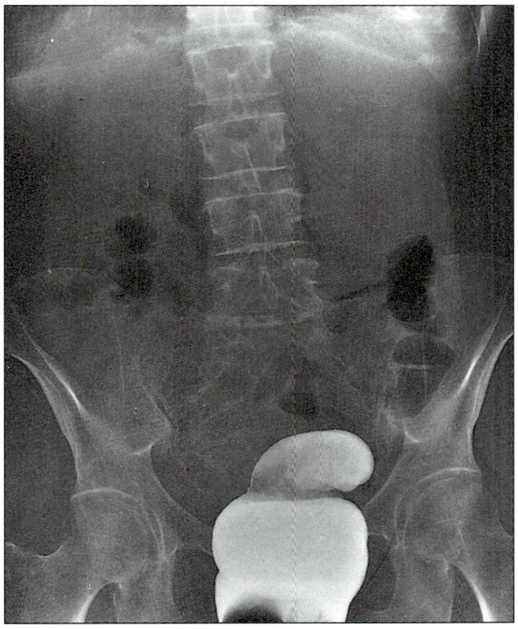

FIGURE 4-62.

A barium enema demonstrates complete retrograde obstruction at the rectosigmoid junction. No etiology is apparent. Usually, sigmoidoscopy (rigid or flexible) is deferred until the acute process has subsided with treatment, but in this case, sigmoidoscopy can help exclude a cancer and can assess the status of the distal rectum, which is essential information to obtain before proceeding with emergency laparotomy. When sigmoidoscopy is performed during the acute phase of diverticular disease, the endoscopist must be careful to use minimal or no insufflation of air to avoid colonic perforation.

HIRSCHSPRUNG'S DISEASE AND OTHER MOTILITY PROBLEMS

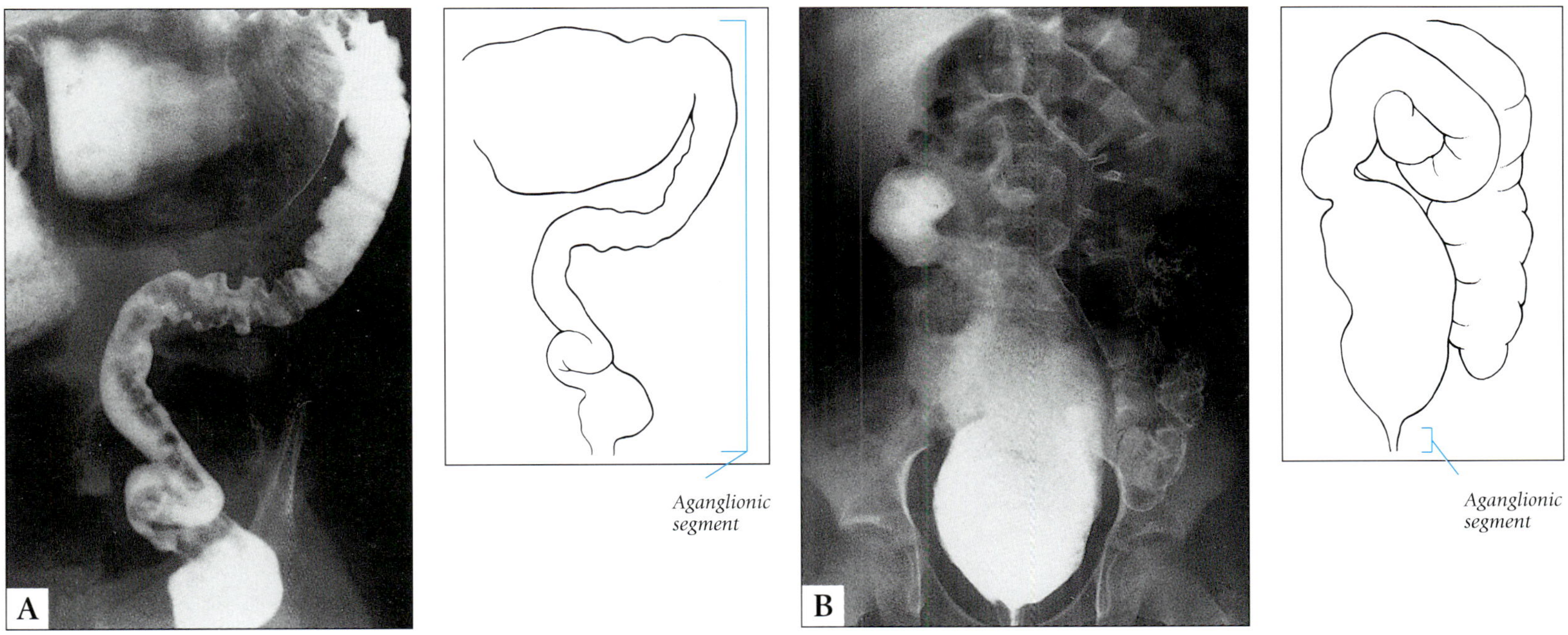

FIGURE 4-63.

In patients with Hirschsprung's disease (congenital aganglionosis), varying lengths of distal bowel receive no enteric innervation. The aganglionic bowel is narrowed and spastic, whereas the normally innervated proximal bowel is dilated and filled with fecal material. In cases of suspected aganglionosis, it is preferable not to cleanse the colon prior to barium studies in order to accentuate the transition zone from aganglionic to normally innervated bowel. **A**, Barium enema in a patient with aganglionosis to the splenic flexure. **B**, Patient with involvement of only the distal 1 to 2 cm of the rectum, *ie*, short segment disease. It is important to remove the insertion catheter used to instill barium in order to avoid missing short segment disease. (*From* Wald [22]; with permission.)

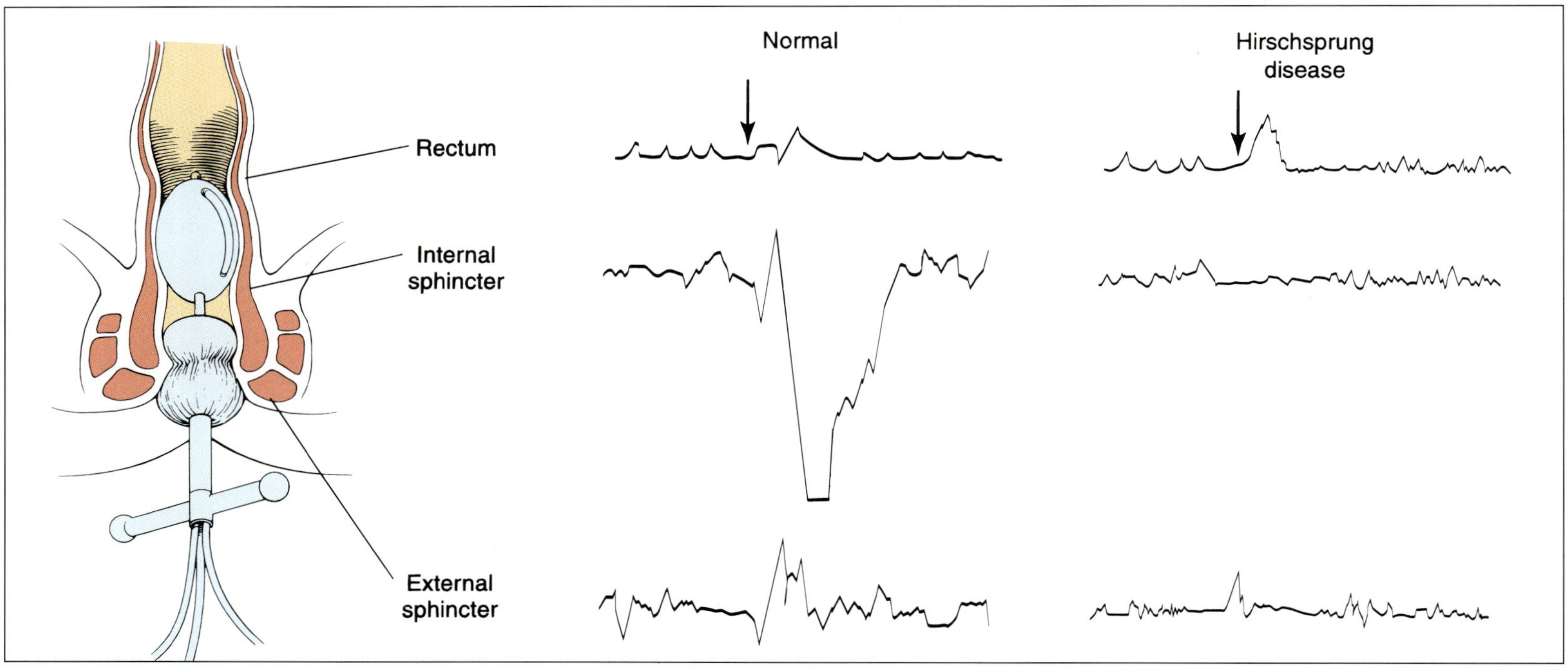

FIGURE 4-64.

Balloon manometry. Internal anal sphincter responses to rectal distension in a patient with Hirschsprung's disease are compared with those in a normal subject using the Schuster-type balloon manometer. In contrast to normal relaxation of the internal anal sphincter following rectal distension (*arrows*), no such relaxation occurs in a patient with Hirschsprung's disease. Thus, the presence of internal anal sphincter relaxation excludes Hirschsprung's disease from consideration. However, failure to detect internal sphincter relaxation is not specific for Hirschsprung's disease, and the diagnosis should be confirmed using histologic or neurohistochemical assessment of biopsy material. (*From* Wald [22]; with permission.)

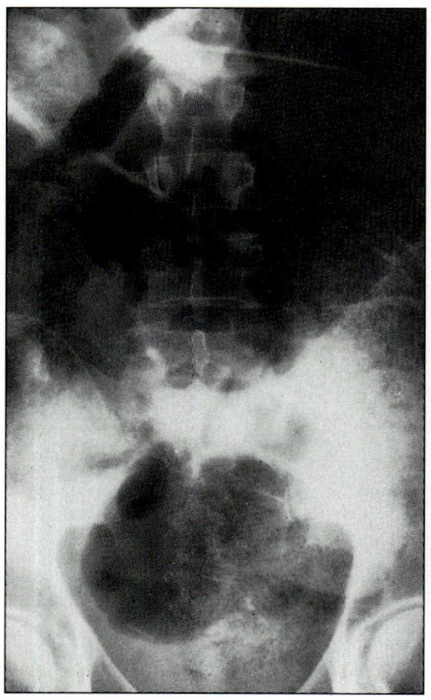

FIGURE 4-65.

Idiopathic megacolon. A large amount of retained stool in the distal colon and considerable distension with air of the transverse colon is depicted. The stool in the rectum suggests that this is not a mechanical obstruction, but an examination of the rectum to exclude a low-lying stricture would be wise.

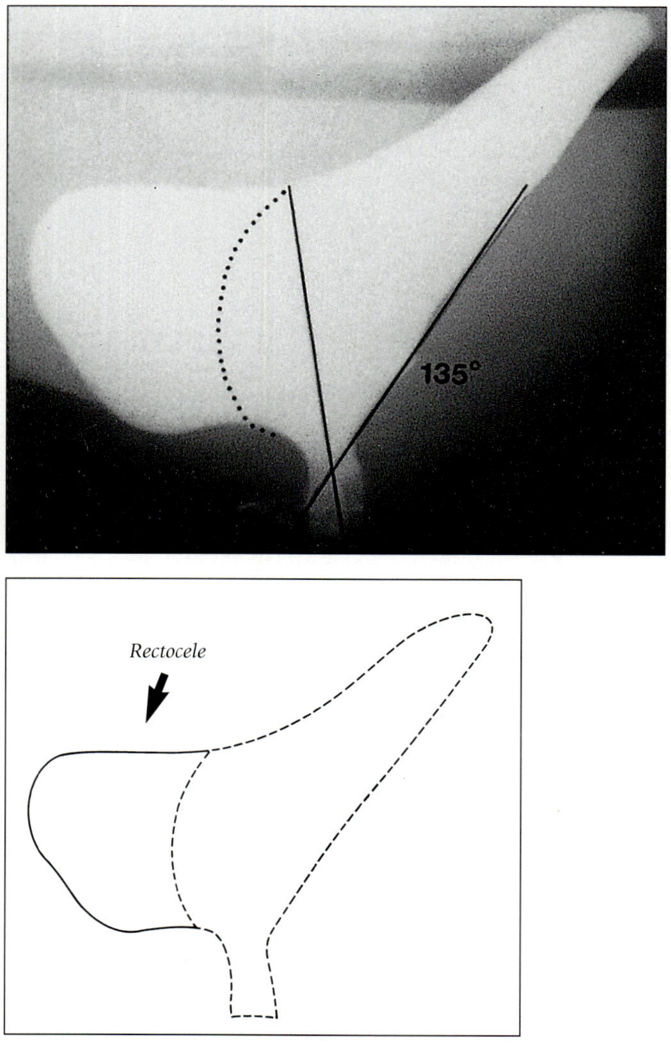

FIGURE 4-66.

Rectocele. During expulsion, a large anterior rectocele fills with barium (*arrow*), but expulsion of contrast appears normal. Several studies have demonstrated that rectoceles are common in women without defecation complaints so that caution is necessary before implicating a rectocele as the cause of defecation difficulty. (*Courtesy* of D. Bauman, Pittsburgh, PA)

DIAGNOSTIC OR ROME CRITERIA FOR IRRITABLE BOWEL SYNDROME

At least 3 months of continuous or recurrent symptoms of:

- Abdominal pain or discomfort
  - Relieved with defecation and/or
  - Associated with change in stool frequency and/or
  - Associated with change in stool consistency
- Two or more of the following symptoms at least 1/4 of the time
  - Altered stool frequency (<3/wk or >3/day)
  - Altered stool form (hard or loose)
  - Altered stool passage (staining, urgency, incomplete evacuation)
  - Passage of mucus
  - Bloating/abdominal distension

FIGURE 4-67.

Irritable bowel syndrome is considered a disorder of gastrointestinal function manifested by abdominal pain and altered bowel habits that occur in chronic or recurrent fashion at times of life stress and emotional tension. Symptom patterns include lower abdominal (occasionally other locations) pain and altered bowel habits, *ie*, constipation, diarrhea, or both. The presence of organic disease that can produce similar symptoms must be excluded. However, a precise, reproducible, and objective definition of this syndrome remains elusive and is particularly problematic for clinicians and investigators. An international committee has put forth a definition of irritable bowel syndrome that uses symptomatic criteria, known as the *Rome Criteria* (shown).

The three major hypotheses put forth to explain the etiology of symptoms in irritable bowel syndrome are 1) patients have an underlying disorder of intestinal motility; 2) emotional tension and psychological factors lead to gastrointestinal symptoms and health seeking behavior; and 3) individuals with irritable bowel syndrome have a low tolerance for pain or an excessive response to normal signals from the gastrointestinal tract. (*From* Drossman *et al.* [23]; with permission.)

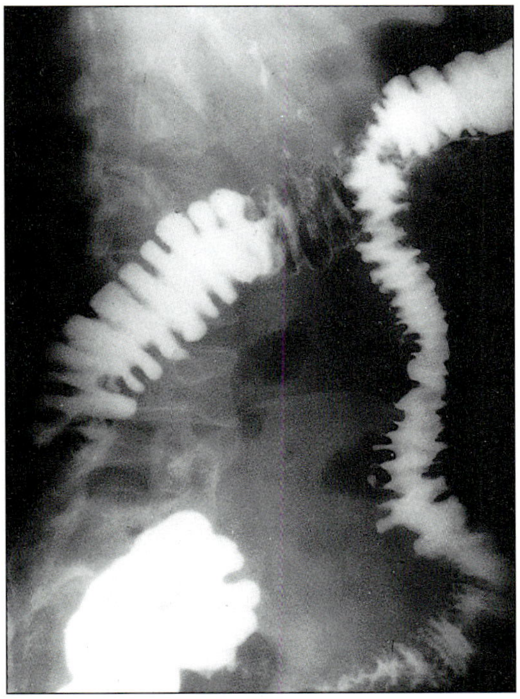

FIGURE 4-68.

Barium enema in an irritable bowel syndrome patient. The extreme hypercontractility of the left and sigmoid colon is indicative of excessive segmenting motor activity. Current evidence suggests that disordered basal motor activity is unlikely and that the exaggerated colonic motor responses to certain stimulants requires more rigorous analysis. Several studies report a high frequency of hysteria, somatization disorder, depression, and anxiety in patients with irritable bowel syndrome. Other studies suggest that laboratory stressors can alter gastrointestinal motility.

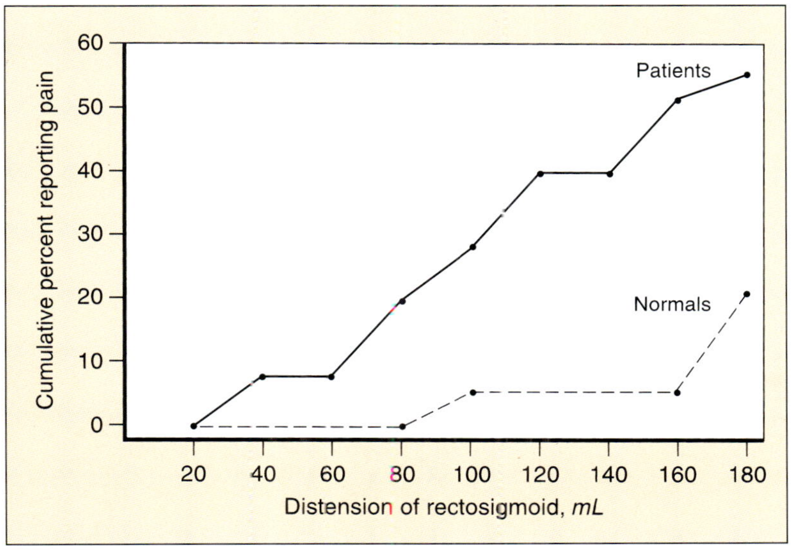

FIGURE 4-69.

Visceral sensations in irritable bowel syndrome. The graph depicts rectosigmoid balloon distension studies in 28 irritable bowel syndrome patients and 20 healthy control subjects. The rectosigmoid balloon was distended in a stepwise fashion by injecting an additional 20 mL of air every 2 minutes up to a total of 180 mL of air. Compared with the control subjects, the incidence of pain complaints was greater in irritable bowel syndrome patients. At maximum balloon distention, 60% of the irritable bowel patients compared with only 20% of the volunteers complained of rectal pain ($P<0.05$). This leftward shift of the pain curve confirmed the presence of an altered visceral pain threshold in the patients with irritable bowel syndrome. (*From* Whitehead *et al.* [24]; with permission.)

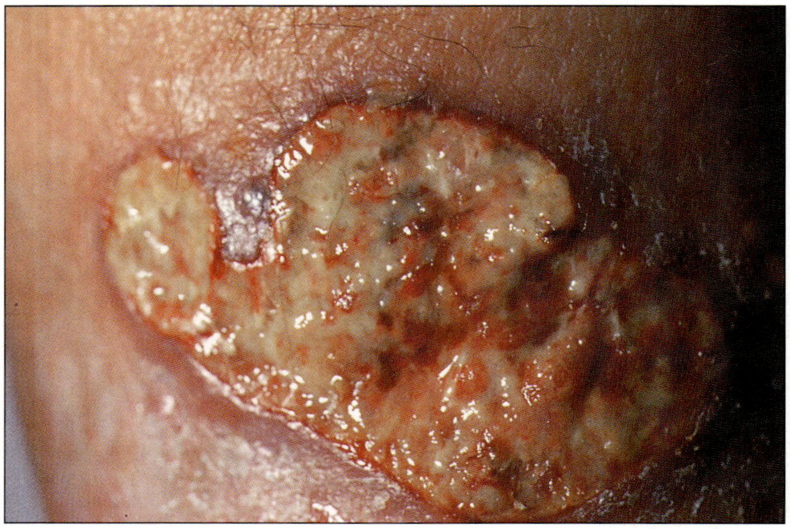

FIGURE 4-70.

Pyoderma gangrenosum first presents as erythematous papules, which rapidly form pustules and vesicles. These lesions coalesce to form large hemorrhagic bullae with dusky, raised edges. The bullae then rupture, leaving behind an enlarging, indurated ulcer with raised edges and a yellowish exudate as seen in this patient. The lesions are most common on the legs but may occur anywhere. Trauma may give rise to a lesion. Ulcerative colitis is the most common underlying cause of pyoderma gangrenosum and is present in 50% of all patients with these lesions. Although Crohn's disease may be associated with this condition, it is much less common. Therapy involves corticosteroids, with or without other immunosuppressive drugs.

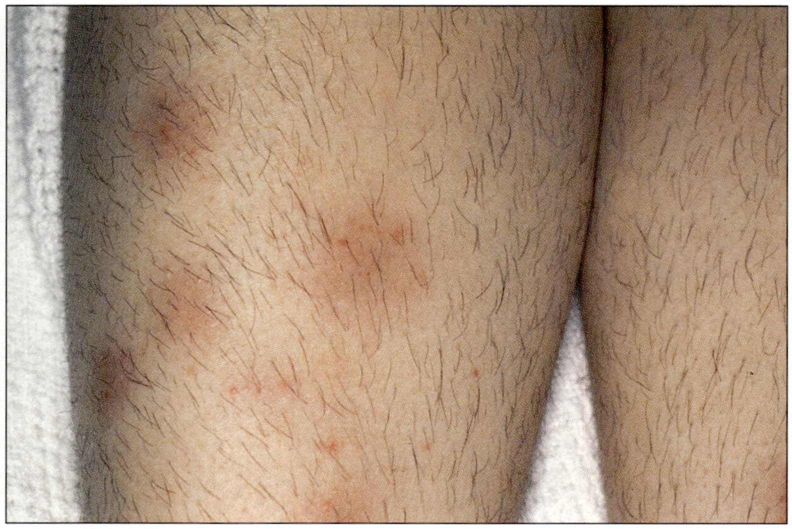

FIGURE 4-71.

Red nodules of erythema nodosum in the pretibial area. Lesions are usually tender, poorly circumscribed, and located deep within the subcutaneous fat. Their appearance is usually accompanied by an exacerbation in the underlying inflammatory bowel disease. Erythema nodosum occurs in about 4% of patients with ulcerative colitis and in 2% of patients with Crohn's disease. Treatment includes bed rest, systemic or intralesional steroids, nonsteroidal anti-inflammatory agents, potassium iodide, colchicine, and dapsone.

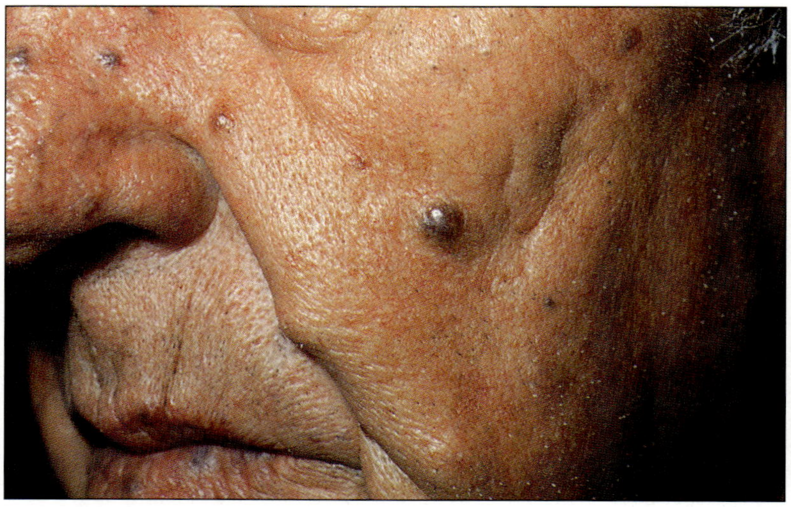

FIGURE 4-72.

A patient with multiple, soft, rubbery, bluish nodules on the nose and cheek caused by the blue rubber bleb nevus syndrome. This syndrome usually occurs sporadically, although autosomal dominant forms have been reported. Cutaneous lesions may be soft and compressible or punctate, flat, and painful. The bluish color is characteristic of this condition. Gastrointestinal lesions in this syndrome consist of cavernous hemangiomas and can be found throughout the gastrointestinal tract, although the large and small intestines are the most common locations.

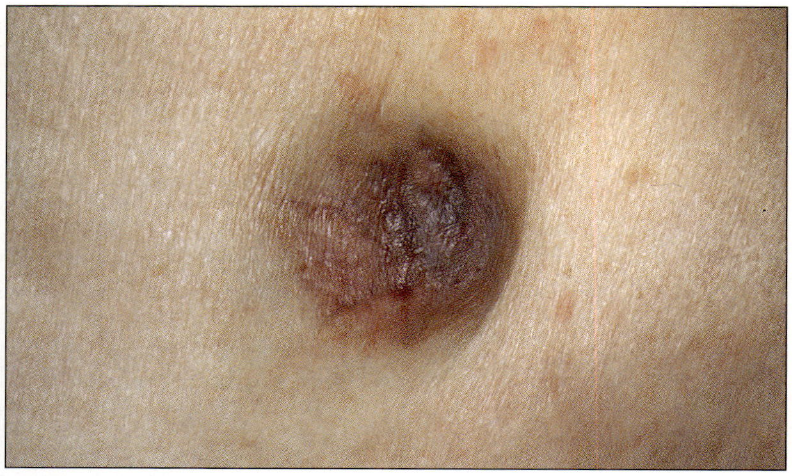

FIGURE 4-73.

Metastatic adenocarcinoma of the colon. A firm nodule, fixed to the underlying tissue, with several overlying large telangiectasias is seen here on the abdomen. The abdominal skin is the most common location for gastrointestinal tract metastases. Colonic adenocarcinomas are the most common cause, followed by gastric carcinomas. The lesions are usually nontender and may range from flesh colored to plum colored. They usually occur in advanced disease states.

REFERENCES

1. Irving MH, Catchpole B: ABC of colorectal diseases: anatomy and physiology of the colon, rectum, and anus. *BMJ* 1992, 304:1106–1108.
2. St. John DJB, Young GP, Alexeyeff MA, *et al.*: Evaluation of new occult blood tests for detection of colorectal neoplasia. *Gastroenterology* 1993, 104:1661–1668.
3. Ahlquist DA, Wieand HS, Moertel CH, *et al.*: Accuracy of fecal occult blood screening for colorectal neoplasia. *JAMA* 1993, 269:1262–1267.
4. Bresalier RS, Kim YS: Malignant neoplasms of the large intestine. In *Gastrointestinal Disease: Pathophysiology, Diagnosis, Management*, ed 5. Edited by Sleisenger MH, Fordtran JS. Philadelphia: WB Saunders; 1993:1449–1493.
5. Moertel CG, O'Fallon JR, Go VLW, *et al.*: The preoperative carcinogenic antigen test in the diagnosis, staging and prognosis of colorectal cancer. *Cancer* 1986, 58:603–610.
6. Podolsky DK: Gastrointestinal Oncology, Unit 22. American Gastroenterological Association; 1989.
7. Moertel CG, Fleming TR, MacDonald JS, *et al.*: Levamisole and fluorouracil for adjuvant therapy of resected colorectal carcinoma. *N Engl J Med* 1990, 322:352–358.
8. Krook JE, Moertel CG, Gunderson LL, *et al.*: Effective adjuvant therapy for high risk carcinoma. *N Engl J Med* 1991, 324:705–715.
9. Shepherd NA: Pathological mimics of chronic inflammatory bowel disease [Review]. *J Clin Pathol* 1991, 44:726–733.
10. Forde KA: Lower gastrointestinal bleeding: The magnitude of the problem. In *Gastrointestinal Bleeding*. Edited by Sugawa C, Schuman BM, Lucas CE. New York: Igaku-Shoin; 1992:13–25.
11. Waye JD: Diagnostic endoscopy in lower intestinal bleeding. In *Gastrointestinal Bleeding*. Edited by Sugawa C, Schuman BM, Lucas CE. New York: Igaku-Shoin; 1992:230–241.
12. Marshall JB: Acute gastrointestinal bleeding: a logical approach to management. *Postgrad Med* 1990, 87:63–70.
13. Jensen DM, Machicado GA: Diagnosis and treatment of severe hematochezia: the role of urgent colonoscopy after purge. *Gastroenterology* 1988, 95:1569–1574.
14. Rex DK, Weddle RA, Lehman GA, *et al.*: Flexible sigmoidoscopy plus air contrast barium enema versus colonoscopy for suspected lower gastrointestinal bleeding. *Gastroenterology* 1990, 98:855–861.
15. Foutch PG: Angiodysplasia of the gastrointestinal tract. *Am J Gastroenterol* 1993, 88:807–818.
16. Deal SE, Zfass AM, Duckworth PF, *et al.*: Arteriovenous malformation (AVMs). Are they concealed by meperidine [Abstract]? *Am J Gastroenterol* 1991, 86:1351.
17. Abdulian JD, Santoro MJ, Chen YK, *et al.*: Dieulafoy-like lesion of the rectum presenting with exsanguinating hemorrhage: successful endoscopic sclerotherapy. *Am J Gastroenterol* 1993, 88:1939–1941.
18. Hyland JMP, Taylor I: Does a high fiber diet prevent the complications of diverticular disease? *Br J Surg* 1980, 67:771–779.
19. Woods RJ, Lavery IL, Fazio VW, *et al.*: Internal fistulas in diverticular disease. *Dis Colon Rectum* 1988, 31:591–596.
20. Reinus JF, Brandt LJ: Vascular ectasias and diverticulosis. Common causes of lower intestinal bleeding. *Gastroenterol Clin North Am* 1994, 23:1–20.
21. Dietzen CD, Pemberton JH: Diverticulitis. In *Atlas of Gastroenterology*. Edited by Yamada T. Philadelphia: JB Lippincott; 1992:279–285.
22. Wald A: Anorectum: In *Atlas of Gastrointestinal Motility*. Edited by Schuster MM. Baltimore: Williams and Wilkins; 1993:29–249.
23. Drossman DA, Thompson WG, Talley NJ, *et al.*: Identification of sub-groups of functional gastrointestinal disorders. *Gastroenterology International* 1990, 3:159–172.
24. Whitehead WE, Engel BT, Schuster MM: Irritable bowel syndrome. Physiological psychological differences between diarrhea-predominant and constipation-predominant patients. *Dig Dis Sci* 1980, 25:404–413.

Chapter 5

Disorders of the Liver

EDITOR

Willis C. Maddrey

CONTRIBUTORS

Ignacio Aiza
Bruce R. Bacon
David Bernstein
Laurence Blendis
Joseph R. Bloomer
Robert S. Brown, Jr.
Peter C. Buetow
Harold O. Conn
Albert J. Czaja
Adrian M. Di Bisceglie
Raymond S. Koff
Ann M. Kools
John R. Lake
William M. Lee
Charles S. Lieber
Milton G. Mutchnick
Eugene R. Schiff
Florence Wong

JAUNDICE

UNCONJUGATED HYPERBILIRUBINEMIA	CONJUGATED HYPERBILIRUBINEMIA
A. Increased bilirubin production	A. Intrahepatic disorder
1. Hemolysis	1. Hepatocellular disease of any cause (*eg*, viral hepatitis)
a. Erythrocyte abnormality (*eg*, hereditary spherocytosis, G-6-PD deficiency)	2. Cholestatic disease of any cause (*eg*, primary biliary cirrhosis)
b. Extracellular abnormality (*eg*, hypersplenism, immunohemolytic anemia)	3. Metabolic disorder
2. Ineffective erythropoiesis (*eg*, thalassemias)	a. Dubin-Johnson syndrome
3. Hematoma breakdown	b. Rotor syndrome
B. Decreased hepatic bilirubin clearance	c. Benign recurrent intrahepatic cholestasis
1. Neonatal hyperbilirubinemia	d. Cholestasis of pregnancy
2. Fasting	B. Extrahepatic disorder
3. Gilbert's syndrome	1. Biliary tract pathology (*eg*, tumor or stricture)
4. Crigler-Najjar syndromes	2. Pancreatic pathology (*eg*, carcinoma)

FIGURE 5-1.

Classification of jaundice according to the serum bilirubin measurement. Jaundice may be detected clinically when the serum bilirubin concentration exceeds 2.0 to 3.0 mg/dL. In this situation the separate quantitation of the serum unconjugated bilirubin concentration (indirect-reacting fraction) and conjugated bilirubin concentration (direct-reacting fraction) can be used to classify jaundice into two general categories that direct further evaluation. Conjugated hyperbilirubinemia is diagnosed when the direct-reacting fraction of serum bilirubin is increased. Because the diazo reaction does not precisely separate conjugated bilirubin from unconjugated bilirubin, some direct-reacting bilirubin will be measured even in normal individuals. Thus conjugated hyperbilirubinemia is present if the direct-reacting fraction of serum bilirubin exceeds 0.3 mg/dL when the total serum bilirubin level is below 2.0 mg/dL or is greater than 15% of the total serum bilirubin concentration when the level exceeds 2.0 mg/dL. Pure unconjugated hyperbilirubinemia is the diagnosis when the direct-reacting fraction of serum bilirubin is normal and the indirect-reacting fraction exceeds 1 mg/dL. The unconjugated bilirubin level may also be increased in those disorders that cause conjugated hyperbilirubinemia (*eg*, hemolysis from hypersplenism in cirrhosis).

JAUNDICE RELATED TO DRUGS

HEPATOCELLULAR PATTERN	CHOLESTATIC PATTERN	MIXED PATTERN
Isoniazid	Chlorpromazine (Geneva Pharmaceuticals, Broomfield, CO)	Sulfonamides
Methyldopa	Erythromycin estolate	
Acetaminophen	Anabolic steroids	

FIGURE 5-2.

Medications being taken should always be reviewed when evaluating the jaundiced patient. This table provides some examples of medications that have caused jaundice. Careful inquiry into use of over-the-counter medications, health foods, and nontraditional remedies, such as folk medicines, is important. Components of herbal teas such as germander or comfrey have caused liver disease and jaundice in unsuspecting patients. If in doubt as to whether a medication, health food, or remedy is causing the jaundice, the best course is to stop the suspected medication and follow-up with the patient. Improvement in liver chemistries is usually seen in 1 to 2 weeks if the discontinued medication is the offending agent.

ETIOLOGY OF JAUNDICE IN THE CRITICALLY ILL PATIENT

Hepatocellular pattern	Cholestatic pattern	Hyperbilirubinemia only	Mixed pattern
Liver ischemia	Parenteral nutrition	Transfusions Hematoma Hemolysis	Multiple coincidental factors
Congestive heart failure	Sepsis	Sepsis	Sepsis
Drugs	Drugs	Drugs	Drugs

Figure 5-3.

The differential diagnosis of jaundice in the critically ill patient is different from that of a patient presenting to the clinic with jaundice as the primary complaint [1]. Most often the critically ill patient has several reasons to be jaundiced. A careful history and physical examination are useful but most important is a careful review of the patient's hospital course. Particular attention should be directed to surgical procedures and the intraoperative course, episodes of hypotension, sepsis, medications, transfusions, evidence of heart failure, and feeding route. Any of these factors, alone or in combination, can cause jaundice. The jaundice is usually a marker of the severity of the underlying illness and not a sign of liver failure. Treatment is supportive and if the patient recovers from the primary illness, the jaundice will clear.

VIRAL HEPATITIS, FROM A THROUGH E

THE HUMAN HEPATITIS VIRUSES

Feature	HAV	HBV	HCV	HDV	HEV
Family	Picornavirus	Hepadnavirus	Flavivirus	Satellite	Alpha-like supergroup
Genome	RNA	DNA	RNA	RNA	RNA
Virion size, *nm*	27	42	55	35	32
Enveloped	No	HBsAg	Yes	HBsAg	No
Enteric transmission	Yes	No	No	No	Yes
Carrier state	No	Yes	Yes	Yes	No
Chronic hepatitis	No	Yes	Yes	Yes	No

Figure 5-4.

Human hepatitis viruses. The five known agents of viral hepatitis belong to distinct, and unrelated, classes of viruses. Four of the five viruses (hepatitis A virus [HAV], hepatitis C virus [HCV], hepatitis D virus [HDV], and hepatitis E virus [HEV]) are RNA-containing viruses whereas the fifth virus, hepatitis B virus (HBV), is a DNA-containing agent. The two nonenveloped agents, HAV and HEV, are characteristically transmitted through enteric routes of spread, and neither is associated with a carrier state of chronic hepatitis. In contrast, the enveloped viruses (HBV, HDV, and HCV) may lead to persistent infection and chronic hepatitis. HBsAg—hepatitis B surface antigen.

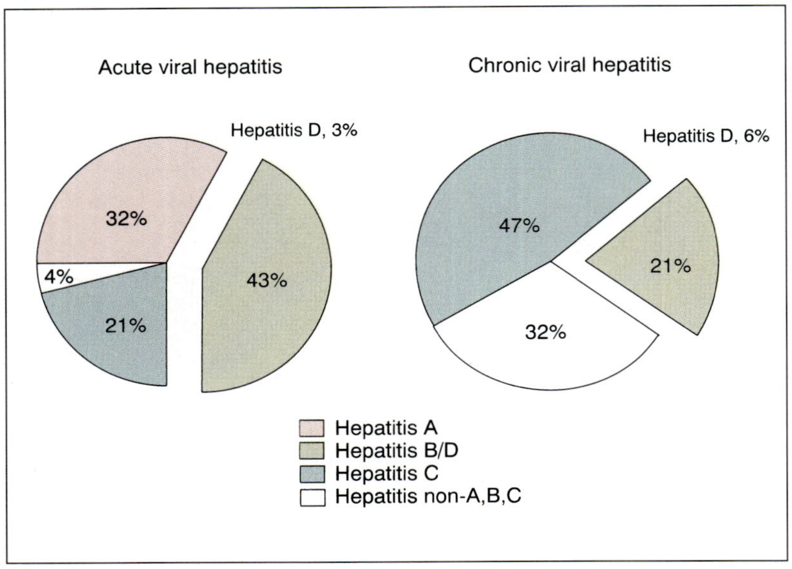

Figure 5-5.

Acute and chronic viral hepatitis proportioned by agent. These figures provide an overview of the relative contributions of each of the agents to acute and chronic viral hepatitis in the United States. Hepatitis E is not shown in the acute hepatitis pie chart because only a handful of cases of this imported infection are reported annually in the United States. The etiology of the small proportion of cases of acute hepatitis, labeled non-A,B,C, remains uncertain. As shown in the chronic viral hepatitis diagram, hepatitis A plays no role. Non-A,B,C is considerably more prevalent in chronic than acute hepatitis, but just as in the case of acute hepatitis, the responsible agent or agents remains to be identified. (*Adapted from* Alter and Hadler [2]; with permission.)

Hepatitis A

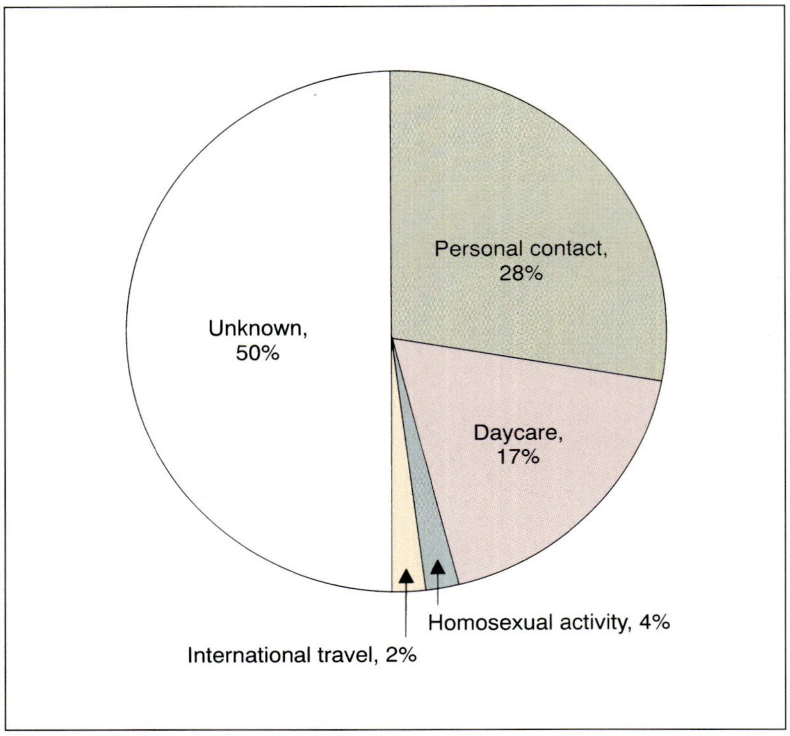

Figure 5-6.

Risk factors of acute hepatitis A virus infection. This diagram demonstrates results of an analysis of certain risk factors (sources of exposure) associated with hepatitis A in cases reported in four sentinel counties of the United States in 1992. Personal contact, usually with an infected household contact, was found in 28% of cases and an association with a day care center in 17%. Homosexual activity and international travel were less important factors. As shown, no risk factors could be identified in half of the cases. (*Adapted from* McQuillan *et al.* [3]; with permission.)

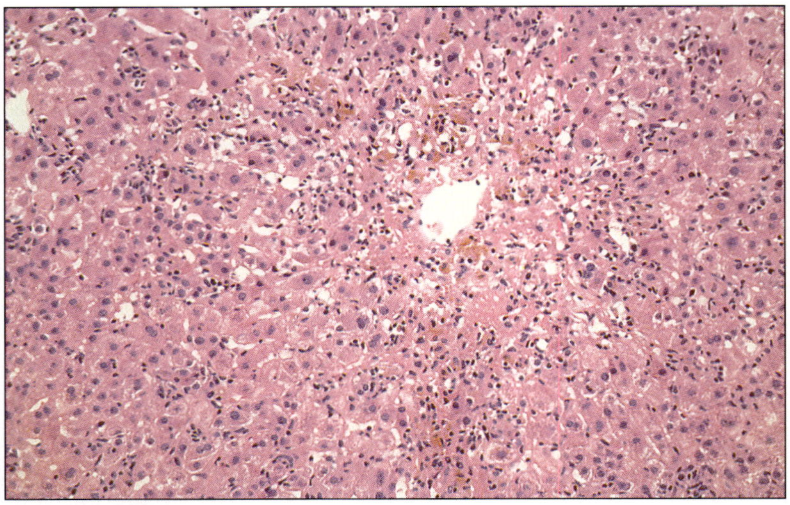

Figure 5-7.

Typical biopsy findings in viral hepatitis. Diffuse hepatocellular necrosis with marked histiocytic reaction and infiltration with polymorphonuclear cells and mononuclear cells. Areas of necrosis and inflammation are intermingled. Hematoxylin and eosin. (*Courtesy of* Z. Goodman, Washington, D.C.)

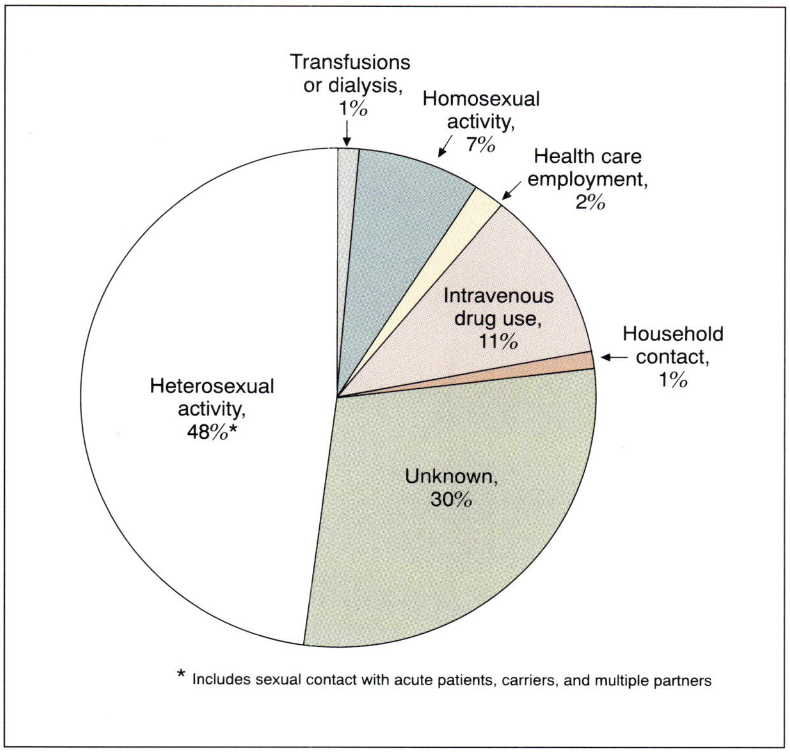

FIGURE 5-8.

Risk factors for infection with hepatitis B virus (HBV). This diagram depicts an analysis of risk factors (sources of exposure) associated with HBV in cases reported in four sentinel counties of the United States in 1992. The importance of sexual activity as a probable source of infection is reflected in the very large proportion of cases in which patients had heterosexual contact with acute cases, HBV carriers, and multiple sex partners. Homosexual activity was reported in 7% of cases and intravenous drug use in 11%. A small percentage of patients reported blood transfusion, dialysis, health care employment, or nonsexual household contact with known HBV cases. In 30% of cases, however, no known risk factors could be identified. (*Adapted from* McQuillan *et al.* [3]; with permission.)

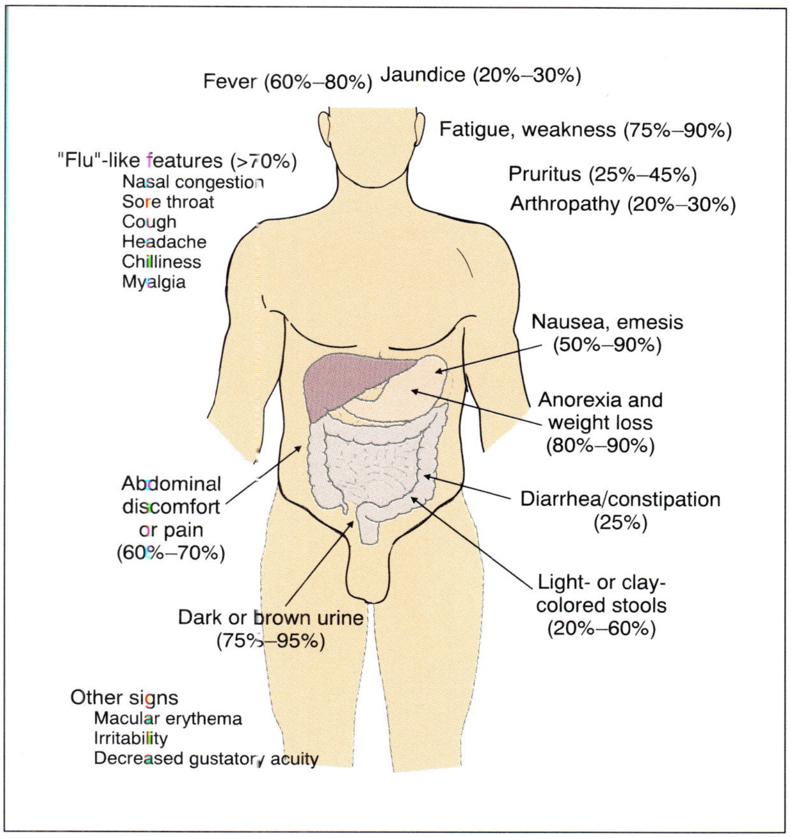

FIGURE 5-9.

Constellation of symptoms reported by patients with acute hepatitis B. Most patients experiencing an acute HBV infection will have a nonicteric or asymptomatic illness [4]. The frequency of recognized acute hepatitis B is correlated to age at the time of infection as shown in Figure 4-8. Adults are more likely to manifest evidence of illness, whereas infants and children rarely do. Patients who do not have icterus in the presence or absence of symptoms are at higher risk for developing chronic disease [5]. Although only a quarter of patients will become clinically jaundiced [6], a larger proportion will report evidence consistent with a cholestatic process by describing changes in color of urine and stool. Most symptoms experienced by patients are protean and frequently attributed to a nonspecific "viral" syndrome.

DIAGNOSTIC INTERPRETATIONS OF HBV MARKERS

HBV Marker	Description	Implications
HBsAg	Noninfectious component of viral coat	Considered the *sine qua non* for acute and chronic infection; it may, however, also be present in the absence of HBV replication, produced by cells with integrated HBV DNA coding for HBsAg; loss of HBsAg accepted as hallmark of recovery
Anti-HBs	Antibody response to HBsAg	Usually indicates recovery and immunity to HBV; it is the protective antibody resulting from vaccination with HBsAg material; also may be present in acute disease or as an inconstant finding in nearly a third of patients with chronic infection [45]
HBeAg	Soluble antigen that correlates with HBV replication and infectivity	Presence in serum signals high level of infectivity because it parallels viral replication; may disappear before or after loss of serum HBV DNA with disease remission; sustained loss of HBeAg in the presence or absence of Anti-HBe with continuing viral replication (HBV DNA) may presage emergence of an HBeAg–negative "mutant" virus
Anti-HBe	Antibody response to HBeAg; not considered protective	Presence suggests decreasing levels of viral replication and HBV DNA and also indicates move towards disease remission or resolution
HBcAg	Found in core of virus	No practical purpose for detecting in serum; HBeAg and HBV DNA are surrogate markers
Anti-HBc IgM	Nonprotective antibody to the HBcAg	Present in recent HBV infection; may recur in reactivation of a chronic hepatitis
Anti-HBc IgG	As above	Presence indicative of acute, chronic, or remote HBV infection; however, titers can decline over many years to undetectable levels; not present in individuals immunized to HBV
HBV DNA	Replicative genetic material of HBV; infectious agent	Presence in serum (by non-PCR methodologies) correlates to viral replication and continued infection; disappears with complete resolution of disease; may become undetectable in disease remission only to emerge once again with disease activation; the significance of its presence in serum as detected only by PCR is unclear

FIGURE 5-10.

A detailed medical history and complete physical examination are key for interpreting the significance of test results for hepatitis B virus (HBV) components (HBV DNA, hepatitis B surface antigen [HBsAg], hepatitis B e antigen [HBeAg], hepatitis B core antigen [HBcAg]) or host immune responses to the virus (antibodies to HBsAg [Anti-HBs], antibodies to HBeAg [Anti-HBe], antibodies to HBcAg [Anti-HBc]) in patients suspected to be infected with HBV. Positive test results for one or several HBV markers may indicate an acute process or raise suspicion of a chronic infection [7]. For example, very recent vaccination for HBV might yield a positive test for HBsAg, suggesting acute disease or a carrier state. Discovery of a HBsAg–negative and Anti-HBs–positive status does not confirm a previous HBV infection but could indicate past HBV vaccination. Clarification of this issue would be achieved by taking an immunization history and a negative test for Anti-HBc immunoglobulin G (IgG). The potential implications associated with the identification of specific HBV markers are shown. IgM—immunoglobulin M; PCR—polymerase chain reaction.

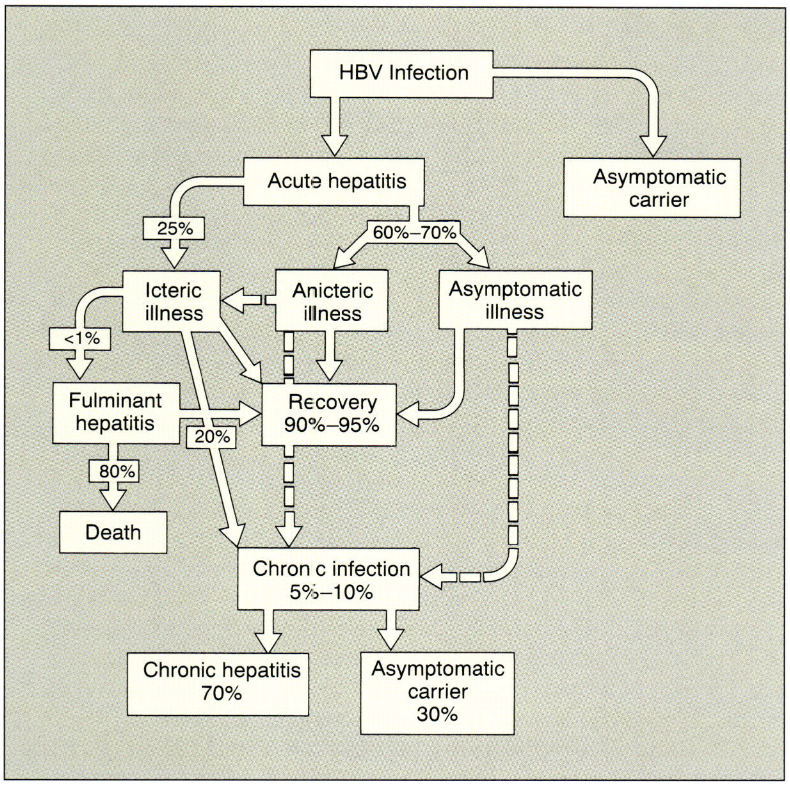

FIGURE 5-11.

Consequences of infection with hepatitis B virus (HBV). Most individuals who are exposed to the HBV will develop acute hepatitis. Those who become icteric are readily diagnosed; many who are anicteric but still display symptoms of illness may be identified. An additional asymptomatic group of patients exists who have abnormalities of one or several biochemical tests but do not exhibit symptoms and thus escape initial detection. The proportion of asymptomatic cases of acute HBV is problematic. Although patients with anicteric or asymptomatic hepatitis bear increased risk for progressing to chronicity [5], the overwhelming majority of patients with acute hepatitis recover without sequelae. A small proportion of patients experience a particularly effective immune clearance of infected hepatocytes that can result in fulminant disease. Although the survival rate is dismal in the absence of orthotopic liver transplantation, survival rates are highest when patients are less than 45 years of age [4]. Most patients with chronic infection have a chronic hepatitis, whereas a smaller proportion of chronically infected individuals manifest an asymptomatic carrier state.

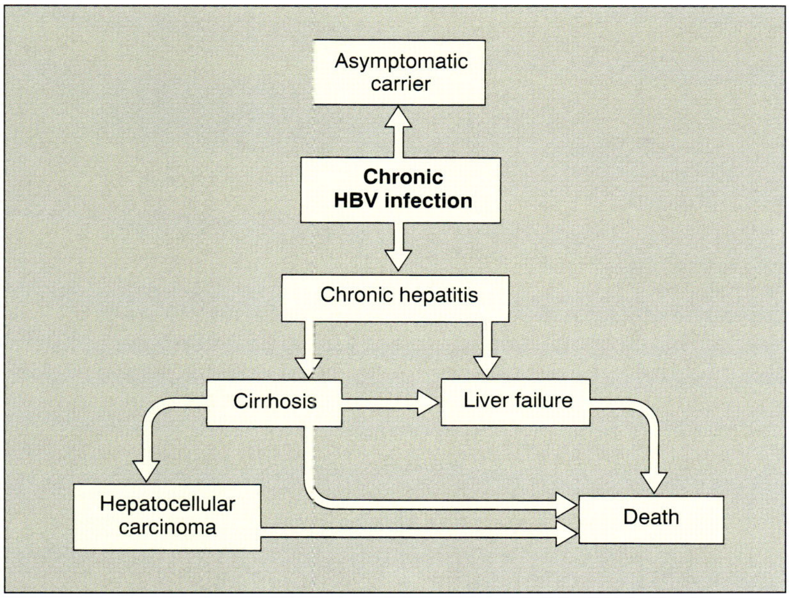

FIGURE 5-12.

Consequences of chronic hepatitis B. Chronic infection with HBV can result in the development of a chronic carrier state with little or no evidence of liver injury or progression to a chronic necroinflammatory condition. Chronic hepatitis may lead to hepatic failure over a relatively short time interval in the presence or absence of cirrhosis [8]. Alternatively, cirrhosis may result with subsequent development of hepatocellular carcinoma or hepatic failure [5].

DIFFERENTIAL DIAGNOSIS OF CHRONIC HEPATITIS

Viral hepatitis
- Hepatitis B
- Hepatitis C
- Hepatitis D
- Hepatitis non-A, non-B, non-C?

Autoimmune liver disease

Drug induced
- Wilson's disease

Cryptogenic

Chronic liver disease–not considered chronic hepatitis
- Primary biliary cirrhosis
- Primary sclerosing cholangitis
- Hemochromatosis
- α_1-Antitrypsin deficiency

FIGURE 5-13.

Patients displaying serologic evidence suggestive of hepatitis B virus (HBV) infection are at a comparable risk for developing other forms of acute or chronic liver disease to that seen in HBV–negative individuals. Admittedly, an index of suspicion is necessary to justify additional evaluation of patients who satisfactorily fulfill the diagnostic criteria for chronic HBV. The etiology to account for chronic hepatitis remains undetermined in 10% to 25% of patients and is referred to as "cryptogenic" [9,10]. Nonetheless, consideration must be given to concomitant extant diseases and, where indicated, appropriate assessment must be undertaken. A group of hepatic disorders such as primary biliary cirrhosis and primary sclerosing cholangitis exist, which may share features with the syndrome of chronic hepatitis but are not considered examples of that syndrome.

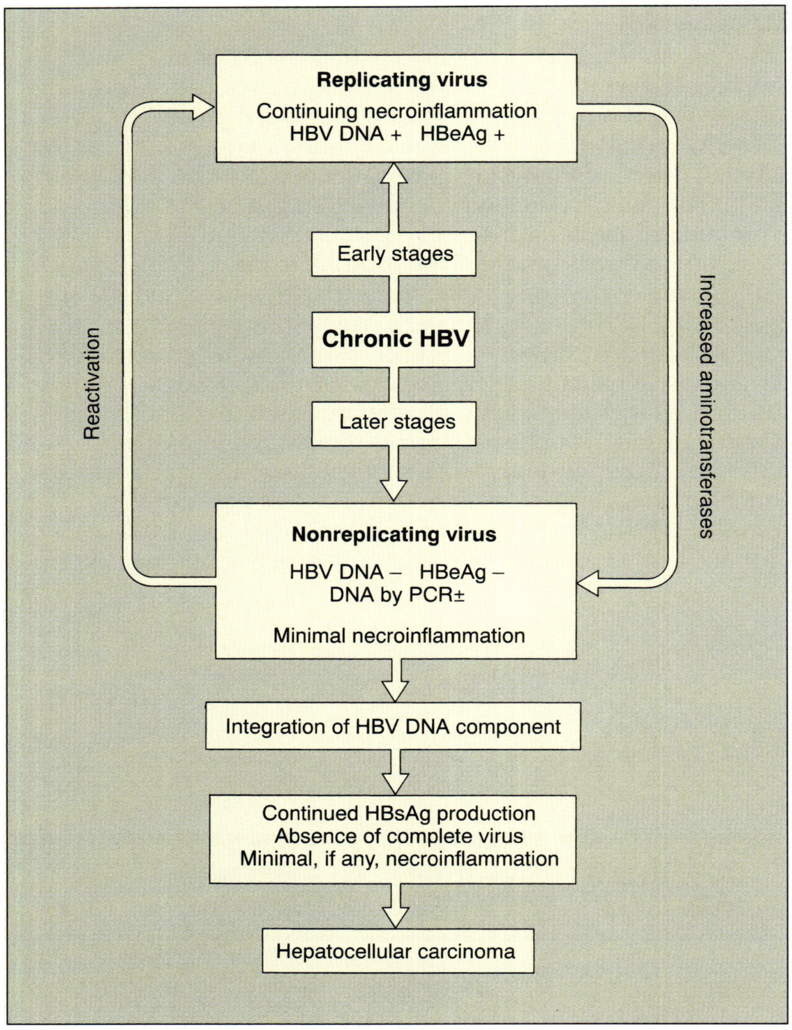

FIGURE 5-14.

Natural history of chronic hepatitis B. With the advent of effective therapy, changes in the natural history of chronic hepatitis can be predicted, and although indications exist that such alterations have taken place in patients responding to treatment, accurate information on the nature and extent of disease modification will require many years of follow-up. Review of data from the preinterferon era has provided information on the long-term consequences of chronic hepatitis B virus (HBV) infection. In the early stages of disease characterized by viral replication and necroinflammation, continuing injury to the liver may result in irreversible damage in the presence, or absence, of cirrhosis. In time, the virus may lose the ability to replicate, usually signalled by loss of hepatitis B e antigen (HBeAg) and HBV DNA and accompanied by a transient increase in necroinflammation [11]. Some of these patients will harbor small quantities of HBV DNA detectable only by polymerase chain reaction (PCR) technology. Such individuals will, after variable time intervals and for undetermined reasons, reactivate their disease once again, thus producing HBeAg and larger amounts of HBV DNA. This relapse can result in additional liver damage which can lead to hepatic failure [11–13]. Other patients in the nonreplicating phase of disease may integrate part of the HBV genome resulting in the production of hepatitis B surface antigen (HBsAg) only, with no concomitant viral replication [14]. In such a setting there is little inflammation, however, the risks of developing hepatocellular carcinoma are increased [14,15].

CONSENSUS FINDINGS OF THERAPEUTIC TRIALS WITH INTERFERON

- Loss of serum HBV DNA and HBeAg in approximately one-third of patients
- Response associated with improvement in liver histology
- Response associated with improvement in aminotransferases
- Successful response requires treatment for a minimum of 3 months
- Dosages of 5 to 10 MU are sufficient to suppress viral replication
- Dosages of 1 or 2 MU are inadequate
- Three times weekly administration of IFN is effective for suppressing viral replication and is better tolerated than daily administration

FIGURE 5-15.

Interferon (IFN) treatment of chronic hepatitis B. IFN-α is at present the most effective treatment for chronic hepatitis B. It is the only drug approved for use in the United States, based in part on the landmark randomized controlled trial wherein IFN-α_{2b} was proven of benefit in the treatment of chronic hepatitis B [16]. A recent meta-analysis [17], which reviewed treatment outcomes in 16 prospective, randomized, controlled studies (including that of Perillo and coworkers [16]), showed that IFN-α was beneficial with loss of hepatitis B surface antigen observed 6% more often in treated patients than in controls. Loss of hepatitis B virus (HBV) replication (hepatitis B e antigen [HBeAg], HBV DNA) occurred 20% more often and normalization of alanine transaminase values was seen at a significantly higher frequency in IFN-treated patients [17]. Numerous therapeutic trials conducted between 1985 and 1990 permit a consensus of findings [18]. The overall treatment response rates were remarkably similar among the listed studies. Various types of IFN-α were used—recombinant as well as natural forms.

ADVERSE EFFECTS OF INTERFERON

Fatigue, malaise, chills	Suppression of bone marrow elements
Alopecia	Autoantibodies
Anorexia, nausea	Interferon neutralizing antibodies
Significant depression, difficulty sleeping	Infections
Emotional lability	Decreased libido

FIGURE 5-16.

Almost all patients receiving interferon will experience some type of adverse effect. Most of these individuals will tolerate these difficulties, motivated by the desire to be rid of the disease. Modification in dose may be necessary, particularly if symptoms become debilitating or if compliance with treatment is threatened. Some patients must discontinue therapy when hematologic problems arise [18,19].

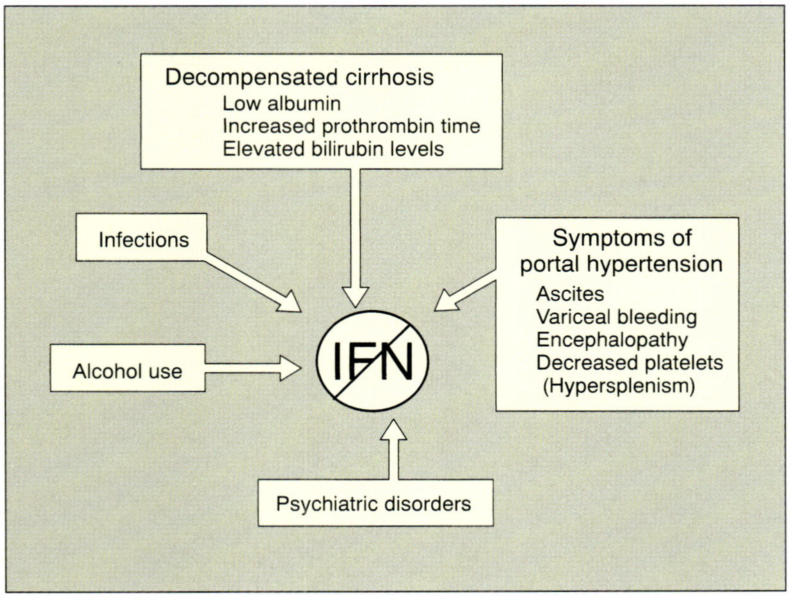

FIGURE 5-17.

Contraindications for engaging in interferon (IFN) therapy. There are patients at increased risk of suffering a calamitous experience when undergoing standard IFN therapy for chronic hepatitis B. Patients with decompensated cirrhosis [20] have little hepatic reserve to sustain what may represent a major inflammatory process that is instrumental in clearance of the virus. Evidence of a predisposition towards liver failure include findings of low albumin levels, increased prothrombin time, and elevated bilirubin. Signs of portal hypertension portend danger when ascites, encephalopathy, episodes of esophageal or gastric variceal bleeding, and hematologic abnormalities are present. Use of IFN in such patients may also promote severe infections particularly if leukocyte counts are low. Continued consumption of alcohol is also a contraindication either when starting treatment or for continuing therapy when informed of the alcohol intake. Finally, clinically relevant psychiatric dysfunction may be aggravated by IFN.

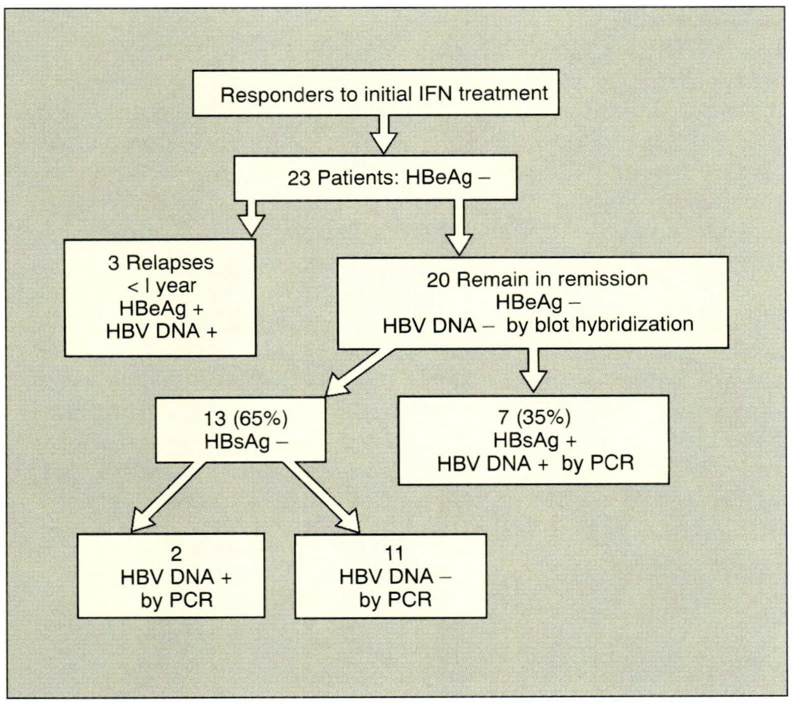

FIGURE 5-18.

Long-term outcomes for responders to interferon (IFN). Most of the clinical trials to assess IFN efficacy have evaluated patients over the course of 1 to 2 years. Recurrence of hepatitis B virus (HBV) replication has been reported in 5% to 50% of responders within the 1st year and in 10% to 20% of patients during the 2nd year of follow-up [18,21]. Furthermore, despite seroconversion to a hepatitis B surface antigen (HBsAg)–negative and antibodies to HBsAg–positive condition in patients, low levels of HBV DNA can be identified indefinitely in liver tissue [22]. Although traces of the HBV DNA can be retained for long periods in the liver, the significance of this observation remains unknown. What is clear is that patients responding to IFN are not likely to reactivate nor to demonstrate findings of chronic inflammation in the liver. Clearly, the disease in such responders has entered a stage of remission (forever, it is hoped) and such people behave as if they are free of disease. Twenty three (36%) of 64 patients responding to IFN and followed for a mean of 4.3 years at the National Institutes of Health (NIH) are presented [23]. As shown, 65% of patients with sustained loss of hepatitis B e antigen (HBeAg) lost HBsAg. Other studies from Spain report a 24% seroconversion to HBsAg–negative status and in a study of Chinese patients, no patients lost HBsAg during a follow-up period similar to that of the NIH study [24,25]. PCR—polymerase chain reaction.

Hepatitis D

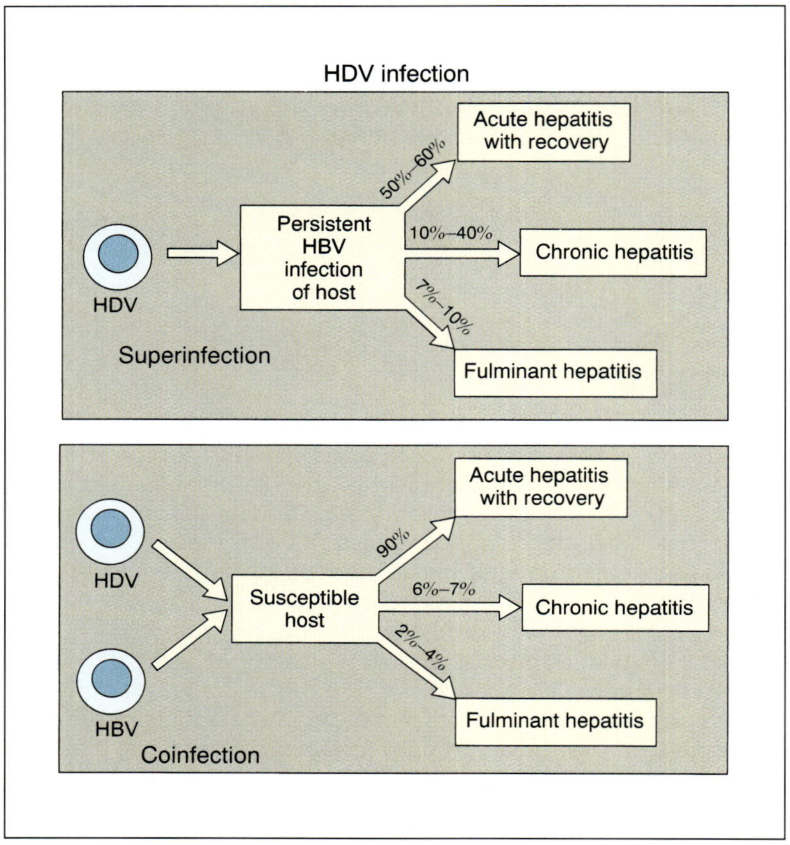

FIGURE 5-19.

Hepatitis D virus (HDV). The virus superinfects patients with hepatitis B infection or coinfects the host together with hepatitis B. In general, the sequelae of HDV infection are more serious when superinfection of the host with persistent hepatitis B virus (HBV) infection occurs. As shown in the *upper panel*, superinfection is associated with a risk of chronic hepatitis in 10% to 40% of patients; fulminant disease is seen in 7% to 10%. In contrast, as shown in the *lower panel*, HDV and HBV coinfections are less often associated with grave outcomes. Only 6% to 7% coinfections lead to chronic hepatitis and only 2% to 4% end with fulminant hepatitis. (*Adapted from* Conjeevaram and DiBisceglie [26]; with permission.)

Hepatitis C

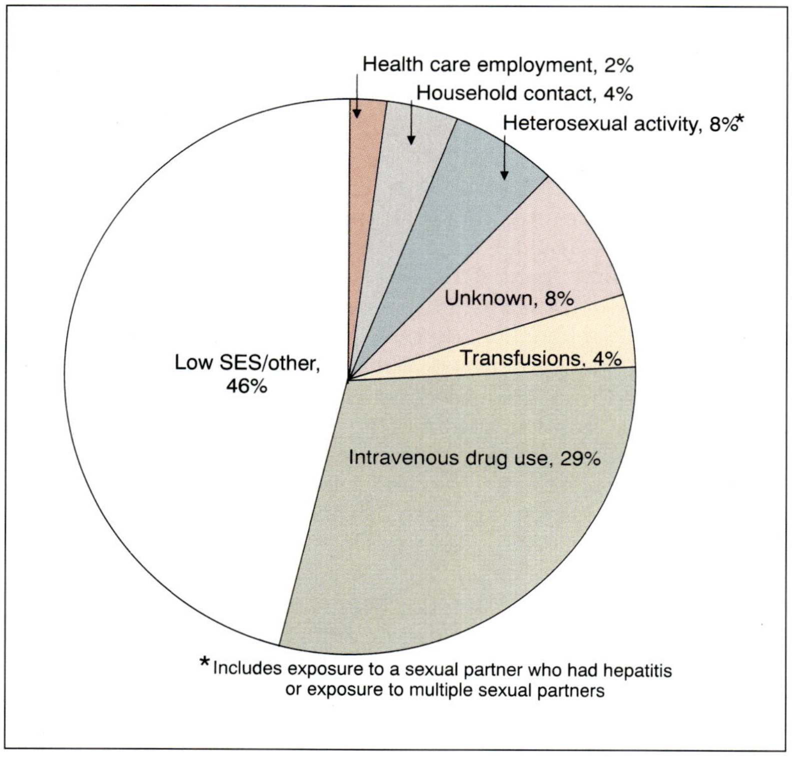

FIGURE 5-20.

Risk factors associated with acute hepatitis C virus (HCV). As shown in this diagram, based on data collected by the Centers for Disease Control and Prevention in their four sentinel county study in 1992, 29% of reported acute HCV infections were associated with intravenous drug use and 4% were associated with blood transfusion. Thus, a third of reported cases could be linked with bloodborne modes of transmission. Twelve percent could be linked with either heterosexual activity or household contact, which includes exposure to a sexual partner or household member with hepatitis or with exposure to multiple sexual partners. Health care employment was identified in 2% of cases. Although only 6% had no distinguishing risk factor or exposure history, nearly half of reported cases were in patients from low socioeconomic status (SES) levels or who reported so-called "high-risk" behaviors or contacts, but not in the 6 months before the onset of illness. The significance of low SES and high-risk indicators remains to be established. (*Adapted from* McQuillan *et al.* [3]; with permission.)

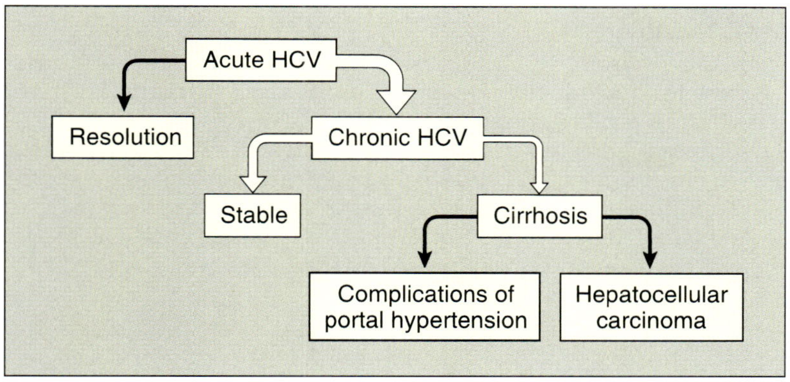

FIGURE 5-21.

Evolution of acute hepatitis. The natural history of hepatitis C virus (HCV) is not fully known. At least 80% of infected patients will develop chronic disease. Cirrhosis occurs in 20% to 40% of chronic HCV patients and in 16% to 32% of all patients infected with HCV. Complications of cirrhosis and hepatocellular carcinoma develop in 4% to 8% of infected patients. The time course to the development of cirrhosis and its complications is highly variable [27–30].

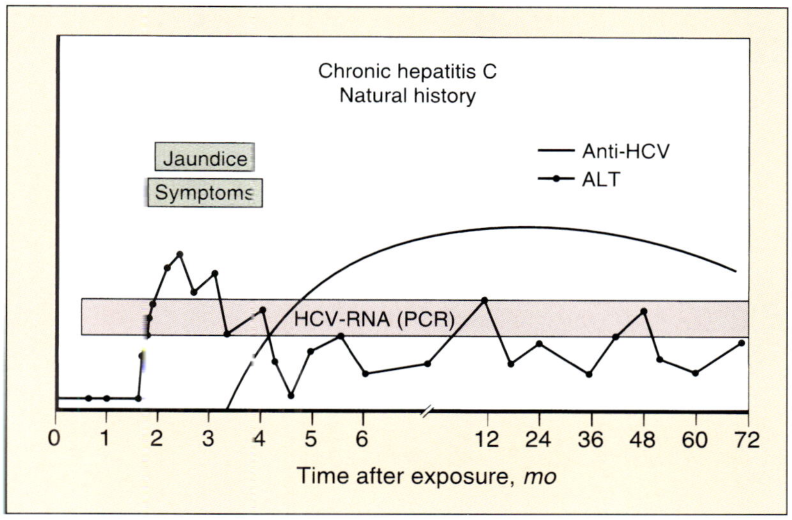

FIGURE 5-22.

Serologic sequence in chronic hepatitis C virus (HCV). HCV-RNA appears approximately 2 to 4 weeks after exposure. Symptoms and jaundice may appear 6 to 24 weeks after exposure. Antibody to HCV (Anti-HCV) appears 12 to 14 weeks after exposure and its presence is lifelong. Anti-HCV does not denote chronicity or active infection. HCV-RNA denotes active disease. Nevertheless, most patients do not present during the acute phase of the illness but instead are diagnosed years later with chronic HCV [31,32]. ALT—alanine aminotransferase; PCR—polymerase chain reaction. (*Adapted from* Hoofnagle [33]; with permission.)

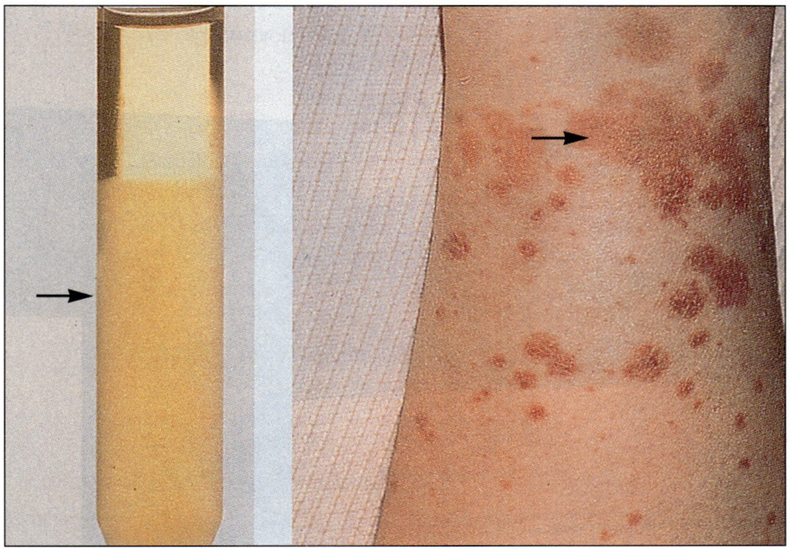

FIGURE 5-23.

Vasculitis and cryoglobulinemia related to hepatitis C virus. Mixed essential cryoglobulinemia has been associated with many chronic liver diseases. However, there appears to be an abnormally high prevalence of cryoglobulinemia in patients with hepatitis C. The figure on the **right** depicts an area of palpable purpura approximately 2 by 3 cm on the medial aspect of the lower extremity of a patient with hepatitis C (*arrow*). The photograph on the **left** shows uncentrifuged serum after 48 hours at 4°C with the *arrow* indicating cryoprecipitate [34–36].

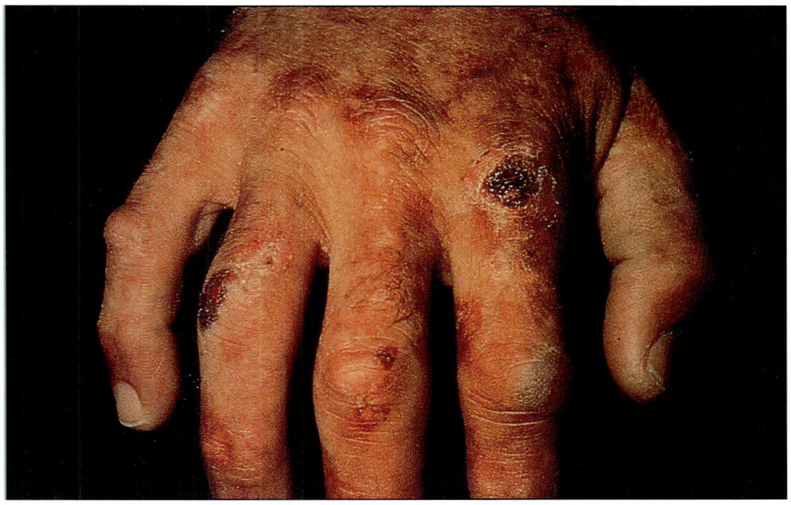

FIGURE 5-24.

Porphyria cutanea tarda. Fifty percent of cases of porphyria cutanea tarda in the United States are positive for antibodies to hepatitis C virus. Furthermore, many cases of chronic hepatitis C have histologic evidence of increased iron depositions in the liver. Preliminary studies suggest that iron overload impedes interferon therapy for chronic hepatitis [37–39].

PREDICTORS OF RESPONSE
Serum HCV-RNA levels
Genotype 1b
Hepatic iron concentration
Cirrhosis
Duration of illness
? Total dose of interferon

FIGURE 5-25.

Predictors of response. Factors associated with a favorable response to interferon include the presence of a low serum hepatitis C virus (HCV)-RNA level, genotype other than 1b, normal hepatic iron concentration, the absence of cirrhosis, and a relatively short duration of chronic hepatitis. Treatment regimens with higher doses or longer durations of interferon therapy than the licensed regimen in the United States (3 MU three times a week for 6 months) have been associated with more favorable response rates [40–43].

AUTOIMMUNE HEPATITIS

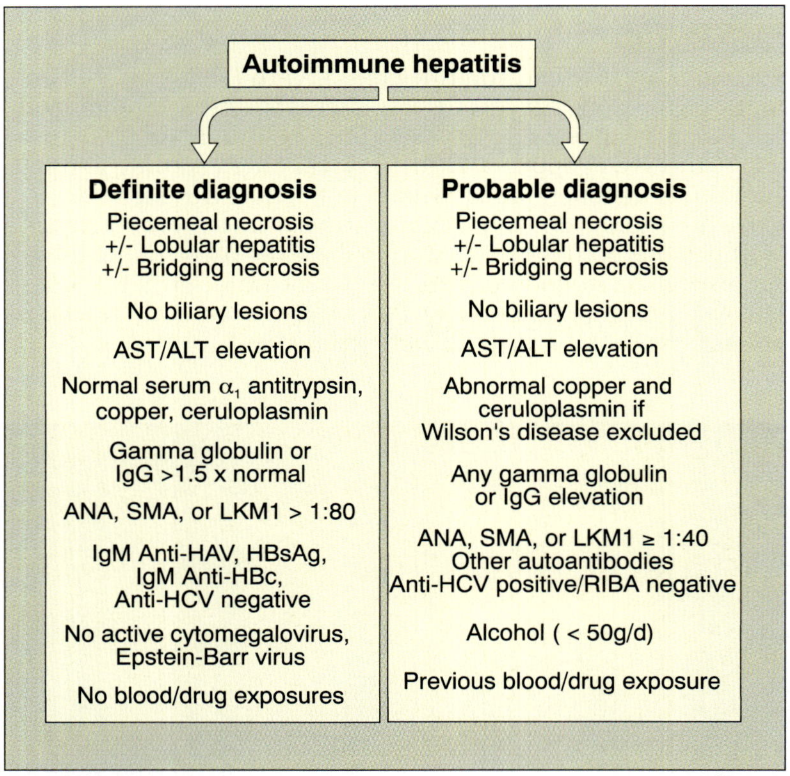

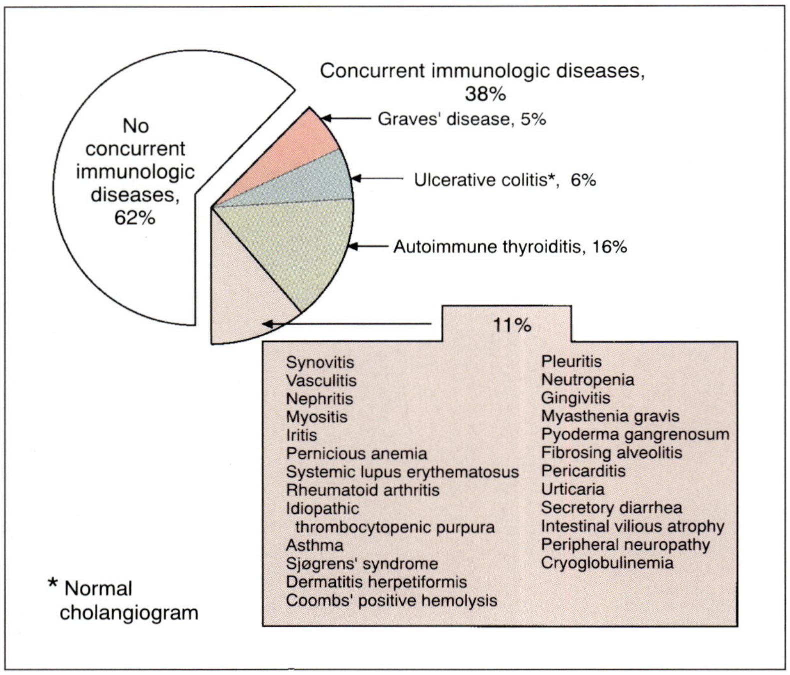

FIGURE 5-26.

Diagnostic criteria for autoimmune hepatitis. The International Autoimmune Hepatitis Group met for the first time in Brighton, England, in June 1992. This panel formulated the criteria for a definite and probable diagnosis of autoimmune hepatitis [44]. The 6-month criterion of disease activity to establish chronicity was waived. Levels of significant hypergammaglobulinemia and autoantibody titer were described, and elimination factors were strictly defined [60]. Lobular hepatitis was accepted within the spectrum of the disease. Laboratory and histologic features of cholestasis precluded the definite diagnosis as did markers of true viral infection [60]. The criteria recognized the possibility of an acute, even fulminant, onset of the disease and permitted the diagnosis even in those patients without conventional immunoserologic markers [60]. ALT—alanine aminotransferase; ANA—antinuclear antibodies; Anti-HAV—antibodies to hepatitis A virus; Anti-HBc—antibodies to hepatitis B core antigen; Anti-HCV—antibodies to hepatitis C virus; AST—aspartate aminotransferase; HBsAg—hepatitis B surface antigen; IgG—immunoglobin G; IgM—immunoglobin M; LKM1—liver-kidney microsome type 1; RIBA—recombinant immunoblot assay; SMA—smooth muscle antibodies.

FIGURE 5-27.

Concurrent immunologic diseases in type 1 autoimmune hepatitis. Autoimmune thyroiditis is the most common associated immune disease [45–47]. The presence of ulcerative colitis does not compel the diagnosis of primary sclerosing cholangitis (PSC), but it does mandate the performance of cholangiography [48]. Forty-two percent of patients with type 1 autoimmune hepatitis and ulcerative colitis have cholangiographic features of PSC and recalcitrance to corticosteroid therapy [48]. Patients with concurrent immunologic diseases commonly have the HLA DR4 [47,49].

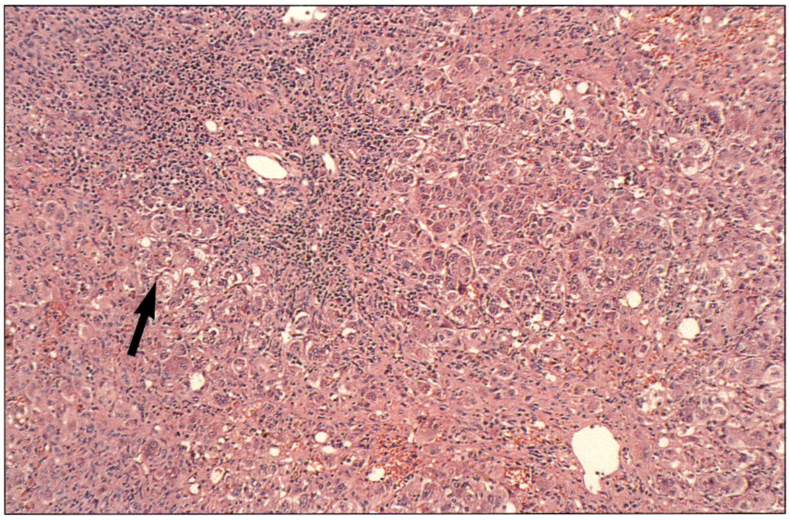

FIGURE 5-28.

Histologic findings of periportal hepatitis and bridging necrosis in severe type 1 autoimmune hepatitis (hematoxylin and eosin; original magnification, ×100). The histologic hallmark of autoimmune hepatitis is periportal hepatitis (piecemeal necrosis), which is the *sine qua non* of the disease [50]. It is defined as disruption of the limiting plate of the portal tract by inflammatory infiltrate (*arrow*). Gamma globulin deposits were found in hepatic mesenchymal cells in association with lymphocytes, plasma cells, histocytes, and proliferated bile ductules, and the character of the lesion suggested an immunologically mediated cytodestructive process [51]. The specificity of piecemeal necrosis for autoimmune hepatitis is no longer recognized [44]. Extension of the inflammatory activity between portal tracts (portal–portal bridging necrosis) or between portal tracts and central vein (portal–central bridging necrosis) connotes a more severe lesion with a greater propensity for progression to cirrhosis [50]. Portal–central bridging has a higher predilection for cirrhosis than portal–portal bridging, but in most instances the lesions are of mixed character or indeterminate because of sampling variation [50].

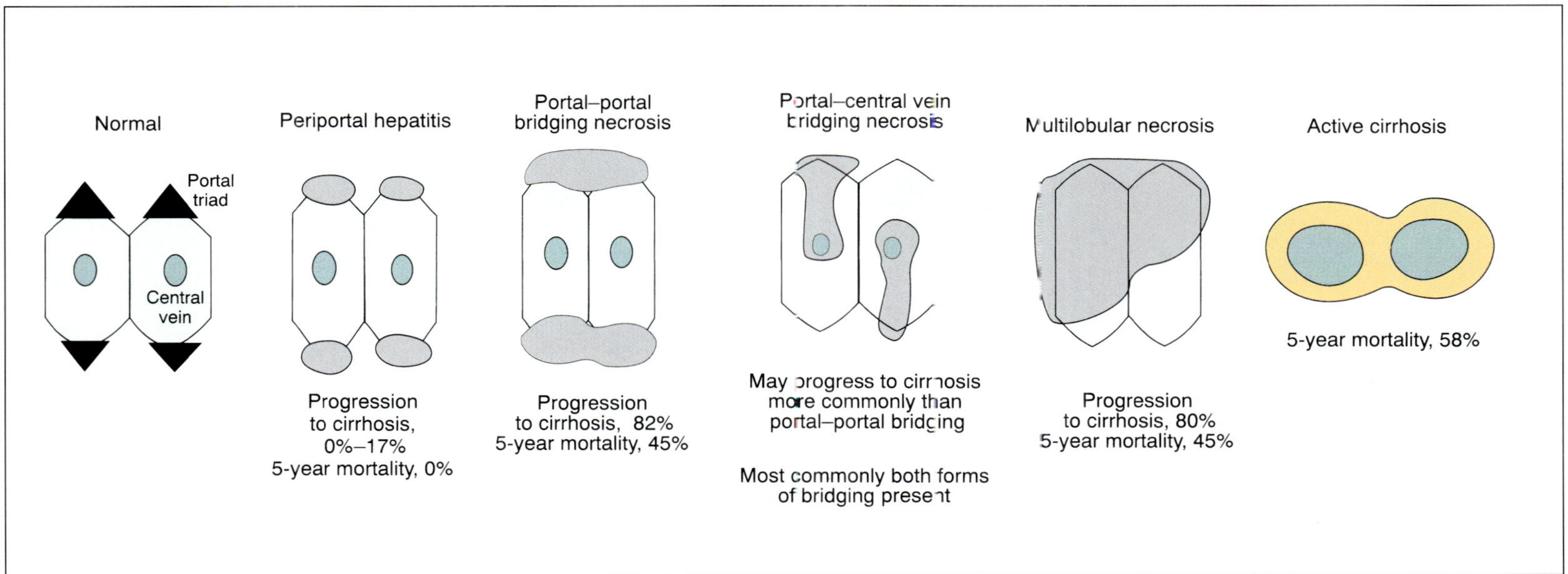

FIGURE 5-29.

Prognoses of initial histologic patterns in untreated type 1 autoimmune hepatitis. The severity and aggressiveness of the inflammatory process can be estimated by the histologic pattern at presentation [50,52]. The type and degree of hepatic inflammation can be assessed by needle biopsy with 90% accuracy [50]. Sampling variation and intraobserver interpretive error limit the ability of needle biopsy to evaluate cirrhosis [50]. Portal–portal and portal–central bridging necrosis are frequently mixed findings or are difficult to distinguish. Periportal hepatitis, which is the hallmark lesion of autoimmune hepatitis, typically has a benign prognosis and does not require therapy per se [50,53]. Transitions can occur between the various histologic patterns spontaneously or during therapy [50,53].

RECOMMENDED PREDNISONE TREATMENT SCHEDULES FOR AUTOIMMUNE HEPATITIS

	Daily doses alone, *mg*	Daily doses with 50 mg azathioprine
Week 1	60	30
Week 2	40	20
Week 3	30	15
Week 4	30	15
Until endpoint	20	10

Figure 5-30.

Regimens are designed to control inflammatory activity rapidly with high initial doses. The dose of prednisone is then reduced systematically over a 4-week period until a fixed daily maintenance dose is achieved [50,53–55]. Laboratory tests are performed at the 2-week and 3-month intervals to document disease response [54]. Dose reduction does not have to be monitored by frequent laboratory tests. After 3 months, testing at 6-month intervals is appropriate [54]. The daily maintenance dose should not be reduced until histologic remission is achieved. Treatment failure or major drug toxicity are the only indications for interim dose adjustments [50,55].

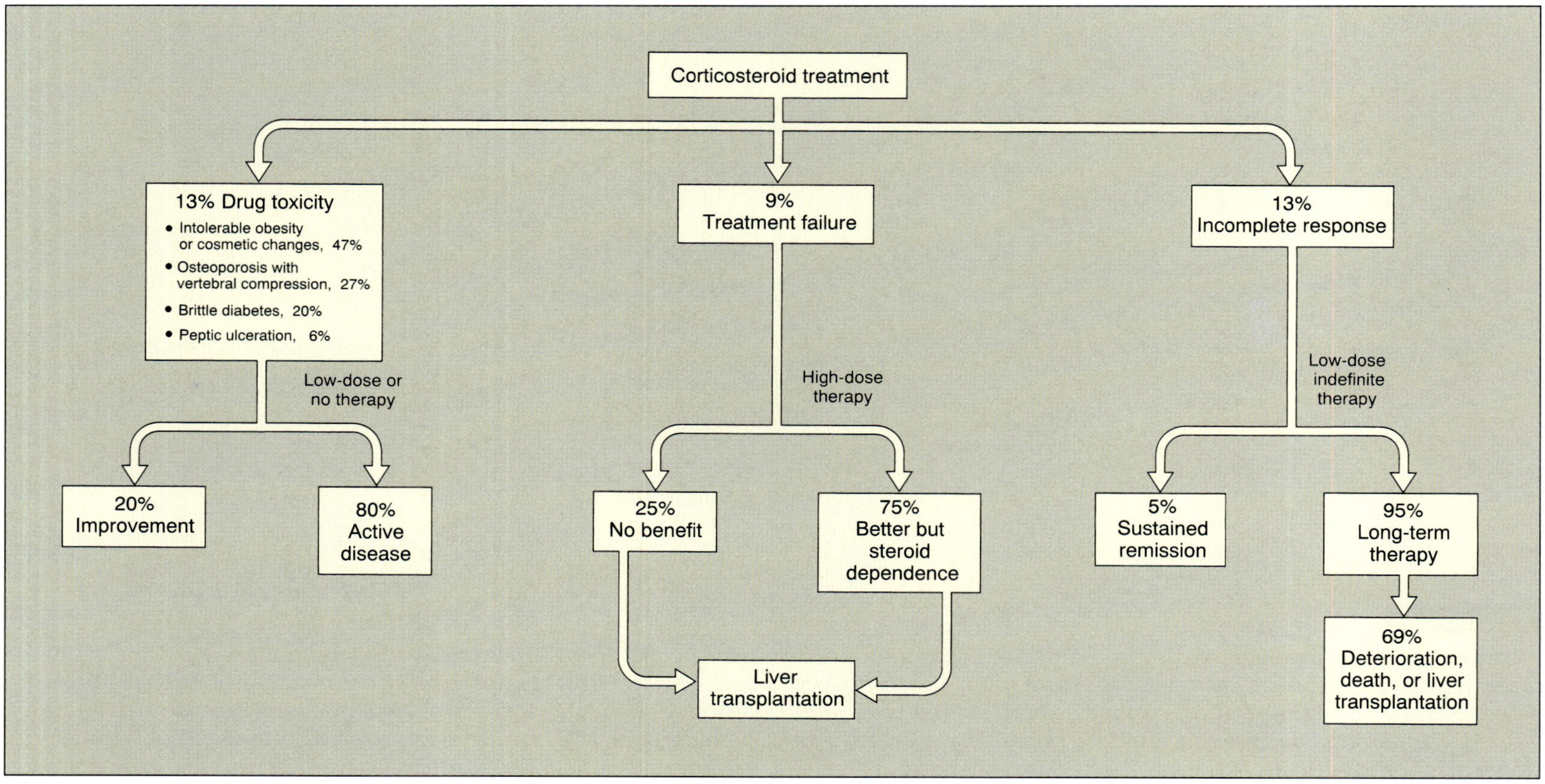

Figure 5-31.

Adverse responses to corticosteroid therapy and treatment strategies. Patients may develop serious drug toxicities, deteriorate despite compliance with the treatment regimen (*ie*, treatment failure), or fail to achieve remission after protracted therapy (*ie*, incomplete response) [50]. These outcomes justify changes in the original treatment strategy. Liver transplantation is an option for the decompensated patient [56].

PRINCIPAL CAUSES OF ACUTE LIVER FAILURE

VIRAL HEPATITIS
A, B, D, E, F, herpes simplex virus

DRUG-RELATED LIVER INJURY
Acetaminophen, idiosyncratic drug reactions

TOXINS
CCl_4, *Amanita phalloides*, phosphorus

VASCULAR
Ischemic, venoocclusive, heat stroke, malignant infiltration

MISCELLANEOUS
Wilson's disease, acute fatty liver of pregnancy

FIGURE 5-32.

Etiology of acute liver failure is important because it determines prognosis. In many instances, radically differing initial management is required for each. Disease-specific treatments include antidotes to acetaminophen and mushroom poisoning that must be given immediately upon patient admission to the hospital. Identification of severe heart failure as the cause of acute liver failure will lead to proper resuscitation and correction of any fluid balance disturbance. Likewise, recognition of acute fatty liver of pregnancy will lead to consideration of delivery of the mother as the logical treatment for this condition. Patients with fulminant Wilson's disease carry such a bad prognosis that urgent consideration for transplantation must be immediately undertaken after diagnosis is made.

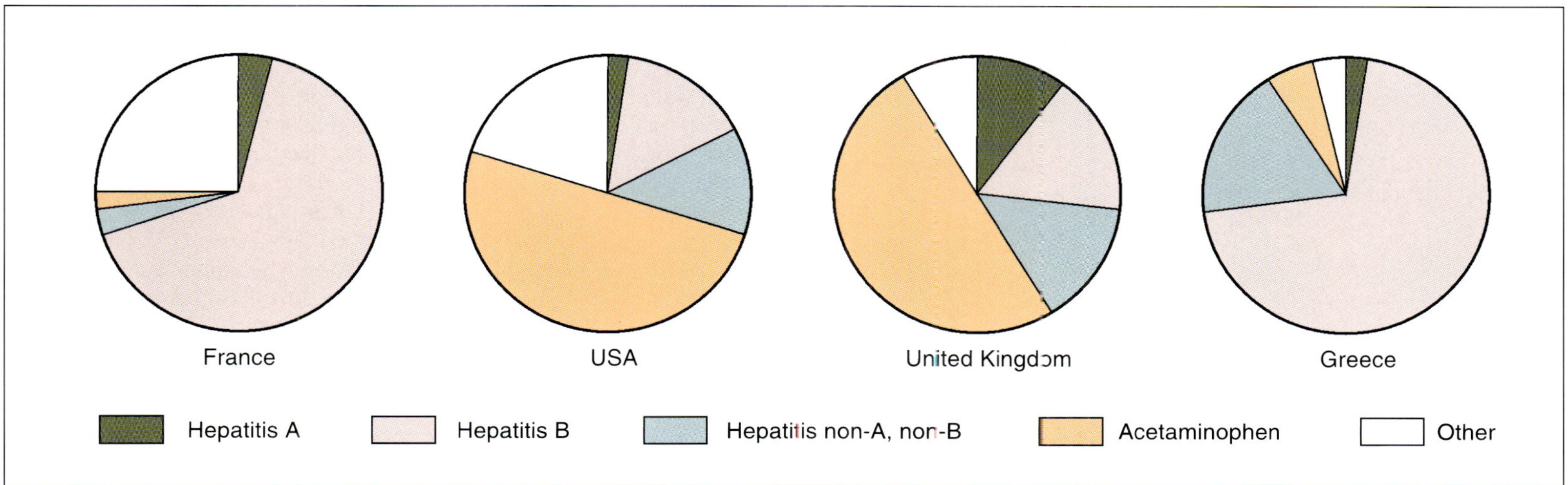

FIGURE 5-33.

Estimated prevalence of the most common causes of acute liver failure worldwide. Great variation is observed between the United Kingdom (high prevalence of acetaminophen toxicity) and Greece (predominantly hepatitis B). Overall, viral hepatitis is the most common cause of acute liver failure outside the United Kingdom. Nevertheless, an increasing number of cases of acetaminophen toxicity is occurring in the United States. Although generally less severe, these cases may account for more than 50% of patient hospital admissions for acute liver failure in certain urban areas [57]. No extensive epidemiologic data concerning this condition are available.

DRUGS IMPLICATED IN IDIOSYNCRATIC LIVER INJURY LEADING TO ACUTE LIVER FAILURE

Infrequent but not rare	Rare	Combination agents with enhanced toxicity
Isoniazid	Carbamazepine	Alcohol-acetaminophen
Valproate	Ofloxacin	Trimethoprim-sulfamethoxazole
Halothane	Ketoconazole	Rifampicin-isoniazid
Phenytoin	Lisinopril	Amoxicillin-clavulanic acid
Sulfonamides	Nicotinic acid	
Propylthiouracil	Labetalol	
Amiodarone	Etoposide (VP-16)	
Disulfiram	Imipramine	
Dapsone	α-Interferon	
	Flutamide	

FIGURE 5-34.

Virtually every drug has been implicated at one time or another as the cause of acute liver injury, but there are also many drugs that have never been associated and still others in which the occasional occurrence of significant liver damage is well known. Frequency of such reactions may vary from one in 100 patients with isoniazid to one in 10,000 patients with halothane and rarer with many other compounds. Implicating a drug requires that the physician make a careful listing of the drugs being taken by the patient, the time period involved, and the quantity ingested. Most examples of hepatotoxicity occur within the first 4 to 8 weeks of beginning use. Combination agents often have enhanced toxicity in comparison to that experienced with either agent alone.

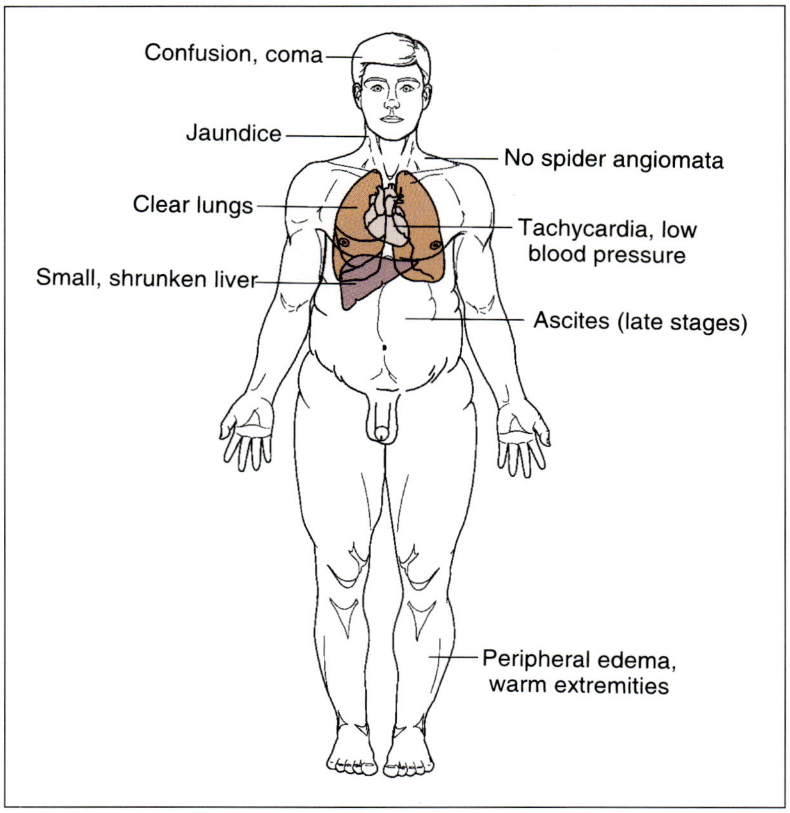

FIGURE 5-35.

Basic physical findings in acute liver failure. Typical features observed in the patient with acute liver failure include confusion, agitation, or even hallucination. Mental status often deteriorates to coma soon after presentation, making history-taking impossible. Most patients will be icteric, although some barely so, and spider angiomata as seen in cirrhotic patients should be absent. Tachycardia, tachypnea, and relative hypotension are common. Asterixis, so commonly observed in chronic hepatic encephalopathy, is rarely seen. *Fetor hepaticus*, a sweet odor caused by mercaptans excreted in the breath, is often observed. Percussion over the rib cage to detect hepatic dullness reveals that the liver span is considerably decreased, and there may be no dullness appreciated, as evidence of the loss of hepatic mass. At autopsy, the normal liver mass of approximately 1600 g may be reduced to as little as 600 g. Edema is not observed initially but may develop in the hospital. Although the extremities are often cold, after resuscitation "warm shock" is the rule.

LABORATORY TESTS IN PATIENTS WITH ACUTE LIVER FAILURE

COMPLETE BLOOD COUNT	
Leukocyte count	Normal unless elevated because of infection
Hemoglobin/hematocrit	Normal unless gastrointestinal bleeding
Platelet count	Low in nearly 80%; frequently less than 100,000/mm^3
SERUM CHEMISTRIES	
Sodium	Normal or low because of excess water intake
Potassium	Usually low because of renal loss of K^+
Chloride	Normal
Carbon dioxide	Low because of central hyperventilation
Blood urea nitrogen	Low
Glucose*	May be dangerously low, causing mental changes
Aspartate aminotransferase	Typically > 1000, may be > 10,000 IU/L
Alanine transaminase	Typically > 1000, may be > 10,000 IU/L
Albumin	Low because of poor synthetic function
Total protein	Low because of poor synthetic function; high globulins suggest chronicity
Ca^{++}	Low because of low albumin
PO_4^-	Often very low requiring replacement
Bilirubin	Typically high; less so in some hyperacute cases; very high in Wilson's disease because of hemolysis or in longstanding disease or renal failure
Alkaline phosphatase	Normal to slightly increased
COAGULATION STUDIES	
Prothrombin time*	Typically at least 4 s prolonged
Partial thromboplastin time	Typically prolonged
ARTERIAL BLOOD GASSES	
pH*	Often 7.5 or greater; acidosis a very bad sign
pCO_2 (partial pressure of carbon dioxide in the artery)	Low because of hyperventilation
pO_2 (partial pressure of oxygen in the artery)	Normal; low also a bad prognostic sign
VIRAL SEROLOGIES	
Hepatitis A IgM	Positive only in acute hepatitis A cases
HBsAg	Positive in many different settings (*see* Table 7-3)
Hepatitis C antibody	Positive test may be seen; rarely causes acute liver failure
Hepatitis D antibody	Order in patients positive for HBsAg
TOXICOLOGY SCREENING TESTS	
Acetaminophen*	Negative; when positive, quantitation useful
Ethanol	Negative; when positive, suspect other agents
Drug screen	Cocaine may cause acute liver failure; positive drug screen also indicates virus exposure (intravenous drug use confirmed)
OTHER ETIOLOGIC TESTS	
Ceruloplasmin*	Should be strikingly low in Wilson's disease; otherwise low normal or normal

FIGURE 5-36.

Usually, these tests are requested by the clinician upon patient's admission to the hospital. Those marked with an *asterisk* are considered to be of utmost diagnostic importance. Initial emergency room tests should include measurement of prothrombin time, glucose, arterial blood gases, complete blood count, a toxicology screen, and a liver profile. Glucose should be given after blood is drawn in the patient with altered mental status until a clear etiology and blood glucose level are determined. HBsAg—hepatitis B surface antigen; IgM—immunoglobulin M.

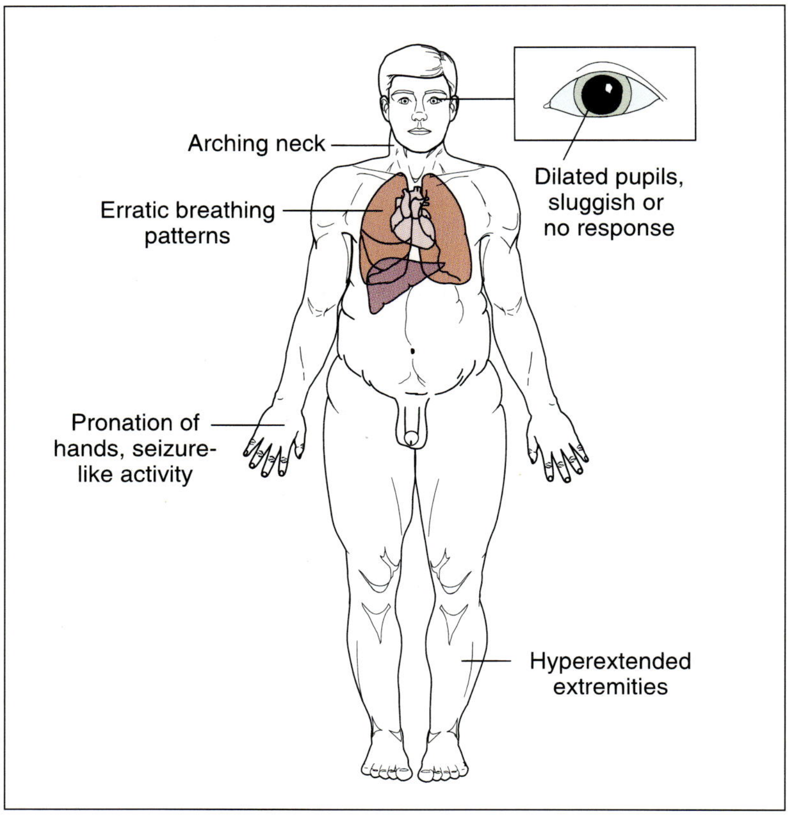

FIGURE 5-37.

Physical findings in patients with advanced hepatic encephalopathy and cerebral edema. Typically, patients will experience a brief period of agitation before the development of coma. Hepatic coma is usually graded as I through IV—grade I is signified by altered personality and subtle changes in cognition; grade II typically demonstrates confusion, slurred speech, and possibly asterixis, but the patient remains able to follow commands; grade III is characterized by deepening coma responsive to strong stimuli with some purposeful movements; grade IV patients are totally unresponsive. Hyperventilation is universal in all stages of hepatic coma. In grade IV coma, decerebrate posturing, changes in breathing patterns, seizures, and pupillary abnormalities all occur in the presence of cerebral edema. These signs, alone or in association with systemic hypertension, warrant immediate intervention with mannitol and pursuit of transplantation, if available. Corticosteroids, hyperventilation, and use of phenobarbital, although recommended for head trauma patients to decrease cerebral edema, are of little benefit in acute liver failure. Diuretics have been used in addition to mannitol but are of uncertain value.

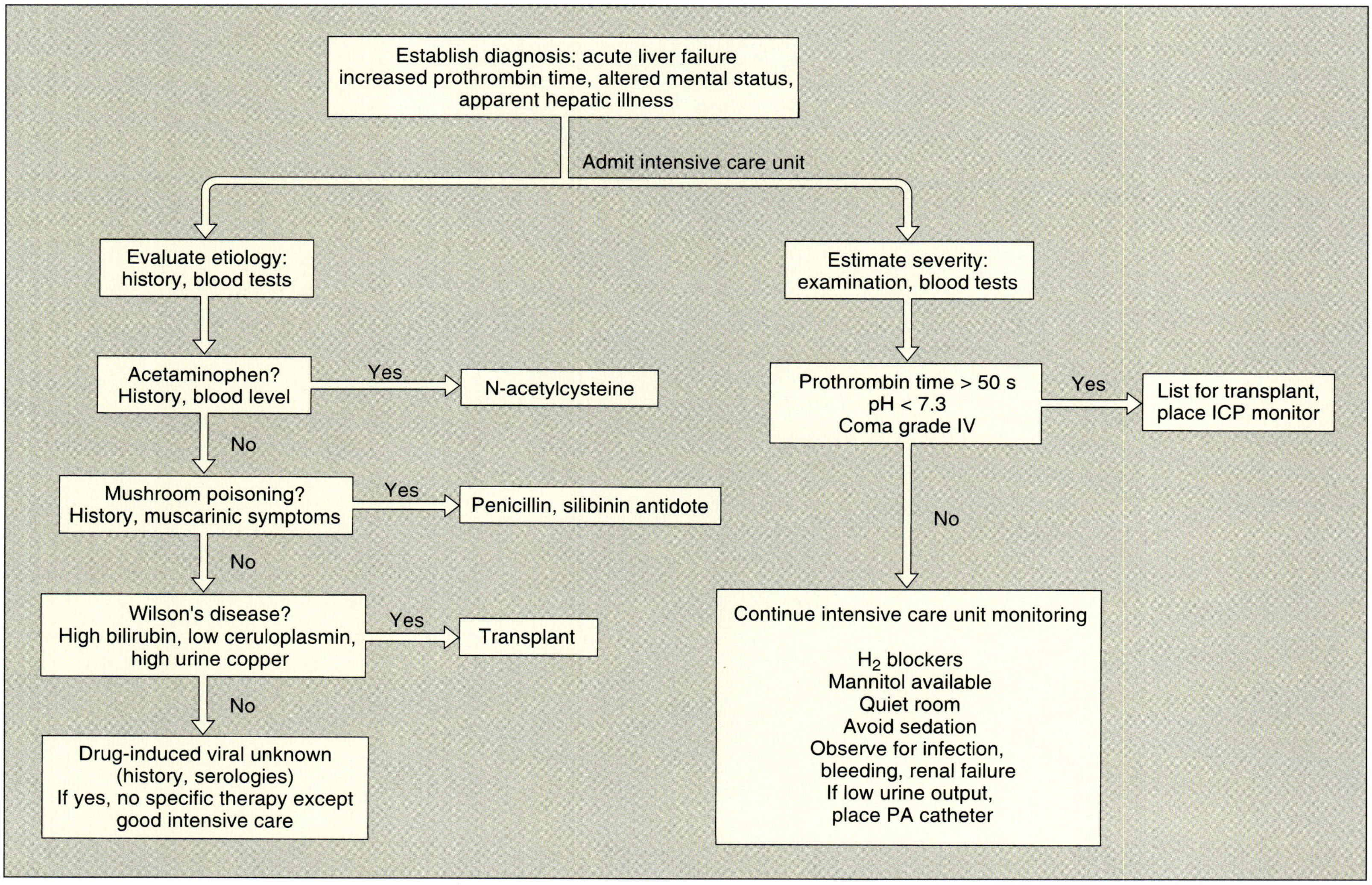

FIGURE 5-38.

Algorithm for triage, diagnosis, and treatment of the patient with acute liver failure. It is first necessary to perform the three E's—*establish* the diagnosis, *evaluate* the etiology, and *estimate* the severity of the illness. ICP—intracranial pressure; PA—pulmonary artery.

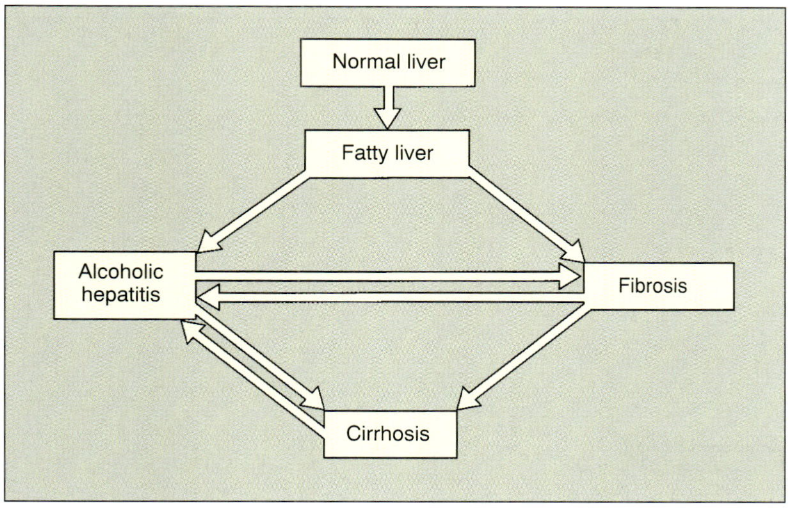

FIGURE 5-39.

As reviewed elsewhere [58], fatty liver invariably develops after heavy alcohol intake; it can progress to alcoholic hepatitis and cirrhosis. In some patients, alcoholic hepatitis is a necessary step in the development of alcohol-induced cirrhosis. However, in some other patients alcohol may stimulate the production of fibrosis and cirrhosis without requiring alcoholic hepatitis as an intermediate lesion. Furthermore, in the alcohol-fed baboon model, fibrosis and cirrhosis also developed in the absence of alcoholic hepatitis [59]. Only a minority of heavy drinkers develop cirrhosis and, experimentally, only one third of baboons fed a high dose of alcohol developed lesions more severe than those of fatty liver. The reason for this individual susceptibility to the development of these more severe complications is not known. Hereditary predisposition may play a role. For the transition of the more benign to the more severe stages of the disease, autoimmune mechanisms have been postulated and cytotoxicity of lymphocytes documented. At present, the mechanism of the transition between fatty liver and alcoholic hepatitis and cirrhosis and the reasons for the difference in individual susceptibility are not settled. It is unclear how alcoholic hepatitis eventually develops into cirrhosis. In addition to fibrogenesis as a response to necrosis and inflammation, it is conceivable that alcohol affects collagen metabolism directly either through increased production or decreased disposition or both, and acetaldhyde has been shown to stimulate collagen production in cultured lipocytes (Ito cells) and myofibroblasts and fibroblasts. At the earliest stages, in the so-called simple or uncomplicated fatty liver, collagen is detectable by chemical means only. When collagen deposition is sufficient to become visible by light microscopy, usually it appears first around the central (also called terminal) hepatic venules, resulting in so-called "pericentral" or "perivenular" fibrosis or sclerosis which extends into the lobule (perisinusoidal and pericellular fibrosis). In cases of alcoholic hepatitis, an increased number of mesenchymal cells and polymorphonuclear leukocytes are present, but even in the absence of alcoholic hepatitis, and prior to any fibrosis, there can be an increased number of mesenchymal cells. Sequential biopsies revealed that, already at the early fatty liver stage, an increased number of myofibroblasts appear in the perivenular areas, and cells transitional between lipocytes and fibroblasts in the perisinusoidal space of Disse. This is eventually accompanied by deposition of abundant collagen bundles, first in the perivenular areas, leading to perivenular, perisinusoidal, and pericellular fibrosis and ultimately to septal fibrosis and cirrhosis. The progression of alcohol-induced injury is not orderly. Alcoholic hepatitis is often found superimposed on already established cirrhosis and the clinical manifestations result both from acute alcoholic hepatitis and from problems arising as complications of cirrhosis. Alcoholic hepatitis is considered at least partially reversible. Alcohol steatosis is considered largely reversible. Even at the stage of alcoholic hepatitis when there is early fibrosis, the possibility exists that some (if not most) of the injury may be reversible. Many patients have coexistence of fatty liver, alcoholic hepatitis, and cirrhosis.

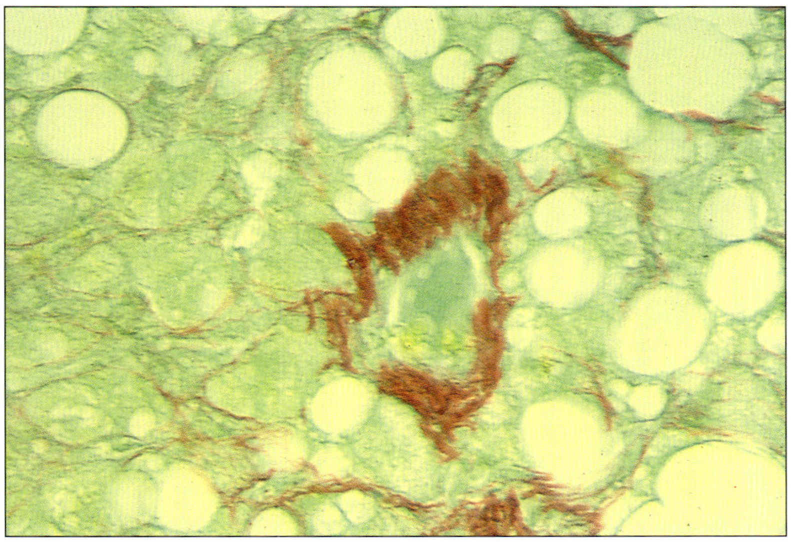

FIGURE 5-40.

Sirius red stain (original magnification × 250) of a liver biopsy from a patient with alcoholic fatty liver without evidence of alcoholic hepatitis. Note the fibrous rim around the terminal hepatic venule (perivenular fibrosis). Some fibrous strands surround the adjacent sinusoids and hepatocytes (perisinusoidal and pericellular fibrosis). This change can contribute to portal hypertension. (*Courtesy of* F. Paronetto, Bronx, NY)

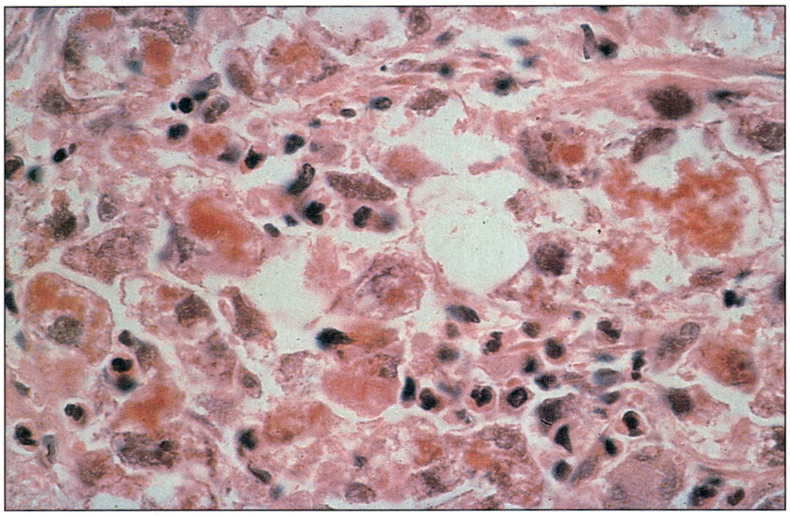

FIGURE 5-41.

Major features found on liver biopsy from a patient with alcoholic hepatitis include marked variation in cell size, evidence of cell necrosis, and variable inflammation with a mixture of polymorphonuclear and mononuclear cells. Pericellular fibrosis is an important feature. In many patients, eosinophilic inclusions (Mallory bodies) are found. The Mallory bodies represent masses of intermediate filaments. Often the most alcoholic-induced injury is in Zone III (centrilobular). Liver biopsy from a patient with active alcoholic hepatitis replete with Mallory bodies (alcoholic hyaline). Hematoxylin and eosin stain. (*Courtesy of* Z. Goodman, Washington, D.C.)

ALCOHOLIC HEPATITIS: CORTICOSTEROID TREATMENT

INDICATIONS

Spontaneous encephalopathy

4.6 (PT-control) + serum bilirubin > 32

CONTRAINDICATIONS

Active gastrointestinal bleeding

Active infection

PREDNISOLONE

40 mg/d (4wk), 20 mg/d (1 wk), 10 mg/d (1 wk)

FIGURE 5-42.

In patients with severe alcoholic liver disease, as indicated by spontaneous encephalopathy or elevated protime and bilirubin (elevated Maddrey's discriminant function), corticosteroid treatment has been shown to be useful [60].

HEMOCHROMATOSIS

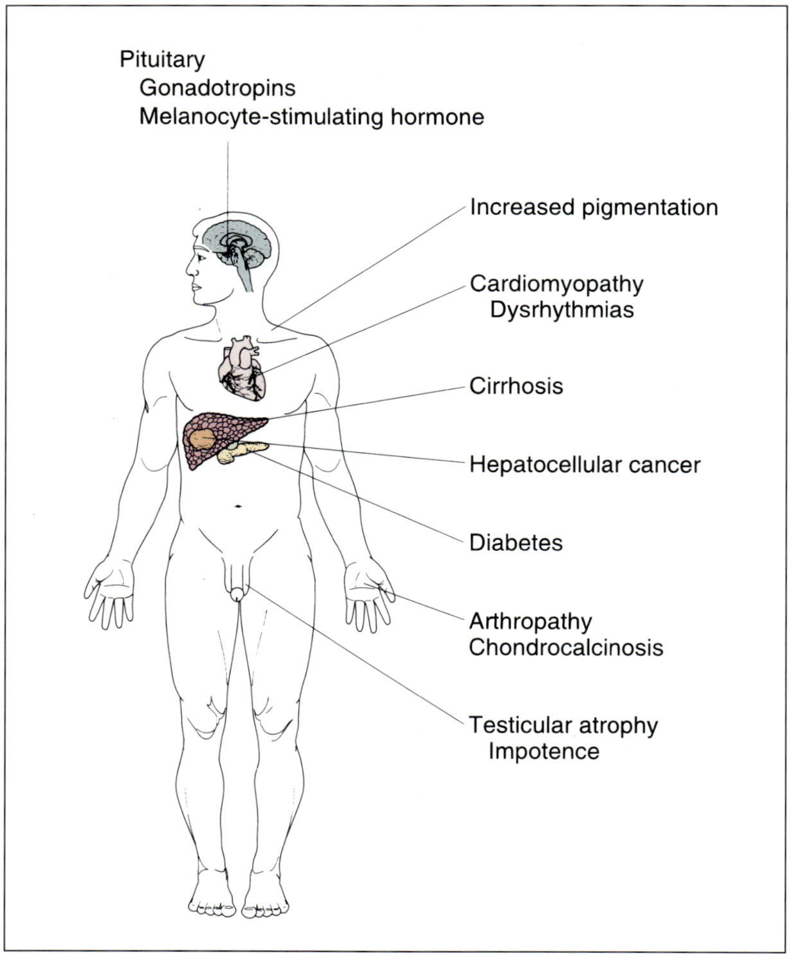

FIGURE 5-43.

Clinical manifestations of hereditary hemochromatosis. The clinical manifestations of hereditary hemochromatosis are protean. The most common abnormalities are found in the liver, and the development of hepatocellular carcinoma is 200 times more common in patients with untreated hemochromatosis than in the general population. In the 1990s, it is distinctly unusual to identify someone with the original triad of pigmentation, cirrhosis, and diabetes. With the advent of screening iron studies on routine chemistry panels, hemochromatosis is now often identified in asymptomatic individuals.

REPRESENTATIVE IRON MEASUREMENTS

	Normal	Hereditary hemochromatosis
Serum iron, *μg/dL*	50–150	180–300
Transferrin, *mg/dL*	250–370	200–300
Transferrin saturation, *%*	20–50	80–100
Serum ferritin, *ng/mL*		
Men	20–300	500–6000
Women	15–250	500–6000

Figure 5-44.

Once the clinician's suspicion is aroused by symptoms and physical findings discussed previously, iron studies should be obtained to determine if any phenotypic expression of the disease exists. Increased transferrin saturation is the most specific abnormality, and a combination of increased transferrin saturation and increased ferritin is both highly specific and highly sensitive. The serum iron concentration is subject to a diurnal variation and is also increased following meals; therefore, iron studies are best obtained in the morning when patients are fasting. All patients with either an elevated transferrin saturation or an elevated ferritin should be further evaluated for hemochromatosis [61].

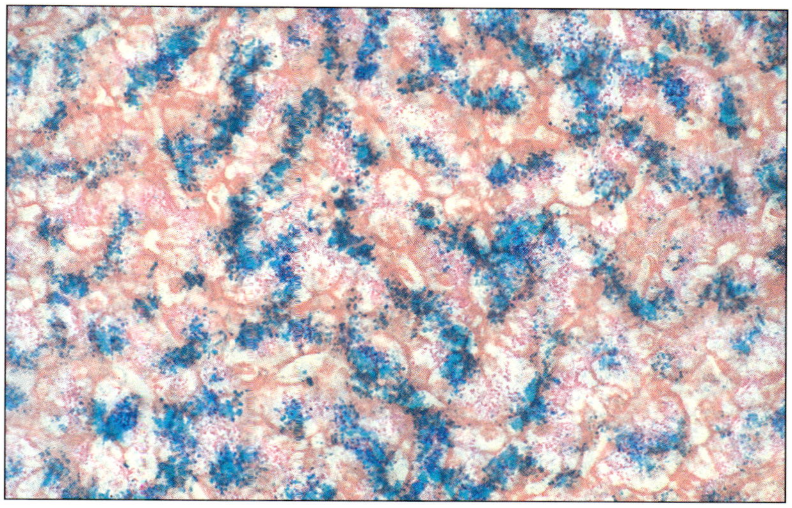

Figure 5-45.

The liver biopsy procedure is essential to establish the diagnosis of hemochromatosis. Histochemical staining with Perls' Prussian blue reagent stains storage iron blue against the counterstain which is red. Shown here is a liver biopsy specimen from a 34-year-old man with newly diagnosed hereditary hemochromatosis. At high power, it is apparent that all iron deposition is in hepatocytes with little or none in reticuloendothelial cells (Kupffer cells). The hepatic iron concentration from this biopsy was 17,350 μg/g dry weight.

WILSON'S DISEASE

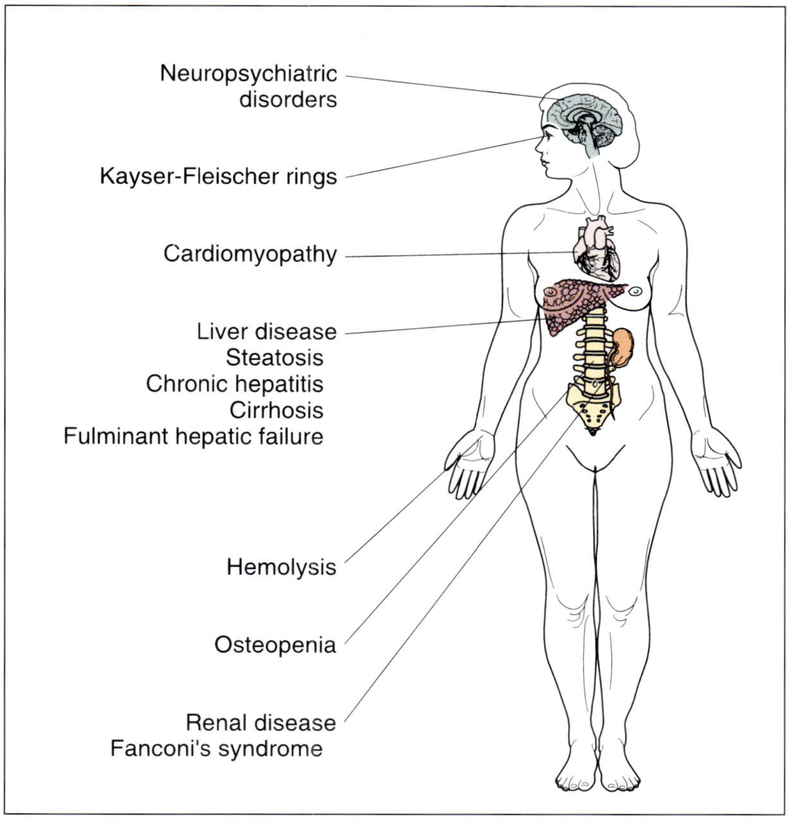

Figure 5-46.

Clinical manifestations of Wilson's disease. There are numerous clinical manifestations of Wilson's disease including the presence of Kayser-Fleischer rings. Many psychiatric symptoms and disorders are typical of Wilson's disease. Rarely, cardiomyopathy ensues. All patients with Wilson's disease have hepatic involvement that can range from fairly mild steatosis to the insidious development of cirrhosis or the often fatal fulminant hepatic failure. The renal disease that occurs in Wilson's disease is comparable with that seen in Fanconi's syndrome. Hemolysis is caused by copper toxicity; many patients have significant osteopenia [62–64].

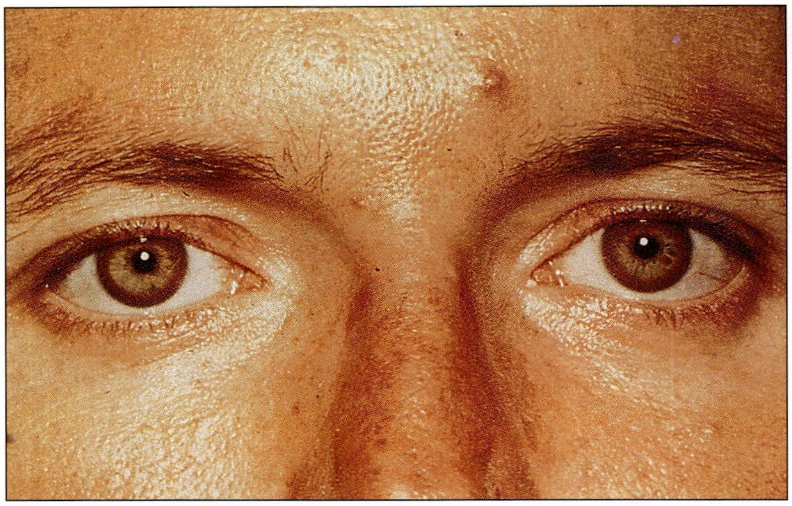

FIGURE 5-47.

Kayser-Fleischer rings. This young man has classical Kayser-Fleischer rings, identified as the golden-brown pigment deposits in Descemet's membrane in the periphery of the iris. These rings can be seen with the naked eye, but occasionally, a slit-lamp examination is necessary to identify them. Another unusual ophthalmologic manifestation of Wilson's disease is sunflower cataracts.

CHARACTERISTIC LABORATORY FEATURES OF WILSON'S DISEASE

	Normal	Wilson's disease
Serum copper, *µg/dL*	80–140	< 80
Urine copper, *µg/24 h*	< 40	> 100
Serum ceruloplasmin, *mg/dL*	20–40	< 20
Hepatic copper concentration, *µg/g dry weight*	15–50	250–3000

FIGURE 5-48.

Characteristic laboratory features of Wilson's disease. Serum copper levels are typically depressed, but this feature is not a highly sensitive and specific laboratory finding. Twenty-four–hour urine copper excretion is the best confirmatory test, along with hepatic copper concentration as determined by liver biopsy. Serum ceruloplasmin levels are depressed in the majority of patients with Wilson's disease but can be depressed in severe malabsorption and malnutrition.

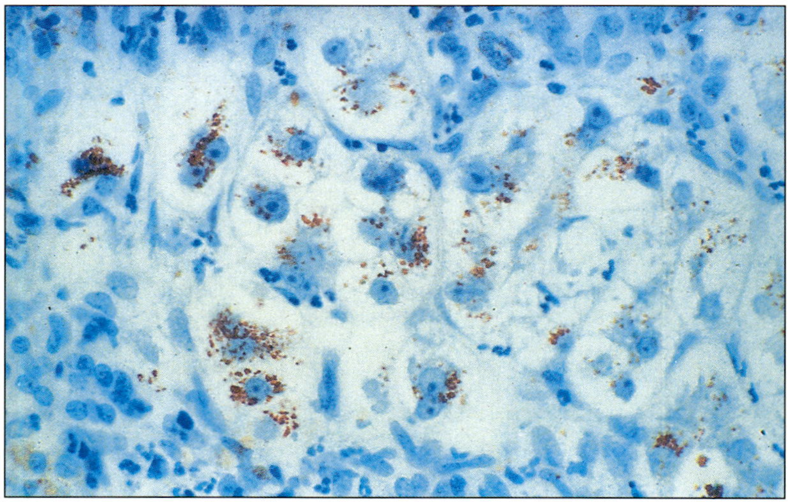

FIGURE 5-49.

A rhodanine stain of a liver biopsy for diagnosis of Wilson's disease. There are several histochemical stains for copper that can be used to help identify Wilson's disease. This figure is an example of a test that stains the copper-associated protein a golden-brown color against the blue counterstain.

Ascites

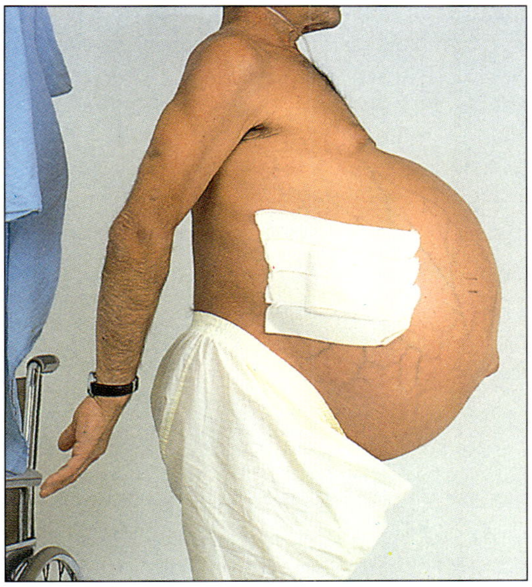

FIGURE 5-50.

Ascites often develops insidiously over the course of months in patients with cirrhosis, and the patient presents with abdominal distension. Ascites may develop suddenly if there is a precipitating cause such as infection, an alcoholic binge, development of a hepatoma, or thrombosis of the hepatic vein. Once ascites becomes clinically obvious, the patient usually is ill with moderate muscle wasting. The umbilicus is everted. Pedal edema is common, partly related to the hypoalbuminemia and partly related to the pressure on the inferior vena cava by the abdominal fluid.

ASCITIC FLUID ANALYSIS
Polymorphonuclear count
> 250/µL is diagnostic of spontaneous bacterial peritonitis
Ascitic fluid albumin concentration
Serum-ascitic fluid albumin gradient > 11 g/L is suggestive of cirrhotic, rather than malignant, ascites

FIGURE 5-51.

Ascitic fluid analysis should include a total polymorphonuclear count and albumin concentration. A serum-ascitic fluid albumin gradient of greater than 11 g/L represents cirrhotic rather than malignant ascites. A high-protein content may be associated with Budd-Chiari syndrome or pancreatic ascites. A total polymorphonuclear count of greater than 250/µL is diagnostic of spontaneous bacterial peritonitis.

DIFFERENTIAL DIAGNOSIS OF ASCITES	
Cirrhosis	Constrictive pericarditis
Hepatoma	Nephrotic syndrome
Tuberculous peritonitis in the malnourished alcoholic	Pancreatitis
Peritoneal carcinomatosis	Malignant chylous ascites, especially lymphoma
Right-sided cardiac failure	

FIGURE 5-52.

Many causes of noncirrhotic ascites exist. Hepatic venous obstruction or Budd-Chiari syndrome must be considered, especially if the protein count of the ascitic fluid is high. Severe right-sided heart failure or constrictive pericarditis is usually clinically obvious and can be confirmed with the characteristic echocardiographic findings. A chest radiograph will also demonstrate the changes of right heart failure or calcification of the pericardium as causes of constrictive pericarditis. Similarly, nephrotic syndrome as a cause of ascites can be easily diagnosed by the presence of generalized edema and proteinuria. Tuberculous ascites should be suspected in the severely malnourished alcoholic cirrhotic. The patient is usually febrile, but fever may be absent in half of the patients. The leukocyte count of the ascitic fluid is usually, but not always, elevated. These leukocytes are usually lymphocytes, but sometimes can be polymorphs. The protein content of the ascitic fluid is usually greater than 3 5 g/L. The ascitic fluid should be stained for acid-fast bacilli, but the smears are rarely positive. Positive culture is found in only half the patients. Malignant ascites is often blood stained and the protein count is high. Cytology of the ascitic fluid is often negative. Chylous ascites suggests metastatic cancer, predominantly lymphoma. Pancreatic ascites can complicate acute pancreatitis but is rarely gross. A high-ascitic amylase level of greater than 1000 U/L is diagnostic of pancreatic ascites.

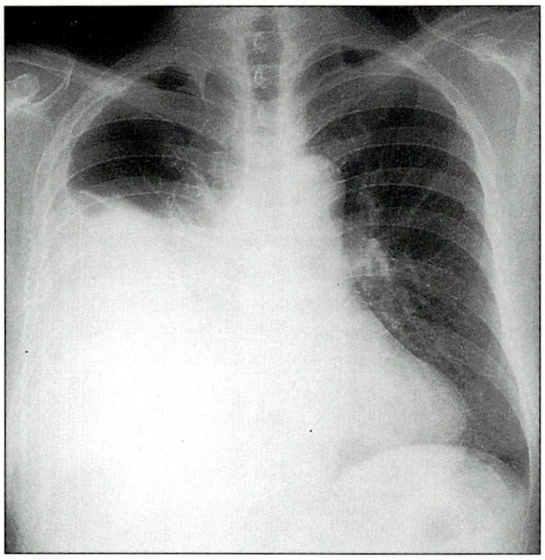

FIGURE 5-53.

Pleural effusion is present in about 6% of patients with ascites and usually is on the right side. This effusion is the result of a defect in the diaphragm that allows the ascitic fluid to pass up into the pleural cavity. In contrast, a left-sided pleural effusion in an ascitic patient may indicate pulmonary pathology. Occasionally, a pleural effusion can be seen in the absence of ascites caused by the negative intrathoracic pressure drawing up the ascitic fluid through the diaphragmatic defect into the pleural cavity. Thoracentesis is followed by rapid refilling of the pleural cavity because of the negative intrathoracic pressure, and control of the pleural effusion can only be achieved with the control of ascites.

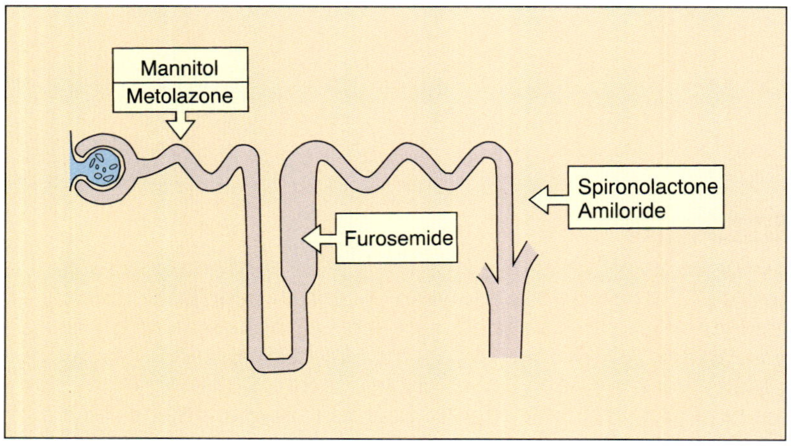

FIGURE 5-54.

Diuretic therapy is usually required in addition to sodium and fluid restriction to control ascites. The aim of diuretic therapy is to block the various renal sodium-retaining mechanisms and thereby increase urinary sodium excretion. Distal diuretics (*eg*, spironolactone, triamterene, amiloride) are relatively weak. The half-life of spironolactone in patients with end-stage cirrhosis is between 10 to 35 hours because of impaired metabolism. There is a lag phase of 2 to 4 days before the onset of action and up to 7 days for offset of action when therapy is discontinued. Therefore, dosages of spironolactone should not be adjusted more often than once every 7 days. Amiloride is preferred because its onset and offset of action are not as long. Loop diuretics are very powerful. They can increase urinary sodium excretion as much as 300%. The onset of action of furosemide is within 30 minutes after oral administration, with a peak effect within 1 to 2 hours and most of the natriuretic activity completed within 3 to 4 hours. The dose-response curve of furosemide is sigmoidal. After a maximal response is reached, administration of higher doses does not produce a further natriuretic response. Diuretics that act on the proximal renal tubule are very potent. They should not be used without careful monitoring because severe intravascular volume depletion leading to renal dysfunction is a common complication. They are generally not recommended as outpatient therapy.

TIPS–PATIENT SELECTION

ABSOLUTE CONTRAINDICATIONS	RELATIVE CONTRAINDICATIONS
Hepatic encephalopathy	Dental sepsis
Cardiac disease	Spontaneous bacterial peritonitis
Renal dysfunction	Hepatocellular carcinoma
Noncompliance with sodium and fluid restrictions	

FIGURE 5-55.

Transjugular intrahepatic portosystemic stent shunt (TIPS) is generally not recommended in refractory ascites if the patient has a prior history of spontaneous hepatic encephalopathy, cardiac or renal disease, and noncompliance with dietary sodium and fluid restriction. Dental and other foci of sepsis and bacterial peritonitis have to be treated before TIPS insertion, because infection of the shunt will be very difficult to eradicate. Similarly, patients with previous spontaneous bacterial peritonitis must remain on prophylactic antibiotic therapy, such as norfloxacin, for life. The presence of a hepatocellular carcinoma is also a relative contraindication. If, however, the prognosis is longer than 6 months and the patient does not have any other contraindications, then TIPS should be used as a treatment for refractory ascites. In the suitable patient, TIPS can significantly improve quality of life.

CLINICAL FEATURES OF SPONTANEOUS BACTERIAL PERITONITIS

Significant fever	Worsening encephalopathy
Chills	Worsening of ascites
Abdominal pain	Hypotension
Abdominal tenderness	Asymptomatic
Reduced bowel sounds	

FIGURE 5-56.

The clinical features of spontaneous bacterial peritonitis are quite variable and the diagnosis requires a high index of suspicion. These features can range from the classical picture of fever, chills, generalized abdominal pain, and absent bowel sound to one of a totally asymptomatic patient. Frequently, patients only present with worsening of liver function or hepatic encephalopathy. (*From* Hoefs and Runyon [65].)

MICROORGANISMS RESPONSIBLE FOR SPONTANEOUS BACTERIAL PERITONITIS

ORGANISMS ISOLATED

GRAM-NEGATIVE BACILLI (70%)	ANAEROBES (5%)	GRAM-POSITIVE ORGANISMS (25%)
E. coli	*Bacteroides*	*Streptococcus viridans*
Klebsiella	*Clostridia*	Group D *Streptococcus*
C. freundii	*Lactobacillus*	*S. pneumoniae*
Proteus		*S. aureus*
Enterobacter		

FIGURE 5-57.

Many cases of spontaneous bacterial peritonitis (SBP) are caused by microorganisms of intestinal origin. Nonenteric organisms are only responsible for 20% of episodes of SBP. Gram-negative bacilli overall account for 70% of all patients, with *Escherichia coli* as the most common pathogen isolated, being found in 50% of patients. Other gram-negative organisms include *Klebsiella* species, *Citrobacter freundii*, *Proteus*, and *Enterobacter*. Gram-positive organisms are responsible for 25% of cases and include *Streptococcus pneumoniae*, *Streptococcus viridans*, group D *Streptococci*, and *Staphylococcus aureus*. Anaerobic organisms are uncommon causes of SBP because the oxygen tension in the ascitic fluid is too high for their survival. Among these, *Bacteroides* species appear to be more common than other anaerobes. A small percentage of cases are polymicrobial, and every effort should be made to look for an underlying cause of the infection in such cases.

TREATMENT FOR SPONTANEOUS BACTERIAL PERITONITIS

Cefotaxime	Less nephrotoxic
	Broad spectrum
	2 g, 8 hourly
Cefoxitine	Enterococcal cover
	1 g, 6 to 8 hourly
Aztreonam	500 mg, 8 hourly
Amoxicillin-clavulanic acid	1 g amoxicillin & 200 mg clavulanic acid, 6 hourly

Do not use aminoglycosides because they can precipitate renal failure

Do not wait for culture results

Prompt treatment reduces mortality

FIGURE 5-58.

Spontaneous bacterial peritonitis (SBP) is a severe infective complication of ascites. If untreated, it has a mortality rate of 50%. Therefore antibiotic therapy should be given immediately after a diagnostic polymorphonuclear count is available without waiting for culture results. Cefotaxime, a new broad-spectrum third generation cephalosporin, is now recognized as the treatment of choice for SBP. It is effective in 85% of patients, and the incidence of nephrotoxicity is negligible with the therapeutic doses used. Its spectrum includes most organisms responsible for SBP. The recommended dose is 2 g every 8 hours. Cefoxitine provides good cover for enterococcal infections, whereas newer antibiotics including amoxicillin-clavulanic combinations and aztreonam are also adequate. The number of patients in the studies assessing the efficacy of these antibiotics is, however, small. Aminoglycosides should never be used in cirrhotic patients, because the risk of nephrotoxicity is high and the development of nephrotoxicity is not related to serum concentrations. The ascitic fluid polymorphonuclear count should decrease rapidly once treatment is given, returning to normal within 48 hours, together with a parallel clinical improvement.

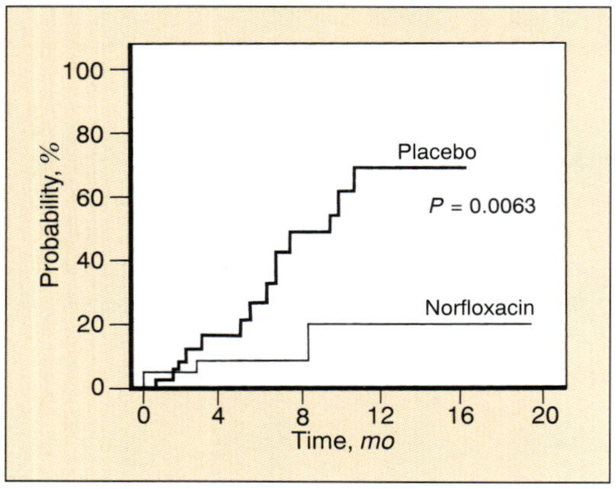

FIGURE 5-59.

Various therapeutic modalities have been tried to reduce the risk of recurrence. Diuretic therapy has been shown to increase ascitic protein content and opsonin activity but not to influence outcome. Selective intestinal decontamination to eliminate aerobic gram-negative bacilli with oral nonabsorbable antibiotics has proved to be effective in reducing the recurrence of spontaneous bacterial peritonitis. Norfloxacin (400 mg daily) has been shown to be significantly better than placebo to reduce the incidence of recurrence of spontaneous bacterial peritonitis. It is the drug of choice, because it has the advantages of rarely causing bacterial resistance and of having a low incidence of side effects when administered long term. (*Adapted from* Gines *et al.* [66].)

Variceal bleeding

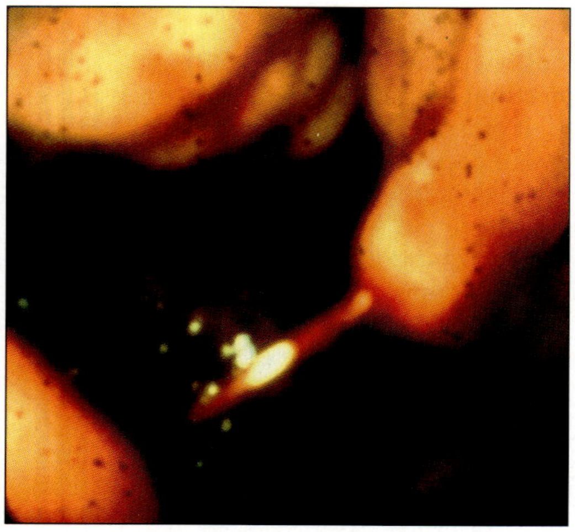

FIGURE 5-60.

Active hemorrhage from an esophageal varix. Pressure within esophageal varices averages almost 30 mm Hg in cirrhotic patients. Coughing, straining, defecation, or lifting may increase variceal pressure to arterial pressure levels. Indeed, bleeding at such high pressures may give rise to arterial jets, as shown in this remarkable endoscopic photograph. Needless to say, large volumes of blood can quickly be lost from such lesions. Therapy includes banding or sclerosing these varices. Varices that continue to bleed despite aggressive therapy can be treated by transjugular intrahepatic portosystemic stent shunt or portosystemic shunt. (*Courtesy of* N. Currey, Rancho Mirage, CA)

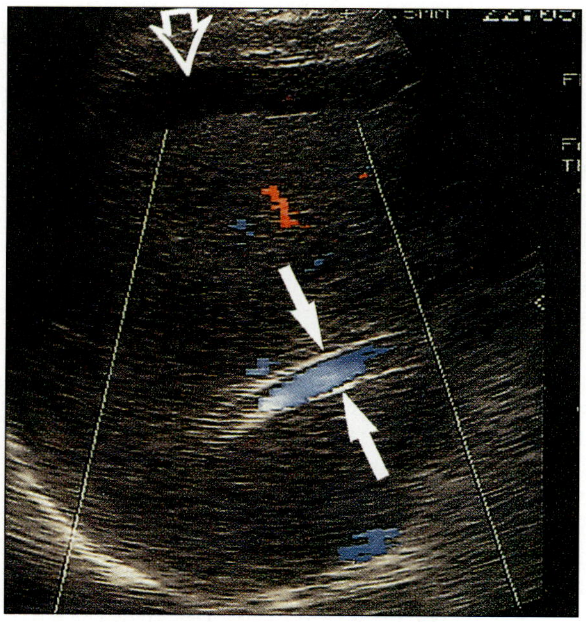

FIGURE 5-61.

Transjugular intrahepatic portosystemic shunt (TIPS). This hepatic Doppler sonogram in a 55-year-old man with alcoholic cirrhosis and portal hypertension shows the position of a patent TIPS [67]. The procedure was performed because of refractory, debilitating ascites. The shunt shows characteristic echogenicity (*solid arrows*) and an intense blue signal caused by shunted blood flow. Ascites (*open arrow*) is present anterior to the liver. After the placement of the shunt, the patient's esophageal varices diminished in size and the ascites began to disappear without further therapy. The patient was awaiting liver transplantation at the time of this ultrasonographic examination. The shunt became occluded 8 months later. (*From* Sadler and Shapiro [67]; with permission.)

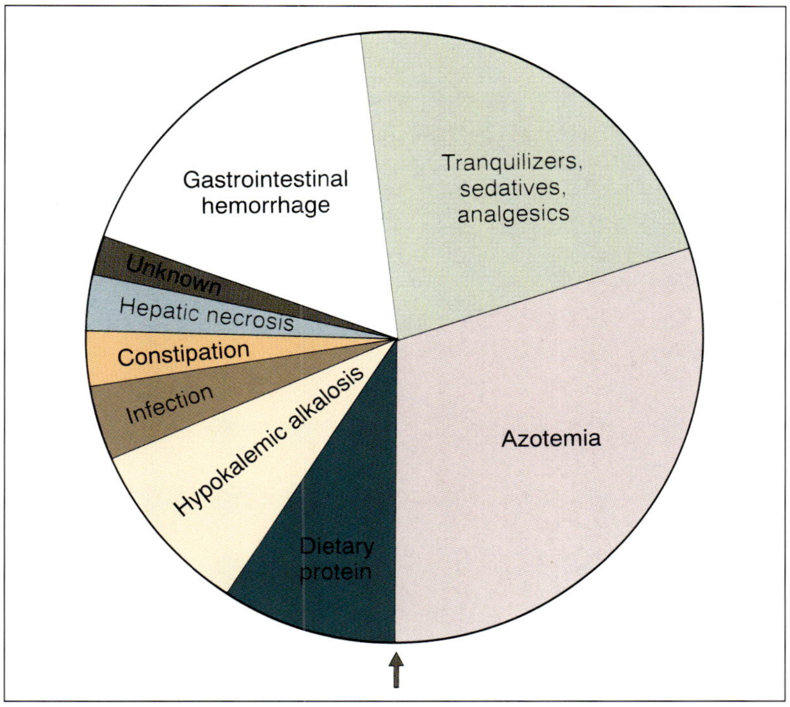

FIGURE 5-62.

Precipitants of hepatic encephalopathy in 100 consecutive patients with hepatic encephalopathy at the West Haven Veterans Administration Hospital, West Haven, Connecticut. The most common precipitant was azotemia, which occurred in one third of the patients [68]. In about half of them the azotemia had been precipitated by diuretic agents such as furosemide. Precipitation of hepatic encephalopathy by tranquilizers, sedatives, or analgesic agents appears to be primarily responsible for induction of impaired mental state in a quarter of the episodes. Ninety-seven episodes had occurred in cirrhotic patients, 13 of whom had portacaval anastomoses. The severity of the encephalopathy tended to be milder in the azotemic and drug-induced patients. Hypokalemic alkalosis, which had been caused by vomiting, diarrhea, or diuretic drugs, was seen in 10% of the patients. Severe encephalopathy occurred in association with gastrointestinal bleeding, infection, or azotemia. (*From* Fessel and Conn [68].)

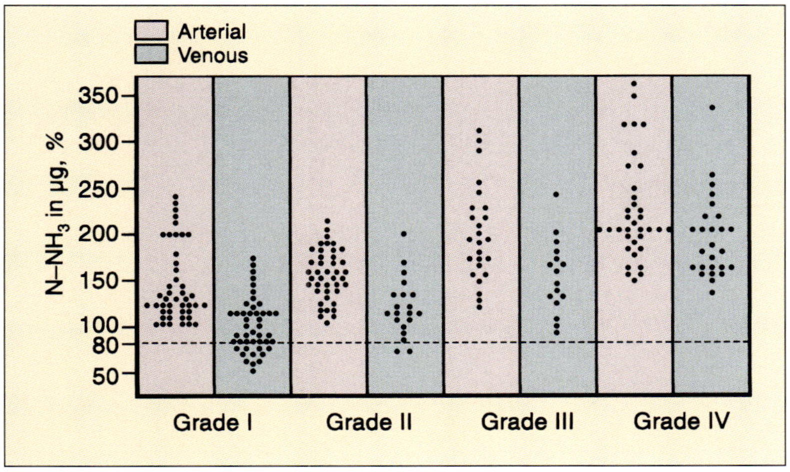

FIGURE 5-63.

Association of blood ammonia concentrations and the grade of hepatic encephalopathy in untreated cirrhotic patients. There is a step-wise progression between the arterial ammonia levels and the degree of portosystemic encephalopathy (PSE) (columns 1, 3, 5, and 7) [69]. There is, however, much overlap in ammonia concentrations between the adjacent grades of PSE. With venous ammonia levels (columns 2, 4, 6, and 8) the same trend is evident, but the degree of overlap is even greater. Arterial ammonia levels correlate much more closely with the degree of hepatic encephalopathy than venous levels. It is not possible to predict these gradients. (*From* Stahl [69]; with permission.)

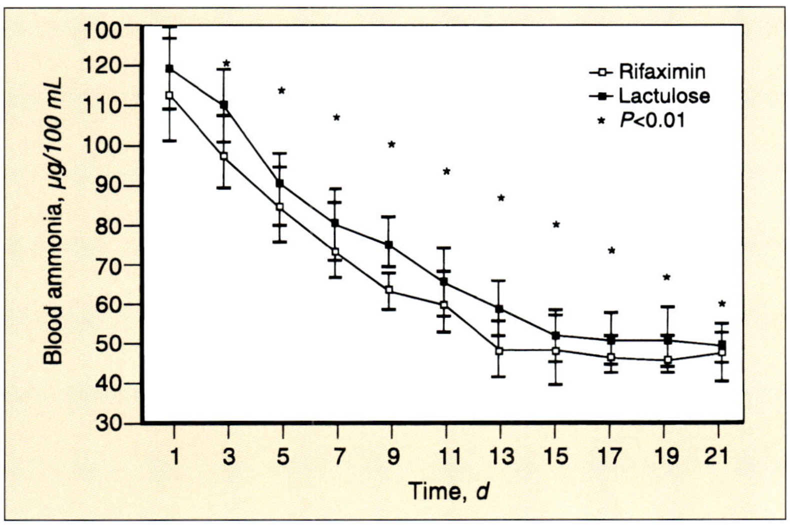

FIGURE 5-64.

Antibiotic therapy with neomycin or related nonabsorbed broad-spectrum antibiotic agents has been a primary form of therapy for hepatic encephalopathy for 20 years. It was frequently toxic, causing renal disease, hearing loss, malabsorption, and other lesions [70]. Rifaximin, a nonabsorbed, nontoxic antibiotic agent, may improve the treatment of hepatic encephalopathy [71]. In a randomized comparison of rifaximin (1200 mg/d) and lactulose (40 g/d), the mean venous blood ammonia concentrations were significantly lower in the rifaximin-treated patients than in those who received lactulose in every determination. This figure suggests that rifaximin may be at least as effective as lactulose in the management of hyperammonemic hepatic encephalopathy. (*From* Bucci and Palmieri [71]; with permission.)

VASCULAR DISORDERS OF THE LIVER

Hepatic vein thrombosis (Budd-Chiari syndrome)

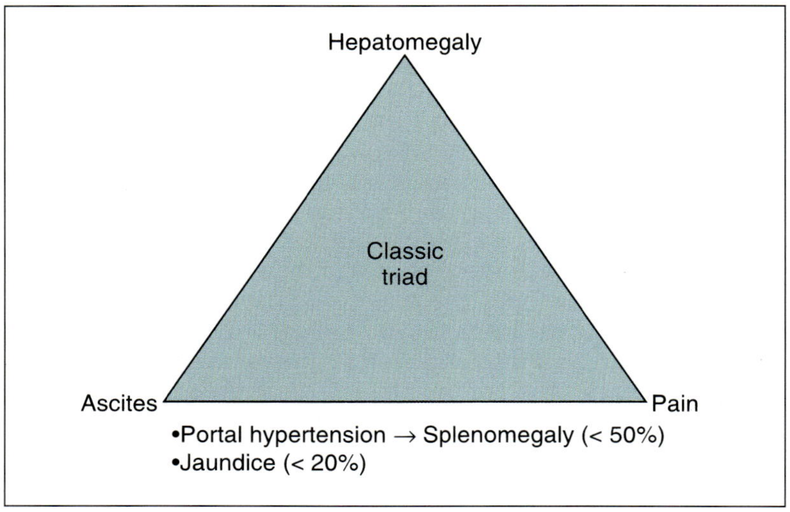

FIGURE 5-65.

Clinical manifestations of Budd-Chiari syndrome. The classic triad of abdominal pain, hepatomegaly, and ascites is present in the majority of patients with Budd-Chiari syndrome. Of these, pain is the least constant finding. Jaundice is rare, occurring in less than 20% of patients. Splenomegaly is found in almost 50%. In some instances, splenomegaly is a consequence of an underlying hematologic disorder, such as polycythemia rubra vera, whereas in others it results from portal hypertension. The remaining clinical signs are those associated with portal hypertension per se.

BUDD-CHIARI SYNDROME

PREDISPOSING FACTORS

Hematologic

Polycythemia rubra vera
Paroxysmal nocturnal hemoglobinuria
Myeloproliferative disorders
Chronic myelogenous leukemia
Hypercoagulable states (lupus anticoagulant, antithrombin III deficiency protein C/protein S deficiency)

Tumors

Hepatocellular carcinoma
Renal cell carcinoma
Adrenal cell carcinoma
Leiomyosarcoma
Choriocarcinoma
Right atrial myxoma

Phlebitis

Trauma

Infectious

Amebic abscess
Aspergillosis
Hydatid cysts

Oral contraceptives

Pregnancy and postpartum

Venal caval web

Radiation

Behcet's disease

Rare causes

Inflammatory bowel disease
Protein-losing enteropathy
Syphilitic gummas
Sarcoidosis

? Cirrhosis

? Previous episodes of hepatitis

FIGURE 5-66.

Etiology of Budd-Chiari syndrome. This table lists the disorders that predispose patients to the development of Budd-Chiari syndrome. The majority of underlying disorders are hematologic with a thrombotic diathesis.

Ischemic hepatitis (formerly, shock liver)

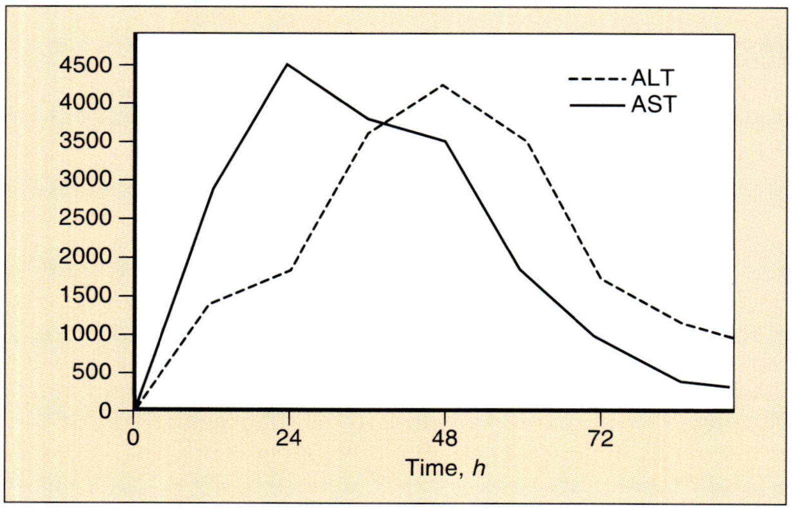

FIGURE 5-67.

Ischemic hepatitis. Transient decreases in arterial flow to the liver may result in ischemic necrosis of the centrilobular perivenular zone of the liver. In some patients, even a brief episode of hypotension is sufficient to cause ischemic injury. Patients with severe heart failure often develop ischemic hepatitis during episodes of ventricular tachycardia. The most common setting for ischemic hepatitis is following or during cardiac bypass. Those patients with preexisting elevation in right atrial pressures, such as is seen in patients with tricuspid regurgitation, appear to be at greatest risk for developing ischemic hepatitis. Laboratory features of ischemic hepatitis are shown in this figure. The most characteristic feature is extreme elevations of the aminotransferase levels. The enzymes usually rise within 12 to 24 hours after the ischemic episode and peak within 48 hours. Thereafter, the levels decline logarithmically. The decreases reflect clearance of the enzymes from the circulation, which is a first-order process. In the majority of instances, the level of aspartate aminotransferase (AST) is higher than the level of alanine aminotransferase (ALT) in the first 2 to 3 days but declines at a more rapid rate, as a result of differences in the serum half-lives of the two proteins.

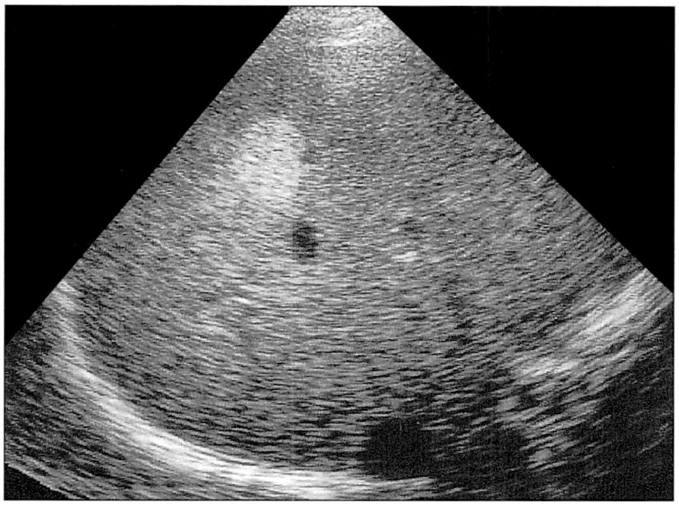

FIGURE 5-68.

Ultrasound in the diagnosis of hepatic hemangiomas. On imaging with ultrasound, hemangiomas appear as single echogenic lesions with well-defined borders. Posterior accustic enhancement is characteristic. This tumor is the most common benign hepatic tumor, found in 3% to 5% of all autopsies. Hemangiomas are usually single and small, but may be multiple and large. The majority of patients are asymptomatic and have normal liver chemistries. Large lesions (larger than 4 cm) may cause symptoms such as a sensation of a mass and abdominal pain.

HEPATIC CYSTS AND ABSCESSES

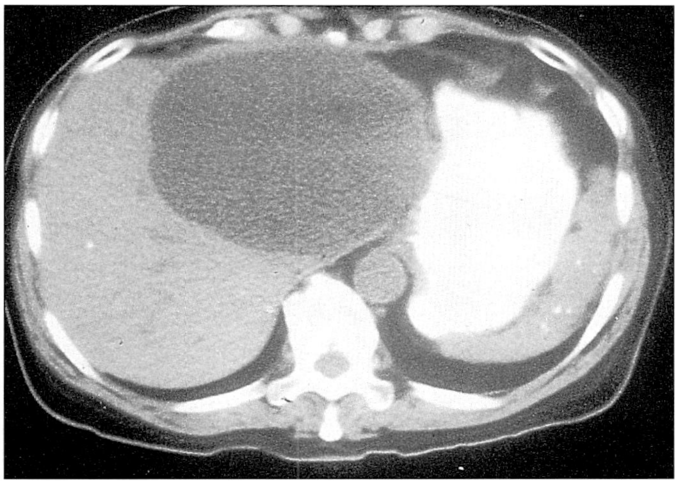

FIGURE 5-69.

Computed tomographic imaging of an hepatic cyst. Intrahepatic cysts are seen on computed tomographic scans as a low-attenuation space-filling lesion. The attenuation coefficient is usually similar to water and always lower than blood. They do not fill with administration of intravenous contrast dye.

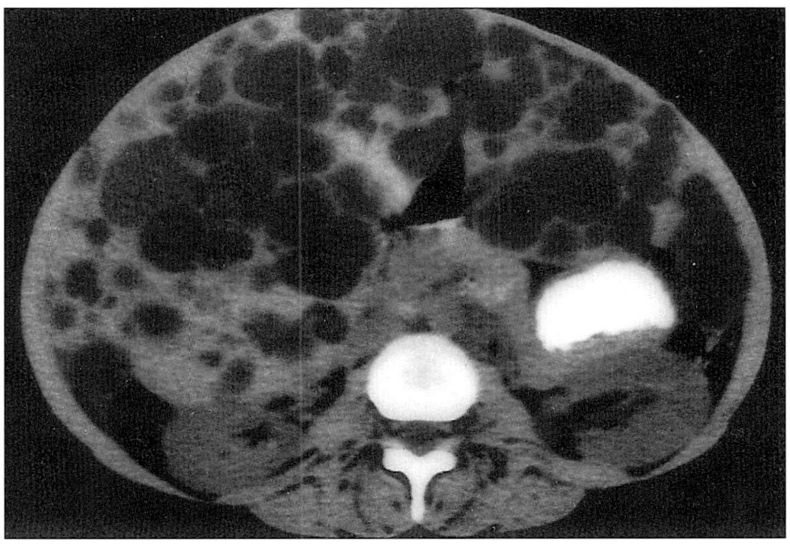

FIGURE 5-70.

Computed tomographic scan of the abdomen showing massive hepatomegaly related to multiple cysts of varying diameter, some as large as 4 to 5 cm. Interestingly, no cysts can be seen in the kidney.

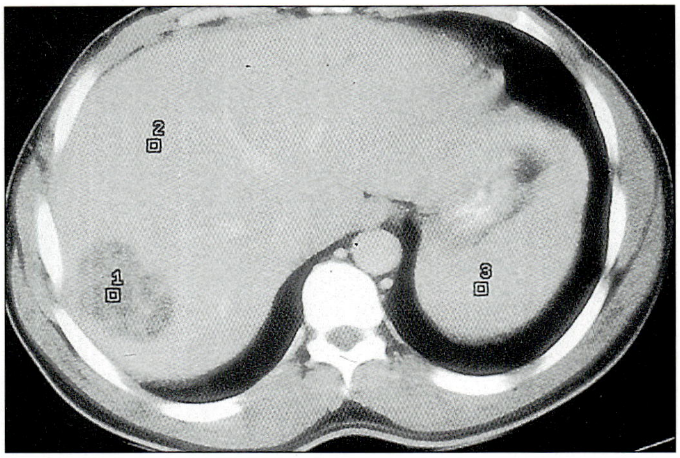

FIGURE 5-71.

Amebic abscesses are the most common type of liver abscesses worldwide. They are more frequently localized in the right lobe superoanteriorly, near the diaphragm. They are usually single, but may also be multiple and involve both lobes. Computed tomographic scan is very sensitive in the detection of amebic abscesses. It is also very useful in detecting extrahepatic involvement such as in the pleural space or lung. Amebic abscesses appear as a hypodense round or oval lesions with irregular borders. Approximately 20% of amebic abscesses may be superinfected by bacteria. Both ultrasound and computed tomographic scan may be used when drainage is indicated and as follow-up after institution of medical therapy.

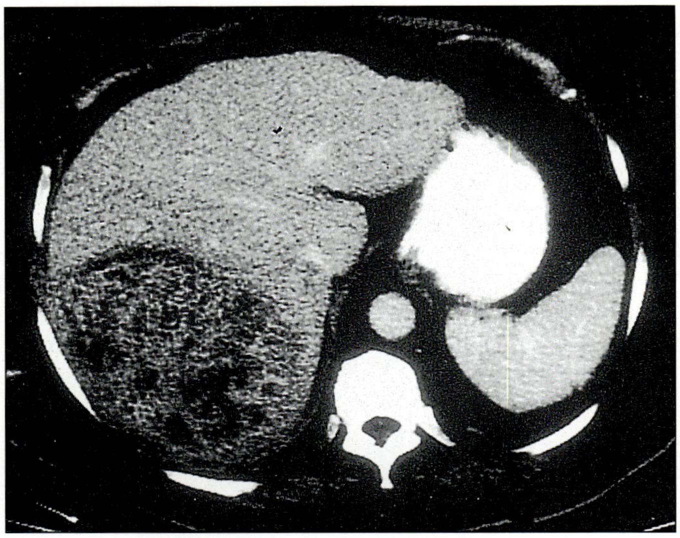

FIGURE 5-72.

Pyogenic abscesses are the most common type found in the United States. They may arise from biliary or hematogenous sources, may be single or multiple, and are more frequently found in the right lobe. The abscess cavities are variable in size and when multiple may coalesce to give a honeycomb appearance. By ultrasound they appear as round or oval hypoechoic lesions with a well-defined border and a variable number of internal echoes. Computed tomographic scan is highly sensitive in the localization of pyogenic liver abscesses. These lesions are hypodense areas that may sometimes show an air-fluid level indicating a gas-producing organism. Both computed tomography and ultrasound may be used in the aspiration of pyogenic abscesses, which can be done for both diagnostic and therapeutic purposes.

MALIGNANT TUMORS OF THE LIVER

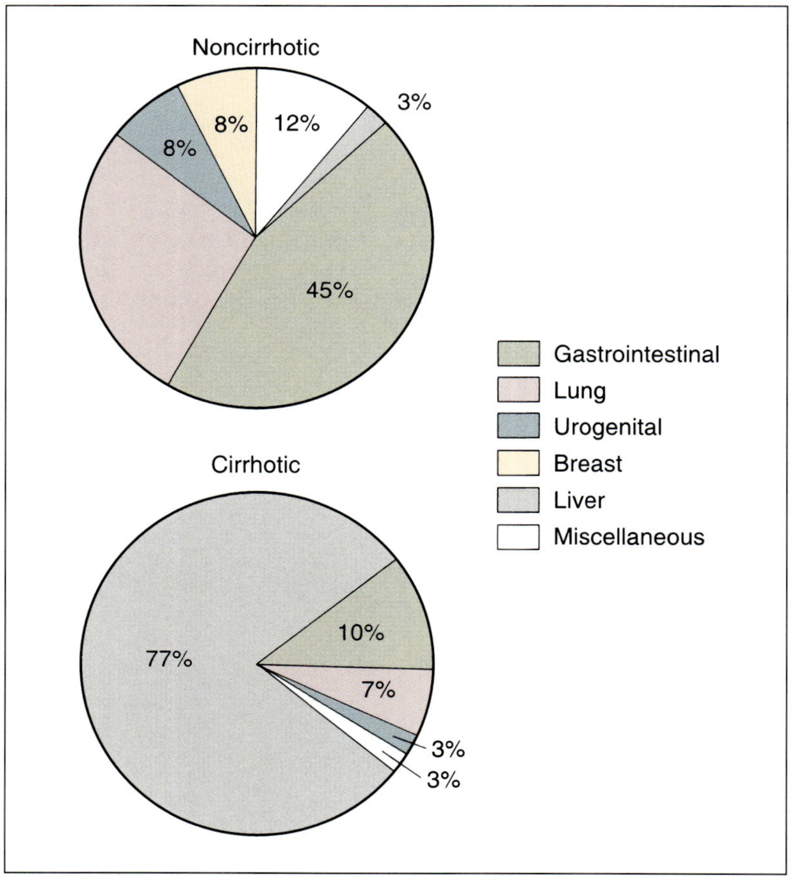

FIGURE 5-73.

The relative frequency of various tumors of the liver. Note that metastases are by far the most frequent, particularly in the developed western world. Among the primary malignant tumors, hepatocellular carcinoma is the most frequent. In the cirrhotic liver, hepatoma is more frequent that metastases.

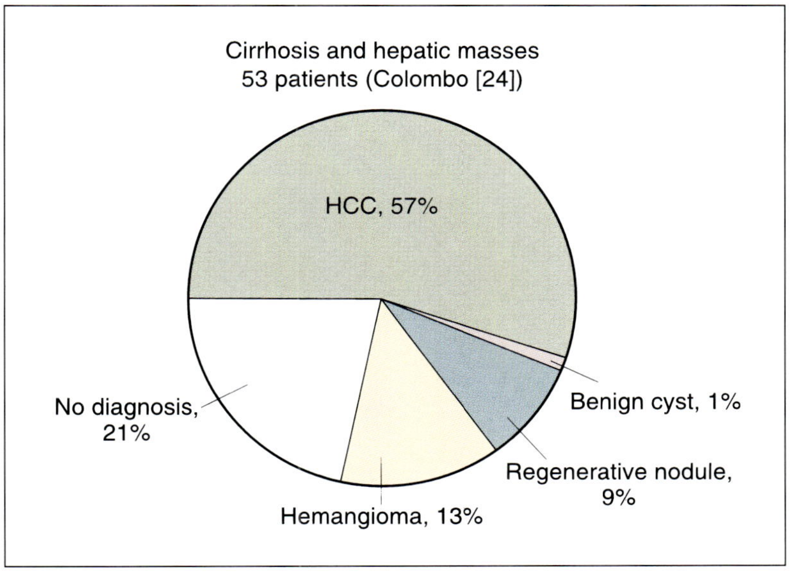

FIGURE 5-74.

Differential diagnosis of a mass found within the liver among cirrhotic patients [72]. Because of the poor prognosis for hepatocellular carcinoma (HCC) and the recognition that this tumor occurs against a background of chronic viral hepatitis and liver disease, attempts have been made to screen for the tumor in asymptomatic patients. In this way, small tumors may be found that are more amenable to therapy. Unfortunately, the presence of a mass within the liver of a patient with cirrhosis is not necessarily synonymous with HCC. This figure indicates that whereas most such masses turn out to be HCC, they may also represent cysts, angiomata, and regenerative nodules. In some cases, no obvious pathology can be found. The significance of regenerative nodules is uncertain, but it seems that the larger ones (greater than 1 cm, macroregenerative nodules) may sometimes lead to the development of HCC. (*Adapted from* Columbo *et al.* [73].)

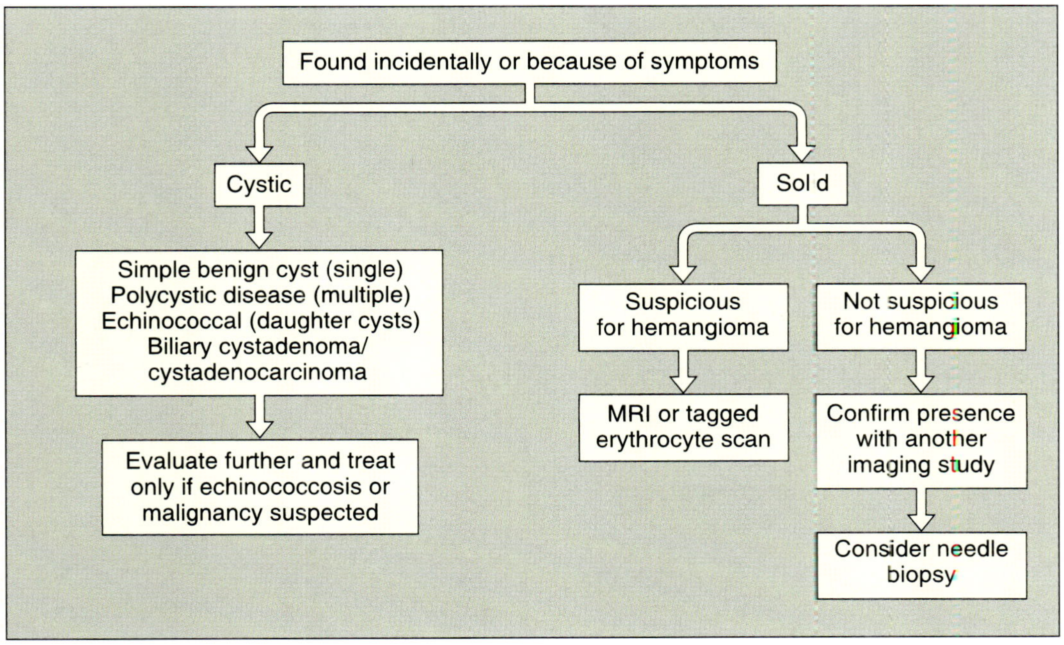

FIGURE 5-75.

Algorithm for evaluation of patients found to have a mass in noncirrhotic liver. The most likely etiology varies depending on whether the masses are found incidentally or if the patient presents with some symptoms referable to the liver. Thus cysts of the liver and hemangiomata are often found incidentally at the time of imaging studies for some other purpose, whereas patients with right upper quadrant pain or discomfort are more likely to have hepatic metastases, hepatocellular adenoma, or some unusual primary malignancy of the liver such as fibrolamellar hepatocellular carcinoma, angiosarcoma, or epithelioid hemangioendothelioma. MRI—magnetic resonance imaging.

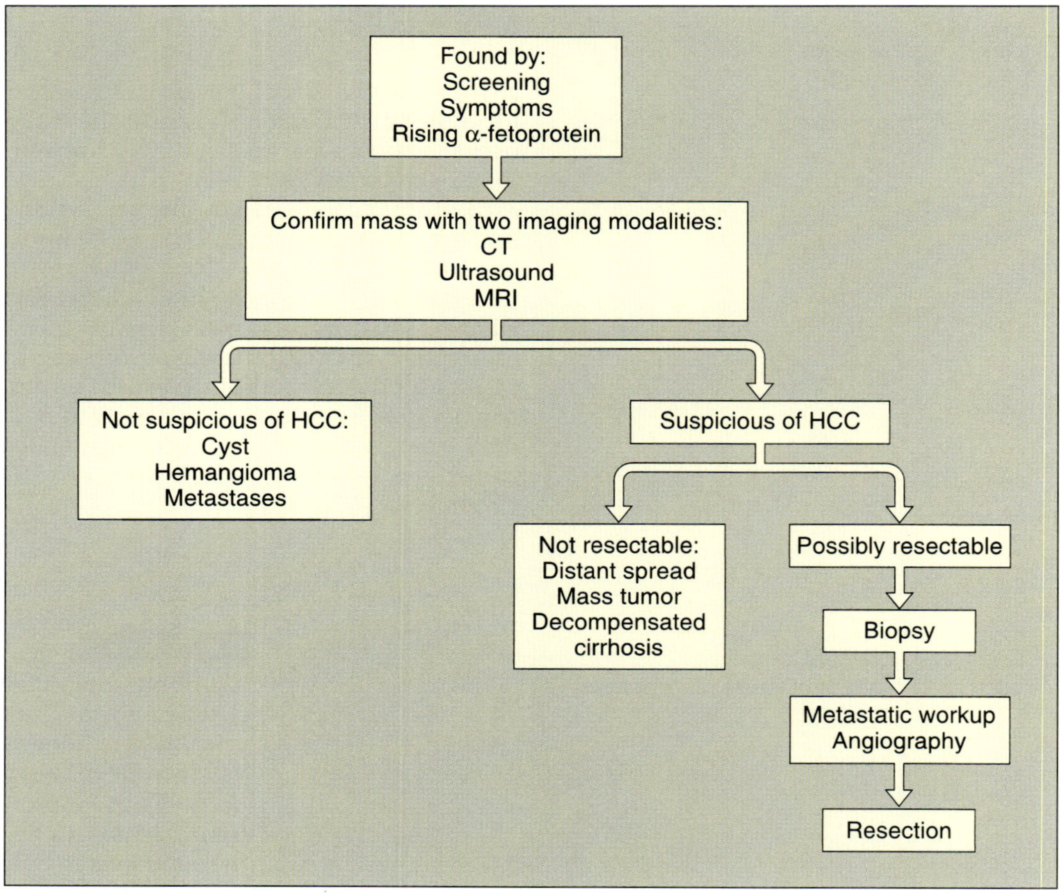

FIGURE 5-76.

An algorithm for evaluating masses in patients known to have cirrhosis where the possibility of hepatocellular carcinoma (HCC) is very much higher. The approach involves confirming the presence of the mass by using at least two imaging modalities which gives some idea of the extent of the tumor and also some preliminary idea of whether it is resectable or not. Definitive therapy usually requires a biopsy of the lesion—this may be done under direction by ultrasound or computed tomography (CT) or at the time of exploratory surgery. MRI—magnetic resonance imaging.

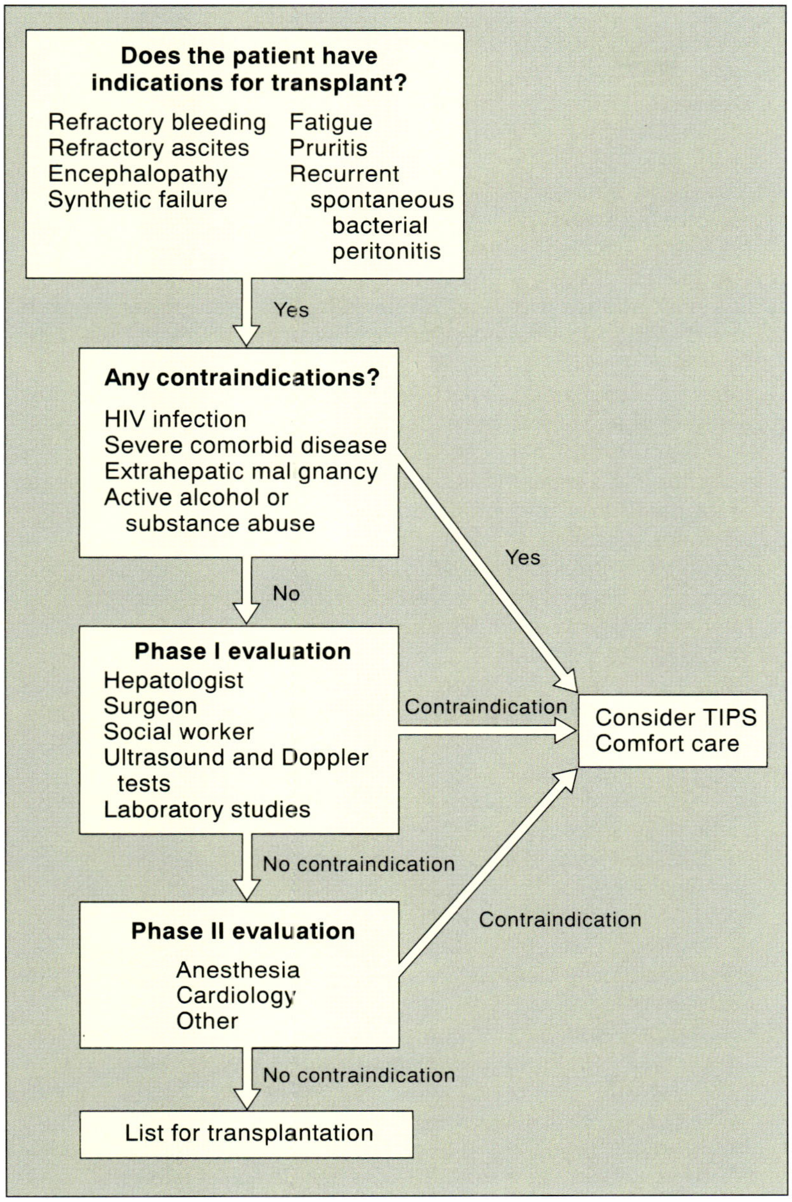

FIGURE 5-77.

The evaluation of patients for liver transplantation represents team efforts including hepatologists, transplantation surgeons, social workers, and consultants. The initial evaluation involves assessing whether indications for orthotopic liver transplantation (OLT) are present, including refractory variceal bleeding, encephalopathy, ascites, and marked impairment of synthetic function. Other unusual indications representing impaired quality of life include pruritus, metabolic bone disease, and xanthomatous neuropathy (seen in cholestatic diseases). Relatively uncommon indications are for correction of metabolic disorders that may (*ie*, α_1-antitrypsin deficiency, Wilson's disease, and tyrosinemia) or may not (hereditary oxalosis, familial hypercholesterolemia, and Crigler-Najjar syndrome) produce liver disease. If the patient has appropriate indications for OLT, comorbidities need to be evaluated. Severe cardiopulmonary disease, severe neurologic disease, extrahepatic malignancy, and HIV infection represent absolute contraindications. A careful cardiac evaluation is particularly important in patients over 50 years of age, who have alcoholic liver disorder or hemochromatosis as the cause of their end-stage liver disease, or if pulmonary hypertension is considered. Psychosocial contraindications include active illicit drug use, active alcohol abuse, and a lack of appropriate social support. Patients need considerable assistance after OLT. Compliance with medical therapy following OLT is also important. Portal vein thrombosis can make OLT technically more difficult but represents a contraindication only if a suitable blood vessel cannot be identified to connect a new liver, or if the thrombosis is secondary to tumor. Hepatitis B viremia (HBV) indicated by the presence of hepatitis B e antigen or HBV-DNA in serum represents a contraindication for many programs because of the high risk of HBV re-infection. The use of high-dose hepatitis B immunoglobulin to prevent re-infection in this group represents an area of active clinical investigation. Selection criteria for patients with a history of substance abuse varies from program to program. In a recent study [74], only 6 months of abstinence was found to predict a low risk of post-OLT recidivism. This process of patient selection is dynamic. Patients may be placed on the waiting list or removed as complications or contraindications develop and are treated. TIPS—transjugular intrahepatic portacaval shunts.

REFERENCES

1. Kools AM, Bloomer JR: Jaundice in the ICU: a bedside approach. In *Perspectives in Critical Care*, vol 2. Edited by Cerra FB. St. Louis: Quality Medical Publishing; 1989:165–177.
2. Alter MJ, Hadler SC: Delta hepatitis and infection in North America. In *Hepatitis Delta Virus*. Edited by Hadziyannis SJ, Taylor JM, Bonino F. New York: Wiley-Liss; 1993:243–250.
3. McQuillan G, Alter MJ, Everhart JE: Viral hepatitis. In *Digestive Diseases in the United States*. Edited by Everhart JE. Bethesda, MD: NIH; 1994:127–156.
4. Koff RS: Viral hepatitis. In *Diseases of the Liver*. Edited by Schiff L, Schiff ER. Philadelphia: JB Lippincott Company, 1993:492–577.
5. Seeff LB, Koff RS: Evolving concepts of the clinical and serologic consequences of hepatitis B infection. *Semin Liver Dis* 1986, 6:11–22.
6. Hoofnagle JB, Schafer DF: Serologic markers of hepatitis B virus infection. *Semin Liv Dis* 1986, 6:1–10.
7. Peters M, Vierling J, Gershwin ME, *et al.*: Immunology and the liver. *Hepatology* 1991, 13:977–994.
8. Hoofnagle JH, Seeff LB: Natural history of chronic type B hepatitis. In *Progress in Liver Diseases*. Edited by Popper H, Schaffner F. New York: Grune & Stratton, 1982:469–479.
9. Jeffers J, Hasan F, deMedina M, *et al.*: Prevalence of antibodies to hepatitis C virus among patients with cryptogenic chronic hepatitis and cirrhosis. *Hepatology* 1992, 15:187–190.
10. Czaja AJ, Carpenter HA, Santrach PJ, *et al.*: The nature and prognosis of severe cryptogenic chronic active hepatitis. *Gastroenterology* 1993, 104:1755–1761.
11. Hoofnagle JH, Davis GL, Hanson RG: Chronic type B hepatitis: clinical course. In *Viral Hepatitis and Delta Infection*. Edited by Verme G, Bonino F, Rizzetto M. New York: Alan R. Liss, 1983:41–53.
12. Davis GL, Hoofnagle JH, Waggoner IG: Spontaneous reactivation of chronic hepatitis B infection. *Gastroenterology* 1984, 86:230–235.
13. Davis GL, Hoofnagle JH: Reactivation of chronic type B hepatitis presenting as acute viral hepatitis. *Ann Intern Med* 1985, 102:762–765.
14. Shafritz DA, Shouval D, Sherman HI, *et al.*: Integration of hepatitis B

virus DNA into the genome of liver cells in chronic liver disease and hepatocellular carcinoma: studies in percutaneous liver biopsies and postmortem tissue specimens. *N Engl J Med* 1981, 305:1067–1073.
15. Brechot C, Nalpas B, Courouce A-M, *et al.*: Evidence that hepatitis B virus has a role in liver-cell carcinoma in alcoholic liver disease. *N Engl J Med* 1982, 306:1384–1387.
16. Perrillo RP, Schiff ER, Davis GL, *et al.*: A randomized controlled trial of interferon alfa-2b alone and after prednisone withdrawal for the treatment of chronic hepatitis B. *N Engl J Med* 1990, 323:295–301.
17. Wong DKH, Cheung AM, O'Rourke K, *et al.*: Effect of α-interferon treatment in patients with hepatitis B and antigen-positive chronic hepatitis B: A meta-analysis. *Ann Intern Med* 1993, 119:312–323.
18. Lok ASF: Treatment of chronic hepatitis B. *J Viral Hepatitis* 1994, 1:105–124.
19. Renault PF, Hoofnagle JH: Side effects of α-interferon. *Semin Liver Dis* 1989, 9:273–277.
20. Kassianides C, DiBisceglie AM, Hoofnagle JH, *et al.*: α-Interferon therapy in patients with decompensated chronic type B hepatitis. In *Viral Hepatitis and Liver Disease*. Edited by Zuckerman A. New York: Alan R. Liss, 1988:840–843.
21. Perrillo RP: The management of chronic hepatitis B. *Am J Med* 1994, 96:34S–40S.
22. Kuhns M, McNamara A, Mason A, *et al.*: Serum and liver hepatitis B virus DNA in chronic hepatitis B after sustained loss of surface antigen. *Gastroenterology* 1992, 103:1649–1656.
23. Korenman J, Baker B, Waggoner J, *et al.*: Long-term remission of chronic hepatitis B after α-interferon therapy. *Ann Intern Med* 1991, 114:629–634.
24. Carreno V, Castillo I, Molina J, *et al.*: Long-term follow-up of hepatitis B chronic carriers who responded to interferon therapy. *J Hepatol* 1992, 15:102–106.
25. Lok ASF, Chung HT, Liu VWS, *et al.*: Long-term follow-up of chronic hepatitis B patients treated with interferon alfa. *Gastroenterology* 1993, 105:1833–1838.
26. Conjeevaram HS, Di Bisceglie AM: Natural history. In *Viral Hepatitis*. Edited by Zuckerman AH, Thomas HC. New York: Churchill-Livingstone; 1993:341–349.
27. Jeffers LJ, Hasan F, de Medina M, *et al.*: Prevalence of antibodies to hepatitis C virus among patients with cryptogenic chronic hepatitis and cirrhosis. *Hepatology* 1992, 15:187–190.
28. Merican I, Sherlock S, McIntyre N, *et al.*: Clinical, biochemical and histological features in 102 patients with chronic hepatitis C virus infection. *Q J Med* 1993, 86:119–125.
29. Puoti M, Zonaro A, Ravagg A, *et al.*: Hepatitis C virus RNA and antibody response in the clinical course of acute hepatitis C virus infection. *Hepatology* 1992, 16:877–881.
30. Resnick RH, Koff R: Hepatitis C related hepatocellular carcinoma. *Arch Intern Med* 1993, 17:S108–S111.
31. Alter HJ, Purcell RH, Shih JW, *et al.*: Detection of antibody to hepatitis C virus in prospectively followed transfusion recipients with acute and chronic non A, non B hepatitis. *N Engl J Med* 1989, 321:1494–1500.
32. Tremolada F, Casarin C, Tragger A, *et al.*: Antibody to hepatitis C virus in post-transfusion hepatitis. *Ann Intern Med* 1991, 114:277–281.
33. Hoofnagle J: Chronic hepatitis. In *Liver Biopsy Interpretation for the 1990's. AASLD Postgraduate Course Syllabus 1991*. Edited by Hoofnagle JH, Goodman Z. Thorofare: Slack Inc; 1991:124.
34. Ferri C, Greco F, Longombardo G, *et al.*: Association between hepatitis C virus and mixed cryoglobulinemia. *Clin Exp Rheumatol* 1991, 9:621–624.
35. Lunel F, Musset L, Cacoub P, *et al.*: Cryoglobulinemia in chronic liver diseases: role of hepatitis C virus and liver damage. *Gastroenterology* 1994, 106:1291–1300.
36. Shakil AO, DiBisceglie AM: Images in clinical medicine: vasculitis and cryoglobulinemia related to hepatitis C. *N Engl J Med* 1994, 331:1624.
37. DeCastro M, Sanchez J, Herrera JF, *et al.*: Hepatitis C virus antibodies and liver disease in patients with porphyria cutanea tarda. *Hepatology* 1993, 17:551–557.
38. Fargion S, Piperno A, Cappellini MD, *et al.*: Hepatitis C virus and porphyria cutanea tarda: evidence of a strong association. *Hepatology* 1992, 16:1322–1326.
39. Olynyk JK, Luxon BA, Jeffrey GP, *et al.*: Predicting phlebotomy requirements in the treatment of iron overload [Abstract]. *Hepatology* 1994, 20:A323.
40. Arber N, Moshkowitz M, Konikoff F, *et al.*: Iron overload in patients with chronic hepatitis C virus infection predicts a poor response to interferon therapy [Abstract]. *Gastroenterology* 1994, 106:A860.
41. Campbell C, Daley PJ, Urdea MS, *et al.*: HCV-RNA in peripheral blood mononuclear cells of chronic hepatitis C patients treated with interferon alfa 2b: Another possible indicator of response [Abstract]. *Gastroenterology* 1994, 106:A871.
42. Lam N, DeGuzman L, Pitrak D, *et al.*: Clinical and histologic predictors of response to α-interferon in patients with chronic hepatitis C viral infection [Abstract]. *Gastroenterology* 1994, 106:A923.
43. Marcellin P, Castelnau C, Milotova V, *et al.*: influence of the dose and of the duration of interferon treatment on the response to therapy according to hepatitis C virus genotype in chronic hepatitis C [Abstract]. *Hepatology* 1994, 20:A155.
44. Johnson PJ, McFarlane IG, Alvarez F, *et al.*: Meeting report: International autoimmune hepatitis group. *Hepatology* 1993, 18:998–1005.
45. Czaja AJ, Carpenter HA, Santrach PJ, *et al.*: Evidence against hepatitis viruses as important causes of severe autoimmune hepatitis in the United States. *J Hepatol* 1993, 18:342–352.
46. Czaja AJ, Davis GL, Ludwig J, *et al.*: Autoimmune features as determinants of prognosis in steroid-treated chronic active hepatitis of uncertain etiology. *Gastroenterology* 1983, 85:713–717.
47. Czaja AJ, Carpenter HA, Santrach PJ, Moore SB: Genetic predispositions for the immunological features of chronic active hepatitis. *Hepatology* 1993, 18:816–822.
48. Perdigoto R, Carpenter HA, Czaja AJ: Frequency and significance of chronic ulcerative colitis in severe corticosteroid-treated autoimmune hepatitis. *J Hepatol* 1992, 14:325–331.
49. Czaja AJ, Carpenter HA, Santrach PJ, Moore SB: Significance of HLA DR4 in type I autoimmune hepatitis. *Gastroenterology* 1993, 105:1502–1507.
50. Czaja AJ: Diagnosis, prognosis, and treatment of classical autoimmune chronic active hepatitis. In *Autoimmune Liver Diseases*. Edited by Krawitt EL, Wiesner RH. New York: Raven Press; 1991:143–166.
51. Czaja AJ: Autoimmune chronic active hepatitis—a specific entity? *J Gastroenterol Hepatol* 1990, 5:343–351.
52. Czaja AJ, Rakela J, Ludwig J: Features reflective of early prognosis in corticosteroid-treated severe autoimmune chronic active hepatitis. *Gastroenterology* 1988, 95:448–453.
53. Czaja AJ: Autoimmune hepatitis: current therapeutic concepts. *Clin Immunother* 1994, 1:413–429.
54. Czaja AJ: Chronic active hepatitis. In *Current Therapy in Allergy, Immunology, and Rheumatology*. Edited by Lichtenstein LM, Fauci AS. St. Louis: Mosby-Year Book; 1992:273–278.
55. Czaja AJ: Treatment of autoimmune hepatitis. In *Autoimmune Hepatitis*. Edited by Nishioka M, Toda G, Zeniya M. Amsterdam: Elsevier Science BV; 1994:283–304.
56. Sanchez-Urdazpal L, Czaja AJ, van Hoek B, *et al.*: Prognostic features and role of liver transplantation in severe corticosteroid-treated autoimmune chronic active hepatitis. *Hepatology* 1992, 15:215–221.
57. Lee WM: Medical progress: acute liver failure. *N Engl J Med* 1993, 329:1862–1874.
58. Lieber CS: *Medical and Nutritional Complications of Alcohol: Mechanisms and Management*. New York: Plenum Press; 1992:579.
59. Lieber CS, Robins SJ, Li J, *et al.*: Phosphatidylcholine protects against bibrosis and cirrhosis in the baboon. *Gastroenterology* 1994, 6:152–159.

60. Ramond MU, Poynard T, Rueff B: A randomized trial of prednisone in patients with severe alcoholic hepatitis. *N Engl J Med* 1992, 326:507–512.

61. Edwards CQ, Griffen LM, Goldgar D, *et al.*: Prevalence of hemochromatosis among 11,065 presumably healthy blood donors. *N Engl J Med* 1988, 318:1355–1362.

62. Scheinberg IH, Sternlieb I: Wilson's disease. In *Major Problems in Internal Medicine Series*. Edited by Smith LH. Philadelphia: WB Saunders; 1984.

63. Sternlieb I: Perspectives on Wilson's disease. *Hepatology* 1990, 12:1234–1239.

64. Stremmel W, Meyerow KW, Niederan C, *et al.*: Wilson's disease: Clinical presentation, treatment, and survival. *Ann Intern Med* 1991, 115:720–726.

65. Hoefs JC, Runyon BA: Spontaneous bacterial peritonitis. *Dis Mon* 1985, 31:1–48.

66. Gines P, Rimola A, Planas R, *et al.*: Norfloxacin prevents spontaneous bacterial peritonitis recurrence in cirrhosis. Results of a double-blind placebo controlled trial. *Hepatology* 1990, 12:716–724.

67. Sadler MA, Shapiro RS: Transjugular portosystemic shunt. *N Engl J Med* 1994:330:182.

68. Fessel JM, Conn HO: An analysis of the causes and prevention of hepatic coma [Abstract]. *Gastroenterology* 1972, 62:191.

69. Stahl J: Studies of the blood ammonia in liver disease. Its diagnostic, prognostic and therapeutic significance. *Ann Intern Med* 1963, 58:1–24.

70. Conn HO, Helzberg J: Complications of portal hypertension. *Current Hepatology* 1986, 6:133–140.

71. Bucci I, Palmieri GC: Double-blind, double-dummy comparison between treatment with rifaximin and lactulose in patients with medium to severe degree hepatic encephalopathy. *Curr Med Res Opin* 1993, 13:109–118.

72. Colombo M, de Franchis R, Del Ninno E, *et al.*: Primary hepatocellular carcinoma. *N Engl J Med* 1991, 325:729–731.

73. Columbo M, de Franchis R, Del Ninno E, *et al.*: Hepatocellular carcinoma in Italian patients with cirrhosis. *N Engl J Med* 1991, 325:675–680.

74. Osario RW, Ascher NL, Avery M, et al.: Predicting recidivism after orthotopic liver transplantation for alcoholic liver disease [Part 1]. *Hepatology* 1994, 20:105–110.

Chapter 6

Disorders of the Gallbladder and Biliary Tract

EDITOR

Nicholas F. LaRusso

CONTRIBUTORS

M. Stanley Branch
David L. Carr-Locke
Wendy Z. Davis
Rita De Vos
Valeer J. Desmet
John H. Donohue
Joanne M. Donovan
Keith D. Lindor
Henry A. Pitt
Tonia Roskams
Alfred D. Roston
Eldon A. Shaffer
Johnson L. Thistle
James Toouli

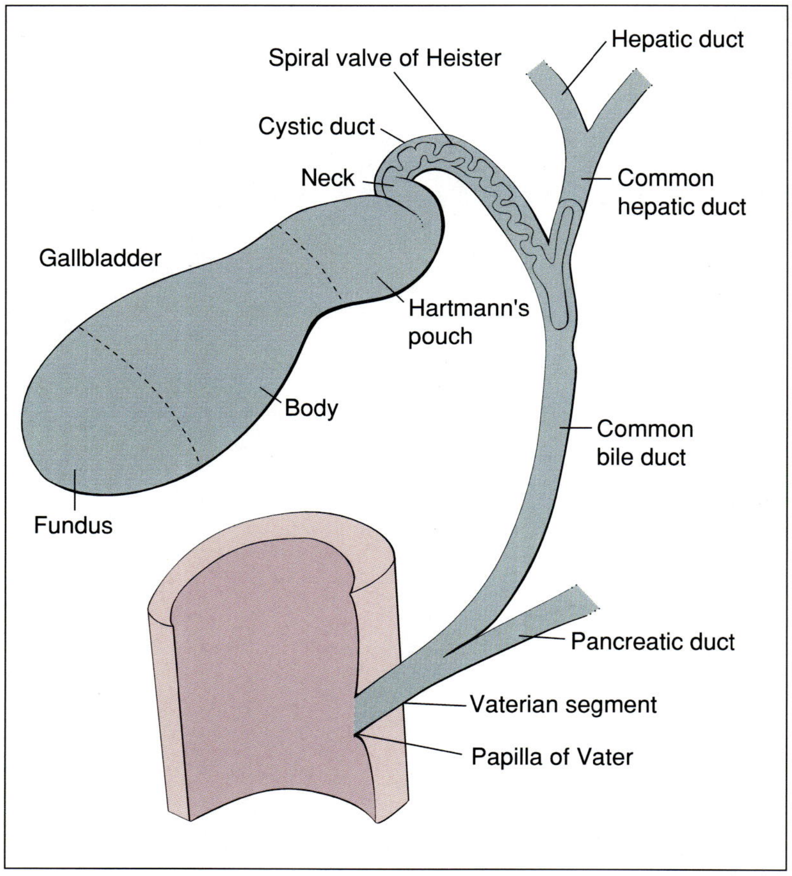

FIGURE 6-1.

The gallbladder is a pear-shaped sac located under the right lobe of the liver lateral to the quadrate lobe; it lies in a depression of the liver surface in contact with the interlobular connective tissue of the liver (facies visceralis). It is covered to a variable extent by peritoneum reflected off the liver. In more than 50% of patients the gallbladder may reach 0.5 to 1 cm beyond the anterior hepatic edge, contacting the anterior abdominal wall. The gallbladder measures up to 10 cm long and 3 to 4 cm wide in adults and has a volume of about 50 mL. It consists of a fundus with a blind end, a central body, and a narrow neck that connects to the cystic duct. The body is the largest segment; it narrows to an infundibulum as it joins the neck. The cholecystoduodenal ligament is a peritoneal fold that attaches the infundibulum to the first portion of the duodenum. In its normal location, the body passes upward and backwards into the neck. Hartmann's pouch is a dilatation in the neck region that may become adherent to the common hepatic duct. It is thought to be a consequence of disease processes and not a normal anatomic configuration [1]. The gallbladder neck is S-shaped, measures 5 to 7 mm in length, and narrows towards its connection with the cystic duct.

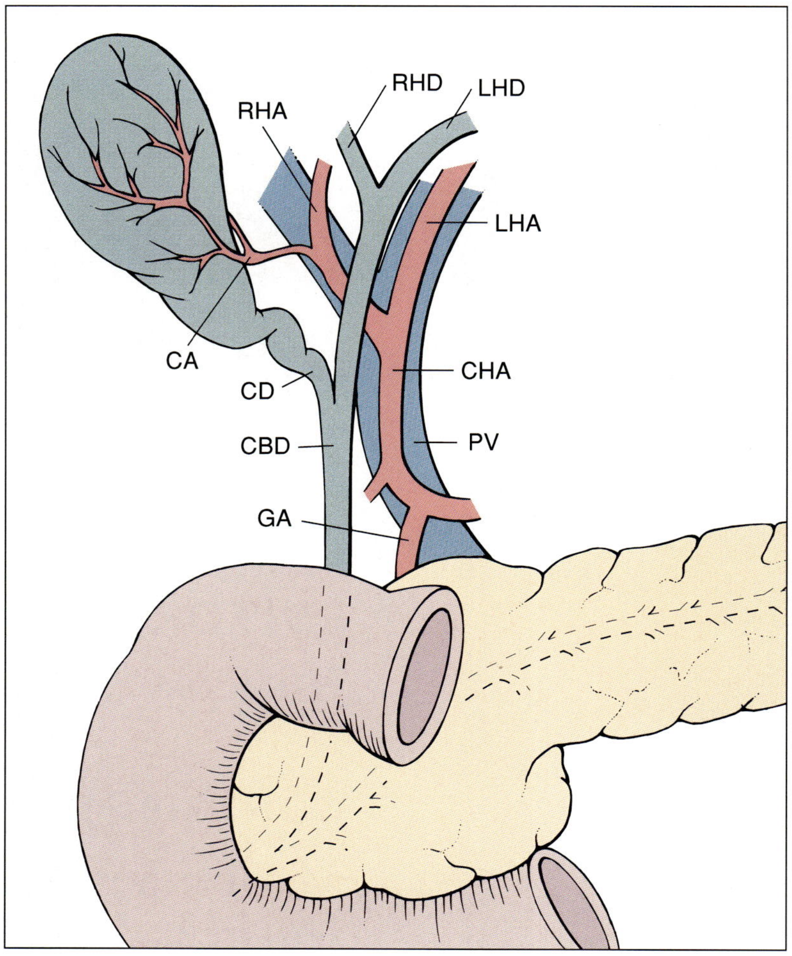

FIGURE 6-2.

The right hepatic duct (RHD) and left hepatic duct (LHD) emerge from the porta hepatis and in most instances join together after about 0.5 to 1 cm to form the common hepatic duct, which further descends in the free edge of the lesser omentum anterior to the foramen of Winslow. At a variable distance (from 1 to 5 cm) the cystic duct (CD) enters to form the common bile duct (CBD) (*see* Fig. 1-4). The latter continues downward in the hepatoduodenal fold of the peritoneum, passes behind the first part of the duodenum and the pancreas, then curves or bends to the right to enter in an oblique way the second part of the duodenum on its posteromedial side [2]. CA—cystic artery; CHA—common hepatic artery; GA—gastroduodenal artery; GB—gallbladder; LHA—left hepatic artery; PV—portal vein; RHA—right hepatic artery. (*Adapted from* Frierson [2].)

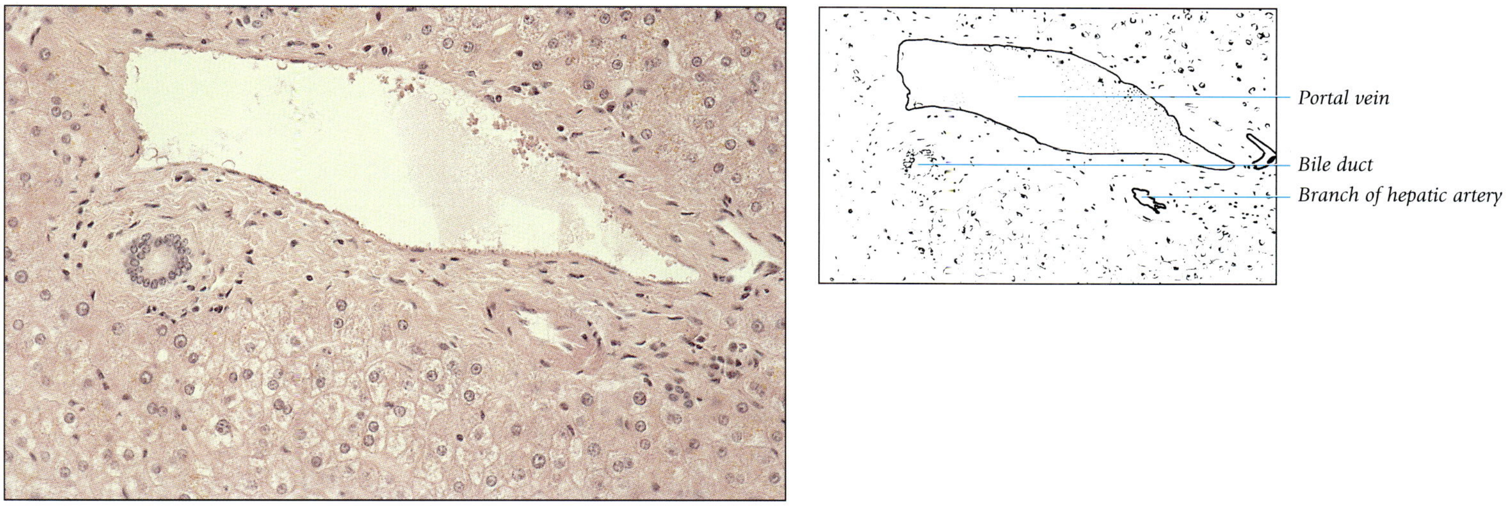

FIGURE 6-3.

Intrahepatic bile ducts. Each medium-sized portal tract usually contains one or two interlobular bile ducts, so that the normal ratio between interlobular bile ducts and portal tracts counted in a microscopic section of normal liver reaches a value between 0.9 and 1.8. This value has importance in diagnosing ductopenia (or paucity of intrahepatic bile ducts), in which case the bile duct to portal space ratio is less than 0.8.

In normal liver, the bile duct is accompanied by a branch of the hepatic artery with an inner diameter roughly equal to the diameter of the duct. Another way of diagnosing ductopenia is the finding of portal tracts with hepatic artery branches that are not accompanied by an interlobular duct ("widowed" arteries) [3]. (Hematoxylin-eosin stain × 125.)

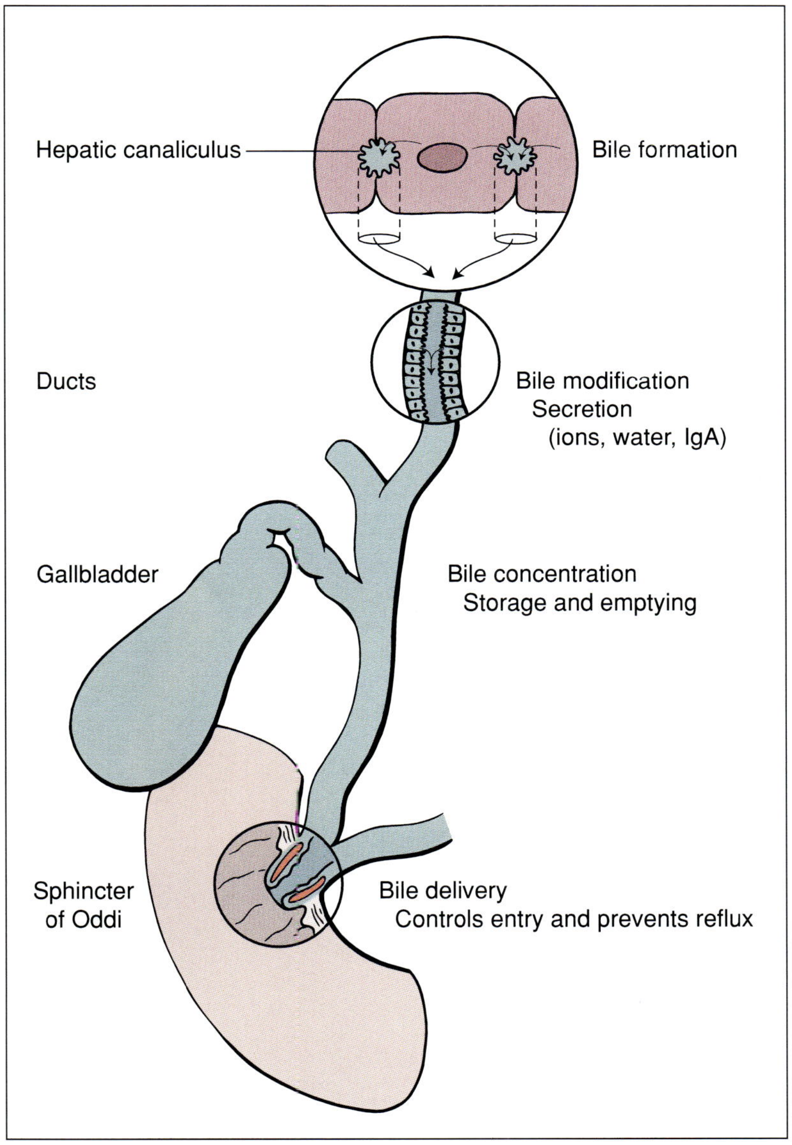

FIGURE 6-4.

Overview of the structure and function of the biliary tract. The biliary tract has four structural and functional components: (1) the hepatic canaliculus, the groove formed between adjoining liver cells, which are responsible for bile formation [4]; (2) the ductal system from the liver to the duodenum, which delivers and modifies bile; (3) the gallbladder, which concentrates, stores, and empties bile when appropriate; and (4) the sphincter of Oddi, which regulates bile delivery to the duodenum and prevents reflux of duodenal contents.

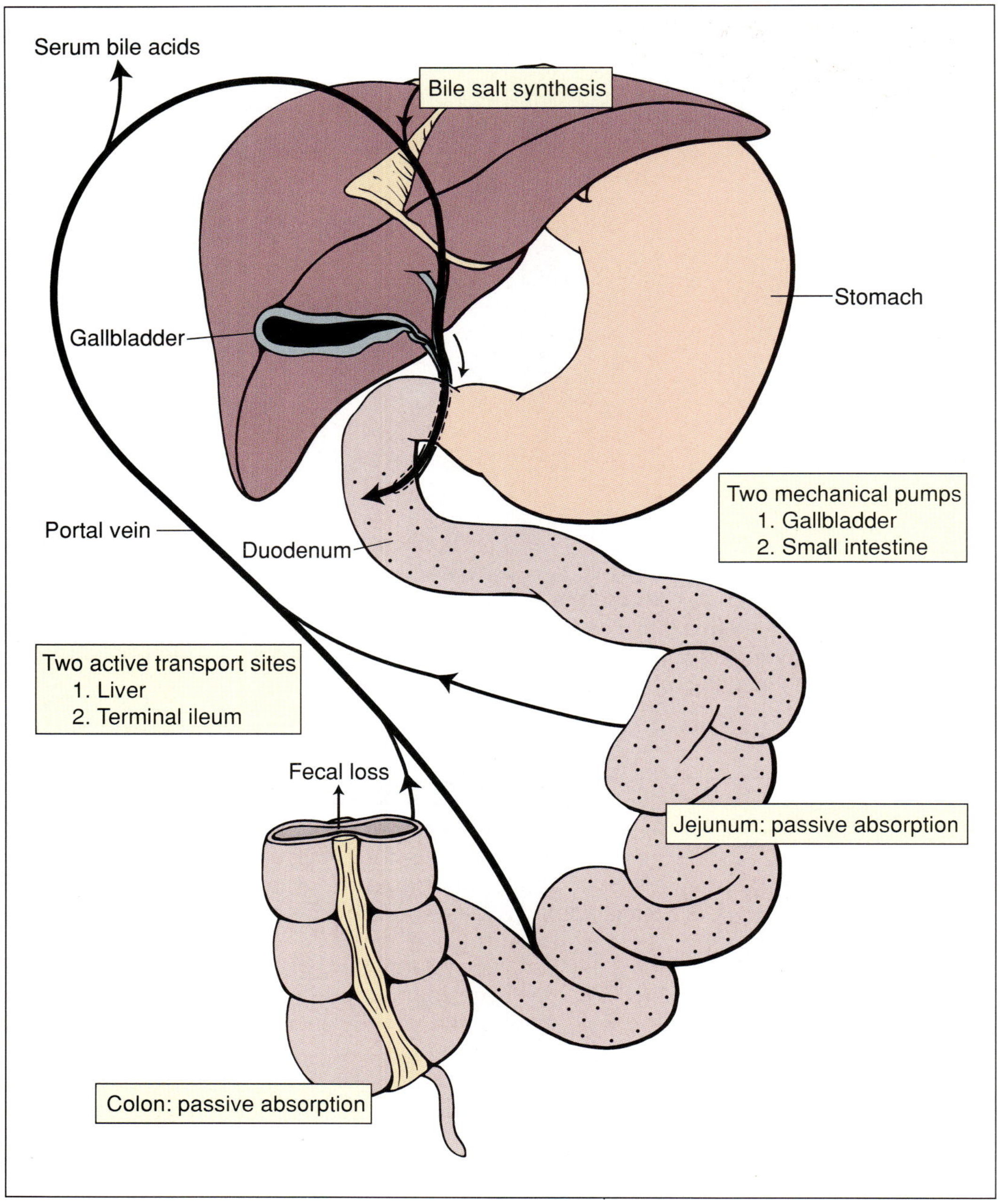

FIGURE 6-5.

Overview of the enterohepatic circulation of bile salts [5]. Bile salts are secreted by the liver then stored in the gallbladder for variable periods of time during the interdigestive period before they enter the duodenum. Absorption is passive in the jejunum and colon but active in the terminal ileum. Bile salts return to the liver via the portal vein to be actively taken up and secreted once again. Bile salts are synthesized from cholesterol only in the liver. The rate of synthesis is determined by the availability of cholesterol and, more importantly, by the returning bile salt pool, which regulates hepatic synthesis of bile salts in a negative feedback manner. Only a small portion of bile salts are lost in each circuit: about 5% are lost from the intestine to exit in feces with each circuit; a very tiny portion enters the blood stream. This enterohepatic circuit is driven by two mechanical pumps, the gallbladder and the small intestine, plus two active transport sites, the terminal ileum and the sinusoidal membrane of the hepatocyte. It has a rapidly flowing conduit, the portal vein. Although this system is very efficient, there are rate-limiting steps in its circuitry, particularly residence time in the gallbladder and transit through the small intestine. The more concentrated sites of the bile salt pool are depicted as a solid in the gallbladder and stippled in the intestine.

GALLSTONES AND THEIR CONSEQUENCES

TYPES OF GALLSTONES

	Cholesterol	Black pigment	Brown pigment
Location	Gallbladder	Gallbladder	Bile ducts
Pathogenesis	Physical-Chemical	Physical-Chemical	Infectious
Composition: Cholesterol	+++	+	++
Calcium and Bilirubin Content	+	+++	++

Figure 6-6.

The three major classes of gallstones—cholesterol stones, black pigment stones, and brown pigment stones—differ in their pathogenesis as well as in their composition [6,7]. Cholesterol and black pigment stones form only in the gallbladder, but brown pigment stones are formed in the bile ducts after bacterial infection of the biliary tree. They are essentially an infectious disease of the biliary tree, and as such, their only major risk factor is mechanical bile stasis because of obstruction or, in some cases, a duodenal diverticula. In contrast, the formation of cholesterol and black pigment stones depends on a physical-chemical problem, that is, the presence of an excess of insoluble constituents of bile. Hence, the composition of these three types of gallstones differs. Cholesterol is the major constituent of cholesterol gallstones, which also contain small amounts of inorganic calcium salts and the calcium salt of bilirubin. Black pigment stones contain large amounts of calcium and bilirubin, whereas brown pigment stones are composed of calcium salts of lipids degraded by bacteria, such as fatty acid soaps, as well as smaller amounts of bilirubin and cholesterol.

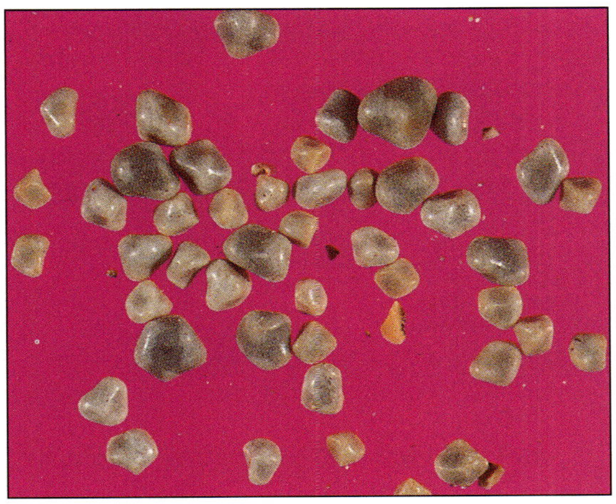

Figure 6-7.

Appearance of gallstones. The type of stone can often be identified visually. Cholesterol stones may be solitary or they may occur as several stones of similar size, suggesting that stone formation occurred at a single instant. Numerous tiny stones may not be individually identified on ultrasound.

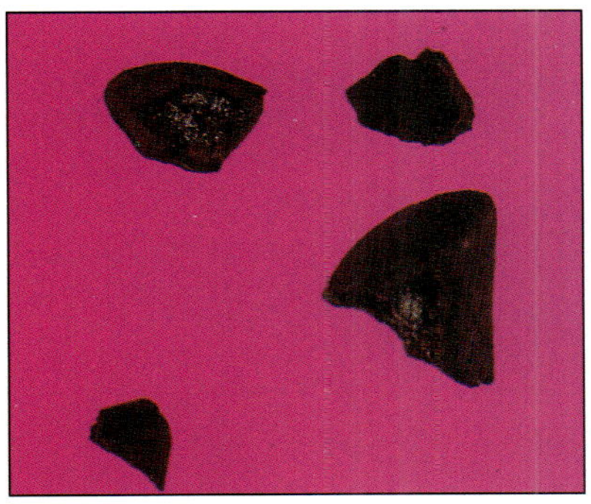

Figure 6-8.

Black pigment stones are amorphous, but may be faceted, a finding consistent with their high content of polymerized bilirubin pigment. Brown pigment stones (not shown) are frequently laminated and occur on a nidus of infection, which may be either a cholesterol or black pigment stone in the Western Hemisphere or frequently a parasite in the Eastern Hemisphere.

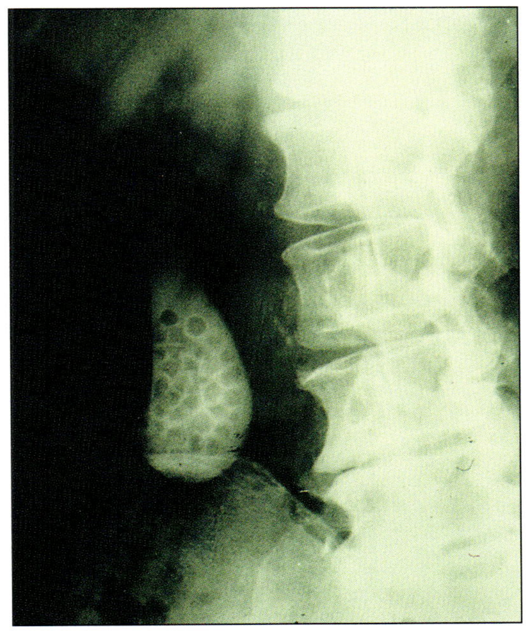

Figure 6-9.

Oral cholecystogram of cholesterol gallstones. Gallstones can be visualized by an oral cholecystogram. Here, the gallbladder is filled with multifaceted lucencies. In contrast to black pigment stones, whose high calcium content renders them radiodense, most cholesterol stones are radiolucent. (*From* Donovan and Carr-Locke [8]; with permission.)

CLINICAL RISK FACTORS FOR CHOLESTEROL GALLSTONE FORMATION

Estrogens:

Pregnancy, Female Sex, Exogenous Administration

Age

Ethnic Origin: Native American

Obesity and Rapid Weight Loss

Hypertriglyceridemia

Gallbladder Stasis:

Spinal Cord Injury, Increased Somatostatin Levels, Vagotomy

FIGURE 6-10.

To summarize the epidemiology of gallstone disease, major risk factors for cholesterol gallstone disease include a high level of endogenous or exogenous estrogen, age, ethnic origin (Native Americans have a higher risk than Europeans, who have a higher risk than Asians and African blacks), obesity, rapid weight loss, hypertriglyceridemia, and gallbladder stasis.

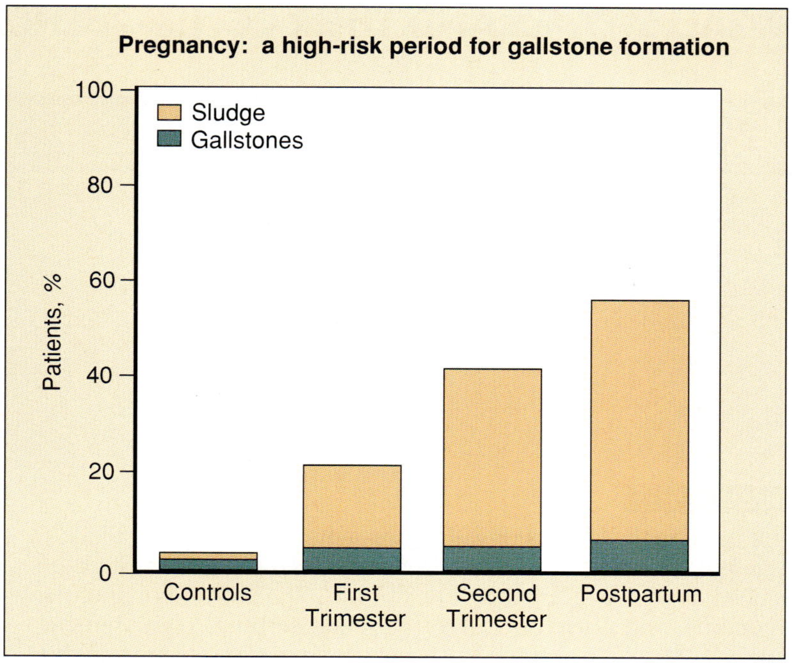

FIGURE 6-11.

Recently, the importance of pregnancy as a high-risk period for gallstone development has emerged. The presence of biliary sludge, the precursor of gallstones, increases throughout pregnancy to reach about 50% in the immediate postpartum period [9]. During pregnancy, about 7% of women develop gallstones, and as many as a third of this group with gallstones or sludge develop symptoms of biliary colic. In the postpartum year, biliary sludge disappears in more than 90% of women, and in a third of patients, small gallstones dissolve or pass spontaneously. Pregnancy is particularly lithogenic because estrogens increase biliary cholesterol saturation and progesterones impair gallbladder motility. (*Data from* Maringhini *et al.* [9].)

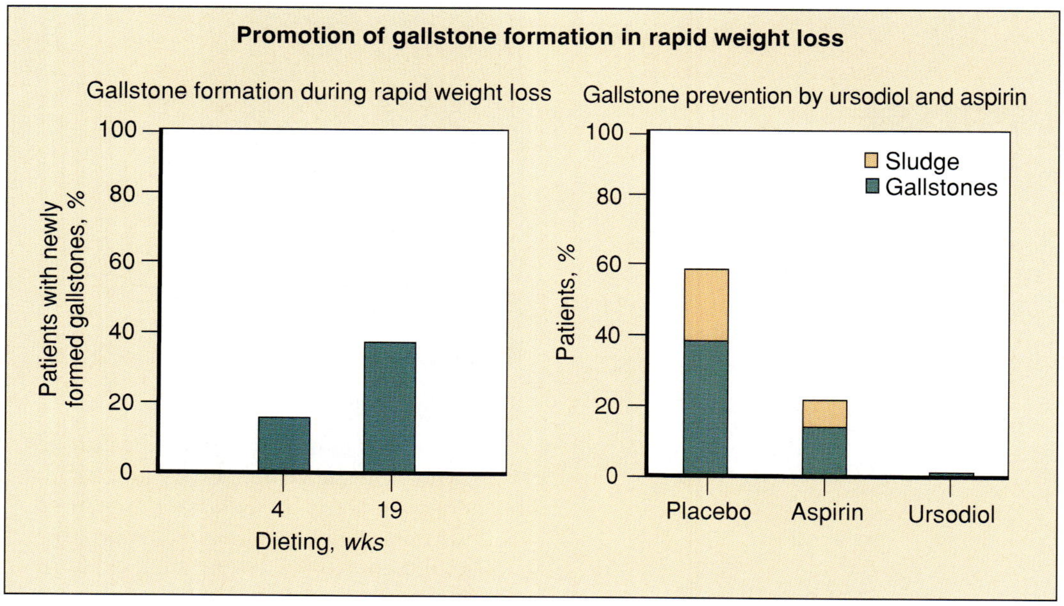

FIGURE 6-12.

Patients undergoing rapid weight loss, either by dieting or after gastric surgery for treatment of morbid obesity, are at high risk of developing gallstones [10,11]. Over several months, about a third developed gallstones. Prophylaxis with the acid form of hydrophilic bile salt ursodeoxycholate has, however, been demonstrated to prevent gallstone formation both in the setting of rapid weight loss, as shown here, and after gastric surgery. Aspirin was also associated with a nonsignificant decrease in gallstone formation. Inhibition of prostaglandin formation may prevent mucin hypersecretion, and consequently, protect against gallstone formation. Ursodeoxycholic acid decreases cholesterol secretion into bile and delays cholesterol crystal formation. (*Data from* Broomfield *et al.* [11].)

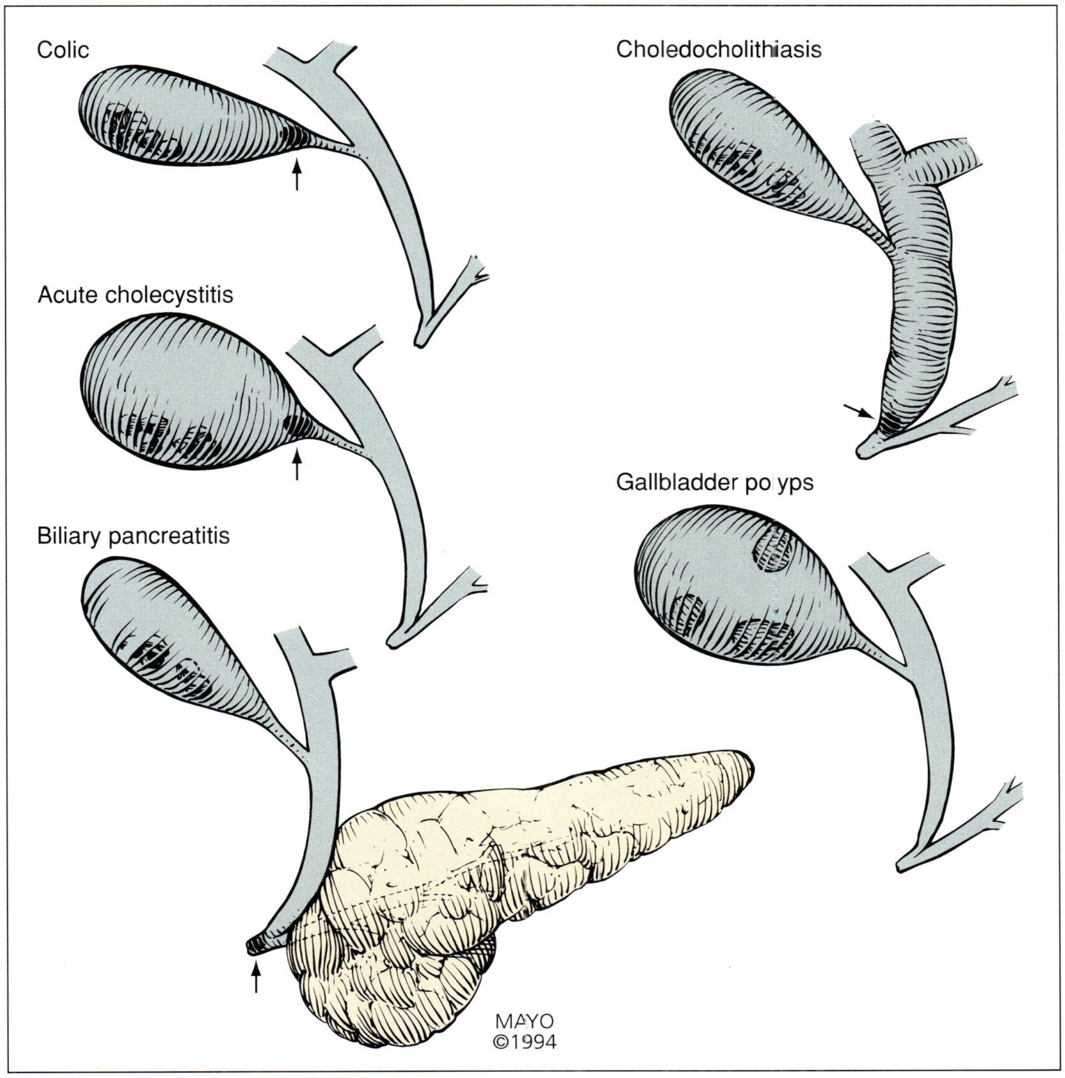

FIGURE 6-13.

The indications for laparoscopic cholecystectomy are comparable to those for open cholecystectomy. Asymptomatic cholelithiasis, even in patients with insulin-dependent diabetes mellitus and other diseases that complicate the management of acute gallbladder disease, is not an appropriate reason for operation [12,13]. Most patients will present with episodic, postprandial pain, incorrectly termed *biliary colic,* and have pathologic findings of mild chronic cholecystitis. Acute inflammatory changes, with or without bacterial infection of the gallbladder, may be treated laparoscopically. The anatomy of the hepatoduodenal ligament may be obscured by edema, scarring, or hemorrhage, however, necessitating conversion to open cholecystectomy more frequently than in patients with chronic symptoms. In many patients with biliary pancreatitis, pancreatic inflammation resolves spontaneously and without complication. Because of the risk of recurrence, these patients should undergo laparoscopic cholecystectomy, preferably as soon as clinical and, ideally, biochemical evidence of pancreatitis has resolved. Urgent endoscopic intervention with sphincterotomy should be performed in the minority of patients whose biliary pancreatitis does not rapidly improve. Similarly, patients with acute cholangitis from choledocholithiasis should undergo initial endoscopic biliary decompression. Patients with nonacute symptoms from common duct stones may be treated laparoscopically to remove both the gallbladder and choledocholithiasis, or these patients may be treated by both laparoscopic and endoscopic procedures. Some patients with biliary tract symptoms will have gallbladder polyps on ultrasound examination. These are sometimes gallstones attached to the gallbladder wall by mucus strands and should be treated as symptomatic cholelithiasis. Because neoplastic polyps may already contain or may become an invasive carcinoma, asymptomatic gallbladder polyps should be excised by laparoscopic cholecystectomy, with the realization that if invasive gallbladder cancer is found, an open, potentially curative, surgical procedure may be indicated. A calcified gallbladder (porcelain gallbladder) and perhaps large (3 cm or more) gallstones that predispose the patient to carcinoma of the gallbladder should be treated prophylactically with cholecystectomy. The intense inflammatory changes around a porcelain gallbladder may preclude its laparoscopic removal. (By permission of Mayo Foundation.)

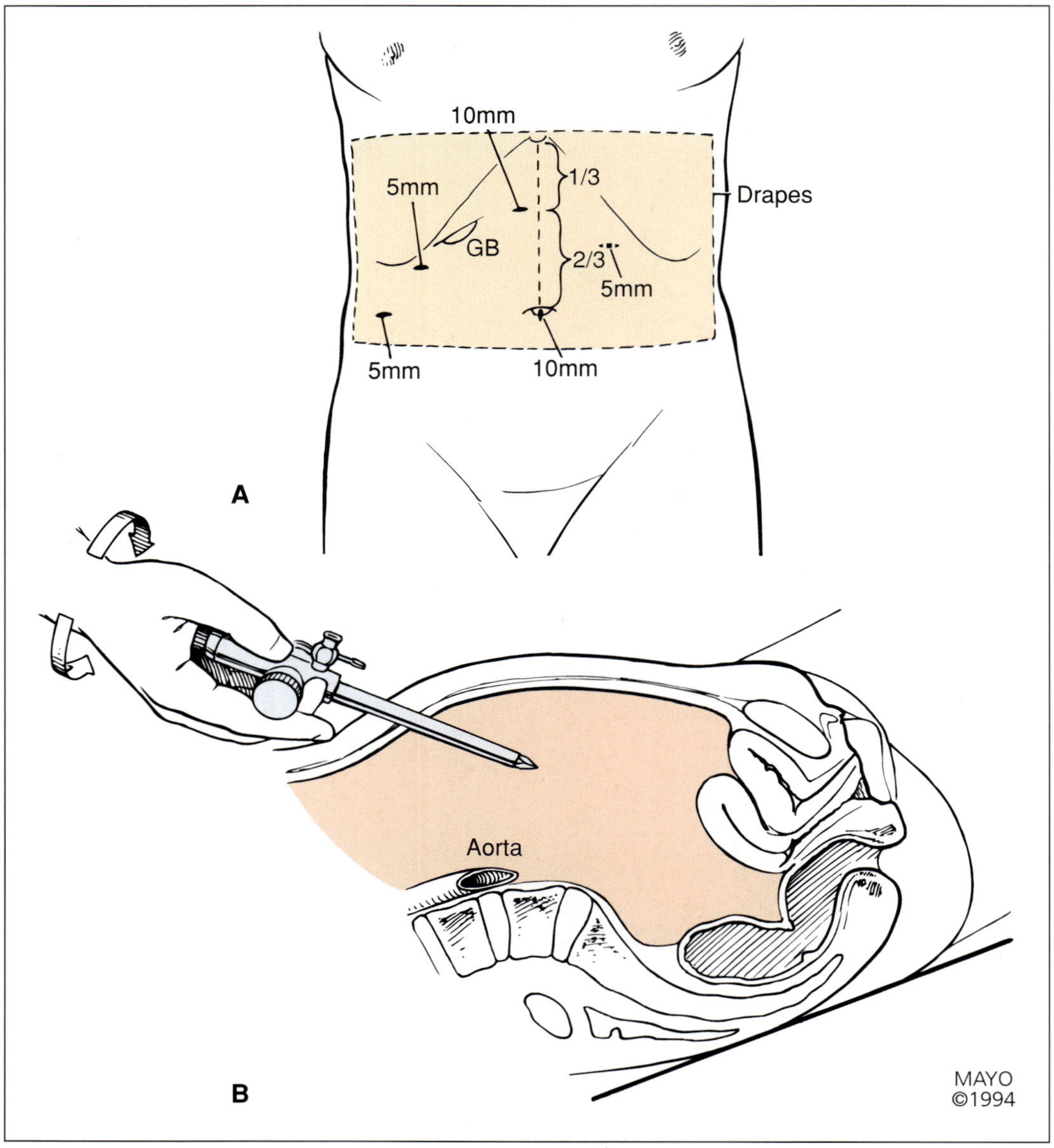

FIGURE 6-14.

A, Most surgeons establish four laparoscopic ports during laparoscopic cholecystectomy. There are two 10-mm instruments. One is inserted at the umbilicus and used for the laparoscope; the other is inserted in the upper midline approximately a third of the distance from the xiphoid process to the umbilicus (primary surgical port). Two 5-mm cannulae are used, one for cephalad retraction of the gallbladder fundus (placed near the anterior axillary line several centimeters below the costal margin) and one for countertraction by the assistant or primary surgeon (usually inserted 2 to 4 cm below the right costal margin near the midclavicular line). **B,** If the closed technique is used for initial trocar placement, it is critical to aim the instrument into the pelvis and use controlled steady pressure to minimize the risk of potentially lethal injuries to abdominal or retroperitoneal structures by the trocar tip. Once the initial port has been inserted, the trocar is removed and the laparoscope is placed via the cannula. The other three instruments can be placed under direct visualization. Occasionally, a fifth instrument port may be needed to retract a ptotic or enlarged left lobe of the liver. A 5-mm instrument in the left hypochondrium is usually adequate for this purpose (**A**). (*From* Donohue *et al.*[14]; by permission of Mayo Foundation for Medical Education and Research.)

POSTOPERATIVE CARE

In the operating room

Remove nasogastric and urinary catheters (if placed)

Extubation by anesthesiologist

In the recovery room

Parenteral narcotic order: morphine sulfate, 1–2 mg IV, prn

Antiemetic order: droperidol, 2.5–5.0 mg IM, prn

Oxygen by face mask

On the nursing unit

Diet: advance to regular as tolerated

Activity: out of bed as tolerated

Medications:

Analgesics: parenteral narcotic (morphine sulfate, (4–8 mg sc q 4 h prn) and oral acetaminophen/narcotic combination (one to two tablets every 6 prn)

Antiemetic: droperidol, 2.5–5.0 mg IM, prn

Muscle relaxant: diazepam, 1–2 mg IM, prn

Miscellaneous: urinary catheterization, prn

Laboratory tests: none routinely

Dismissal: when patient is comfortable, eating regular diet, and voiding spontaneously

After discharge from hospital

Activity as tolerated

Diet of choice

Pain medication: acetaminophen or acetaminophen/narcotic combination, prn

Shower immediately, bathe or swim in 48 hours

Follow-up: check up 7–10 days postoperatively (suture removal, if indicated)

IM = intramuscularly; IV = intravenously; prn = as needed; q = every; sc = subcutaneously.

FIGURE 6-15.

The care of patients after an uneventful laparoscopic cholecystectomy is straightforward, even in most patients with underlying medical problems. Nearly all patients can be extubated in the operating room, and nasogastric and urinary drainage tubes can be removed, if present.

During routine observation of the patient in the recovery room, oxygen is administered and parenteral narcotics and antiemetic medication should be given as indicated. Some patients, particularly young healthy ones, may be dismissed from hospital the day of their operation. They should have stable vital signs, tolerate solid food, be comfortable with only oral analgesics, and be voiding spontaneously before discharge.

The vast majority of patients are ready for dismissal the day following their surgical procedure. Pain medication is generally sparingly required, but both parenteral and oral medications should be available while the patient is in the hospital. Referred phrenic pain is not uncommon after laparoscopy and usually resolves completely within 24 to 48 hours. Postoperative nausea and anorexia are most frequently the reasons for overnight hospitalization. Antiemetic medication should be administered as indicated. Some patients, most often young muscular ones, may complain of abdominal wall spasms related to trauma from trocar insertion. An antispasmatic medication, such as benzodiazepine, is effective in controlling this symptom. Patients should ambulate the day of operation and can be advanced to a regular diet as soon as tolerated (postoperative ileus is nonexistent or minimal with laparoscopic cholecystectomy). No blood tests are taken after a routine laparoscopic cholecystectomy; liver function test results are often abnormal, despite no operative complications [15].

On leaving the hospital, there should be no restrictions on the patient's activity or diet as a result of the surgical procedure. The patient may shower immediately and immersion of the wounds is permissible within 2 days of surgery. Wound herniation is infrequent from laparoscopic incisions; therefore, heavy lifting and straining are not contraindicated postoperatively. Foods high in fat content may cause diarrhea due to loss of the gallbladder's reservoir function, but this usually resolves within several weeks.

Analgesics may be needed as the patient increases activity, but requirements are usually minimal. The average patient should be back to full activity and employment in 1 to 2 weeks after laparoscopic cholecystectomy. (By permission of Mayo Foundation [14].)

RESULTS OF LAPAROSCOPIC CHOLECYSTECTOMY

Country, year of report [Reference]	No. patients	Conversion to laparotomy (%)	Complications (%)	Duct injuries (%)	Mortality (%)	Mean (median) hospital stay in days
Europe, 1991 [16]	1,236	3.6	1.6	0.3	0	(3)
USA, 1991 [17]	1,518	4.7	5.1	0.5	0.07	1.2
USA, 1992 [18]	1,983	4.5	2.1	0.3	0.10	NS
International, 1992 [19]	2,671	3.7	NS	0.2	0.11	NS
Canada, 1992 [20]	2,201	4.3	6.4	0.1	0	(1)
Belgium, 1992 [21]	3,244	6.5	6.4	0.5	0.20	NS
Switzerland, 1992 [21]	1,091	8.1	2.8	0.5	0	NS
France, 1992 [21]	2,955	4.8	3.4	0.6	0.20	NS
France/Belgium, 1992 [21]	6,091	5.3	4.6	0.2	0.20	NS
USA, 1993 [22]	77,604	NS	2.0	0.6	0.04	NS
USA, 1993 [23]	9,597	NS	2.5	0.3	0.04	NS
Switzerland, 1994 [24]	3,722	7.0	4.8	0.6	0.08	4.4
Mexico, 1994 [25]	2,399	4.1	8.9	0.3	0.12	NS

NS = not stated.

FIGURE 6-16.

The outcome of more than 100,000 laparoscopic cholecystectomy patients is summarized. In more than 95% of patients the procedure was completed laparoscopically, conversion to laparotomy being the result of technical considerations or intraoperative complications. Proceeding to celiotomy should not be regarded as a complication, and the incidence of this event depends on the severity of pathologic findings as much as on the skill of the surgeon. The definition of perioperative complications differs among reports but remains in an acceptable range of 2% to 6%. One of the most feared complications of any cholecystectomy is injury to the major extrahepatic biliary tree. The frequency of this serious problem rose with the advent of laparoscopic cholecystectomy, but it seems to be falling with increased experience [26]. Although the mortality of laparoscopic cholecystectomy compares favorably to that of open cholecystectomy, the younger age of patients and the less complex nature of the disease explain some of this discrepancy [27]. A significant rise in the incidence of cholecystectomy have been noted in the United States [27,28], probably because of both patient- and physician-related factors. This increase of approximately 30% has resulted in a comparable total number of deaths after laparoscopic cholecystectomy compared to open cholecystectomy [27]. When hospital stays are compared, it is interesting that the average stay is substantially longer in Europe (3–4 days) compared with North America (1 day), both in the Canadian national health care system and in the United States fee-for-service practices.

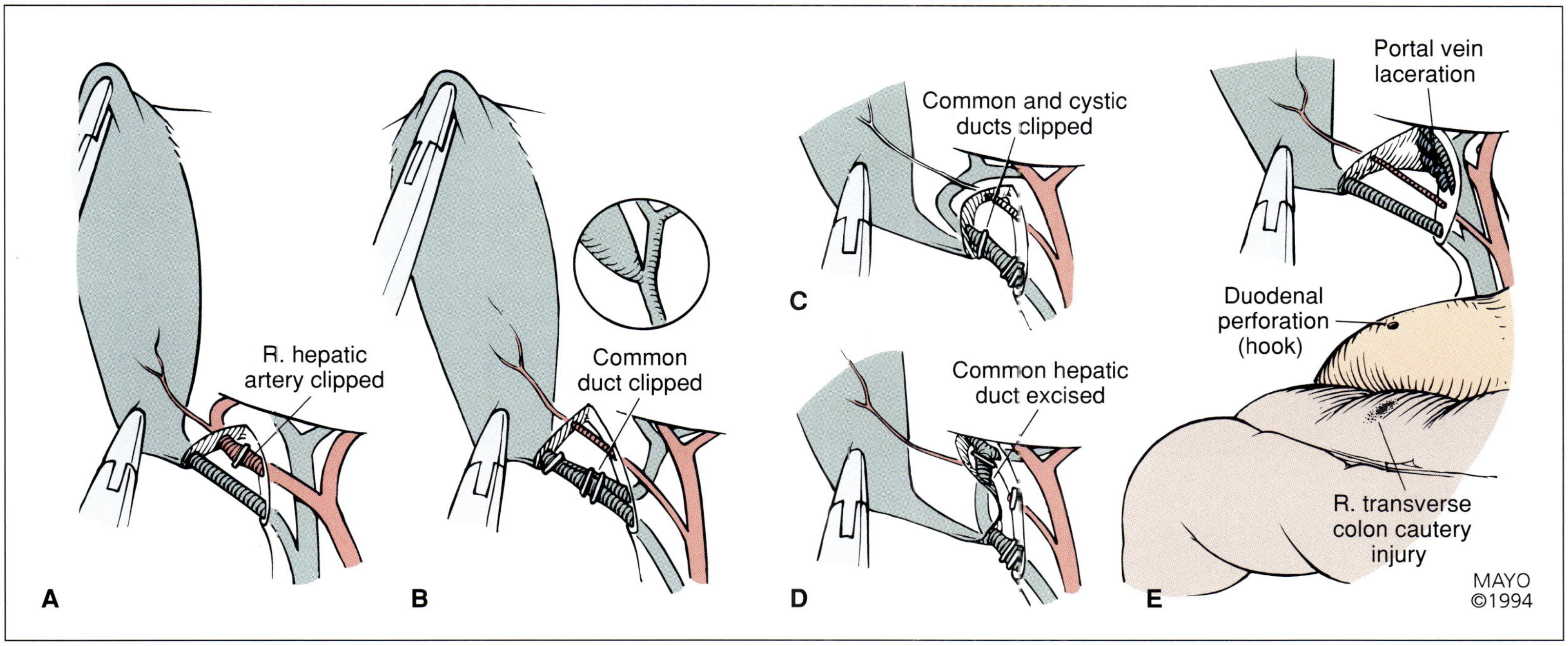

FIGURE 6-17.

Many complications of laparoscopic cholecystectomy are related to instrument placement (wound infection, hematoma or hernia; visceral or vascular injuries) and pneumoperitoneum (respiratory compromise, metabolic acidosis and its sequelae with the use of carbon dioxide, hypotension, and gas embolization). Numerous injuries of structures adjacent to the gallbladder have been seen after laparoscopic cholecystectomy. Vascular injuries, particularly to a tortuous right (R.) hepatic artery (**A**), occur when the dissection plane strays from the gallbladder wall. Portal vein lacerations (*see panel E*) have been reported but are infrequent. Excessive lateral traction on the gallbladder can result in a lateral choledochotomy (not illustrated) or occlusion of the common bile duct if the distal ductal clips are placed without identification of the cystic duct–common hepatic duct confluence (**B**). A short cystic duct (*inset*), a configuration normally present when the gallbladder drains aberrantly into the right hepatic ductal system, is especially prone to this error. Improper identification of the common bile duct, a function of not visualizing the gallbladder cystic duct junction and pursuing a plane of dissection within the hepatoduodenal ligament, has disastrous consequences. Occlusion of the common duct (**C**) resulting from excision of the entire common hepatic duct (**D**) can result from such a mistake. Excessive use of cautery or laser energy around the common bile duct will result in a delayed, ischemic form of ductal stricture. Perforations of both the duodenum and the transverse colon may occur (**E**) as a result of inappropriate manipulation of sharp instruments or cautery, especially when these anatomic structures are outside the field of view of the laparoscope.

Laparoscopic cholecystectomy offers great advantages to patients in terms of faster recovery and less postoperative pain when perioperative complications are minimized and the procedure is appropriately used in patients with symptomatic gallstones. Laparoscopic cholecystectomy has become the treatment of choice for most patients with biliary stone disease without the benefit of randomized, prospective trials. Recent reports of such protocols, however, [19,20] have borne out these benefits. (By permission of Mayo Foundation.)

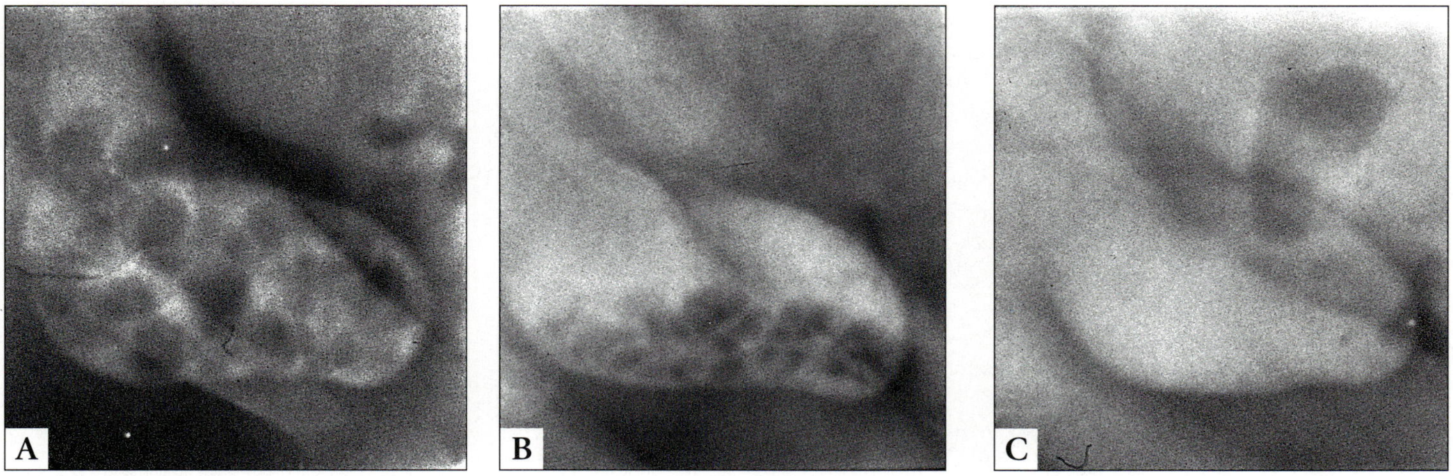

Figure 6-18.

In general, laparoscopic cholecystectomy is the treatment for symptomatic gall stones; but some patients are poor surgical candidates or refuse surgery. When cholesterol stones are carefully selected and the patient complies with a full therapeutic dose of chenodiol or ursodiol, any number of stones 1 cm or less in size can usually be dissolved completely within 1 or 2 years. Very small floating stones may dissolve within 6 months. If no change in size is apparent by oral cholecystography after 12 months of therapy, success is unlikely. A decrease in stone diameter of less than 50% may be difficult to assess ultrasonically, especially if several stones are present. Ultrasound is more accurate, however, for confirming complete dissolution when no residual stones can be detected by oral cholecystography. **Panels A**, **B**, and **C** illustrate progressive dissolution of typical cholesterol stones demonstrated by oral cholecystography.

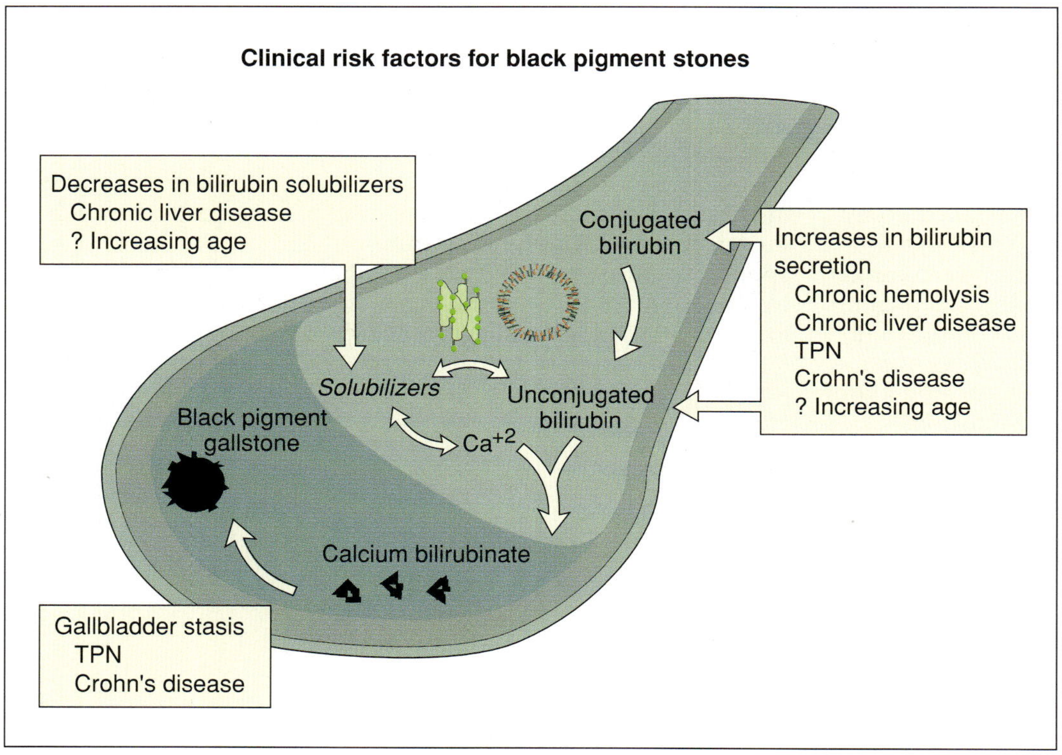

Figure 6-19

Clinical risk factors for black pigment gallstone disease include states in which calcium bilirubinate precipitation is favored—either increased unconjugated bilirubin secretion or impaired secretion of bile salts that solubilize unconjugated bilirubin. Decreased secretion of biliary lipids, particularly bile salts, is observed in chronic liver disease [31]. Black pigment gallstones are associated with situations in which conjugated bilirubin secretion is increased: chronic hemolysis, chronic liver disease, administration of total parenteral nutrition (TPN), and Crohn's disease. The underlying pathophysiologic defect leading to prevalence of black pigment stones with increasing age is unknown. As is found with cholesterol gallstones, gallbladder stasis, such as occurs in patients who receive TPN and in those with extensive Crohn's disease, can further accelerate formation of black pigment gallstones.

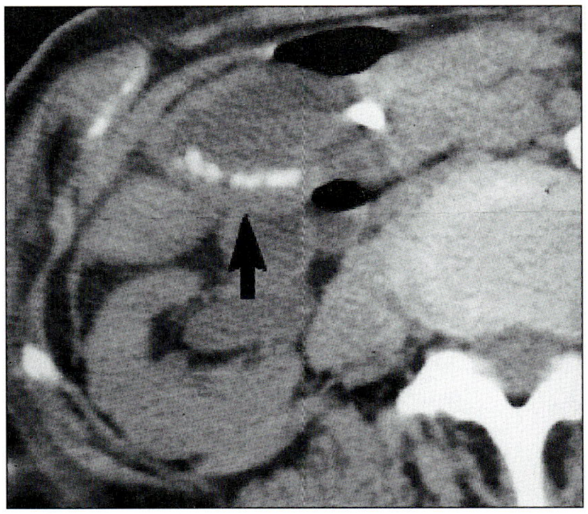

FIGURE 6-20.

Pigment stones are usually detectable on CT scan (*arrow*). If there are only a few small stones, it is important to make thin slices (*eg*, 3 mm) to avoid missing a small part of the gallbladder that may contain all of the stones. Rapid scanning CT allows complete coverage of the gallbladder without respiratory variation. Oral cholecystography radiopaque media may require 10 days to completely clear from the gallbladder and, if retained, may mask or be misinterpreted as stone calcification. Because oral contrast in the duodenum adjacent to the gallbladder also may be confused with stone calcification, avoidance of all contrast is optimal.

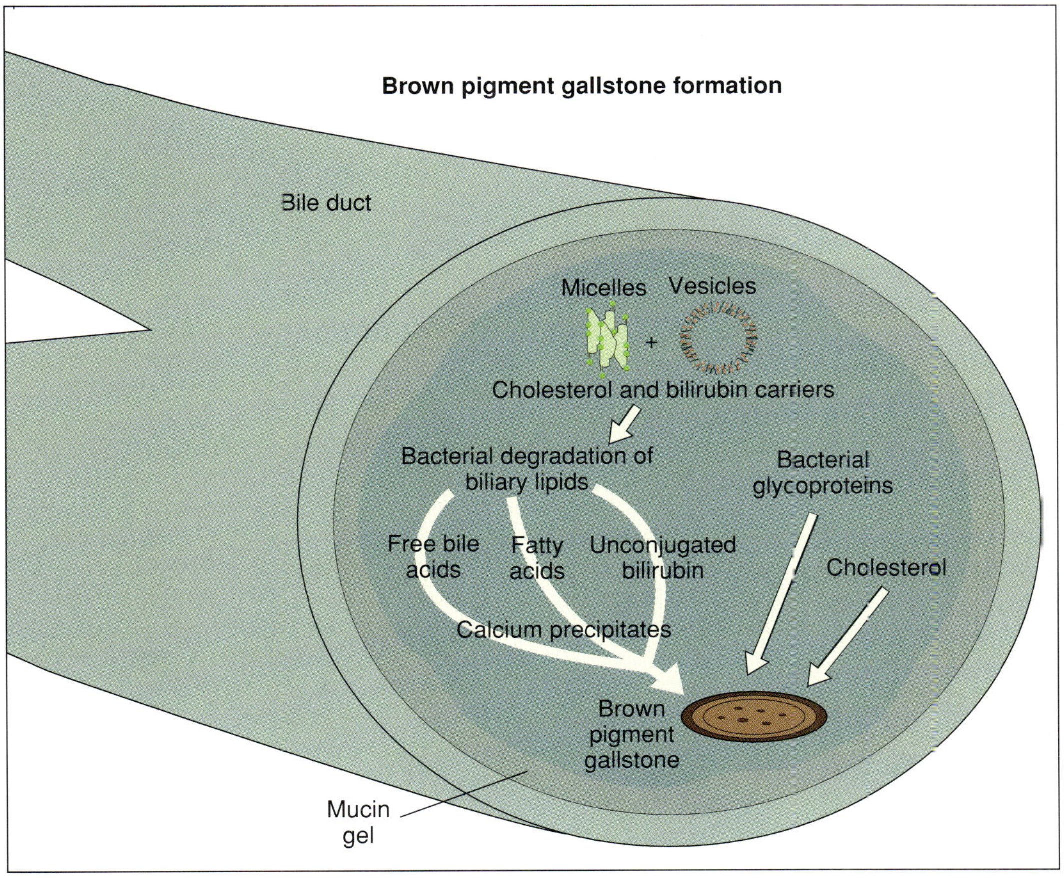

FIGURE 6-21.

Pathophysiology of brown pigment gallstone formation. The initiating event in brown pigment gallstone formation is obstruction of a bile duct and subsequent infection [32,33]. Bacterial enzymes degrade biliary lipids to an insoluble form while depleting the available cholesterol and bilirubin solubilizing agents. Phosphatidylcholine is hydrolyzed by bacterial phospholipase A_2, which forms free fatty acids that precipitate as calcium salts. After bacterial deconjugation, free bile acids can precipitate as either the calcium salts or the protonated bile acid. Bile salts and phosphatidylcholine depletion decrease cholesterol solubility: cholesterol precipitates to form a variable fraction of brown pigment gallstones. Unconjugated bilirubin (UCB) is produced when bacterial β-glucuronidase hydrolyzes conjugated bilirubin. Obstruction of the bile duct by brown pigment gallstones sets up a vicious circle of stasis and further bacterial infection. (*Adapted from* Donovan and Carey [34].)

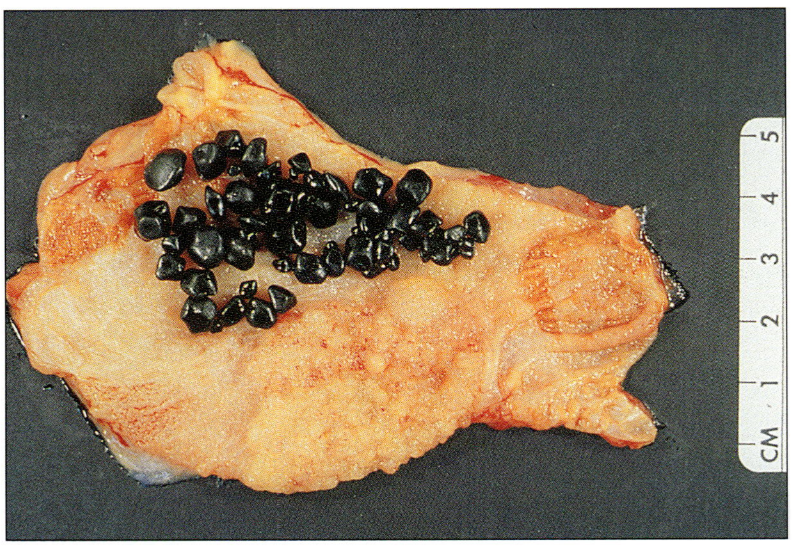

FIGURE 6-22.

Cholesterol stones with a thin surface layer of black pigment, along with an adenocarcinoma in the neck of the gallbladder. Although it is unusual for a neoplasm to exist in addition to stones, this consideration must be kept in mind and the therapeutic plan reassessed if a neoplasm is suspected. Gallstones increase the risk of gall bladder cancer.

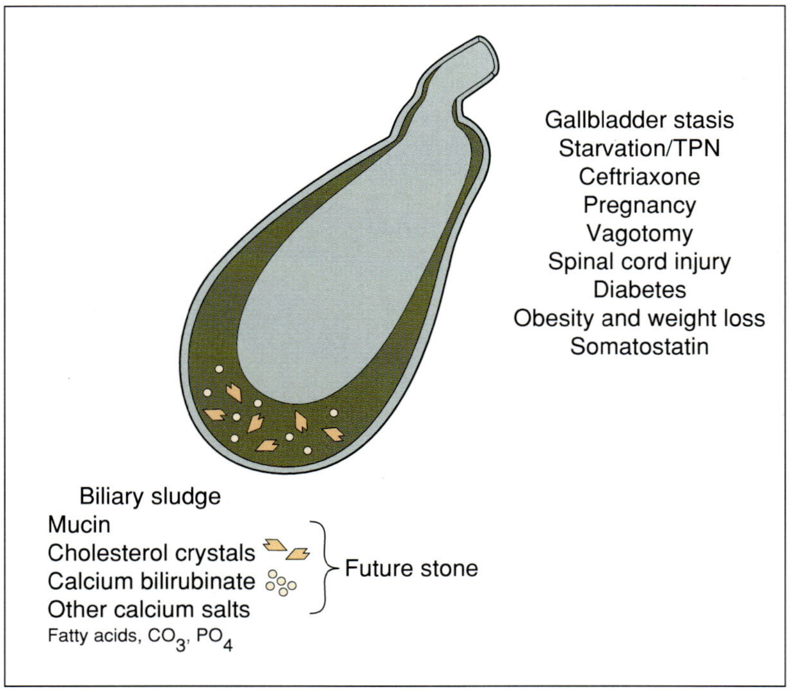

FIGURE 6-23.

Gallbladder stasis, sludge and stone formation. Impaired gallbladder contractility leading to bile stasis and sludge develops in association with starvation and total parenteral nutrition (TPN), ceftiaxtrone therapy in children, pregnancy and female sex hormones (particularly progesterone), vagotomy, sickle hemoglobinopathy, spinal cord injury, diabetes mellitus, obesity, and long-term treatment with the somatostatin analog octreotide. Celiac disease and achalasia are associated with abnormal gallbladder emptying but not with increased gallstone formation. Biliary sludge consists of mucin (a high molecular weight glycoprotein secreted by the gallbladder mucosa), cholesterol microcrystals, calcium bilirubinate, and other calcium salts (*eg*, palmitate, stearate) [35,36]. In some instances sludge may predispose to stone formation [37].

LEVEL OF RISK FOR HARBORING COMMON BILE DUCT STONES

High likelihood (use ERCP)
- Bilirubin > 2 mg/dL
- Alkaline phosphatase > 150 mg/dL
- Jaundice/pancreatitis
- Dilated common bile duct/stone

Intermediate likelihood (use IOC)
- Bilirubin 1.5–2.0 mg/dL
- Alkaline phosphatase 110–150 mg/dL
- Transaminase level more than twice normal
- Remote jaundice/pancreatitis

Low likelihood (no ERCP, no IOC)
- Normal liver function test results
- No ductal dilatation
- No jaundice/pancreatitis

FIGURE 6-24.

The diagnosis and management of choledocholithiasis in the era of laparoscopic cholecystectomy may be facilitated by determination of a patient's likelihood of harboring stones. Risk factors suggesting a high likelihood for common bile duct stones include bilirubin level greater than 2 mg/dL, alkaline phosphatase level greater than 150 units/L, jaundice or severe pancreatitis (or both), a dilated common bile duct or stone visualized on noninvasive imaging, and increasingly high results in serial liver function tests. This group of patients may benefit from endoscopic retrograde cholangiopancreatography (ERCP). Patients with an intermediate likelihood are those with bilirubin levels of 1.5 to 2.0 mg/dL, alkaline phosphatase levels of 110 to 150 units/L, transaminase levels more than twice normal, a remote history of jaundice or pancreatitis, and liver tests showing rapid improvement. This intermediate group may benefit from intraoperative cholangiography (IOC), but decisions about endoscopic stone removal versus laparoscopic or open surgical stone removal are guided by available local expertise. In patients whose liver test results are normal and there is no ductal dilatation, jaundice, or pancreatitis, neither ERCP nor IOC is recommended based on the low probability that common bile duct stones are present.

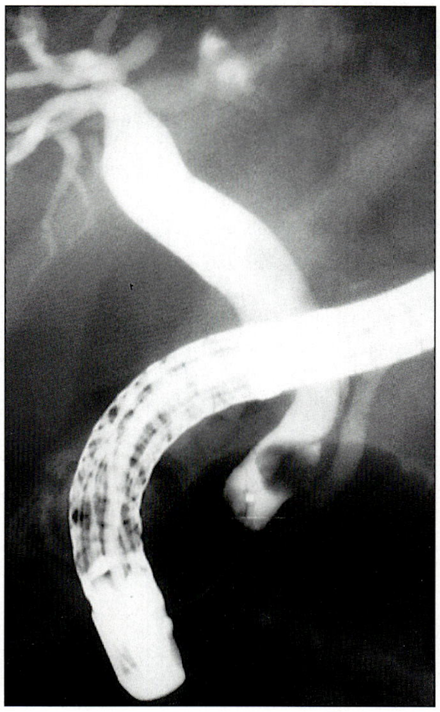

FIGURE 6-25.

Endoscopic retrograde cholangiopancreatography is the most accurate invasive diagnostic modality and can clearly demonstrate intraluminal filling defects as well as ductal dilatation. Other diagnostic modalities, depending on availability and local expertise, include percutaneous cholangiography, intraoperative cholangiography, and common bile duct exploration, performed laparoscopically or by an open approach. Surgical and endoscopic ductal clearance rates are usually reported to be greater than 95%. Mortality rates for surgical series range from 0% to 28%, depending on the patient populations selected, and recurrence rates range from 5% to 21%. In contrast, endoscopic ductal clearance has a published mortality rate ranging from 0% to 3% and a recurrence rate of less than 5%.

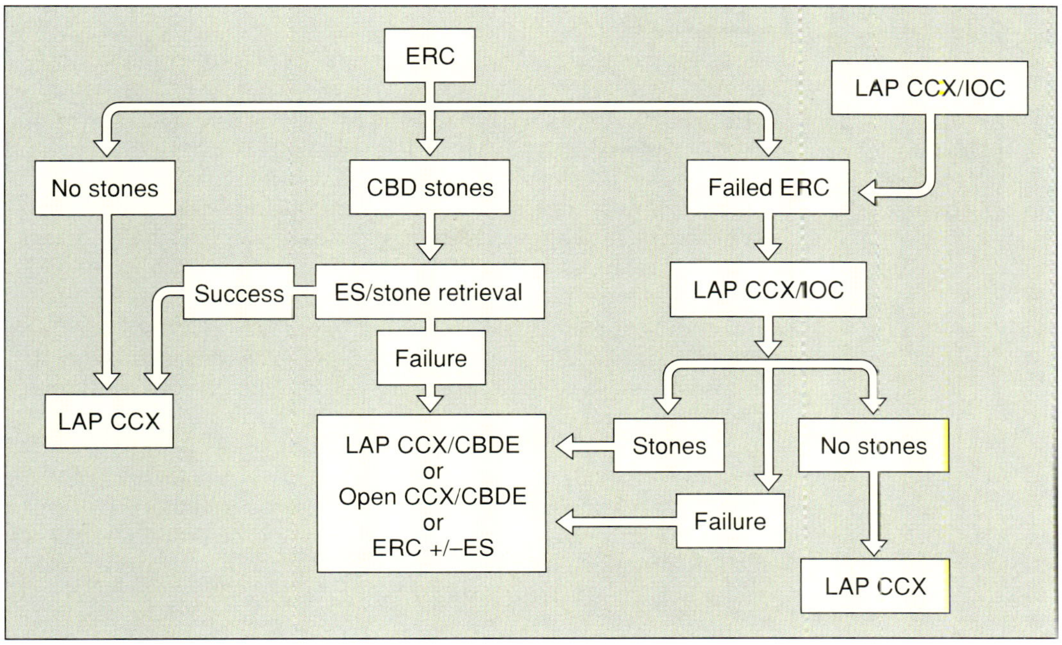

FIGURE 6-26.

An algorithm for management of common bile duct stones in the era of minimally invasive therapy. Entry points into this algorithm are guided by the available local expertise.

If endoscopic retrograde cholangiography (ERC) reveals no stones, the next step is laparoscopic cholecystectomy (LAP CCX). If stones are documented by ERC then successfully removed via endoscopy (usually requiring endoscopic sphincterotomy [ES]), LAP CCX is, again, the next step. If stones are documented but retrieval is unsuccessful, options include LAP CCX with laparoscopic common bile duct exploration (CBDE), open cholecystectomy with bile duct exploration, or referral for more expert endoscopy. If ERC fails, one option is to proceed with LAP CCX and intraoperative cholangiography (IOC). If no stones are documented, the procedure would involve cholecystectomy only. If, however, laparoscopic cholangiography documents stones, the options are to proceed with laparoscopic common bile duct exploration, to perform open cholecystectomy with bile duct exploration, or to remove the gallbladder and refer for ERC. These three options are also applicable if laparoscopic cholangiography fails.

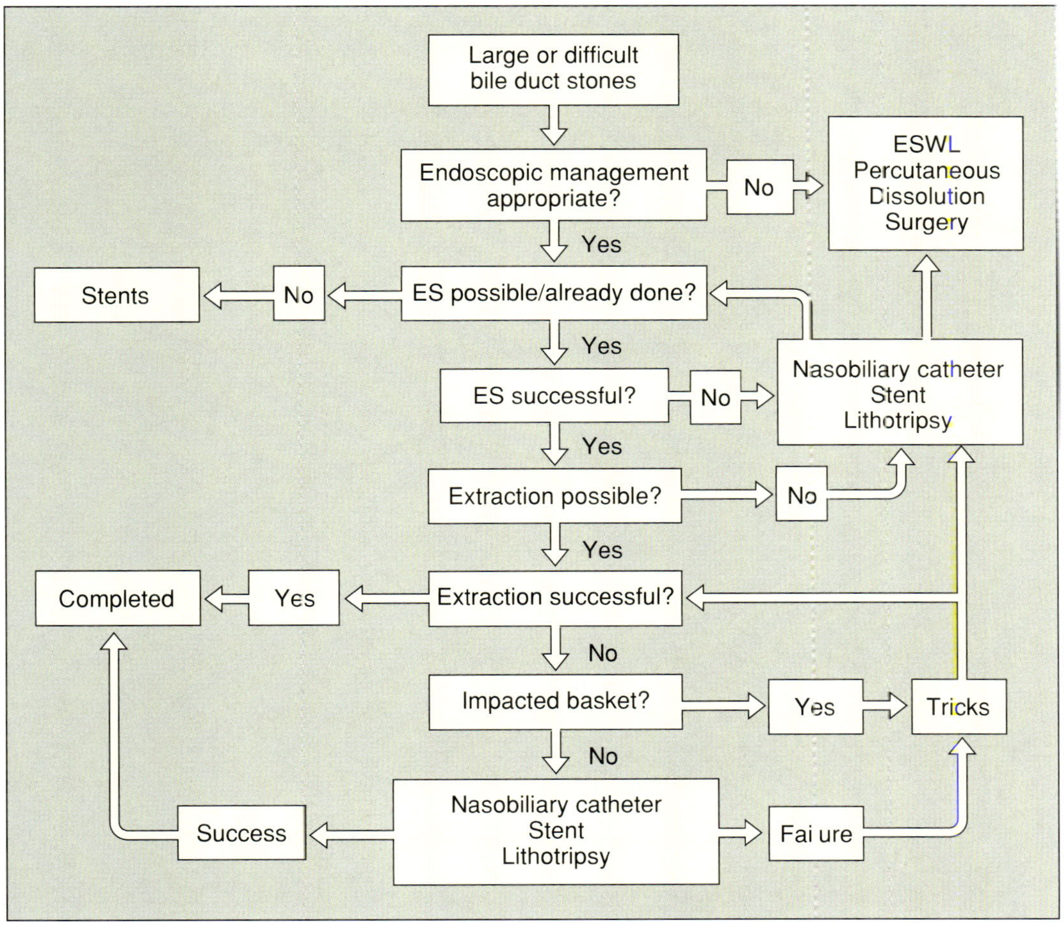

FIGURE 6-27.

Algorithmic approach to the management of difficult bile duct stones. The availability of local expertise and referral centers play an important role. It is imperative to facilitate adequate drainage. ES—endoscopic sphincterotomy; ESWL—extracorporeal shockwave lithotripsy.

COMPLICATIONS OF ENDOSCOPIC SPHINCTEROTOMY
Acute Complications, 6%–10%
Pancreatitis, 2%–3%
Hemorrhage, 2%–3%
Cholangitis, 1%–2%
Perforation, 0.5%–1.5%
Mortality, 0.5%–1.0%
Late Complications, 5%–10%
Sphincter stenosis
Recurrent stones
Cholangitis without obstruction

FIGURE 6-28.

Endoscopic sphincterotomy has an overall rate of acute complications of 6% to 10% that is well documented in the literature [38]. Pancreatitis is defined by its characteristic abdominal pain with elevated amylase and lipase levels. Hemorrhage is defined as any bleeding that results in endoscopic therapy or hospitalization. Cholangitis is defined as fever and elevated liver function test results and leukocyte count. Perforation is pain associated with retroperitoneal air, and the syndrome of "post-endoscopic retrograde cholangiopancreatography (ERCP) pain" characterizes those patients with abdominal pain after undergoing endoscopic retrograde cholangiopancreatography who are admitted to hospital and in whom all laboratory tests are normal. In multivariate analysis, certain risk factors have emerged that contribute to the development of pancreatitis. These risk factors include a previous history of post-ERCP pancreatitis and the number of attempts at ductal cannulation. Late complication rates as high as 5% to 10% result from sphincter stenosis, recurrent stones, and cholangitis without obstruction. Only after careful consideration of the potential risks, as well as the intended benefits, should sphincterotomy be undertaken.

INFECTIONS OF THE BILIARY TREE

BACTERIOLOGY OF ACUTE CHOLANGITIS

	Bile Culture (%)	Blood Culture (%)
Positive Cultures		
Overall	99	29
Unimicrobial	44	77
Polymicrobial	56	23
Types of Bacteria		
Escherichia coli	35	53
Enterococcus spp	16	9
Klebsiella spp	14	11
Proteus spp	12	6
Pseudomonas spp	9	9
Enterobacter spp	5	5
Aerobacter spp	3	1
Staphylococcus aureus	1	3
Anaerobes	1	2
Candida spp	1	1

FIGURE 6-29.

Enteric organisms have consistently been implicated in cholangitis. This table shows the most prevalent bacteria isolated from blood and bile cultures in a large series of patients with cholangitis. With improving culture techniques, anaerobic organisms such as *Bacteroides fragilis* and *Clostridium* spp are also being isolated with increasing frequency [39]. (*Adapted from* Sinanan [39].)

BILE PENETRATION OF ANTIBIOTICS USED FOR ACUTE CHOLANGITIS

	Mean peak biliary level (% serum concentration)				
Patient groups	**Ciprofloxacin**	**Imipenem**	**Cefoperazone**	**Ceftazidime**	**Netilmicin**
Obstructed	85	16	26	23	16
Relieved	198	17	48	22	17
Control	490	16	728	18	18

FIGURE 6-30.

The ideal antibiotic regimen for acute cholangitis would provide excellent gram-negative, anaerobic, and enterococcal coverage. Dooley and colleagues proposed that coverage be initiated with mezlocillin or a cephalosporin in combination with an aminoglycoside and that adjustments be made based on culture results and clinical course [40]. More recent work by Leung and coworkers has emphasized the importance of biliary excretion of antibiotics in the effective treatment of cholangitis [41–43]. As shown in this table, compared with other broad-spectrum antibiotics, ciprofloxacin has superior penetration into bile both before and after relief of obstruction. (*Adapted from* Lee and Leung [41].)

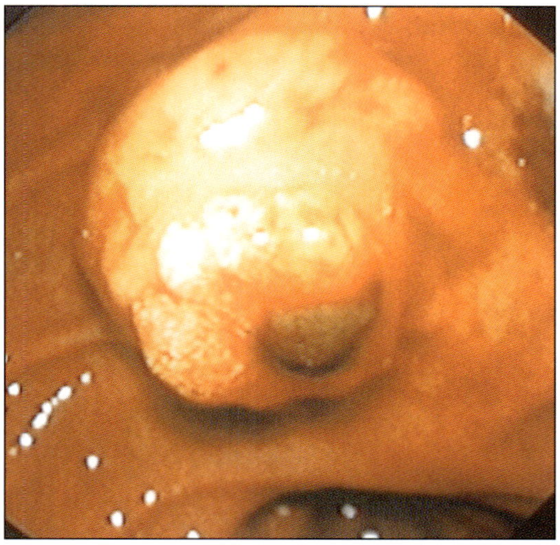

FIGURE 6-31.

Endoscopy in acute cholangitis. Stone disease remains the most common cause of cholangitis in most large series in the United States. Choledocholithiasis occurs in 8% to 15% of patients undergoing cholecystectomy; the incidence in patients more than 60 years of age is even higher, estimated at 15% to 60% in some series [44]. At endoscopy, the obstructing stone is often seen bulging from the papillary orifice, as in this figure. A recent randomized, controlled trial supports early endoscopic examination and intervention in cases of suspected stone-related acute cholangitis [45].

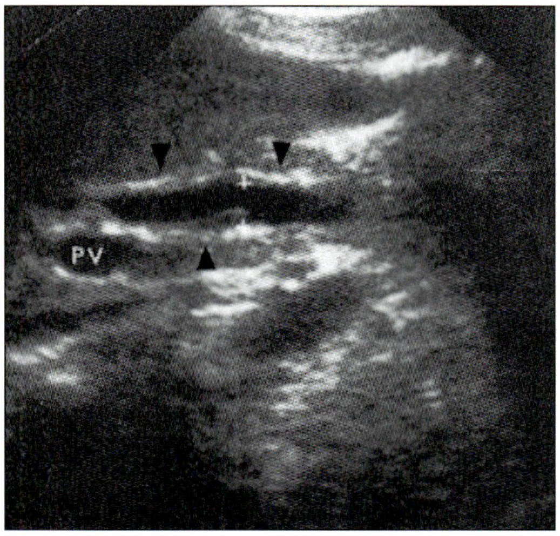

FIGURE 6-32.

Radiographic appearance of AIDS cholangiopathy. Biliary tract disease is being reported with increasing frequency in the AIDS population. Abdominal pain and laboratory evidence of cholestasis are common clinical features that may prompt further investigation. Both ultrasound and CT may demonstrate cholangiographic abnormalities. This ultrasound depicts dilation (13 mm) and thickening (*arrowheads*) of the common bile duct in a case of cholangitis associated with cryptosporidiosis. PV—portal vein. (*From* Teixidor *et al.* [46]; with permission.)

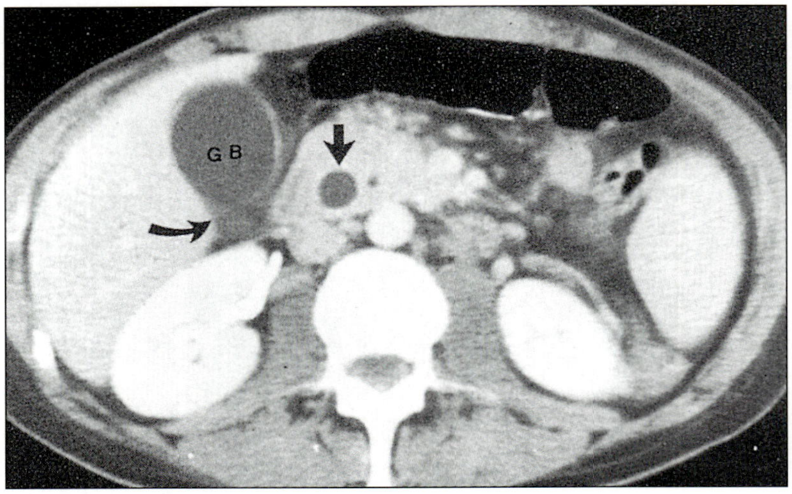

FIGURE 6-33.

AIDS cholangiopathy. This CT scan shows thickening of the gallbladder (GB) wall, pericholecystic fluid (*curved arrow*), and dilation of the common bile duct (*straight arrow*). (*From* Teixidor *et al.* [46]; with permission.)

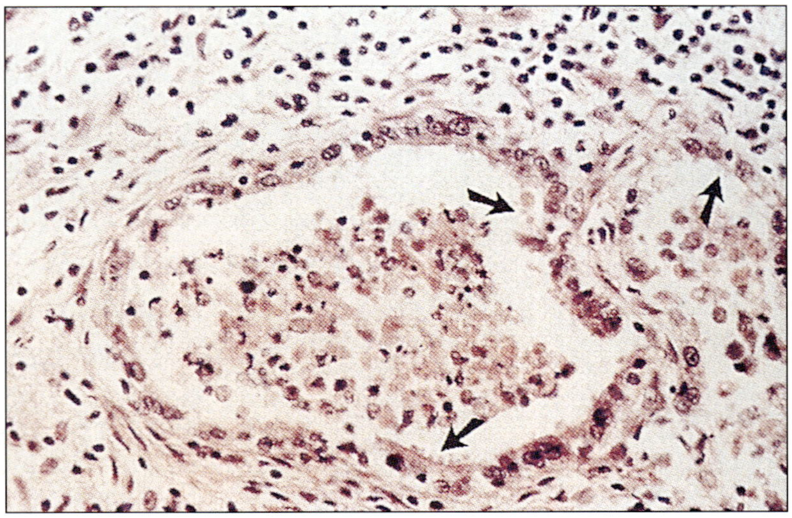

FIGURE 6-34.

Infectious agents in AIDS cholangiopathy. Histologic section reveals dilated periductal glands with neutrophilic infiltrate; *Cryptosporidium* organisms (*arrows*) are seen adhering to the epithelium. Other infectious agents that can cause AIDS cholangiopathy are microsporidia, cytomegalovirus, and mycobacteria avium complex. (*From* Teixidor *et al.* [46]; with permission.)

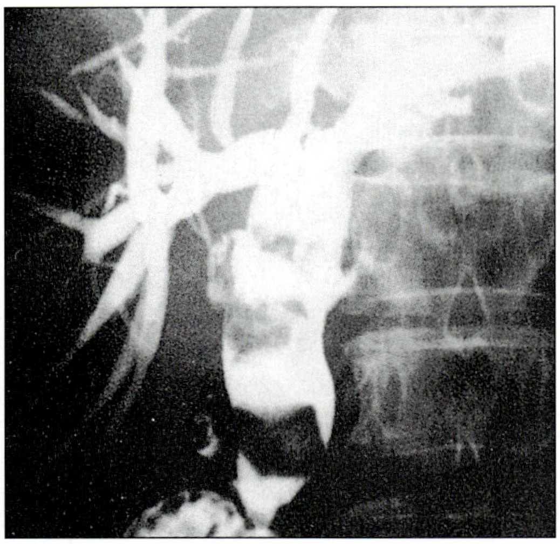

FIGURE 6-35.

Oriental cholangiohepatitis. Oriental cholangiohepatitis, or recurrent pyogenic cholangitis, is defined by recurrent episodes of abdominal pain, fever, and jaundice associated with intrahepatic and extrahepatic bile duct stones. The syndrome is common in Southeast Asia; in Hong Kong, it is the most common disease of the biliary tract [47]. With the influx of Asian immigrants, the disease is being seen with increasing frequency in the United States. The presentation is usually a dramatic illustration of Charcot's triad (fever, jaundice, right upper quadrant pain). Cholangiographic findings may include prominent filling defects and marked dilation of intrahepatic and extrahepatic systems; more peripheral intrahepatic ducts taper abruptly. (*From* Lim [48]; with permission.)

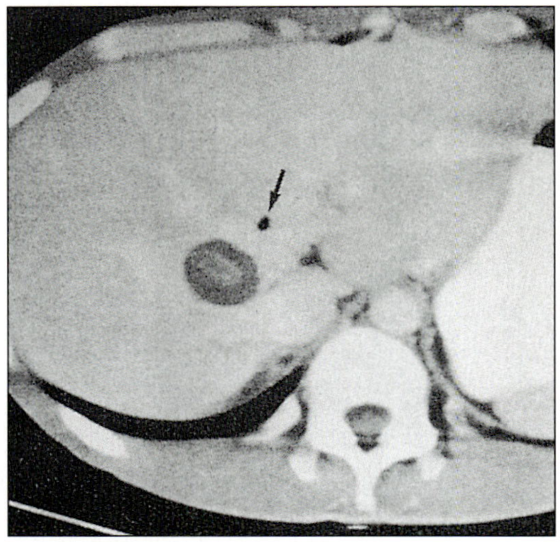

FIGURE 6-36.

Oriental cholangiohepatitis. On CT scan a cystically dilated common duct with indwelling stone is seen; pneumobilia is shown at the *arrow*. Bacteria, flukes, or both may be detected in the bile. (*From* Lim [48]; with permission.)

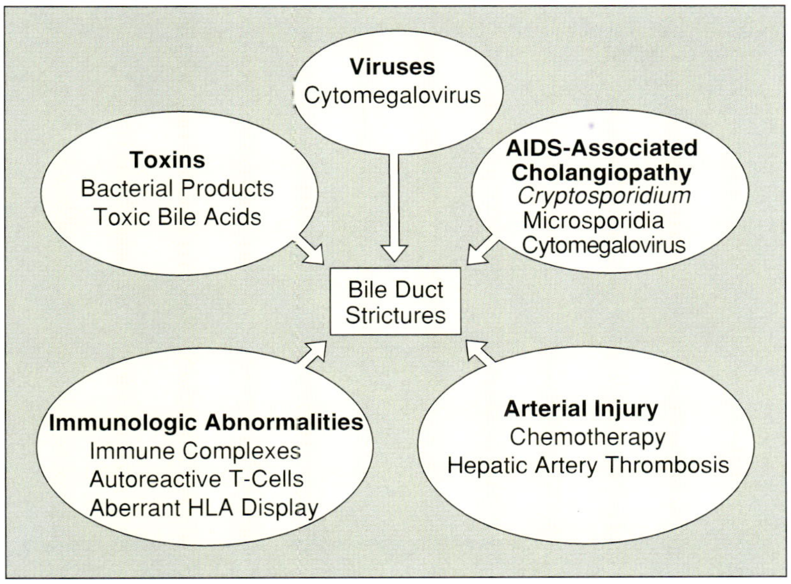

FIGURE 6-37.

Possible causes of bile duct injury are shown. Among the toxins, various bacterial products may serve either as direct mediators leading to damage or stimulate production of various cytokines. Toxic bile acids have been sought but not found. The usual viruses involving the liver have been excluded, although HIV in cytomegalovirus has been shown to lead to damage of intrahepatic bile ducts [39]. Other HIV-associated infections include those due to *Cryptosporidium* spp and microsporidia [49]. Arterial injury, caused either by infusion of chemotherapeutic agents through the hepatic artery leading to arterial damage [50], or by hepatic artery thrombosis after liver transplantation, can lead to ischemic damage of the extrahepatic biliary tree because of the unique vascular supply of this structure. Lastly, immunologic abnormalities have been described in patients with primary sclerosing cholangitis (PSC). These abnormalities include increased concentrations of immune complexes that do not localize to the bile ducts but rather to the small vessels where they may lead to damage of the small intrahepatic artery branches and subsequent ischemic cholangitis [51,52]. Similarly, autoreactive T cells and aberrant expression of HLA class II antigens on bile duct cells that may serve as targets for these T cells have been described [53,54].

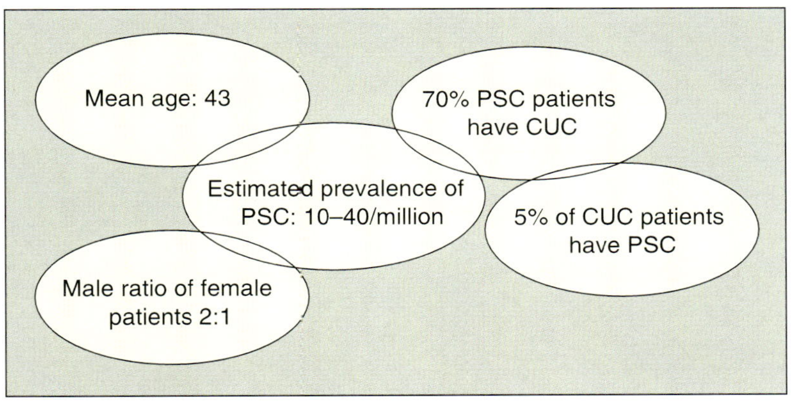

FIGURE 6-38.

Epidemiologic characteristics of primary sclerosing cholangitis (PSC) based largely on Mayo Clinic experience with 100 to 150 patients per year who have this disorder. There is a clear male preponderance. It is estimated that 70% of patients with PSC have coexisting ulcerative colitis (CUC), whereas less than 5% of patients with ulcerative colitis have PSC [55,56]. In no series of ulcerative colitis patients has routine cholangiography been performed. This is noteworthy because some patients with PSC have normal liver biochemistry values, although studies to date relating incidence of PSC to chronic ulcerative colitis have relied on cholangiograms in patients with persistently abnormal liver biochemistry values.

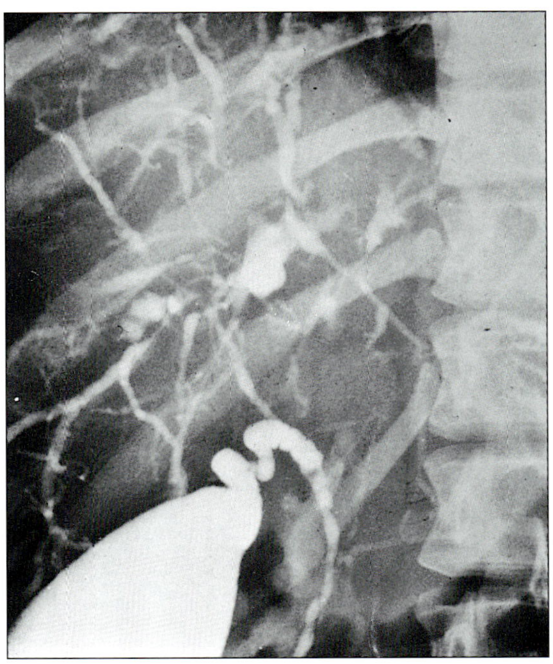

FIGURE 6-39.

Classic cholangiographic appearance of sclerosing cholangitis. Multifocal strictures and intervening cholangiectatic ductal segments are seen.

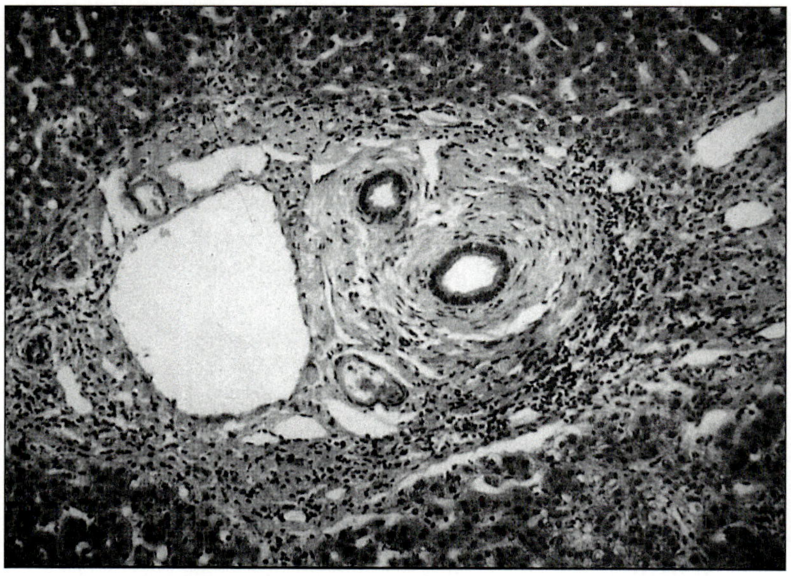

FIGURE 6-40.

A characteristic liver biopsy specimen is shown. Concentric fibrosis (onion skin) is seen around a damaged bile duct with some surrounding inflammatory infiltrate. (*From* Ludwig [57]; with permission.)

DIFFERENTIAL DIAGNOSIS OF PRIMARY SCLEROSING CHOLANGITIS

Primary biliary cirrhosis
Drug-induced cholestasis
Idiopathic adulthood ductopenia
Cholestatic alcoholic hepatitis or chronic viral hepatitis
Abnormalities of bile ducts
- AIDS-related
  - *Cryptosporidium* spp
  - Microsporidia
  - Cytomegalovirus
- Damage to hepatic artery (5 floxuridine infusions)
- Extrahepatic bile duct obstruction from stones
- Surgical strictures
- Choledochal cysts
- Cholangiocarcinoma
- Lymphoma
- Metastatic adenocarcinoma

FIGURE 6-41.

Differential diagnosis of primary sclerosing cholangitis.

CLINICAL FEATURES AT PRESENTATION OF PRIMARY SCLEROSING CHOLANGITIS

Symptom	Patients affected, %
Fatigue	75
Pruritus	60
Jaundice	45
Fever	20
Cholangitis	10
Asymptomatic	25

FIGURE 6-42.

Hepatomegaly and splenomegaly are the most common clinical features at presentation of a patient with primary sclerosing cholangitis. Jaundice occurs in slightly less than 50% of patients.

COMPLICATIONS OF CHOLESTATIC LIVER DISEASE

Complications associated with chronic liver disease
- Portal hypertension
- Variceal bleeding
- Ascites
- Hepatic encephalopathy

Complications specific for cholestasis
- Osteopenia
- Fat-soluble vitamin deficiency
- Hypercholesterolemia

Complications specific for underlying cholangiopathy
- Dominant stricture
- Ascending cholangitis
- Intraductal stones
- Cholangiocarcinoma

FIGURE 6-43.

The complications that must be sought in caring for patients with primary sclerosing cholangitis include those due to advancing liver disease (largely the complications of portal hypertension), those due to chronic cholestasis, and those found nearly exclusively in patients with an underlying cholangiopathy.

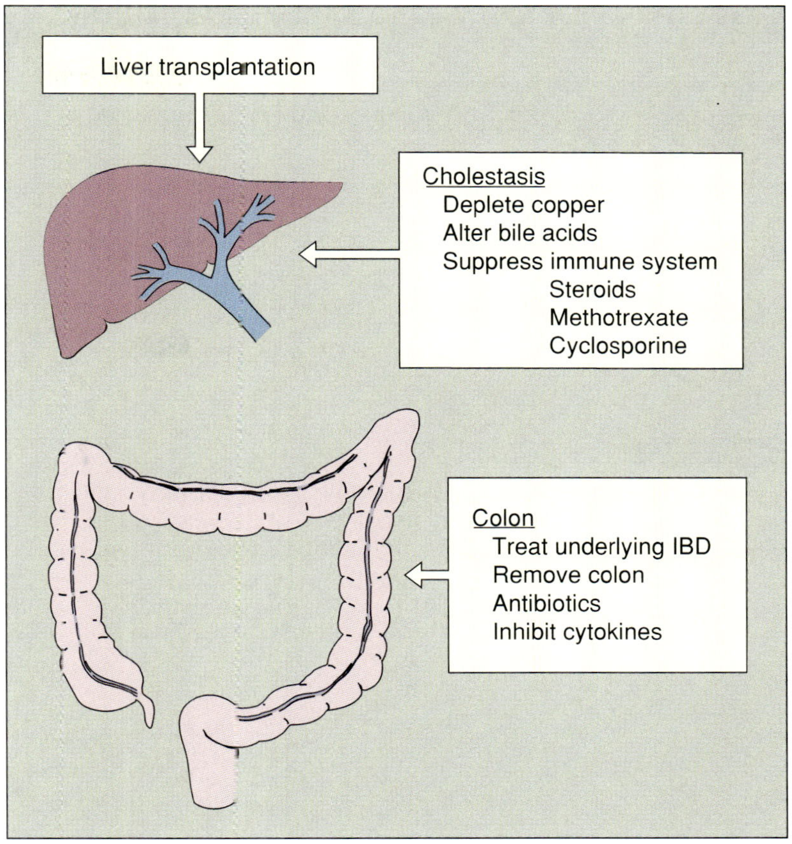

FIGURE 6-44.

Various approaches to the management of primary sclerosing cholangitis (PSC) are shown. Measures directed at the colon include aggressive treatment of the underlying inflammatory bowel disease (IBD), removal of the colon (*eg*, proctocolectomy), or antibiotics to alter the bacterial flora of the colon. None of these so far have been shown to be useful. Inhibition of cytokine production is the basis for ongoing work, but the results of such pilot studies are not yet available. Measures directed at cholestasis, such as depletion of copper, also have been unsuccessful [58]. Alteration of bile acids with agents such as ursodeoxycholic acid is currently undergoing investigation and appears promising [59,60]. Suppression of the immune system with corticosteroids [61], methotrexate [62], or cyclosporine [63] was unsuccessful. Lastly, liver transplantation remains a viable option for patients with advanced PSC. The 2-year survival rate of these patients is approximately 83%, comparable to results found in patients with primary biliary cirrhosis. Retransplantation, however, is more often required in patients with PSC than in those with primary biliary cirrhosis. The University of Pittsburgh's large experience with PSC suggests that patients with this disease have a slightly worse prognosis than patients with primary biliary cirrhosis. A recent study combining data from the Mayo Clinic and the University of Pittsburgh showed an overall 5-year survival rate of 73% after transplantation for PSC [64].

SPHINCTER OF ODDI DYSFUNCTION

BILIARY SPHINCTER OF ODDI DYSFUNCTION: PRESENTATION

Biliary pain

Elevation in liver function tests may or may not occur

Serum amylase level is normal

Codeine association occasionally

FIGURE 6-45.

Characteristic presentation of patients with biliary sphincter of Oddi dysfunction. Patients are usually female and 40 to 50 years old. The condition is fairly rare and difficult to diagnose without refferal to a gastroenterologist with experience in biliary manometry.

CLASSIFICATION OF BILIARY SPHINCTER OF ODDI DYSFUNCTION

TYPE	CLINICAL PRESENTATION
Type 1	Biliary pain Abnormal liver enzyme levels Fixed stenosis on radiograph
Type 2	Biliary pain and Transient elevation of enzyme level and/or Dilated duct and/or Delay in emptying of duct
Type 3	Biliary pain

FIGURE 6-46.

Biliary sphincter of Oddi dysfunction may be subdivided into three types according to clinical presentation. Patients with type 1 sphincter of Oddi dysfunction have a high rate of cure after sphincterotomy. Patients with type 2 or type 3 require further evaluation with sphincter of Oddi manometry and treatment tailored accordingly.

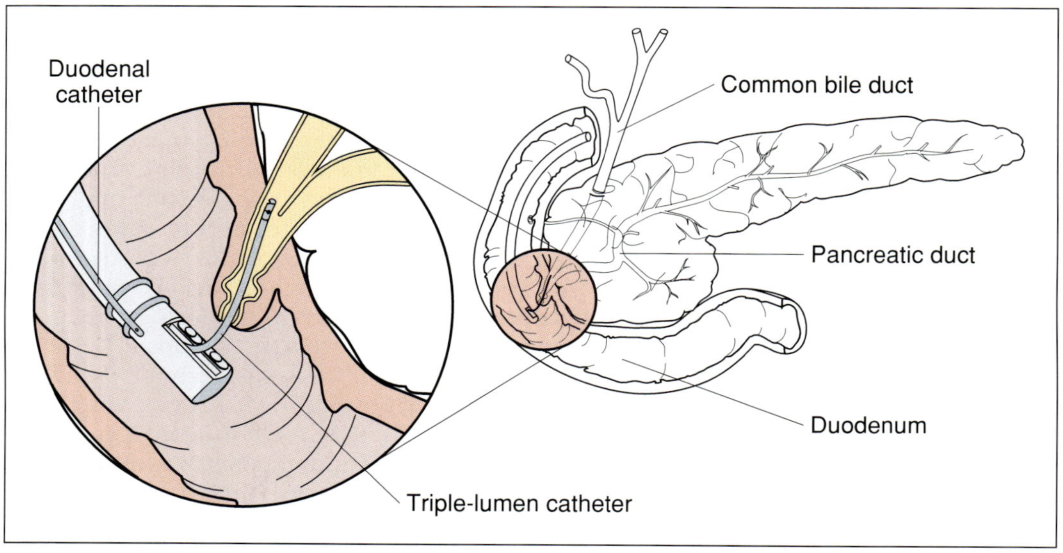

FIGURE 6-47.

Endoscopic manometry is performed with the use of a standard duodenoscope. The manometric catheter is introduced into either the common bile duct or the pancreatic duct to record ductal pressures. It is then withdrawn so that the three recording lumens are situated within the sphincter of Oddi. A separate catheter may simultaneously record duodenal pressure. (*Adapted from* Toouli [65].)

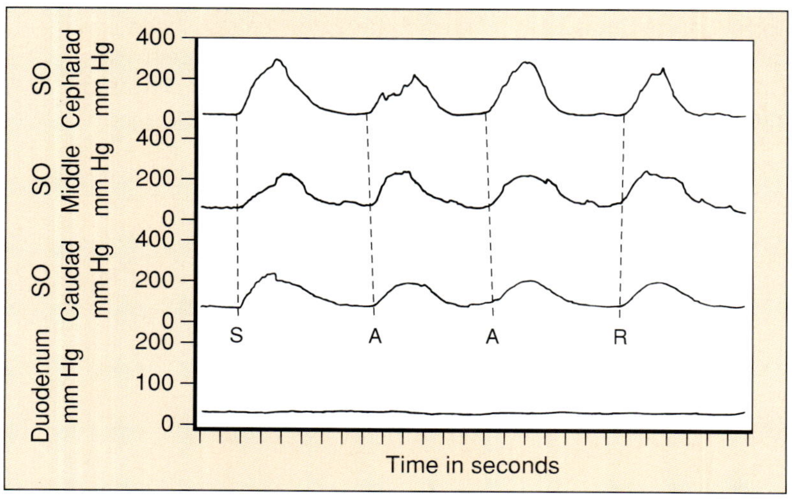

FIGURE 6-48.

This representative tracing shows recordings from the sphincter of Oddi (SO) and duodenum. The sphincter has a low tone on which are superimposed prominent phasic contractions. The contractions are primarily orientated in an antegrade (A) direction. However, in addition, some waves are orientated in a retrograde (R) direction or are simultaneous (S). Simultaneous recording from the duodenum shows that the activity of the sphincter of Oddi is independent of duodenal contractions. (*Adapted from* Toouli [65].)

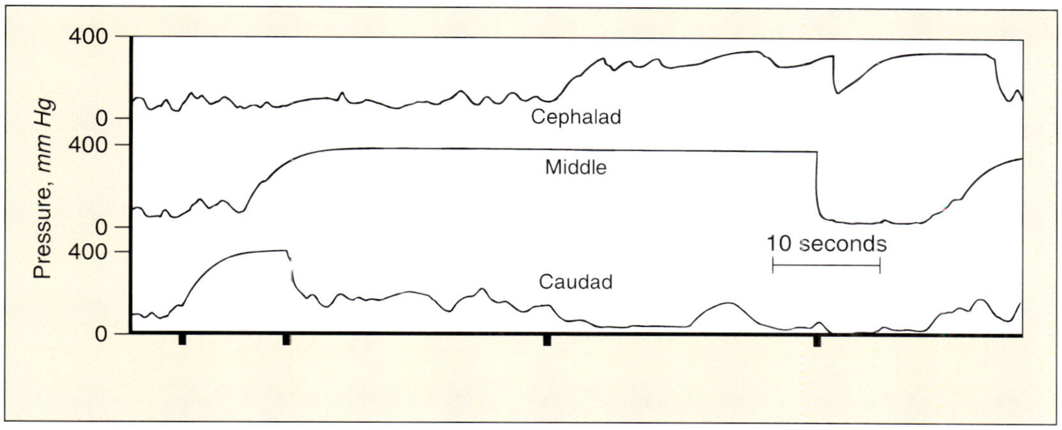

FIGURE 6-49.

Manometric tracing from a patient with stenosis of the sphincter of Oddi. The black rectangles indicate a step-wise pull through of the manometric catheter that has been inserted into either the bile duct or the pancreatic duct. As the catheter is withdrawn through the sphincter of Oddi, the basal pressure is noted to be elevated and peaks at approximately 350 mm Hg. This was reproduced on at least two repeat pull throughs and is consistent with stenosis of the sphincter of Oddi.

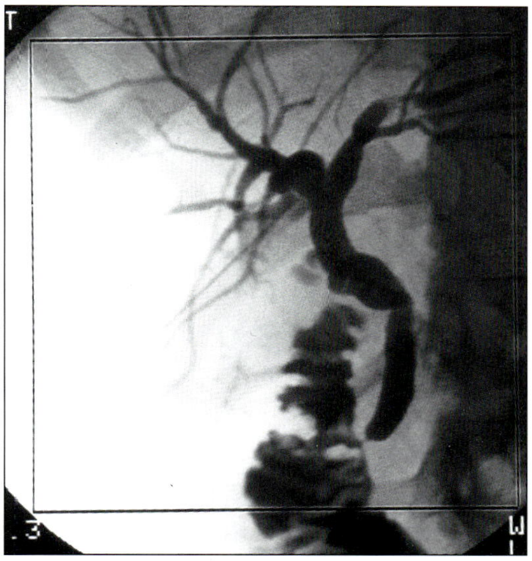

FIGURE 6-50.

Radiograph of a patient who had sphincter of Oddi dysfunction with fixed stenosis of the sphincter. The stenosis is demonstrated by the stricture at the lower end of the bile duct. This patient presented with recurrent pain and abnormal liver enzyme levels. The patient was classified as having type 1 sphincter of Oddi dysfunction and was cured by division of the sphincter.

BILIARY TRACT NEOPLASMS

CLASSIFICATION OF BILIARY TRACT NEOPLASMS

PRIMARY	SECONDARY	RARE
Carcinoma of the gallbladder	Hepatic "embolization"	Granular cell tumor
Cholangiocarcinoma	Hepatocellular carcinoma	Carcinoid tumor
Intrahepatic	Hilar lymph nodes	Cystadenoma
Perihilar	Metastatic tumor	Mucoepidermoid tumor
Distal	Lymphoma	Squamous cell carcinoma
Diffuse	Extension from adjacent organs	Sarcoma

FIGURE 6-51.

The vast majority of biliary tract neoplasms are primary adenocarcinomas of the gallbladder or bile ducts. Among these primary biliary neoplasms, carcinoma of the gallbladder and perihilar cholangiocarcinoma are the most common. Distal bile duct tumors are more common than intrahepatic cholangiocarcinomas, and truly diffuse tumors are rare. Considerable overlap exists, however, so that many of these tumors extend into the adjacent area.

Malignant biliary obstruction may also be secondary to other neoplasms. For example, hepatocellular carcinoma may obstruct intrahepatic or perihilar ducts or may "embolize" into the bile duct lumen [66]. This embolic phenomenon rarely occurs with cancer of the colon or other cancers that have metastasized to the liver. Metastatic tumors may also cause biliary obstruction by involving hilar lymph nodes [67]. Similarly, lymphomas that involve hilar nodes and those around the head of the pancreas may be confused with primary biliary tract tumors [68]. Secondary malignant obstruction may also be caused by tumors in the pancreas, ampulla, duodenum, stomach, and rarely, the colon.

RISK FACTORS FOR GALLBLADDER CANCER

Gallstones	Estrogens
Choledochal cysts	Typhoid carriers
Anomalous duct junction	Porcelain gallbladder
Carcinogens	Gallbladder polyps

FIGURE 6-52.

In most series, more than 90% of patients with gallbladder cancer have gallstones [68]. Gallbladder cancer is more likely to occur in patients with a single large gallstone than in those with multiple gallstones. Patients with choledochal cysts may have carcinomas anywhere in the biliary tree, but a significant proportion of these tumors arise in the gallbladder [69]. Most patients with congenital biliary cysts have an abnormal pancreatobiliary duct junction, and this abnormality has been recently associated with gallbladder cancer in the absence of a choledochal cyst [70].

Carcinogens have been suspected as a cause of biliary tract neoplasms because excretion in the bile is a common mode of clearance of toxic metabolites. Concentration in the gallbladder may be an additional factor in patients who are prone to or have formed gallstones. Obesity and estrogens are additional risk factors that are also associated with gallstone formation [68]. Typhoid carriers are also at risk for all types of hepatobiliary carcinoma [68]. A porcelain (calcified) gallbladder is another rare phenomenon associated with gallbladder carcinoma. Finally, the presence of gallbladder polyps is also a risk factor; polyps larger than 1 cm are more likely to become malignant and are an indication for cholecystectomy.

CHOLANGIOCARCINOMA RISK FACTORS

Hepatolithiasis	Chemicals
Liver flukes	Nitrosamines
Biliary cysts	Drugs
Sclerosing cholangitis	Ulcerative colitis
Radionuclides	

FIGURE 6-53.

Patients with biliary tract disease associated with bile stasis and infection are prone to develop cholangiocarcinoma. Just as gallstones are a risk factor for gallbladder cancer, intrahepatic stones can lead to cholangiocarcinoma. Bile duct malignancies develop in 5% to 10% of patients with hepatolithiasis [71]. An association between cholangiocarcinoma and the liver fluke *Clonorchis sinensis* has been known for more than three decades [68]. Clonorchiasis occurs frequently in east Asia where ingestion of infected raw fish is common. In Thailand the liver fluke *Opisthorchis viverrini* has been associated with a high incidence of cholangiocarcinoma [68]. Although the majority of choledochal cysts present in infancy and childhood, more than 75% of cholangiocarcinomas associated with choledochal cysts have occurred in patients presenting with symptoms as adults [68–70]. Sclerosing cholangitis is another biliary tract disease associated with an increased risk of cholangiocarcinoma [72]. Bile duct tumors have been found at autopsy in up to 40% of patients dying with sclerosing cholangitis and in 10% to 35% of patients undergoing liver transplantation [68]. The majority of patients with sclerosing cholangitis also have ulcerative colitis. Patients with ulcerative colitis are also at increased risk for developing cholangiocarcinoma, and this risk is independent of how the colon has been managed [73].

Several clues suggest that exposure to radiation increases the risk of bile duct malignancies. Development of hepatic and bile duct neoplasms has been clearly documented after exposure to the α-emitting radiocontrast agent Thorotrast [74]. Thorotrast will also cause cholangiocarcinoma in hamsters, and plutonium or americium leads to bile duct malignancies in beagles [75]. In animal models nitrosamines [76] also can cause cholangiocarcinoma. Because nitrosamines are present in high concentrations in cured meats, dietary factors may also contribute to the pathogenesis of bile duct tumors. Dioxin has also been recently implicated as a cause of cholangiocarcinoma [70]. In addition, several drugs (including isoniazid, methyl dopa, and oral contraceptive) have also been implicated [68].

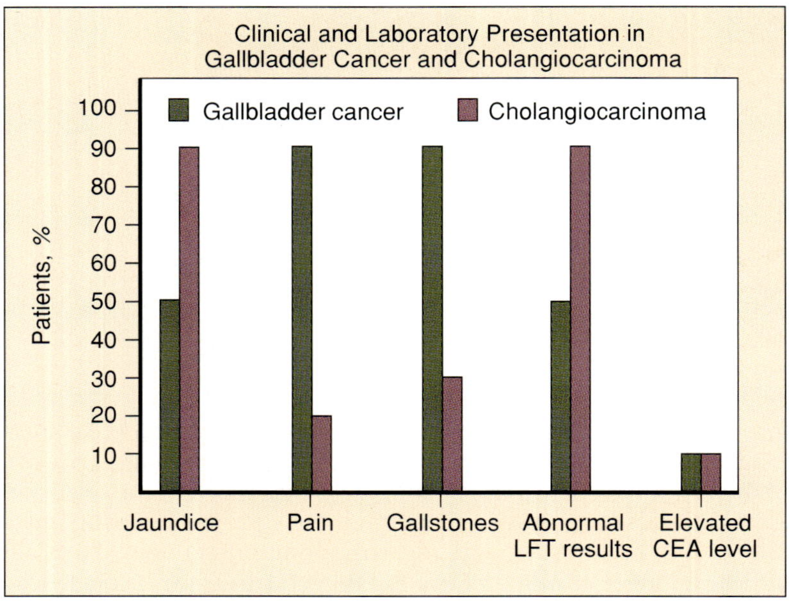

FIGURE 6-54.

The clinical and laboratory presentation of patients with gallbladder cancer and cholangiocarcinoma are somewhat different. The vast majority of patients with gallbladder cancer have a history of right upper quadrant pain and are found to have gallstones; however, clinical jaundice and abnormal liver function test (LFT) results are present in approximately half of the patients in whom the tumor also invades the bile ducts. In contrast, approximately 90% of patients with cholangiocarcinoma will present with clinical jaundice and abnormal LFT results. Pain is an infrequent presenting symptom, and the 30% incidence of gallstones in these patients is similar to their cohort with a mean age in the 60's. Slight elevations of serum CEA occur in only a small minority of patients with gallbladder cancer or cholangiocarcinoma.

ASSESSMENT OF RESECTABILITY

Patient factors	Tumor factors
Age	Liver invasion
Medical condition	Colonic invasion
Cardiopulmonary status	Duodenal invasion
Liver function	Vascular invasion
Renal function	Liver metastases
Nutrition	Peritoneal metastases
Sepsis	Distant metastases

Figure 6-55.

Both patient and tumor factors must be considered in the assessment of resectability of patients with carcinoma of the gallbladder or cholangiocarcinoma. In general, the patient's overall medical condition is more important than the chronologic age. Preexisting cirrhosis may dramatically increase the risk of surgery, especially if portal hypertension is also a problem. In patients with obstructive jaundice a cluster of physiologic abnormalities must also be considered. These alterations include impaired hepatic function, renal function, immune function, hemostasis, cardiopulmonary function, and wound healing and an altered gastrointestinal barrier. Renal function, nutritional status, and underlying sepsis are the best predictors of outcome [77].

Local invasion of the adjacent liver is a common problem that mandates liver resection. Extension of a gallbladder cancer into the right transverse colon can be managed by local colonic resection. In most cases encasement or occlusion of the main portal vein or proper hepatic artery will prevent resection. However, encasement of a portal vein or hepatic artery branch on the same side as the contemplated resection should not preclude exploration. Metastatic disease in the liver, peritoneum, or other distant sites is a contraindication to resection.

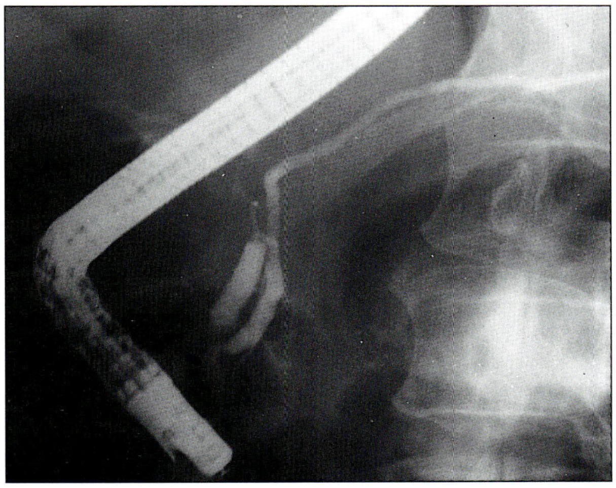

Figure 6-56.

This endoscopic retrograde cholangiopancreatography (ERCP) shows a patent pancreatic duct and an occluded common bile duct in a patient with a distal cholangiocarcinoma. In patients with distal bile duct obstruction, the additional information provided by the pancreatogram may give useful diagnostic information. Thus, ERCP is the diagnostic test of choice when a distal lesion is suspected.

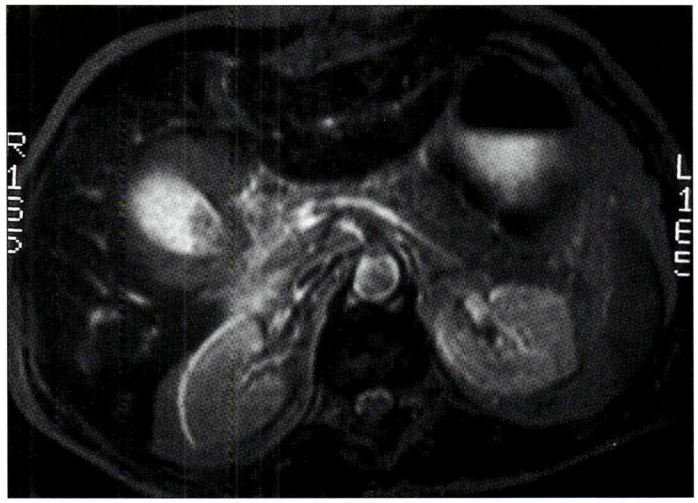

Figure 6-57.

This MR scan, T2 image, shows the gallbladder (*white*) with gallstones and invasion of the adjacent liver (*grey*) and portal structures. MR imaging is better than standard CT scans at demonstrating invasion of the tumor into adjacent structures as well as encasement or occlusion of the portal vein and hepatic artery [78]. Whether newer spiral CT scans will be as useful as MR imaging has yet to be determined. New MR scans can also provide good cholangiographic data.

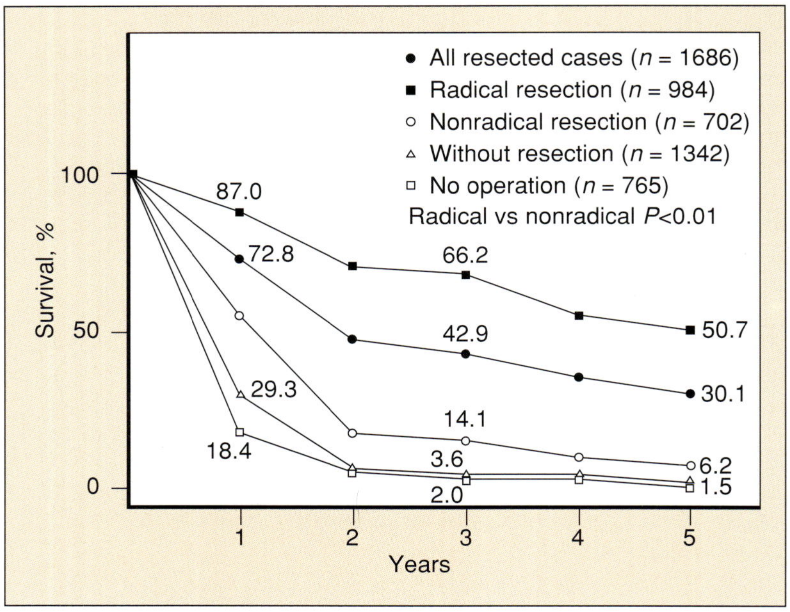

FIGURE 6-58.

This graph demonstrates cumulative survival for a collected series of Japanese patients with gallbladder carcinoma [69]. Patients undergoing radical operations survived longer ($P < 0.01$). These results are among the best that have been reported. Other analyses from North America [80], Europe [81], and Japan [82] all support the concept that more radical operations will improve survival. In general, more than 85% of patients with stage 1 lesions undergoing simple cholecystectomy should have a 5-year survival. More than 65% of patients with stage II tumors managed with extended cholecystectomy may be expected to have survive for 5 years. In comparison, 15% to 25% of patients with stage III and IV gallbladder cancers treated with radical operations may survive for 5 years.

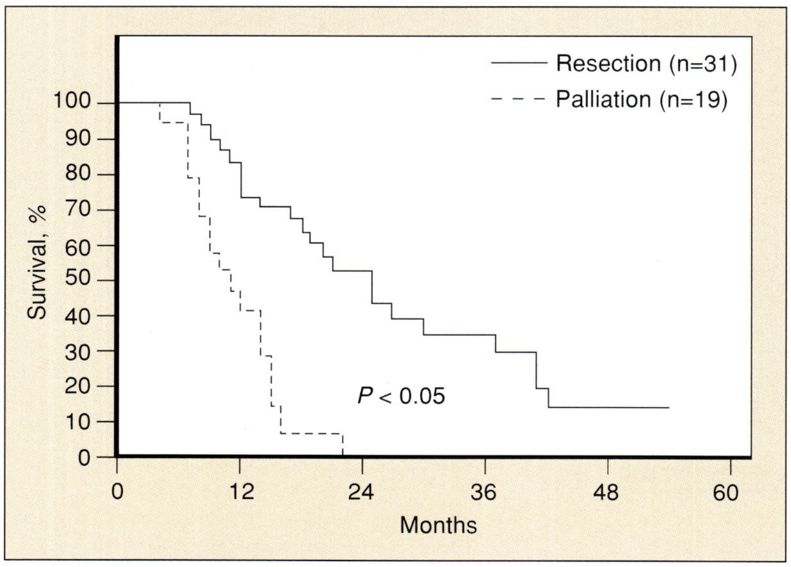

FIGURE 6-59.

This actuarial Kaplan-Meier curve shows survival for patients with operatively staged perihilar cholangiocarcinoma undergoing surgical resection or operative palliation at The Johns Hopkins Hospital [83]. Patients who underwent resection survived significantly ($P < 0.01$) longer. The majority of these patients underwent hilar resection with a low hospital mortality but only a modest (10% to 15%) 5-year survival. These data with respect to hilar resection are better than those in a recent collected series [84] that reported an 8% hospital mortality and only a 7% 5-year survival. In this collected series liver resection was associated with a 15% operative mortality but led to a 17% 5-year survival.

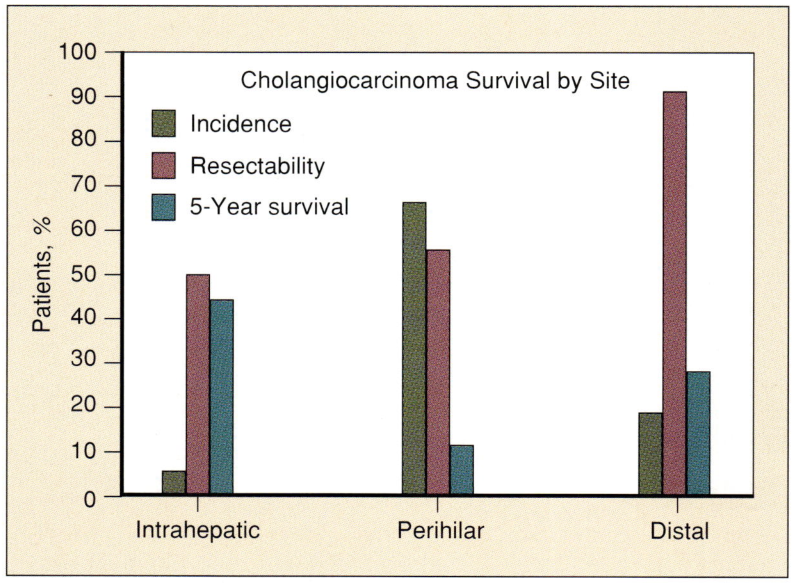

FIGURE 6-60.

This graph depicts the incidence, resectability rate, and 5-year survival for 250 patients with cholangiocarcinoma managed at The Johns Hopkins Hospital over a 20-year period. Intrahepatic tumors were the least common (6%) and had the lowest resectability rate (50%) but resulted in the best survival when resected (50%). Perihilar tumors were most common (67%) and were resected in 58% but resulted in the worst survival (17%). Distal tumors accounted for 27% of the patients and had the highest resectability rate (91%), with an intermediate survival (28%).

REFERENCES

1. Dawson JL, Tan KC: Anatomy of the Liver. In *Wright's Liver and Biliary Disease: Pathophysiology, Diagnosis and Management*, vol 1, ed 3. Edited by Millward-Sadier GH, Wright R, Arthur MJP. London: WB Saunders; 1992:3–11.
2. Frierson HF: The gross anatomy and histology of the gallbladder, extrahepatic bile ducts, Vaterian system, and minor papilla. *Am J Surg Pathol* 1989, 13:146–162.
3. Nakanuma Y, Ohta G: Histometric and serial section observations of the intrahepatic bile ducts in primary biliary cirrhosis. *Gastroenterology* 1979, 76:1326–1332.
4. Erlinger S: Bile flow. In *The Liver: Biology and Pathobiology*. Edited by Arias IM, Boyer JI, Fausto N, *et al.* New York: Raven Press; 1994:769–786.
5. Carey MC: Enterohepatic circulation. In *The Liver: Biology and Pathobiology*. Edited by Arias IM, Boyer JL, Fausto N, *et al.*: New York: Raven Press; 1994:677–718.
6. Carey MC: Pathogenesis of gallstones. *Am J Surg* 1993, 165:410–419.
7. Trotman BW: Pigment gallstone disease. *Gastroenterol Clin North Am* 1991, 20:111–126.
8. Donovan JM, Carr-Locke DL: Gallstones. In *Primary Care of Women*. Edited by Carlson K, Eisenstat S. St. Louis: CV Mosby, 1995:86–97.
9. Maringhini A, Ciambra M, Baccelliere P, *et al.*: Biliary sludge and gallstones in pregnancy: Incidence, risk factors, and natural history. *Ann Intern Med* 1993, 119:116–120.
10. Shiffman ML, Sugerman HJ, Kellum JM, *et al.*: Gallstone formation after rapid weight loss: a prospective study in patients undergoing gastric bypass surgery for treatment of morbid obesity. *Am J Gastroenterol* 1991, 86:1000–1005.
11. Broomfield PH, Chopra R, Sheinbaum RC, *et al.*: Effects of ursodeoxycholic acid and aspirin on the formation of lithogenic bile and gallstones during loss of weight. *N Engl J Med* 1988, 319:1567–1572.
12. National Institutes of Health Consensus Development Conference Statement on gallstones and laparoscopic cholecystectomy. *Am J Surg* 1993, 165:390–398.
13. American College of Physicians. Guidelines for the treatment of gallstones. *Ann Intern Med* 1993, 119:620–622.
14. Donohue JH, Grant CS, Farnell MB, *et al.*: Laparoscopic cholecystectomy: Operative technique. *Mayo Clin Proc* 1992, 67:441–448.
15. Halevy A, Gold-Deutch R, Negri M, *et al.*: Are elevated liver enzymes and bilirubin levels significant after laparoscopic cholecystectomy in the absence of bile duct injury? *Ann Surg* 1994, 219:362–364.
16. Cuschieri A, Dubois F, Mouiel J, *et al.*: The European experience with laparoscopic cholecystectomy. *Am J Surg* 1991, 161:385–387.
17. The Southern Surgeon's Club: A prospective analysis of 1518 laparoscopic cholecystectomies. *N Engl J Med* 1991, 324:1073–1078.
18. Larson GM, Vitale GC, Casey J, *et al.*: Multipractice analysis of laparoscopic cholecystectomy in 1,983 patients. *Am J Surg* 1992, 163:221–226.
19. Airen M, Appel M, Berci G, *et al.*: Retrospective and prospective multi-institutional laparoscopic cholecystectomy study organized by the Society of American Gastrointestinal Endoscopic Surgeons. *Surg Endosc* 1992, 6:169–176.
20. Litwin DEM, Girotti MJ, Poulin EC, *et al.*: Laparoscopic cholecystectomy: Trans-Canada experience with 2201 cases. *Can J Surg* 1992, 35:291–296.
21. Perissat J: Laparoscopic cholecystectomy: the European experience. *Am J Surg* 1993, 165:444–449.
22. Deziel DJ, Millikan KW, Economou SG, *et al.*: Complications of laparoscopic cholecystectomy: A national survey of 4,292 hospitals and an analysis of 77,604 cases. *Am J Surg* 1993, 165:9–14.
23. Deveney KE: The early experience with laparoscopic cholecystectomy in Oregon. *Arch Surg* 1993, 128:627–632.
24. Schlumpf R, Klotz HP, Wehrli H, *et al.*: A nation's experience in laparoscopic cholecystectomy. Prospective multicenter analysis of 3722 cases. *Surg Endosc* 1994, 8:35–41.
25. Mucio M, Felemovicius J, De la Concha F, *et al.*: The Mexican experience with laparoscopic cholecystectomy and common bile duct exploration. *Surg Endosc* 1994, 8:306–309.
26. Woods MS, Traverso LW, Kozarek RA, *et al.*: Characteristics of biliary tract complications during laparoscopic cholecystectomy: a multi-institutional study. *Am J Surg* 1994, 167:27–34.
27. Steiner CA, Bass EB, Talamini MA, *et al.*: Surgical rates and operative mortality for open and laparoscopic cholecystectomy in Maryland. *N Engl J Med* 1994, 330:403–408.
28. Legorreta AP, Silber JH, Costantimo GN, *et al.*: Increased cholecystectomy rate after the introduction of laparoscopic cholecystectomy. *JAMA* 1993, 270:1429–1432.
29. Barkun JS, Barkun AN, Sampalis JS, *et al.*: Randomized controlled trial of laparoscopic versus minicholecystectomy. *Lancet* 1992, 340:1116–1119.
30. McMahon AJ, Russell IT, Baxter JN, *et al.*: Laparoscopic versus minilaparotomy cholecystectomy: A randomized trial. *Lancet* 1994, 343:135–138.
31. Alvaro D, Angelico M, Gandin C, *et al.*: Physico-chemical factors predisposing to pigment gallstone formation in liver cirrhosis. *J Hepatol* 1990, 10:228–234.
32. Kaufman HS, Magnuson TH, Lillemoe KD, *et al.*: The role of bacteria in gallbladder and common duct stone formation. *Ann Surg* 1989, 209:584–591.
33. Malet PF, Takabayashi A, Trotman BW, *et al.*: Black and brown pigment gallstones differ in microstructure and microcomposition. *Hepatology* 1984, 2:227–234.
34. Donovan JM, Carey MC: Physical-chemical basis of cholesterol and pigment gallstone information. *Gastroenterol Clin North Am* 1991, 20:47–66.
35. Lee SP, Nicholls JF: Nature and composition of biliary sludge. *Gastroenterology* 1986, 90:677–686.
36. Lee SP, Maher K, Nicholls JF: Origin and fate of biliary sludge. *Gastroenterology* 1988, 94:170–176.
37. Carey MC, Cahalane MJ: Whither biliary sludge? *Gastroenterology* 1988, 95:508–523.
38. Cotton PB, Lehman G, Vennes J, *et al.*: Endoscopic sphincterotomy complications and their management: an attempt at consensus. *Gastro ntest Endosc* 1991, 37:383–393.
39. Sinanan MN: Acute cholangitis. *Infect Dis Clin North Am* 1992, 6:571–599.
40. Dooley JS, Hamilton Miller JM, Brumfit W, *et al.*: Antibiotics in the treatment of biliary infection. *Gut* 1984, 25:988–998.
41. Lee JG, Leung JW: Endoscopy and gallstones. In *Annual of Gastrointestinal Endoscopy*. Edited by Cotton PB. London: Current Science; 1993:97–106.
42. Leung JWC, Chan CY, Lai CW, *et al.*: Effect of biliary obstruction on the hepatic excretion of imipenem-cilastatin. *Antimicrob Agents Chemother* 1992 36:2057–2060.
43. Leung JWC, Venezuela RR: Cholangiosepsis: endoscopic drainage and antibiotic therapy. *Endoscopy* 1992, 23:220–223.
44. NIH Consensus Conference Statement. *Am J Surg* 1993, 165:337–548.
45. Lai ECS, Mok FPT, Tan ES, *et al.*: Endoscopic biliary drainage for severe acute cholangitis. *N Engl J Med* 1992, 326:1582–1586.
46. Teixidor HS, Godwin TA, Ramirez EA: Cryptosporidiosis of the biliary tract in AIDS. *Radiology* 1991, 180:51–56.
47. Khuroo MS, Dar MY, Yattoo GN, *et al.* Serial cholangiographic appearances in recurrent pyogenic cholangitis. *Gastrointest Endosc* 1993, 39:674–679.
48. Lim JH: Oriental cholangiohepatitis: Pathologic, clinical, and radiologic features. *AJR Am J Roentgenol* 1991, 157:1–8.
49. Bonacini M: Hepatobiliary complications in patients with human immunodeficiency virus infection. *Am J Med* 1992, 92:404–411.

50. Ludwig J, Kim CH, Wiesner RH, *et al.*: Floxuridine-induced sclerosing cholangitis: an ischemic cholangiopathy. *Hepatology* 1989, 9:215–218.
51. Bodenheimer HC Jr, LaRusso NF, Thayer WR Jr, *et al.*: Elevated circulating immune complexes in primary sclerosing cholangitis. *Hepatology* 1983, 3:150–154.
52. Garred P, Lyon H, Christoffersen P, *et al.*: Deposition of C3, the terminal complement complex and vitronectin in primary biliary cirrhosis and primary sclerosing cholangitis. *Liver* 1993, 13:305–310.
53. Lindor KD, Wiesner RH, LaRusso NF, *et al.*: Enhanced autoreactivity of T-lymphocytes in primary sclerosing cholangitis. *Hepatology* 1987, 7:884–888.
54. Chapman RW, Kelly PMA, Heryet A, *et al.*: Expression of HLA-DR antigens on bile duct epithelium in primary sclerosing cholangitis. *Gut* 1988, 29:422–427.
55. Lindor KD, Wiesner RH, MacCarty RL, *et al.*: Advances in primary sclerosing cholangitis. *Am J Med* 1990, 89:73–80.
56. Broome U, Glaumann H, Hellers G, *et al.*: Liver disease in ulcerative colitis: an epidemiological and follow-up study in the county of Stockholm. *Gut* 1994, 35:84–89.
57. Ludwig J: Surgical pathology of the syndrome of primary sclerosing cholangitis. *Am J Surg Pathol* 1989, 13:43–49.
58. LaRusso NF, Wiesner RH, Ludwig J, *et al.*: Prospective trial of penicillamine in primary sclerosing cholangitis. *Gastroenterology* 1988, 95:1036–1042.
59. O'Brien CB, Senior JR, Arora-Mirchandani R, *et al.*: Ursodeoxycholic acid for the treatment of primary sclerosing cholangitis: a 30-month pilot study. *Hepatology* 1991, 14:838–847.
60. Beuers U, Spengler U, Kruis W, *et al.*: Ursodeoxycholic acid for the treatment of primary sclerosing cholangitis: a placebo-controlled trial. *Hepatology* 1992, 16:707–714.
61. Lindor KD, Wiesner RH, Colwell LJ, *et al.*: The combination of prednisone and colchicine in patients with primary sclerosing cholangitis. *Am J Gastroenterol* 1991, 85:57–61.
62. Knox TA, Kaplan MM: A double-blind controlled trial of oral-pulse methotrexate therapy in the treatment of primary sclerosing cholangitis. *Gastroenterology* 1994, 106:494–499.
63. Wiesner RH, Steiner B, LaRusso NF, *et al.*: A controlled clinical trial evaluating cyclosporine in the treatment of primary sclerosing cholangitis [abstract]. *Hepatology* 1991, 14:63.
64. Abu-Elmagd KM, Malinchoc M, Dickson ER, *et al.*: Efficacy of hepatic transplantation in patients with primary sclerosing cholangitis. *Surgery* 1993, 177:335–343.
65. Toouli J: Sphincter of Oddi. In *Surgery of the Biliary Tract.* Edited by Toouli J. New York: Churchill Livingstone; 1993:267–278.
66. Prinz RA, Ko TC, Maltz SB, *et al.*: Common bile duct obstruction by free floating tumor. *HPB Surg* 1993, 6:319–323.
67. Webb TH, Lillemoe KD, Pitt HA, *et al.*: Pancreatic lymphoma: is surgery mandatory for diagnosis or treatment? *Ann Surg* 1989, 209:25–30.
68. Pitt HA, Dooley WC, Yeo CJ, *et al.*: Malignancies of the biliary tree. *Curr Probl Surg* 1995, 32:1–90.
69. Iwai N, Yanagihara J, Tokiwa K, *et al.*: Congenital choledochal dilatation with emphasis on pathophysiology of the biliary tract. *Ann Surg* 1992, 215:27–30.
70. Tanaka K, Nishimura A, Yamada K, *et al.*: Cancer of the gallbladder associated with anomalous junction of the pancreatobiliary duct system without bile dilatation. *Br J Surg* 1993, 80:622–624.
71. Chijiiwa K, Ichimiya H, Kuroki S, *et al.*: Late development of cholangiocarcinoma after the treatment of hepatolithiasis: immunohistochemical study of mucin carbohydrates and core proteins in hepatolithiasis and cholangiocarcinoma. *Int J Cancer* 1993, 55:82–91.
72. Rosen CB, Nagorney DM, Wiesner RH, *et al.*: Cholangiocarcinoma complicating primary sclerosing cholangitis. *Ann Surg* 1991, 213:21–25.
73. Mir-Madjlessi SH, Farmer RG, Sivak MV Jr: Bile duct carcinoma in patients with ulcerative colitis: Relationship to sclerosing cholangitis. *Dig Dis Sci* 1987, 32:145–152.
74. Ito Y, Kojiro M, Nakashima T, *et al.*: Pathomorphologic characteristics of 102 cases of Thorotrast-related hepatocellular carcinoma, cholangiocarcinoma and hepatic angiosarcoma. *Cancer* 1988, 62:1153–1158.
75. Taylor GN, Lloyd RD, Mays CW, *et al.*: Plutonium- or americium-induced liver tumors and lesions in beagles. *Health Phys* 1991, 61:337–347.
76. Kinami Y, Ashida Y, Seto K, *et al.*: The effect of incomplete bile duct obstruction in diisopropanolnitrosamine-induced cholangiocarcinoma. *HPB Surg* 1991, 3:117–125.
77. Pitt HA, Cameron JL, Postier RG, *et al.*: Factors influencing mortality in biliary tract surgery. *Am J Surg* 1981, 141:66–72.
78. Fan ZM, Yamashita Y, Harada M, *et al.*: Intrahepatic cholangiocarcinoma: spin-echo and contrast-enhanced dynamic MR imaging. *Am J Roentgenol* 1993, 161:313–317.
79. Ogura Y, Mizumoto R, Isaji S, *et al.*: Radical operations for carcinoma of the gallbladder: present status in Japan. *World J Surg* 1991, 15:337–343.
80. Gagner M, Rossi RL: Radical operations for carcinomas of the gallbladder: present status in North America. *World J Surg* 1991, 15:344–347.
81. Gall FP, Kockerling F, Scheele J, *et al.*: Radical operations for carcinoma of the gallbladder: present status in Germany. *World J Surg* 1991, 15:328–336.
82. Tsukada K, Yoshida K, Aono T, *et al.*: Major hepatectomy and pancreatoduodenectomy for advanced carcinoma of the biliary tract. *Br J Surg* 1994, 81:108–110.
83. Pitt HA, Nakeeb A, Abrams RA, *et al.*: Perihilar cholangiocarcinoma: postoperative radiotherapy does not improve survival. *Ann Surg* 1995, 221:788–798.
84. Boerma EJ: Research into the results of resection of hilar bile duct cancer. *Surgery* 1990, 108:572–580.

Chapter 7

Disorders of the Pancreas

EDITOR

Phillip P. Toskes

CONTRIBUTORS

Christopher Forsmark
James H. Grendell
Amy M. Kusske
Thomas O'Dorisio
Rodney V. Pozderac
Howard A. Reber
William M. Steinberg
Mark Toyama

ACUTE PANCREATITIS

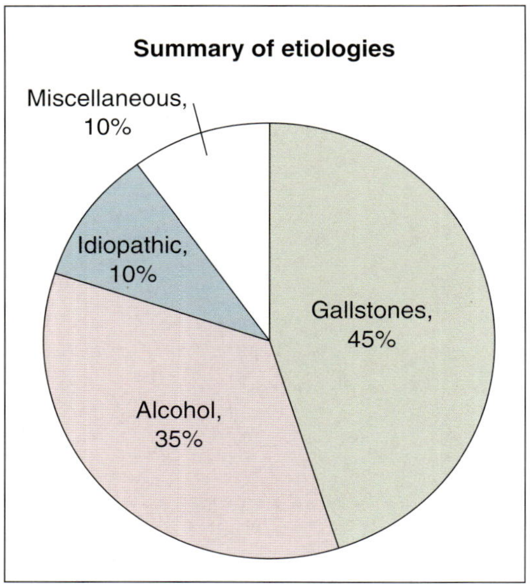

FIGURE 7-1.

Summary of the main etiologies for acute pancreatitis. A compilation of many studies from around the world reveals that gallstones account for 45% of cases, alcoholism for 35% of cases, miscellaneous causes for 10% of cases, and idiopathic for 10% of cases. Miscellaneous causes are listed in Figs. 7-2–7-6.

OBSTRUCTIVE CAUSES OF PANCREATITIS
Gallstones
Ampullary/pancreatic cancer
Worms in pancreatic duct—ascaris
Choledochocele
Periampullary duodenal diverticula
Foreign body obstructing duct
Pancreas divisum with obstruction of accessory papilla
Hypertensive sphincter of Oddi

FIGURE 7-2.

Obstructive causes of acute pancreatitis. Besides gallstones, these causes include ampullary or pancreatic cancer, worms, such as *Ascaris*, choledochocele, periampullary duodenal diverticula, foreign body obstructing the pancreatic duct, pancreas divisum with obstruction of the minor papilla, and hypertensive sphincter of Oddi. By far, the most common cause is gallstones.

TOXINS CAUSING PANCREATITIS
Ethyl alcohol
Methyl alcohol
Scorpion toxin
Organo-phosphorus insecticides

FIGURE 7-3.

Toxins causing acute pancreatitis. Besides ethyl alcohol, these causes include scorpion toxin, and organophosphorous insecticides. By far, the most common cause is ethyl alcohol (ethanol).

MAJOR DRUGS THAT CAUSE PANCREATITIS

With rechallenges	With consistent latencies
Alpha methyl dopa	Acetaminophen
5-Aminosalicylate	dDI
Azathioprine/6 mercaptopurine	Estrogens
Cimetidine	
Furosemide	
Metronidazole	
Pentamidine	
Sulfa drugs	
Sulindac	
Tetracycline	
Valproic acid	

FIGURE 7-4.

Drugs that can cause acute pancreatitis. These can be divided into two groups. The first group includes those in whom a positive rechallenge with the drug has led to recurrent pancreatitis. Examples of these include azathioprine, pentamidine, and valproic acid.

The second group does not have a positive rechallenge reported, but does have a consistent latency (period of time between exposure of the drug and episode of pancreatitis). Examples in this second group are dideoxyinosine (dDI), acetaminophen, and estrogens. Estrogens may cause pancreatitis by inducing hypertriglyceridemia.

METABOLIC CAUSES OF PANCREATITIS

Hypercalcemia
Hypertrigliceridemia
- Type I
- Type IV
- Type V

FIGURE 7-5.

Metabolic causes of acute pancreatitis. These are due to hypercalcemia (from whatever cause) and familial or acquired hypertriglyceridemia (triglyceride levels > 1000 mg/dL).

INFECTIOUS CAUSES OF ACUTE PANCREATITIS

Viruses
- Mumps, cytomegalovirus
- Herpes, hepatitis A, B, C

Bacteria
- *Mycobacteria* (tuberculosis, mycobacterium-avium complex)
- Leptospirosis

Fungi
- *Cryptococcus, candida,* coccidiomycosis

Parasites
- *Ascaris, clonorchis, pneumocystis*

FIGURE 7-6.

Infectious causes of pancreatitis. These are rare in industrialized countries, and can be divided into those caused by viruses (*eg,* mumps, cytomegalovirus, etc.); bacteria (tuberculosis, mycobacteria-avium complex [MAC], and leptospirosis); fungi, such as *cryptococcus,* which can cause microabscesses in the pancreas; and parasites, such as ascariasis, which are a common source of pancreatitis in underdeveloped countries, where these parasites are highly prevalent.

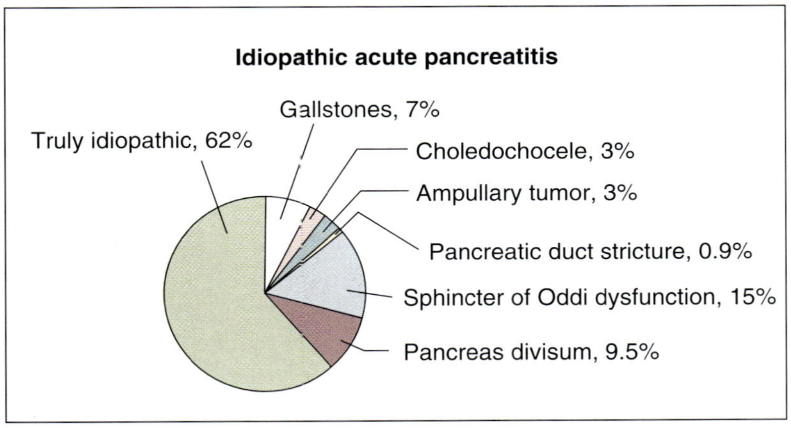

FIGURE 7-7.

"Idiopathic" acute pancreatitis. Final etiologies of cases of idiopathic pancreatitis referred to the Medical College of Wisconsin. After endoscopic retrograde cholangiopancreatography and sphincter of Oddi manometry were performed, 38% of cases were no longer classified as idiopathic, but 62% remained in this category. (*Data from* Venu *et al.* [1].)

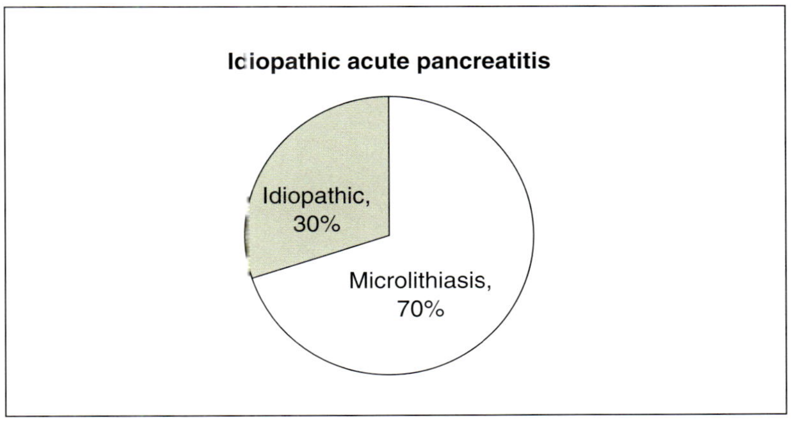

FIGURE 7-8.

Biliary drainage of idiopathic acute pancreatitis. In two series of consecutive patients with idiopathic pancreatitis—one from Seattle, the other from Spain—in which biliary drainage was performed, the majority of patients had microlithiasis as the probable cause of pancreatitis. These patients responded to ursodeoxycholic acid (Ursodiol), endoscopic sphincterotomy, or cholecystectomy, with a reduction in the frequency of attacks of pain [2,3].

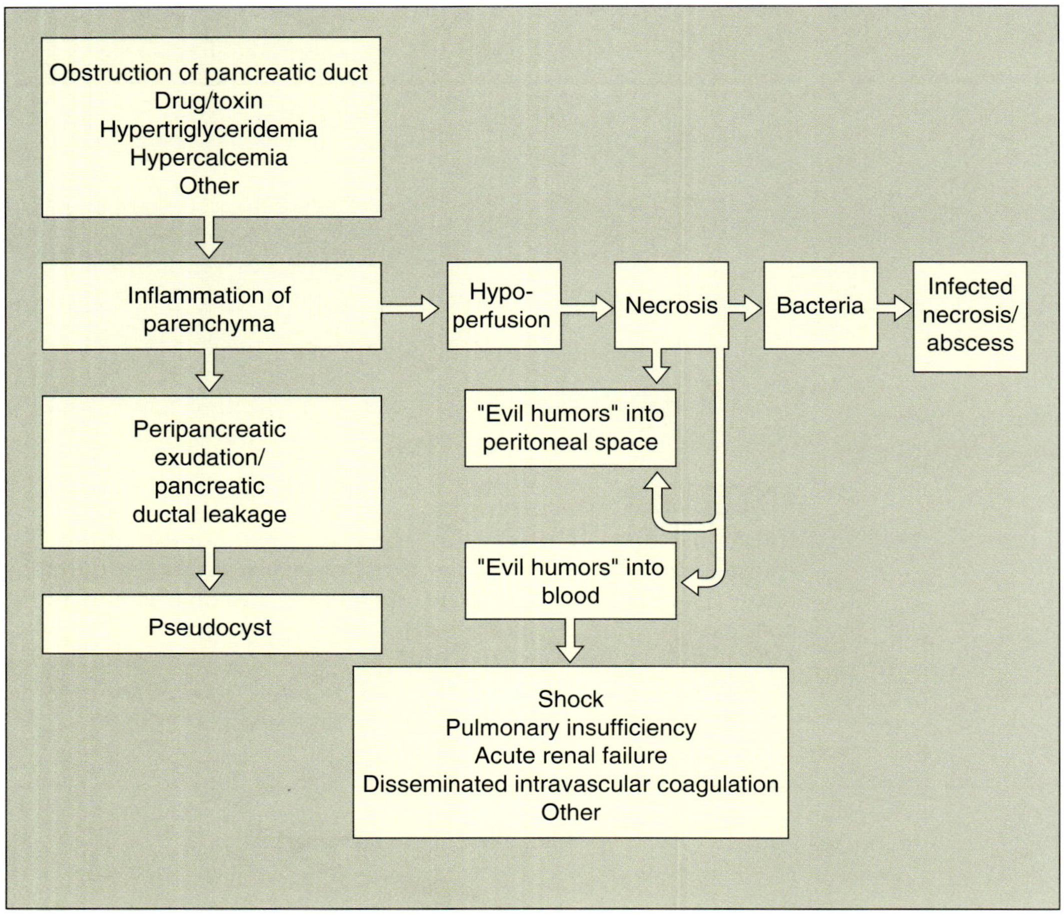

FIGURE 7-9.

Possible pathogenetic sequence of acute pancreatitis. After the acinar cell is triggered, it provokes an intense inflammatory response in the pancreas. Weeping of pancreatic juice into the peripancreatic space or microperforations of the pancreatic ductal system can lead to pseudocyst formation. Subsequent hypoperfusion to the gland can convert mild edematous/interstitial pancreatitis to necrotizing pancreatitis. At this point, release of toxic factors into the systemic circulation, such as trypsin, elastase, or phospholipase A_2, can lead to cardiovascular and pulmonary collapse. The necrotic pancreas can become secondarily infected from hematogenous or transperitoneal sources [4].

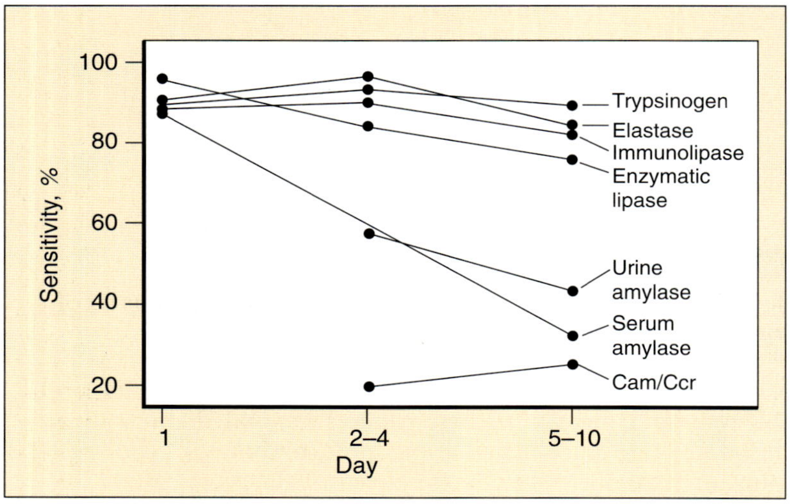

FIGURE 7-10.

Diagnosis of acute pancreatitis. A composite of several studies comparing the sensitivity of diagnostic blood and urine tests in diagnosing acute pancreatitis, depending on the day of presentation to the hospital. On day 1 of abdominal pain, all diagnostic markers are very sensitive. On day 2 and beyond, the serum amylase level drops to normal faster than the lipase of the immunologic markers—immunolipase, tryspinogen, or immunoelastase. The urinary diagnosis of acute pancreatitis—timed urine amylase collection or the amylase to creatinine clearance ratio (Cam/Ccr)—offers no advantages to the serological diagnosis. (*Adapted from* Steinberg *et al.* [5].)

RANSON CRITERIA FOR SEVERITY OF ACUTE PANCREATITIS

	Non-gallstone pancreastits (*eg,* alcohol)	Gallsone pancreatits
On admission		
Age, *y*	>55	>70
WBC *mm^{-3}*	>16,000	>18,000
Blood glucose *mg/dL*	>200	>220
Serum LDH *IU/mL*	>350	>400
Serum AST *IU/mL*	>250	>250
At 48 hours		
Hematocrit ↓%	>10	>10
BUN ↑ *mg/dL*	>5	>2
Serum Ca^{++} *mg/dL*	<8	<8
pO_2 *mmHg*	<60	—
Base deficit *mEq/L*	>4	>5
Fluid requirements *L*	>6	>4

FIGURE 7-11.

Ranson criteria. There are two lists used to predict severity and outcome: one for nongallstone pancreatitis (Ranson 1974) and one for acute gallstone pancreatitis (Ranson 1979). Three or more risk factors are associated with an increased probability of severe disease [6,7].

COMPLICATIONS OF ACUTE PANCREATITIS

Local	Systemic
Necrosis	Shock
Pseudocysts	Respiratory failure
Abcess	Renal failure
Ileus	Metabolic—hypocalcemia, hyperglycemia
Gastrointestinal obstruction	Coagulopathy—disseminated intravascular coagulation
Fistulization	
Gastrointestinal hemorrhage—pseudoaneurysm	

FIGURE 7-12.

Complications of acute pancreatitis can be divided into local and systemic. Complications can also be divided into two groups—early (occurring in the first week, such as pulmonary, renal, and cardiovascular failure) and late (occurring mostly after the first week, such as infected necrosis, pseudocyst, and abscess.)

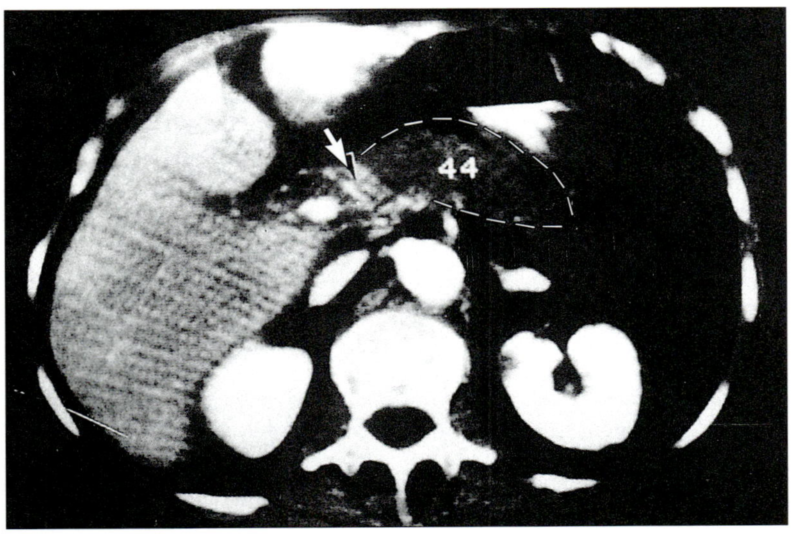

FIGURE 7-13.

Bolus contrast computed tomography (CT) in severe acute pancreatitis. A major unsettled issue in the pathophysiology of acute pancreatitis is why most cases are mild and self-limited whereas some progress to the more severe, potentially lethal end of the spectrum of disease. Impairment of the pancreatic microcirculation leading to tissue ischemia may be an important factor in determining the extent of injury and necrosis of the pancreas and the ultimate severity of the disease process. A clinical correlate of this tissue ischemia may be failure of the pancreas to enhance its density on CT after intravenous injection of a bolus of radio contrast agent in patients with more severe acute pancreatitis. (*Arrowhead*—Normally enhancing tissue in neck of pancreas; *outlined area*—Nonenhancing body and tail of the pancreas.)

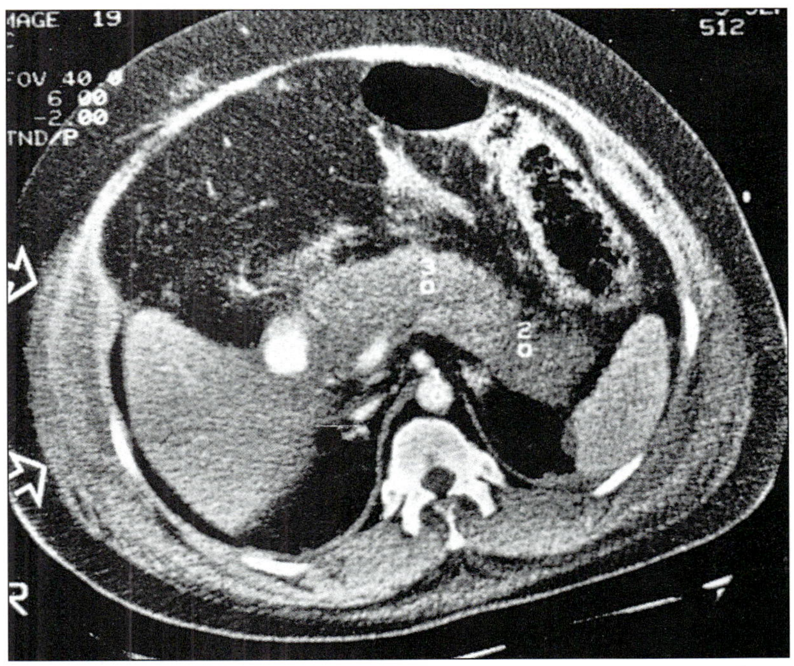

FIGURE 7-14

Dynamic computed tomography (CT) scan of the pancreas peformed by injecting large doses of intravenous contrast rapidly (bolus injection) and scanning the pancreas with thin cuts. This CT scan shows poor perfusion of the pancreas. The presence of poor perfusion on CT scan has about a 90% predictive value of predicting necrosis at surgery; however, only about 60% of patients with necrosis on CT scan have a severe course clinically [8,9].

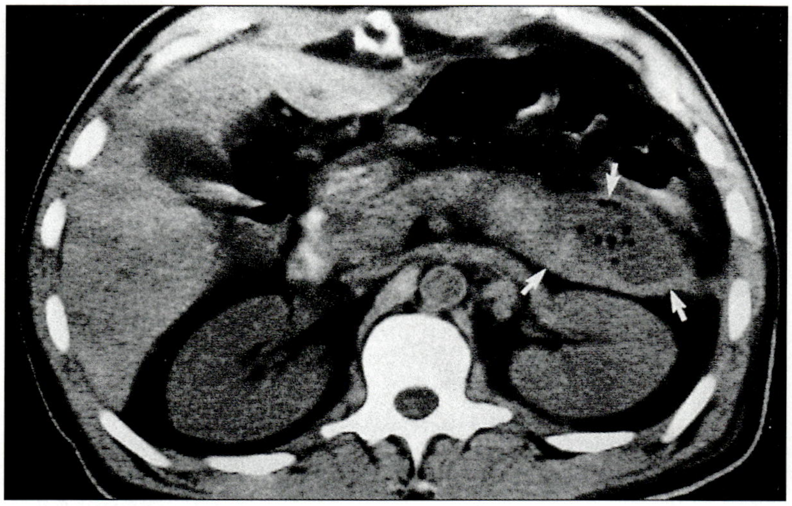

FIGURE 7-15.

A computed tomography (CT) scan of the pancreas indicating gas bubbles within the substance of the pancreas. This suggests pancreatic abscess secondary to gas-producing organisms; however, sterile necrosis with microcommunication with the gut can lead to this CT finding. Only with a fine-needle aspirate can one diagnose an abscess with assurance. (*From* Freeny and Lawson [10]; with permission.)

PRINCIPLES OF TREATMENT OF ACUTE PANCREATITIS

Intravascular volume
Analgesia
Put pancreas to "rest"
Nothing by mouth, nasogastric tube only for ileus or vomiting
Treat complications—Pulmonary, shock, renal, metabolic
Remove obstructing gallstone in severe gallstone pancreatitis
Antibiotics for severe disease
Percutaneous aspiration of pancreas to document infection in patient who fails to respond.

FIGURE 7-16.

The principles of treatment of acute pancreatitis are summarized here. Hospitalization is required, and in severe cases, therapy should be administered in an intensive care unit.

ENDOSCOPIC RETROGRADE CHOLANGIOPANCREATOGRAPHY IN ACUTE GALLSTONE PANCREATITIS

	Emergency	Conservative	P value
All patients	*N*=97	*N*=98	
Complications	18%	29%	0.07
Mortality	5%	9%	0.400
Biliary stone patients	*N*=64	*N*=63	
Complications	16%	33%	0.030
Cholangitis	0%	12%	0.001
Mortality	2%	8%	0.090

FIGURE 7-17.

This Hong Kong study randomized 195 patients to emergency endoscopic retrograde cholangiopancreatography (ERCP) within 24 hours of admission versus no emergency ERCP, although most patients in this group received a subsequent ERCP. If a stone was found, it was removed. About two thirds of the total group had gallstones as the etiology. In this subgroup of patients with biliary stones, removing gallstones by emergency ERCP reduced complications, especially cholangitis. Mortality was also reduced, but this was not statistically significant. This study indicated that it is relatively safe to perform emergency ERCP in acute pancreatitis. Proven utility of ERCP is in the removal of suspected gallstones in patients with severe pancreatitis or in those in whom cholangitis is suspected; however, a more recent study suggests that ERCP may not necessarily improve outcome in biliary pancreatitis [11]. Thus, additional studies are needed to settle this issue.

IMIPENEM AND NECROTIZING PANCREATITIS

	Imipenem	No Imipenem	P
Pancreatic sepsis	13.0%	30.0%	< .01
Nonpancreatic sepsis	14.0%	48%	< .01
Death	7.3%	12.1%	Not significant

FIGURE 7-18.

In a randomized study from Italy, 74 patients with necrotizing pancreatitis were randomized within 72 hours of admission to receive imipenem 0.5 g/ 7 d (n=41) versus no antibiotics (n=33). Patients randomized to imipenem had significantly fewer pancreatic and nonpancreatic infections. There was a trend toward lower mortality in the antibiotic group, but it was not statistically significant. This study documents improved outcome in patients with severe pancreatitis who receive a broad-spectrum antibiotic.

ROLE OF SURGERY IN ACUTE PANCREATITIS

Debride necrosis
  Infected/? sterile
Drain abscess/pseudocyst
When diagnosis is in doubt
  Perforated viscus
  Small bowel obstruction/infarction

FIGURE 7-19.

The current indications for surgery in acute pancreatitis are delineated here. The timing and the role of surgical débridement in sterile and infected pancreatic necrosis is debated.

CHRONIC PANCREATITIS

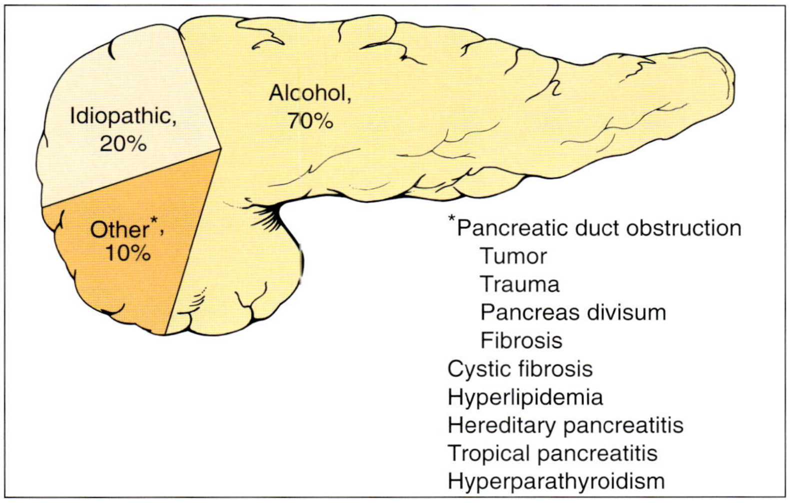

FIGURE 7-20.

Classification of chronic pancreatitis by etiology. Chronic pancreatitis may also be classified by its presumed cause. Chronic alcoholism accounts for approximately 70% of all cases of chronic pancreatitis. Prolonged and substantial abuse is generally required to produce chronic pancreatitis, and most (but not all) patients who present with an episode of acute pancreatitis caused by alcohol consumption already have chronic pancreatic damage. Chronic obstruction of the pancreatic duct may also produce chronic pancreatitis, such as that caused by tumors, trauma, pseudocysts, inflammation and fibrosis (such as after a severe episode of acute pancreatitis), pancreas divisum (with associated minor papilla stenosis), and even after prolonged endoscopic stenting of the the pancreatic duct. After traumatic injury to the pancreatic duct (such as after a motor vehicle accident or a stab wound), chronic pancreatitis may develop within a few months. Pancreas divisum commonly occurs as a normal variant (in 10% of the affected population), and most patients remain asymptomatic. This variant occurs after nonfusion of the two pancreatic buds during development, so that most pancreatic secretion in the dorsal segment drains through the minor papilla rather than the major papilla. A small subset of patients have both pancreas divisum and obstruction at the minor papilla, which may produce both acute relapsing pancreatitis or, more rarely, chronic obstructive pancreatitis. Hyperlipidemia, particularly when the serum triglycerides are above 1000 mg/dL, may produce both acute and chronic pancreatitis. Tropical chronic pancreatitis, probably caused by malnutrition and toxic products in the diet, is rare in the United States. Cystic fibrosis is an important cause of chronic pancreatitis in children, although with improved pulmonary care these patients may live to adulthood. Despite careful evaluation, about 20% of patients (in some studies as high as 30%) have no specific identifiable etiology, and are thus classified as having idiopathic chronic pancreatitis.

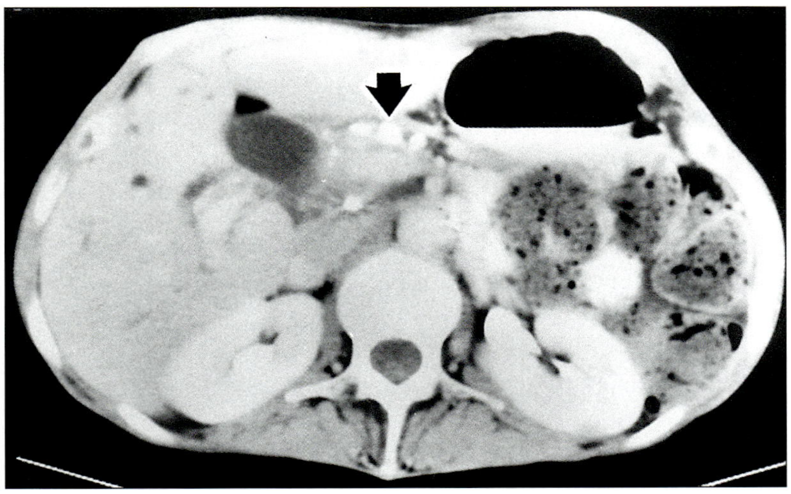

FIGURE 7-21.

Pathophysiology of chronic pancreatitis. The specific mechanism by which alcohol produces chronic pancreatitis is unknown, but it does appear to require substantial alcohol ingestion over at least 6 to 12 years. Various physiologic abnormalities have been documented in both animal models and in humans, including a direct toxic effect of pancreatic acinar cells, stimulation of pancreatic secretion, interference with normal intracellular protein trafficking, and the promotion of the formation of protein plugs within the ductal system. These plugs often become calcified, producing pancreatic ductal stones. Whether these stones contribute to the pathogenesis of alcoholic chronic pancreatitis by obstructing the pancreatic ducts is unknown. They may merely be a marker of alcoholic chronic pancreatitis rather than its cause. Multiple calcified stones within the pancreatic duct on a computed tomography scan (*arrow*).

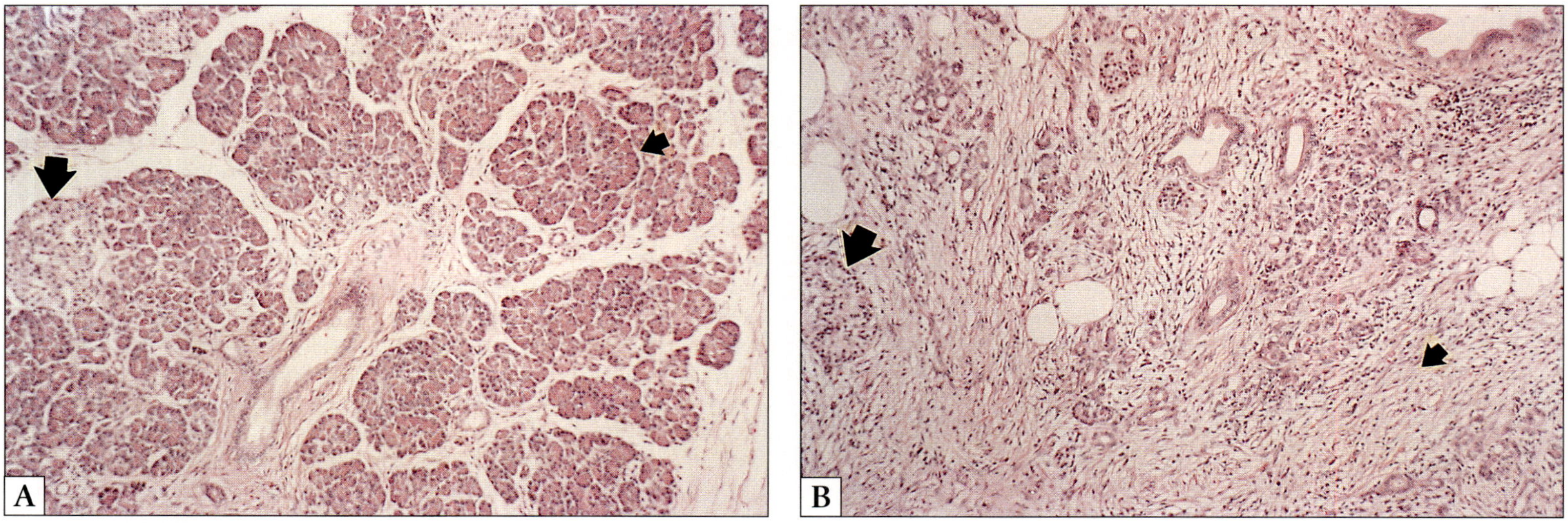

FIGURE 7-22.

Histology of chronic pancreatitis. Regardless of the specific cause of chronic pancreatitis, the histologic result is similar. Pancreatic inflammation, together with progressive fibrosis, leads to destruction of the acinar cells either focally or diffusely, producing exocrine insufficiency and steatorrhea. Intraductal concretions and stones may form, which may block the flow of pancreatic secretions and augment the damage. Inflammation involving pancreatic nerves is also commonly found. The endocrine tissue (the islets of Langerhans) is typically spared until late in the disease process, making diabetes mellitus a late complication. **A**, Normal pancreatic tissue is demonstrated with a normal acinar architecture (*small arrow*) and islets of Langerhans (*large arrow*). **B**, Changes of chronic pancreatitis include destruction of acinar tissue with replacement by fibrosis (*small arrow*), but the islets remain intact (*large arrow*).

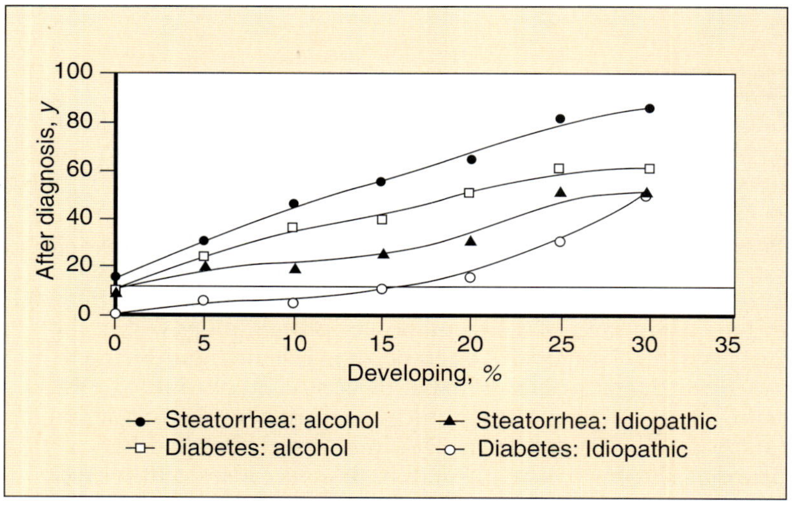

FIGURE 7-23.

Endocrine insufficiency (diabetes mellitus) is a later occurrence than exocrine insufficiency in chronic pancreatitis. Up to 60% to 70% of patients with alcoholic pancreatitis may ultimately develop diabetes mellitus after 20 years of disease, at which time most will have diffuse pancreatic calcifications. Ketoacidosis is unusual, but frequent treatment-associated episodes of hypoglycemia may be a problem. Complications of diabetes mellitus, such as neuropathy and retinopathy, occur as frequently as in other forms of diabetes if incidence is corrected for disease duration. (*Adapted from* Layer *et al.* [12].)

DIAGNOSTIC TESTS IN CHRONIC PANCREATITIS

FUNCTION	STRUCTURE
Direct hormonal stimulation tests	Endoscopic retrograde pancreatography (ERP)
Bentiromide test	Computed tomography
Serum trypsin-like immunoreactivity	Endoscopic ultrasound
Fecal chymotrypsin or fecal elastase	Magnetic resonance imaging
Quantitative fecal fat	Ultrasonography
Blood glucose	Plain abdominal radiograph

Tests are listed in order of decreasing sensitivity

FIGURE 7-24.

Diagnostic tests in chronic pancreatitis. The diagnosis of chronic pancreatitis is most reliably based on the demonstration of consistent histologic abnormalities, but pancreatic tissue is difficult and risky to obtain, and therefore is not available in most patients. Commonly used diagnostic tests rely on abnormalities of either morphology or function. The available diagnostic tests are listed in this table in order of decreasing sensitivity. As chronic pancreatitis progresses, obvious abnormalities develop that make diagnosis straightforward, such as diffuse pancreatic calcifications, a markedly dilated duct, and complications such as a pseudocyst, steatorrhea, and diabetes. Most tests will provide a diagnosis in patients with this far-advanced disease; however, only the most sensitive tests have the potential of identifying the large group of patients with less-advanced disease states.

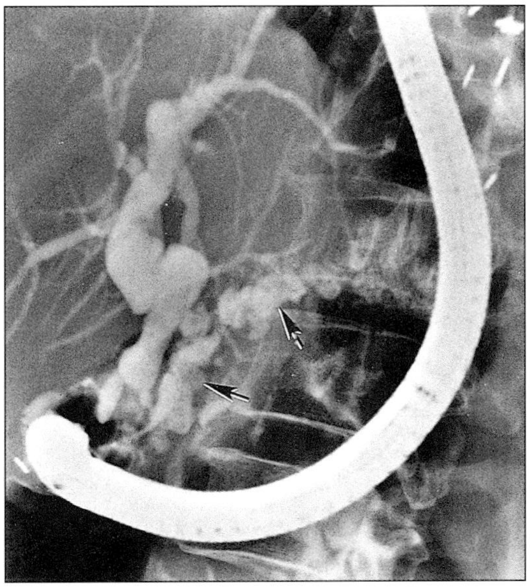

FIGURE 7-25.

Advanced chronic pancreatitis on endoscopic retrograde pancreatography (ERP) with a characteristic "chain-of-lakes" appearance of the pancreatic duct (*arrows*). Substantial evidence now exists that a significant proportion of patients with histologically proven chronic pancreatitis will have normal or only minimally abnormal results of pancreatograms. In addition, various other conditions may mimic the pancreatographic changes of chronic pancreatitis, including normal aging, a recent attack of acute pancreatitis, pancreatic carcinoma, and findings after pancreatic duct stenting. The reported sensitivity of ERP for chronic pancreatitis is 67% to 93%, with specificities ranging from 89% to 100% [13]. These results are generated from studies evaluating patients with more advanced disease, so they are clearly overestimates of true sensitivity and specificity. ERP may also be used to develop therapeutic rather than diagnostic information. In particular, ERP can document main-duct dilation, which is a prerequisite for consideration of surgical duct decompression (Peustow's procedure). ERP can also be useful in differentiating pancreatic malignancy from chronic pancreatitis, both by morphologic criteria and by obtaining cytology from pancreatic duct strictures.

In addition to the abnormalities already described, ERP may document pancreas divisum. This variant anatomy, wherein the bulk of pancreatic secretion drains through the minor papilla, occurs in 10% of the population; in the vast majority of patients, it does not lead to pancreatic disease. In a small minority of patients, obstruction to flow at the minor papilla may produce either acute pancreatitis or chronic pancreatitis. This can be definitively established if the dorsal ductal system is dilated or has changes of chronic pancreatitis, or if a hormonal stimulation test is abnormal. In the absence of these diagnostic criteria, it should not be assumed that this variant is producing the chronic abdominal pain.

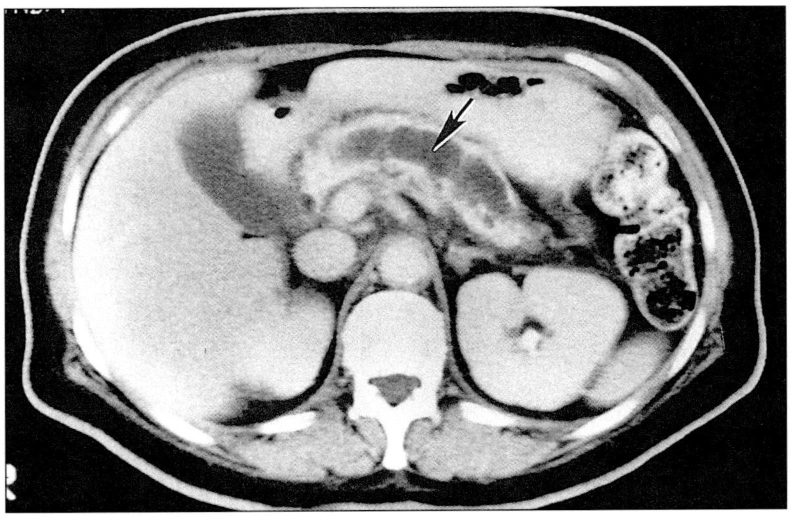

FIGURE 7-26.

Findings on CT that suggest chronic pancreatitis include diffuse calcification, ductal dilation, gland atrophy, irregular contour, and associated pseudocysts. CT is less accurate than endoscopic retrograde pancreatography for the diagnosis of chronic pancreatitis, although the new spiral CT technology allows improved resolution of small structures, such as the pancreatic duct, and appears more accurate than earlier scanning methods. Markedly dilated pancreatic duct (*arrow*) with atrophy of the pancreas.

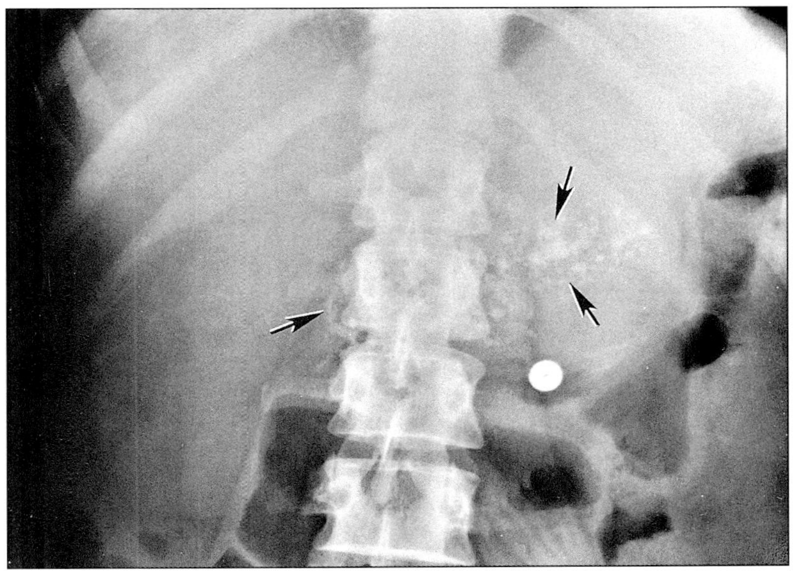

FIGURE 7-27.

Plain abdominal radiograph. The finding of diffuse pancreatic calcification is a specific marker of chronic pancreatitis, but it is only seen in far-advanced disease. Focal calcification is not diagnostic of chronic pancreatitis, and may be seen in a number of other diseases. Although patients with alcoholic chronic pancreatitis will commonly develop diffuse calcifications (70% of patients after 15 years of observation), patients with idiopathic pancreatitis do so only rarely (20%–40% after 15 years of follow-up). The low sensitivity of plain radiographic limits their use as a diagnostic tool. This figure demonstrates diffuse pancreatic calcification (*arrows*).

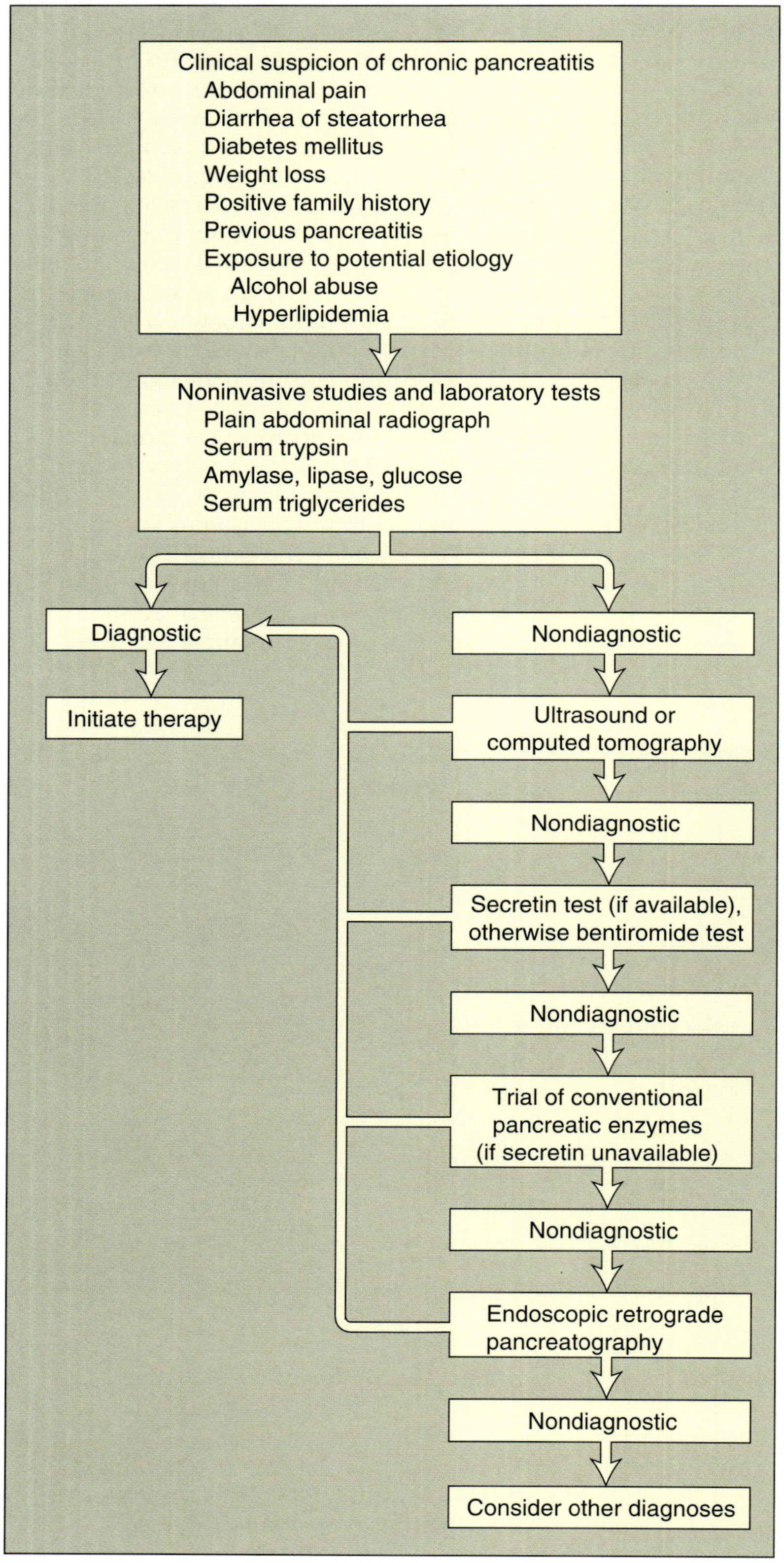

FIGURE 7-28.

Strategy for diagnosis of chronic pancreatitis. The overall diagnostic strategy should take into account the relative accuracy, cost, and risks of each diagnostic test. In its advanced form, chronic pancreatitis can be confirmed by a variety of diagnostic tests, so that overall cost and risk of diagnostic tests should be the major concern. In patients with less advanced disease, the accuracy, and in particular, the sensitivity of the diagnostic test become more important. All of this must be tempered by the availability of the variety of diagnostic tests, in particular, the fact that direct hormonal stimulation tests are not universally available. In centers where direct hormonal stimulation tests are not available, a trial of conventional (*ie*, nonenteric-coated) pancreatic enzymes should be considered as a therapeutic trail in patients without major abnormalities of the pancreatic duct because all other diagnostic tests are less sensitive.

TREATMENT OF PAIN IN CHRONIC PANCREATITIS

- Remove inciting process
- Discontinue consumption of alcohol
- Treat hyperlipidemia
- Treat complications
  - Pseudocyst
  - Duodenal obstruction
  - Common bile duct obstruction
- Analgesics
  - Non-narcotic
  - Narcotic
- Suppress pancreatic secretion
  - Pancreatic enzymes
  - Investigational agents
- Modify neural transmission
  - Celiac plexus block
- Relieve pancreatic ductal obstruction
  - Endoscopic stents (?)
  - Surgery
- Remove pancreas through partial or complete surgery

FIGURE 7-29.

Treatment of pain in chronic pancreatitis. Cessation of consumption of alcohol is a prudent step in patients with alcoholic chronic pancreatitis, but the effect on pancreatic damage is quite variable. Although stopping alcohol consumption may allow for recovery of some pancreatic function, in many patients the disease progresses despite sobriety, albeit possibly at a slower pace. Analgesics are usually required, and many patients require narcotics. The risk of addiction to such drugs is present, and is a particular problem in patients with a history of addictive behavior (chronic alcoholism or drug abuse) and in patients with little social support. Despite the risk of addiction (< 20% overall), adequate pain control should be the primary concern.

Treatments that reduce pancreatic secretion may relieve pain by reducing pancreatic pressure or by other as yet unknown mechanisms. These form the basis for medical therapy of pain, and are discussed in detail in the following figures. Attempts to block neural transmission by celiac axis block are generally ineffective in chronic pancreatitis or are of only short-lived duration, making this technique of little utility for the long-term management of these patients. The effectiveness of surgical therapy in selected patients is discussed in subsequent figures.

PANCREATIC ENZYMES AND PAIN RELIEF IN CHRONIC PANCREATITIS

Criteria	Conventional	Enteric-coated
Release of proteases in duodenum?	Yes	No
Lower cholecystokinin level?	Yes	No
Decrease pancreatic secretion?	Yes	No
Reduce pain?	Yes	No

FIGURE 7-30.

Use of pancreatic enzymes to relieve pain. Conventional pancreatic enzymes (nonenteric-coated) are the only formulations that release their contents in the feedback-sensitive duodenum. Two randomized trials have demonstrated the efficacy of these agents for pain control. This should not be surprising, inasmuch as these release their enzymes in the more distal small bowel, which is not involved in pancreatic feedback regulation. Indeed, some of these enteric-coated preparations may even stimulate pancreatic secretion! Not all patients treated with conventional enzymes responded; certain subsets appear to respond best. These subsets include patients with less-advanced disease (small-duct disease), women, and patients with idiopathic chronic pancreatitis. Overall, up to 75% of carefully selected patients respond to conventional enzymes. In one study, those patients with elevated cholecystokinin (CCK) levels responded best. Although it has not yet become standard to measure CCK levels in patients with chronic pancreatitis, this may well be the most accurate way to select patients for therapy aimed at reducing secretion.

PANCREATIC ENZYMES FOR THE TREATMENT OF STEATORRHEA OR PAIN IN CHRONIC PANCREATITIS

Conventional Enzyme Preparations		Enteric-Coated Enzyme Preparations	
Brand Name	**Units of lipase/pill**	**Brand Name**	**Units of lipase/pill**
Lipase (Viokase)	8000	Pancrelipase (Cotazym-S)	5000
Pancrelipase (Cotazym)	8000	Enteric-coated pancrelipase (Pancrease MT4, MT10, MT16)	4000, 10,000, 16,000, respectively
Amylase (Ku-Zyme HP)	8000	Porcine pancreatic enzyme (Creon)	10,000
		Ultrase MT6, MT12, MT18, MT20	6,000, 12,000, 18,000, 20,000, respectively

FIGURE 7-31.

Enzyme use for pain. Conventional enzymes are required for the treatment of pain, but all commercially available preparations are of relatively low potency. The potency is reflected in the relative units of lipase per pill. Large numbers of pills must therefore be taken (on average, eight pills with meals and at bedtime). Because these conventional enzymes are destroyed by gastric acid, concomitant therapy with an H_2-receptor antagonist or omeprazole is usually required. Enteric-coated preparations are the treatment of choice for steatorrhea because they are of much higher potency and do not require suppression of gastric acid.

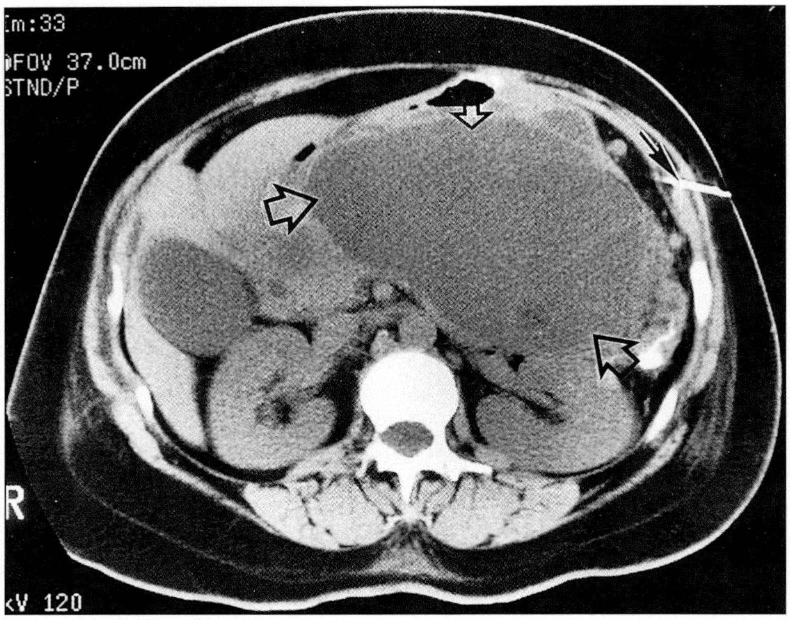

FIGURE 7-32.

Pseudocysts in chronic pancreatitis. A large pseudocyst (*open arrows*), which is being percutaneously drained (*closed arrow*). Pseudocysts that develop in chronic pancreatitis are most commonly caused by duct obstruction, with the formation of a "retention" cyst in the upstream duct or side branch. Unlike the pseudocysts associated with acute pancreatitis, these pseudocysts do not contain activated enzymes, and are usually not a reflection of a necrotizing inflammatory process. These pseudocysts are less likely to produce complications than those associated with acute necrotizing pancreatitis, but they are paradoxically also less likely to resolve. Many of these pseudocysts remain asymptomatic, but they may be complicated by infection, rupture or leak, bleeding, or obstruction of a neighboring hollow viscus (*eg*, duodenum, bile duct, colon, or ureter, among others). Pseudocysts may also worsen chronic pain or even initiate a wasting syndrome.

Recent clinical experience suggests that in patients with pseudocysts smaller than 6 cm, if there is a mature pseudocyst wall on radiographic imaging that does not resemble a cystic neoplasm, minimal symptoms, and no evidence of active alcohol abuse, the risk of complications is extremely small (< 10%). These patients may be safely observed with little risk of serious complication [14,15]. Even larger asymptomatic pseudocysts can be considered for expectant management in this group of patients. Symptomatic pseudocysts or those producing complications require therapy.

Surgical decompression remains the standard criterion for symptomatic pseudocysts with low mortality and little recurrence. Surgical therapy also allows the differentiation of true pseudocysts from cystic pancreatic neoplasms. Percutaneous drainage of symptomatic pseudocysts is usually successful in the short-term, but pseudocyst recurrence is common (although the recurrent pseudocyst may remain asymptomatic!). Percutaneous drainage seems to be particularly effective for infected pseudocysts; however, it is usually ineffective for other complications, such as bleeding, rupture, or leak. Bleeding is a rare event, but carries substantial mortality, often because the bleeding source is a medium-sized artery that has formed a pseudoaneurysm.

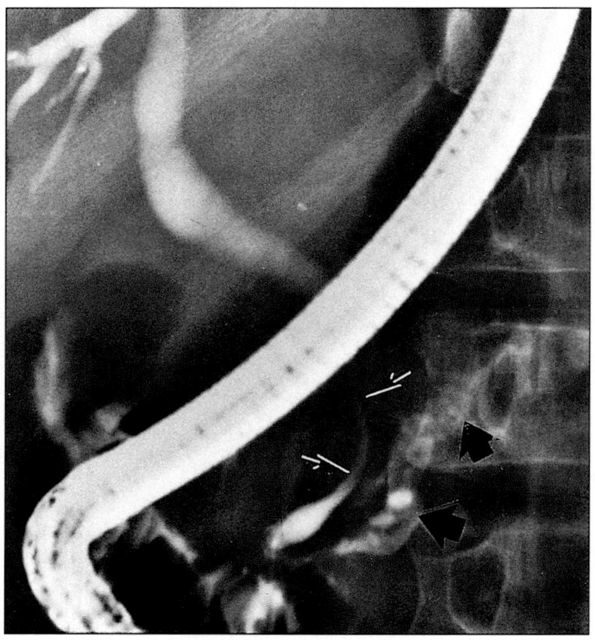

FIGURE 7-33.

Common bile duct stricture in chronic pancreatitis. Common bile duct stricture may develop as a consequence of compression by an adjacent pseudocyst or by progressive fibrosis of the head of the pancreas. This figure demonstrates an endoscopic retrograde cholangiopancreatography with changes of chronic pancreatitis (*thick arrows*) and a coexistent smooth stricture of the intrapancreatic common bile duct (*thin arrow*). Symptomatic obstruction of the bile duct usually requires surgical biliary bypass, usually in conjunction with a Peustow procedure.

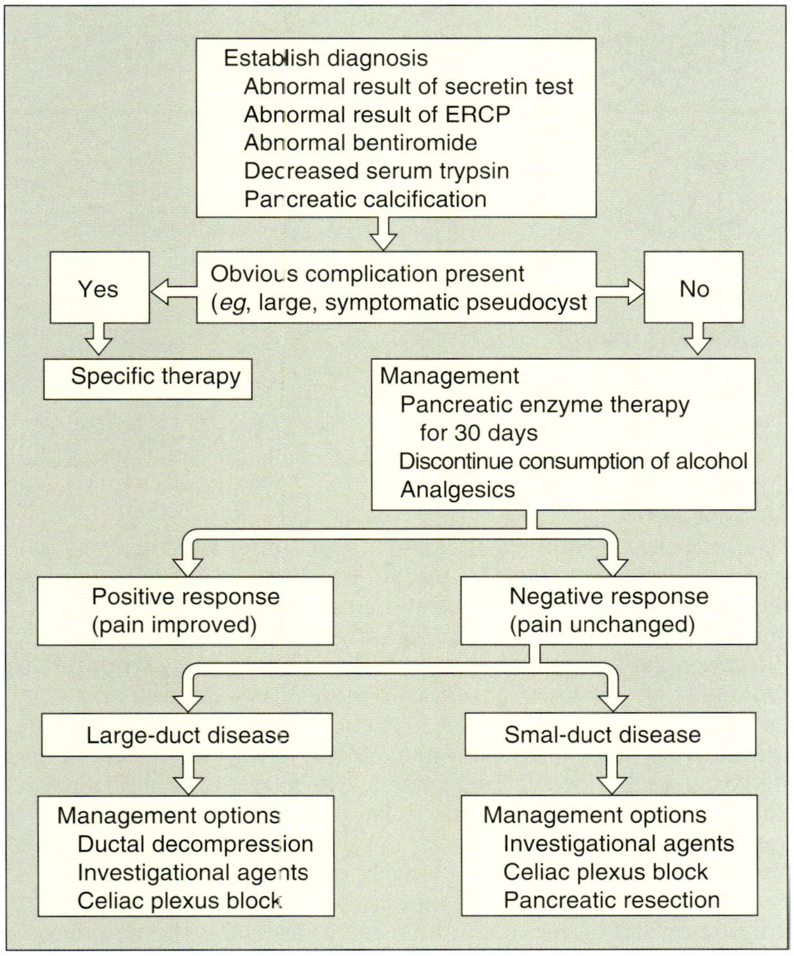

FIGURE 7-34.

Management strategy in chronic pancreatitis. Overall management of chronic pancreatitis requires that the diagnosis first be established. Initial evaluation should focus on defining the presence of obvious complication and in differentiating pancreatic carcinoma from chronic pancreatitis if necessary. All patients with alcoholic chronic pancreatitis should be encouraged to stop drinking alcohol, nutritional deficiencies should be corrected, and diabetes should be treated if present. Analgesics are usually required; the least potent formulation should be tried first.
A trial of conventional enzymes should usually be attempted if patients suffer from pain; although patients with advanced disease are less likely to respond to this therapy, it is without significant side-effects, and may be helpful in a subset of these patients. If medical therapy for pain is ineffective, attempts should be made to differentiate patients with small-duct disease from those with large duct disease. Patients with dilated pancreatic ducts should be considered for surgical therapy, in particular, lateral pancreaticojejunostomy. In patients who do not respond to these therapies, consideration can be given to pancreatic resection, referral to a pancreatic center, or experimental therapies (*ie*, octreotide). ERCP—endoscopic retrograde cholangiopancreatography.

PANCREATIC CANCER

EPIDEMIOLOGIC CHARACTERISTICS OF PANCREATIC CANCER

Factors associated with increased risk of pancreatic cancer	Factors associated with a decreased risk of pancreatic cancer
Age	Fruit and vegetable consumption
Male sex	Allergic disease
Greatest among blacks in U.S.	Tonsillectomy
Urban setting	
Low socioeconomic class	
Tobacco smoking	
Alcohol consumption (?)	
Pancreatitis	
Coffee consumption	
Tea consumption	
Dietary factors	
Meat consumption	
Fat consumption	
Occupational factors	
Radiation exposure	
Chemical exposure	
Previous history of gastrectomy	
Diabetes	

FIGURE 7-35.

Although specific causes have not yet been elucidated, a variety of factors is associated with the development of pancreatic cancer. Age-specific incidence rates show that the disease is uncommon before age 45 and increases steadily thereafter. More than 80% of all cases occur in the 60- to 80-year-old age group; it is more common in males. A variety of dietary factors, such as a high consumption of fat, low consumption of fruit and vegetables, and high coffee and alcohol consumption have been potentially linked to pancreatic cancer development. The strongest epidemiologic association is with tobacco consumption, where there is a two- to threefold increased risk of development. The mechanism by which tobacco consumption increases the risk of pancreatic cancer is unclear. It is possible that carcinogens in the smoke are secreted in bile, reflux into the pancreatic duct from the duodenum, or reach the pancreas through the bloodstream.

CANCER OF THE PANCREAS: GENETIC ALTERATIONS

Codon 12 mutation, K-*ras* oncogene (85%–90%)

p 53 tumor-suppressor gene

DCC gene

APC gene

CD44 gene (may be related to metastatic potential)ll carcinoma

FIGURE 7-36.

As with other tumors, a number of different genetic alterations have been observed in pancreatic cancer. The most common is a single point mutation at codon 12 of the K-*ras* oncogene, present in 85% to 90% of pancreatic cancers. Analysis for this mutation in aspiration pancreatic biopsy specimens, pancreatic or duodenal juice, or possibly, peripheral blood, may ultimately provide a sensitive and specific means of diagnosing early pancreatic cancers. Although less common than K-*ras* mutations, mutation in the p53 tumor supressor gene, the deleted colon cancer (DCC) gene, the adenomatous polyposis (APC) gene, and the gene expressing the glycoprotein CD44 (a putative adhesion molecule), have all been described in cancers of the pancreas, and may play roles in local disease progression, and in the case of CD44, the tendency to metastasize [16].

PRESENTING SYMPTOMS IN PANCREATIC CARCINOMA

SYMPTOM	PATIENTS, %
Weight loss	91
Pain	83
Jaundice	71
Anorexia, nausea	44
Malaise	34
Vomiting	13

FIGURE 7-37.

The three most common symptoms of pancreatic cancer are weight loss, pain, and jaundice. The weight loss that occurs may be quite severe (*ie*, up to 10 kg). The greater and the more rapid the loss, the greater is the likelihood that the tumor will *not* be resectable. Painless jaundice, often regarded as a classical presenting symptom, is actually relatively uncommon. Pain alone is usually dull and located in the midepigastrium. Depending on the location and spread of the tumor, the pain may radiate to the back or either subcostal area. A persistent backache can signify retroperitoneal invasion and a very poor prognosis. Jaundice, when it occurs, is often the symptom that initiates a patient's evaluation. Periampullary tumors often present with jaundice relatively early, and therefore have a better rate of cure; however, jaundice occurring with body or tail tumors can signify hepatic or hilar metastases, and therefore inoperability. Uncommon symptoms or findings include migratory thrombophlebitis, sciatica (caused by retroperitoneal nerve infiltration), or enlarged supraclavicular (Virchow's) or periumbilical (Sister Mary Joseph's) nodes. (*Adapted from* Trede and Carter [17].)

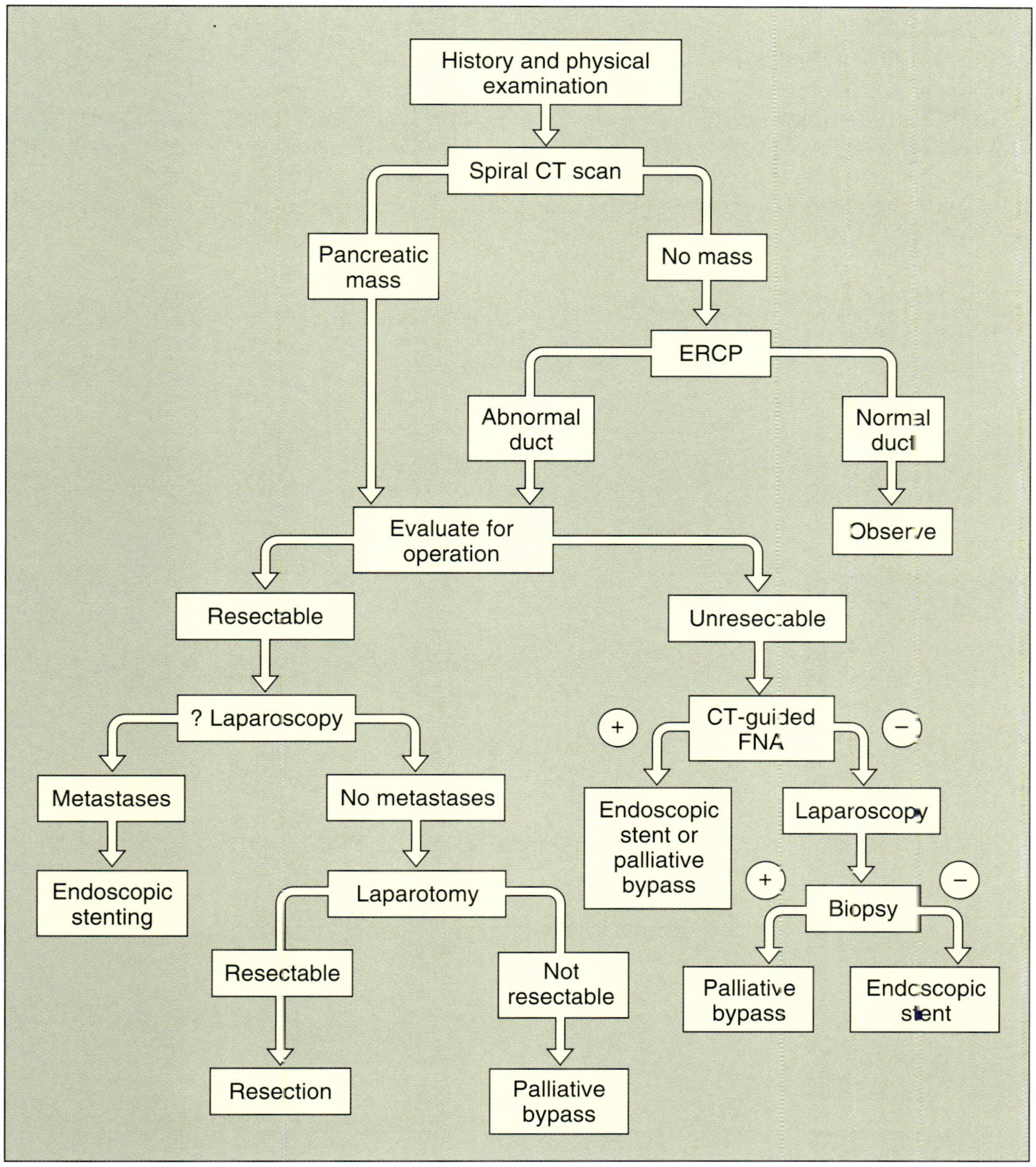

FIGURE 7-38.

Diagnosis of pancreatic cancer. When the history and physical examination suggest the possibility of pancreatic cancer, the first diagnostic test the authors use a spiral computed tomography (CT) scan. If a pancreatic mass is detected, then the patient is evaluated for operation. If no mass is seen on CT scan, then the patient will undergo an endoscopic retrograde cholangiopancreatography (ERCP). If the ERCP demonstrates normal pancreatic and common bile ducts, then the patient may be observed with close follow-up. If the duct anatomy is abnormal, then the patient is evaluated for operation. Some endoscopists may also obtain endoscopic needle aspiration or duct brushings at this point as well.

Patients are evaluated for operation on the basis of CT evidence for resectability and presence of metastases. If the CT scan demonstrates metastases or definite involvement of the major vessels (*eg*, portal vein or superior mesenteric artery) by tumor, the patient's diseases is classified as unresectable. Other factors that may influence whether or not a patient is an operative candidate are their ages and general overall medical condition.

In patients determined to be candidates for operation, the use of laparoscopy as a first step is controversial. Advocates perform laparoscopy to determine if there are any peritoneal or liver metastases present that were not detected by the CT scan. If metastases are present, laparotomy is avoided and the patient may undergo endoscopic stenting. If no metastases are detected by laparoscopy, the patient will undergo laparotomy. Intraoperative determination of resectability will then determine whether or not the patient is a candidate for a resection of the tumor or a palliative bypass procedure.

If a patient is *not* an operative candidate, tissue confirmation of pancreatic cancer is the next step; this is done using CT- or ultrasound-guided fine-needle aspiration. Endoscopic fine-needle aspiration, biopsy, or brushings are also options. If the biopsy is positive, then the patient can undergo endoscopic stenting or be re-evaluated for a palliative bypass. If the biopsy is negative, the patient can undergo laparoscopy and biopsy. If the biopsy is positive, the patient is a candidate for a palliative bypass. If the biopsy is negative, endoscopic stenting can be done.

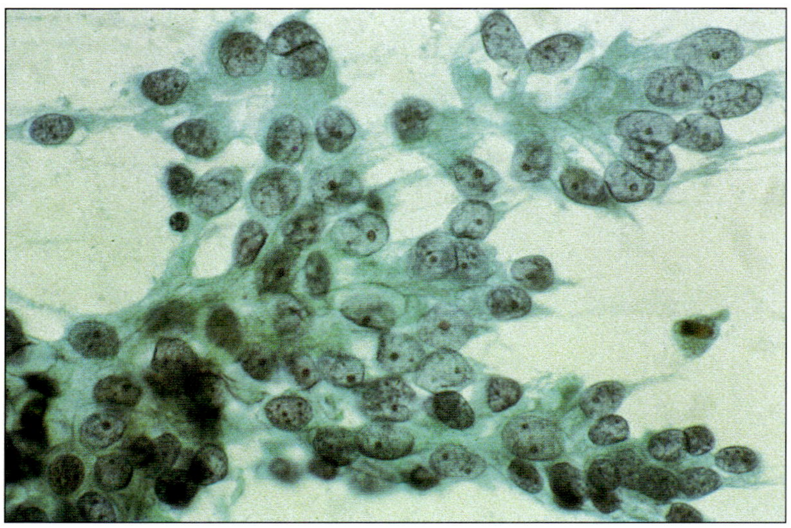

FIGURE 7-39.

Computed tomography (CT) can direct a needle aspiration to obtain a tissue diagnosis from a pancreatic mass. Atypical cells, as seen on this CT-guided needle aspiration sample, signify the presence of pancreatic carcinoma. This procedure plays an important role in patients who are not operative candidates either because their tumors are not resectable or they are in poor medical condition. Confirmation of pancreatic cancer with tissue involvement can initiate palliative procedures, such as endoscopic stenting, chemotherapy, or re-evaluation for an operative bypass.

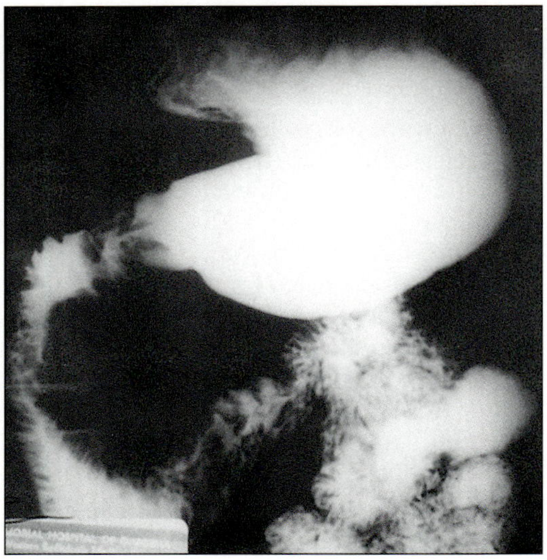

FIGURE 7-40.

Barium studies of the gastrointestinal (GI) tract are not often used to evaluate patients with suspected pancreatic cancer. Because many of these patients present with nonspecific gastrointestinal symptoms, however, an upper GI may be obtained. Findings on upper GI that suggest pancreatic cancer include extrinsic compression, displacement or encasement of the C-loop, mucosal invasion (nodularity or spiculation), or Frostberg's reversed '3' sign. Widened duodenal sweep and the suggestion of compression of part of the duodenal loop is demonstrated here.

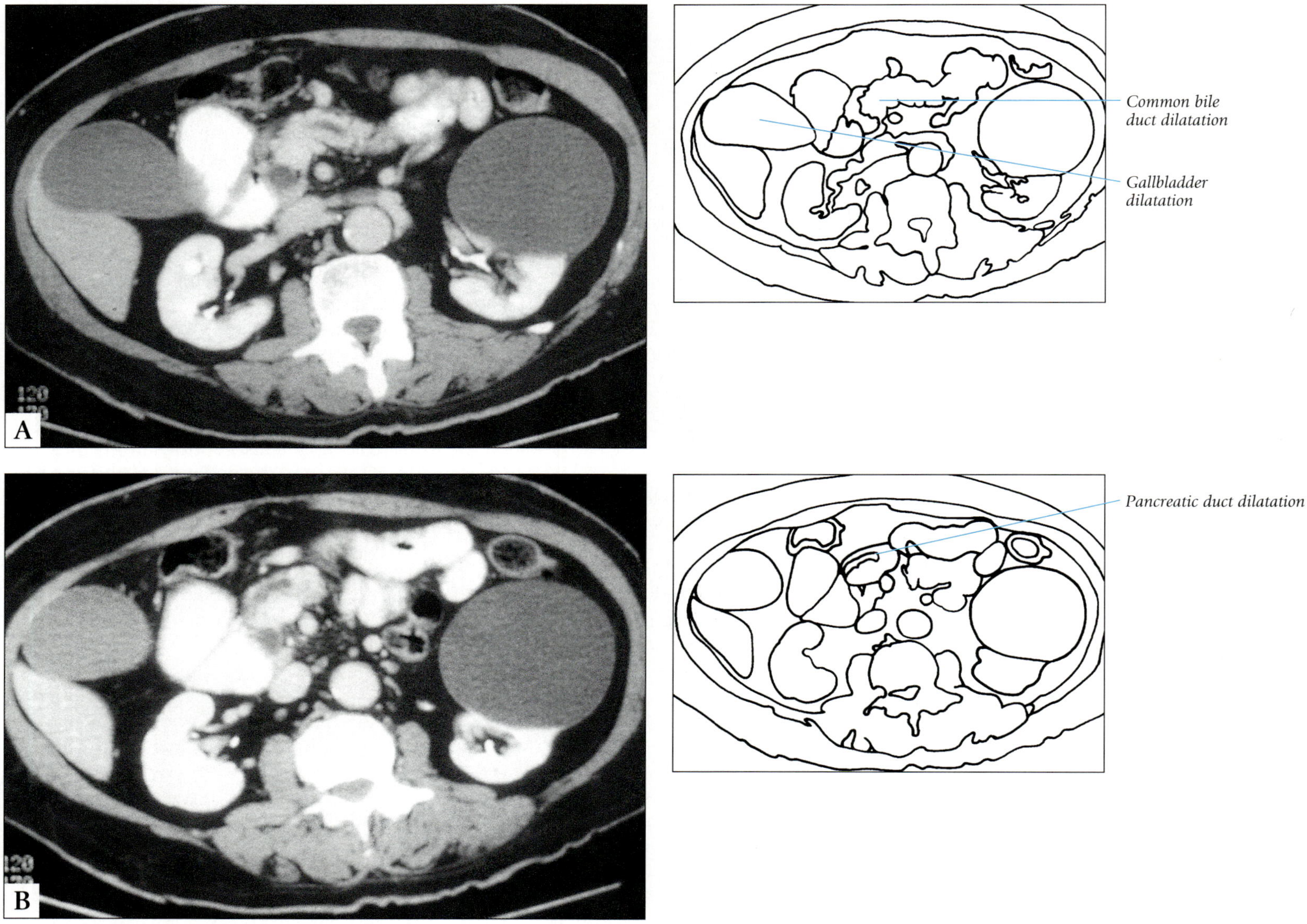

FIGURE 7-41.

A–B, Computed tomography scan demonstrating common bile duct and gallbladder dilatation (*panel A*); pancreatic duct dilatation is also evident (*panel B*).

(*continued on next page*)

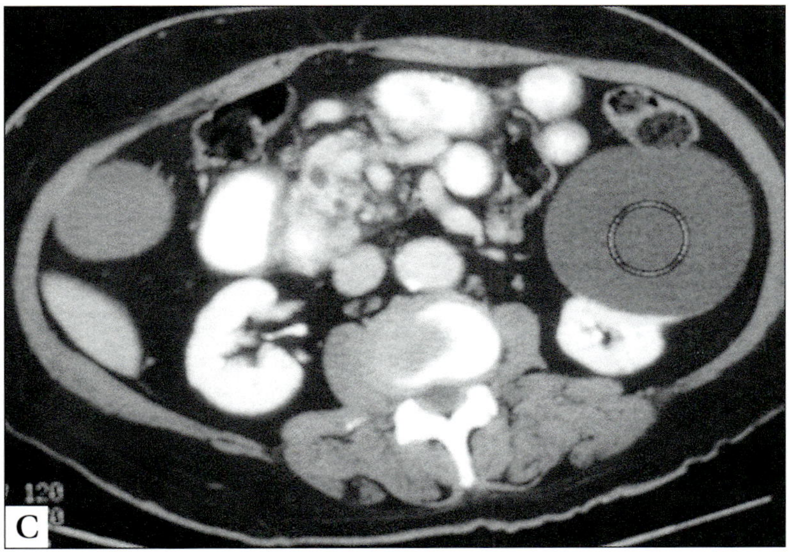

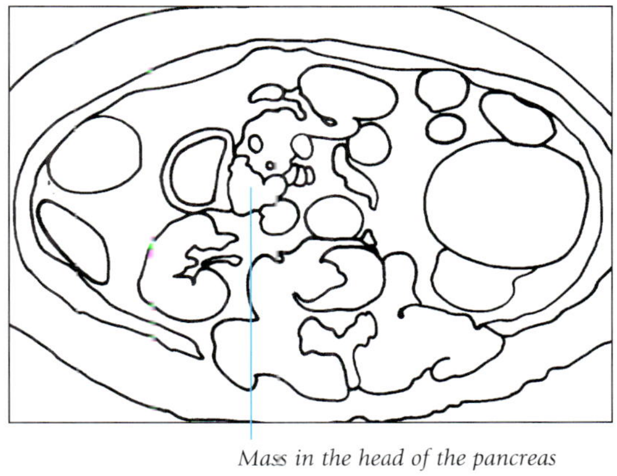

FIGURE 7-41. CONTINUED

C, Mass in the head of the pancreas. Note the presence of a left renal cyst in all three panels.

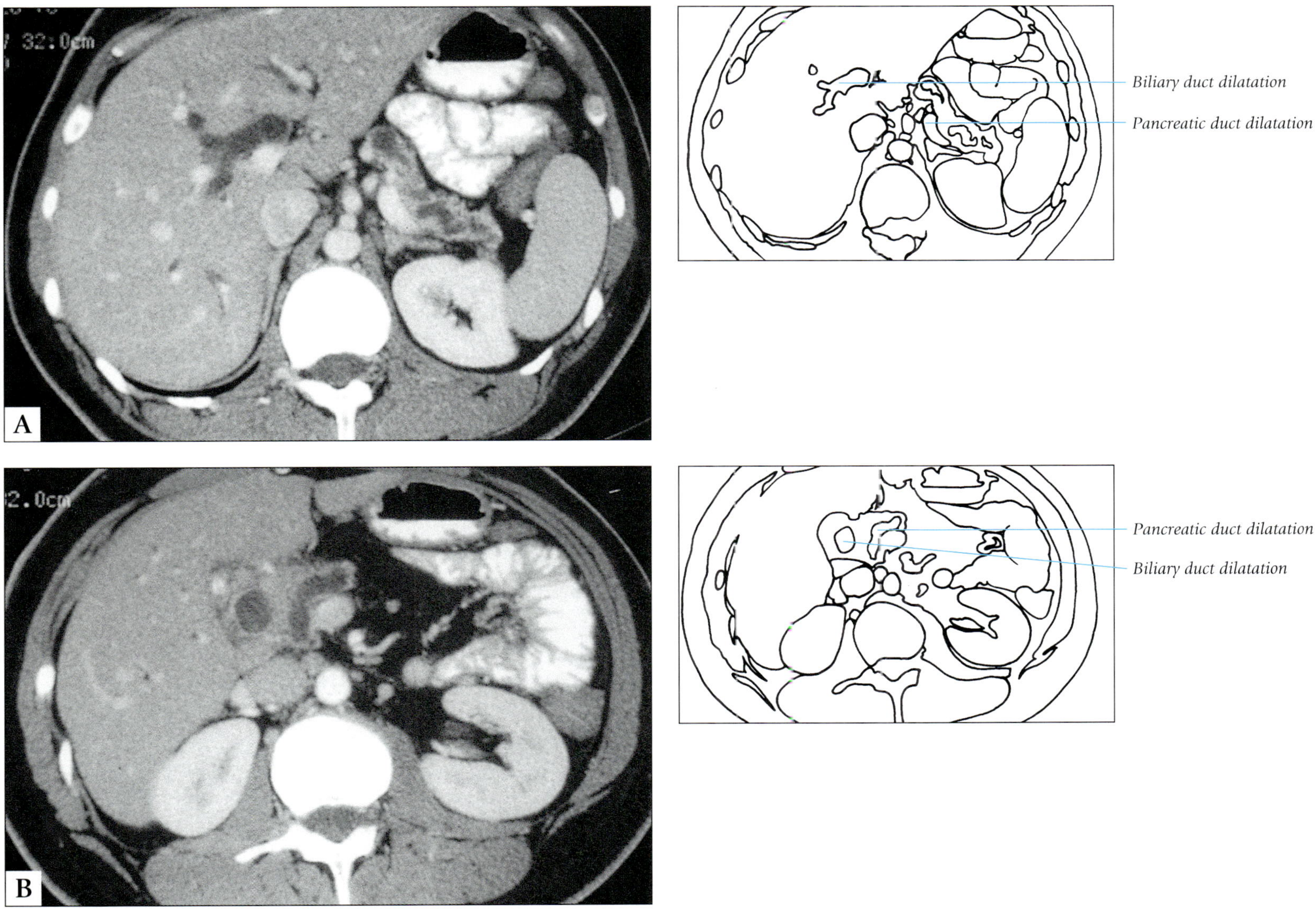

FIGURE 7-42.

A, Computed tomography scan demonstrates intrahepatic biliary duct and pancreatic duct dilatation. **B**, Extrahepatic bile duct and pancreatic duct dilation. (*Courtesy of* Dr. Barbara Kadell, UCLA Department of Radiology.)

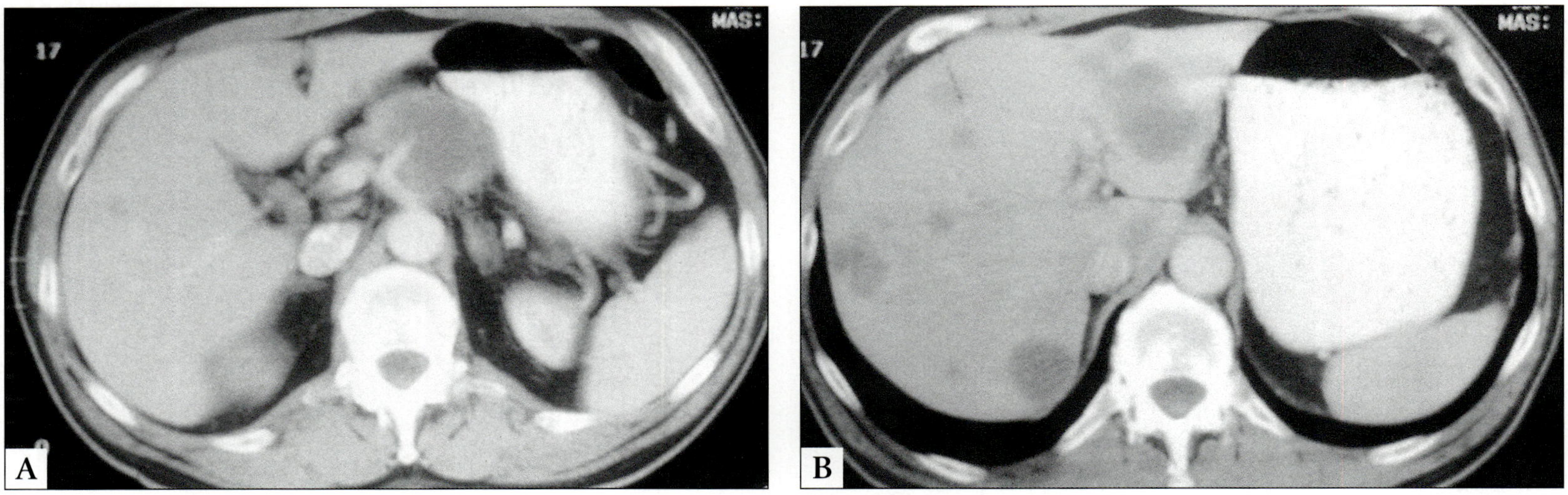

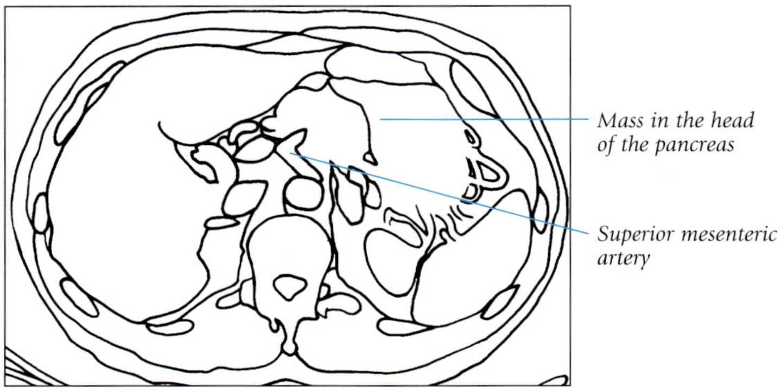

FIGURE 7-43.

A, Computed tomography (CT) scan demonstrates encasement of the superior mesenteric artery by a mass in the head of the pancreas. **B**, CT scan of the liver in the same patient showing the presence of multiple liver metastases. This patient's tumors would not be resectable because of involvement of a major vascular structure and the presence of metastatic disease.

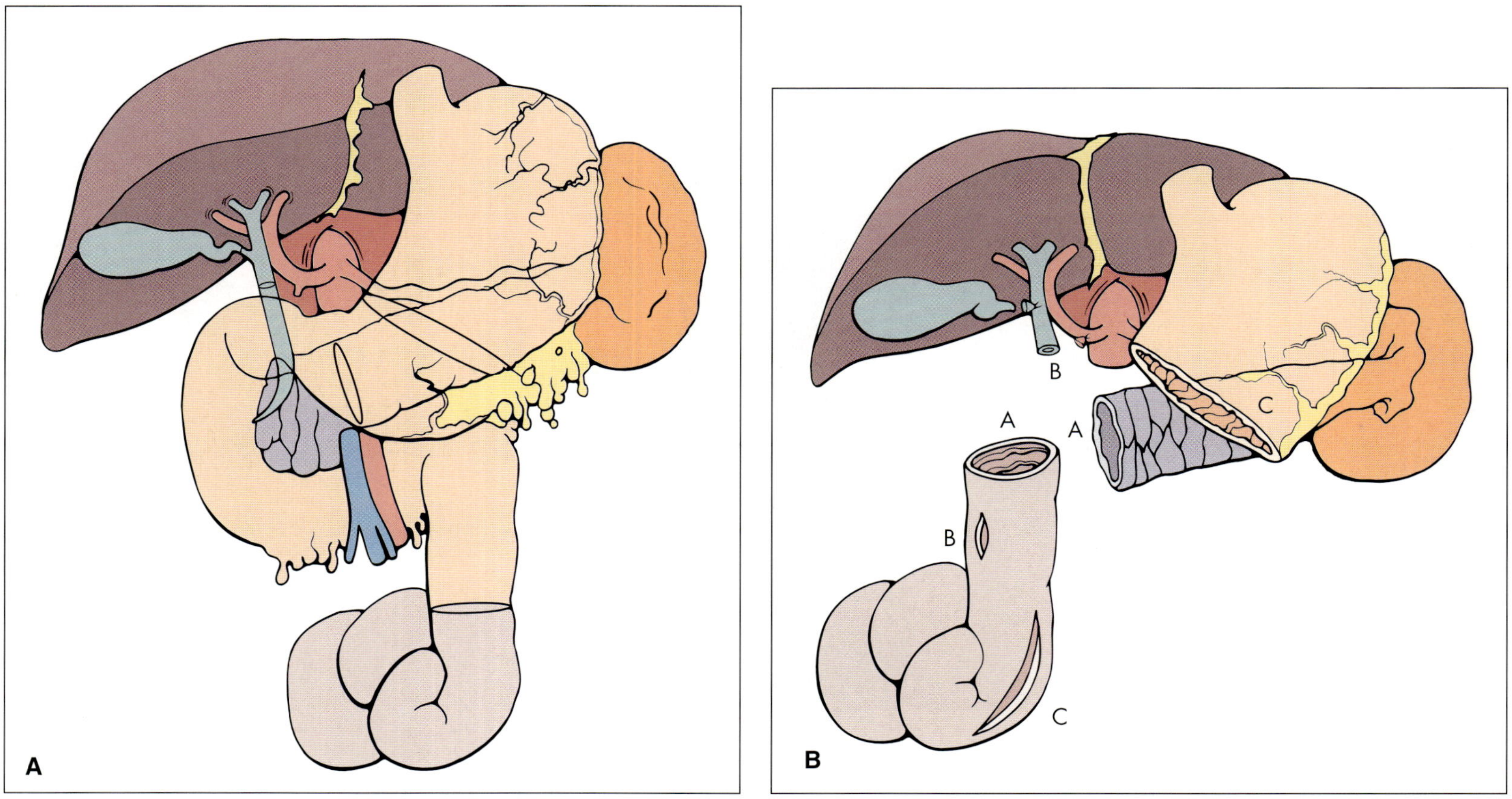

FIGURE 7-44

The standard Whipple operation for pancreatic cancer, which involves resection of the common bile duct, the gallbladder, the duodenum, and the pancreas to the level of the midbody. **A**, Lines of resection.

B, Anatomy after resection and before reconstruction. (A-A—pancreaticojejunosomy; B-B—choledochojejunostomy; C-C—gastrojejunostomy.)

(*continued on next page*)

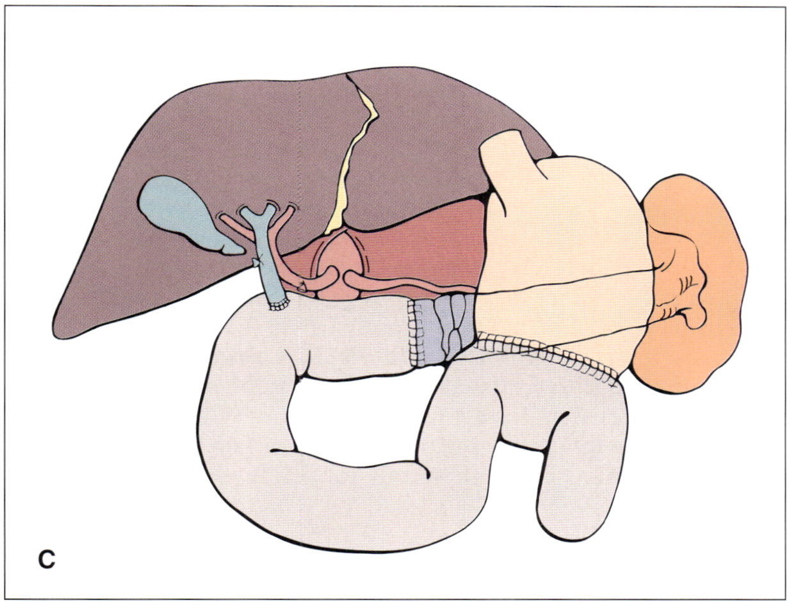

FIGURE 7-44. CONTINUED

C, Anatomy after reconstruction. Pancreatic resection for pancreatic cancer is appropriate only if all gross tumor can be removed with standard resection. The lesion is considered resectable if the following areas are free of tumor: the hepatic artery near the origin of the gastroduodenal artery; the portal and superior mesenteric veins as they pass in front of the uncinate process and behind the body of the pancreas: the superior mesenteric artery, where it courses under the body of the pancreas; the liver and regional lymph nodes. About 20% of cancers of the head of the pancreas can be resected, but because of local and distant spread, this is rarely possible for lesions of the body and tail.

LONG-TERM SURVIVAL RATES AFTER WHIPPLE OPERATION FOR PANCREATIC CANCER

AUTHOR	INSTITUTION	PATIENTS, *NO.*	5-YR SURVIVAL RATE, *%*
Cooperman, 1981	Columbia	70	7.1
van Heerden, 1981	Mayo Clinic	44	2.3
Jones, 1985	Toronto	28	7.0
Grace, 1986	UCLA	37	3.0
Connolly, 1987	Universiy of Chicago	89	3.4
Crist and Cameron, 1989	Johns Hopkins	50	18.0

FIGURE 7-45.

Long-term survival rates for patients with pancreatic cancer remain approximately 5%. There is no difference in long-term survival between patients undergoing total pancreatectomy versus partial pancreatectomy; therefore, the Whipple operation remains preferable to more radical total pancreatectomy. (*Adapted from* Trede [18].)

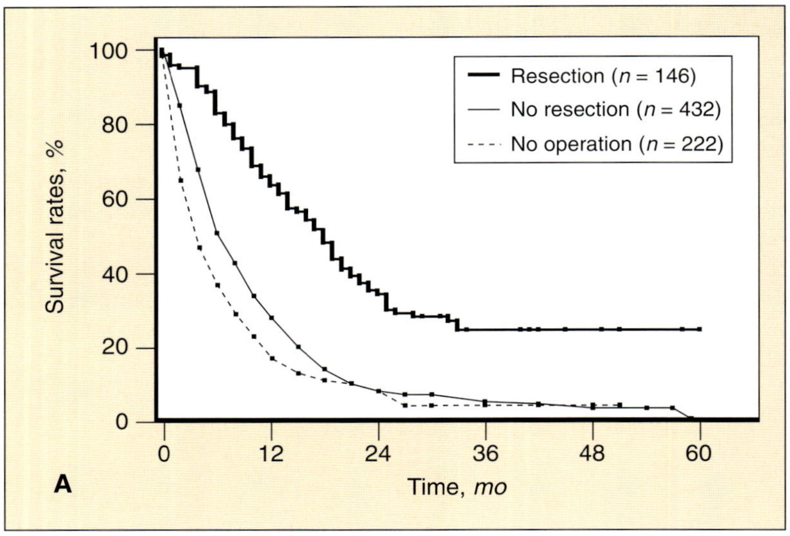

FIGURE 7-46.

A, Survival rates in patients with pancreatic carcinoma treated in various ways. **B**, Survival rates in patients with pancreatic carcinoma based on tumor differentiation. **C**, Survival rates in patients with pancreatic carcinoma based on the presence or absence of lymph node metastases. These results demonstrate some important considerations in treatment. Overall survival rates are poor despite improvements in patient care. However, patients who had a resection had a significant improvement in 5-year survival rates. Tumor differentiation influenced survival as well. Those with poorly differentiated tumors had significantly worse survival rates that those with better differentiated tumors. This is not unexpected because the less differentiated tumors tend to be more aggressive, invasive, and resistant to therapy. The presence of lymph node metastases also influences the overall survival rate. (*Adapted from* Geer and Brennan [19]; with permission.)

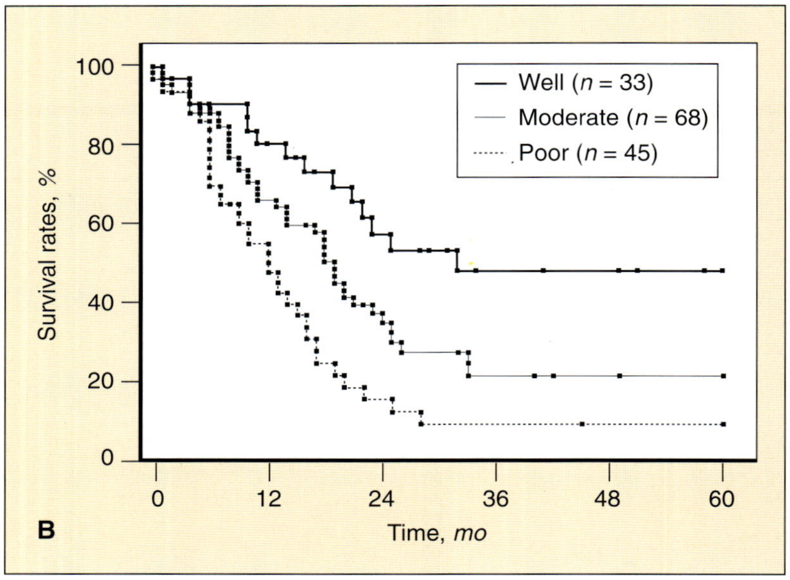

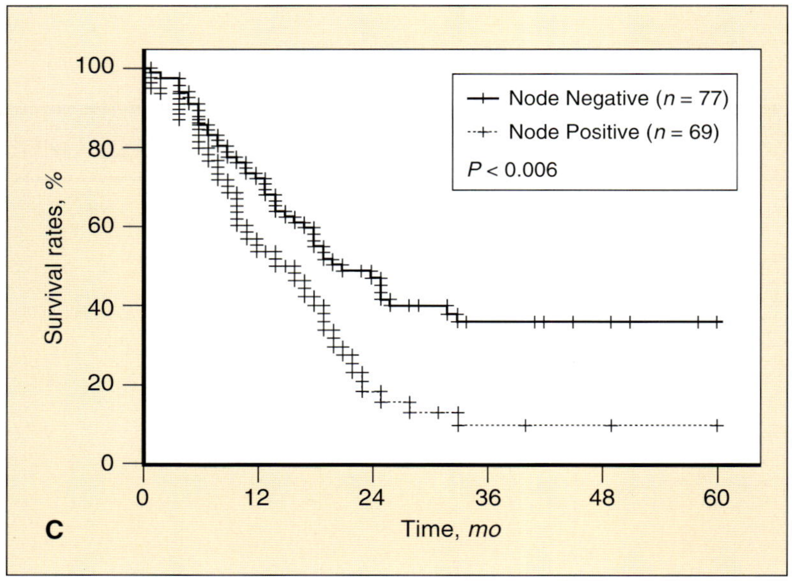

NONSURGICAL THERAPY OF PANCREATIC CARCINOMA: OPTIONS

Radiotherapy

- External beam radiation of the upper abdomen, usually in conjunction with chemotherapy
- Intraoperative radiation therapy—Iodine 125, usually in conjunction with chemotherapy and external beam radiation

Hormonal—tamoxifen

Chemotherapy

- 5-fluorouracil
- Combination chemotherapy

Immunotherapy

FIGURE 7-47.

Nonsurgical options for the treatment of pancreatic carcinoma are limited. Local radiotherapy combined with chemotherapy (5-fluorouracil) has been shown in a study from the Gastrointestinal Tumor Study Group [20,21] to increase survival by 6 to 8 months. Long-term survival is unusual, but occasionally occurs. Pancreatic cancer has been considered to be relatively "radioresistant." Irradiation is made more difficult by the deep location of the pancreas and its proximity to areas that are sensitive to radiation (intestine, spinal cord, liver, kidneys).

Hormonal therapy has not been shown to be of value in unresectable pancreatic carcinoma. Although immunotherapy with monoclonal antibodies has shown some initially promising results, this treatment is new and requires further study.

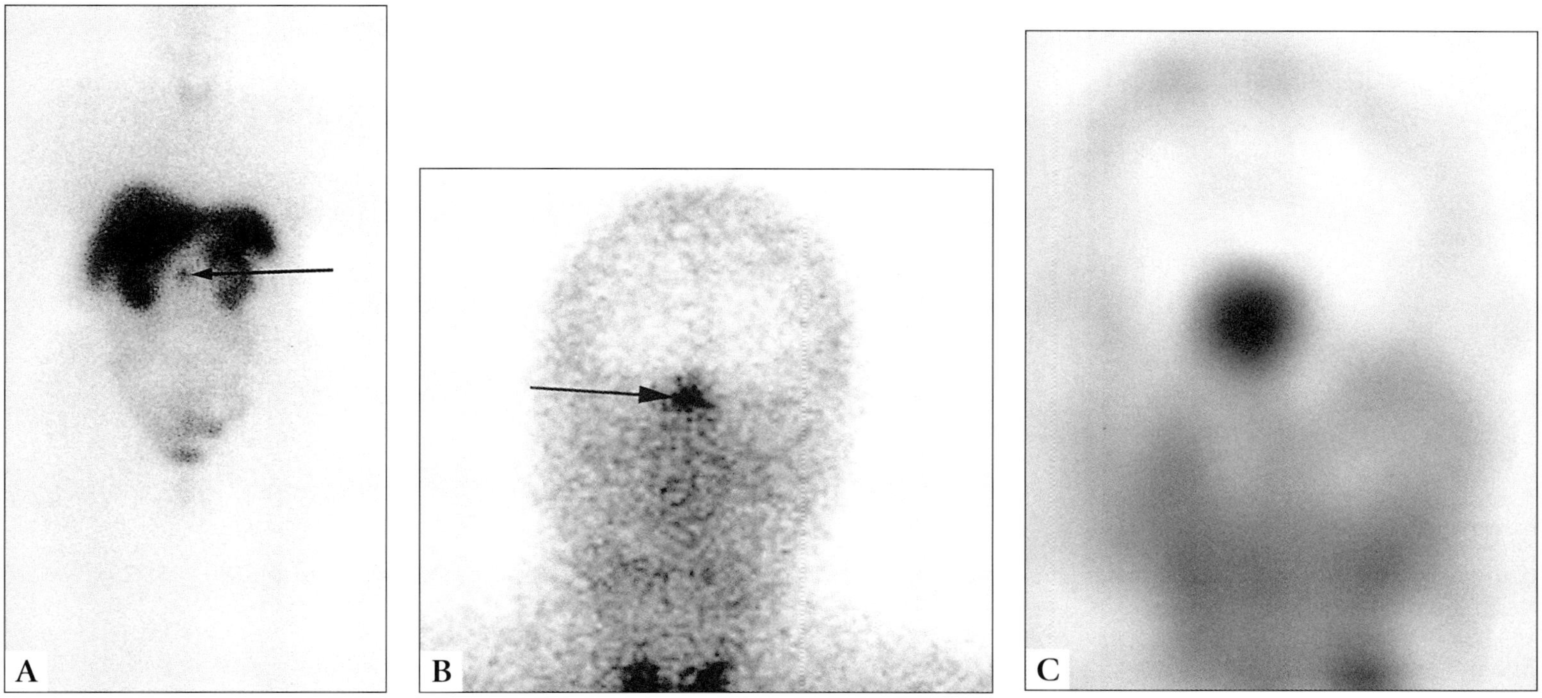

FIGURE 7-48.

This patient is a 46-year-old woman with multiple endocrine neoplasia-1 syndrome who previously underwent partial parathyroidectomy. **A**, Indium (In)-111 pentetreotide anterior whole-body scintigraphy revealed focal abnormally increased activity (*arrow*) in the midline of the upper abdomen. Laparotomy showed this to be a gastrinoma in the body of the pancreas. **B**, Planar anterior and lateral views of the head demonstrated increased pituitary activity (*arrows*), which was also well delineated by SPECT imaging (*panel C*). Subsequent craniotomy and immunohistology revealed the pituitary lesion to be a 2-cm prolactinoma. Approximately 90% of gastrinomas are visualized by scintigraphy. Although MR imaging and computed tomography remain the preferred modalities for evaluation of the pituitary and hypothalamic region, a high percentage of hyperfunctioning thyroid-stimulating hormone-producing, growth hormone-producing, and prolactin-producing anterior pituitary adenomas are visualized by In-111 pentetreotide scintigraphy. Hyperfunctioning adrenocorticotropic hormone-producing anterior pituitary adenomas and posterior pituitary tumors are reportedly not visualized by In-111 pentetreotide scintigraphy.

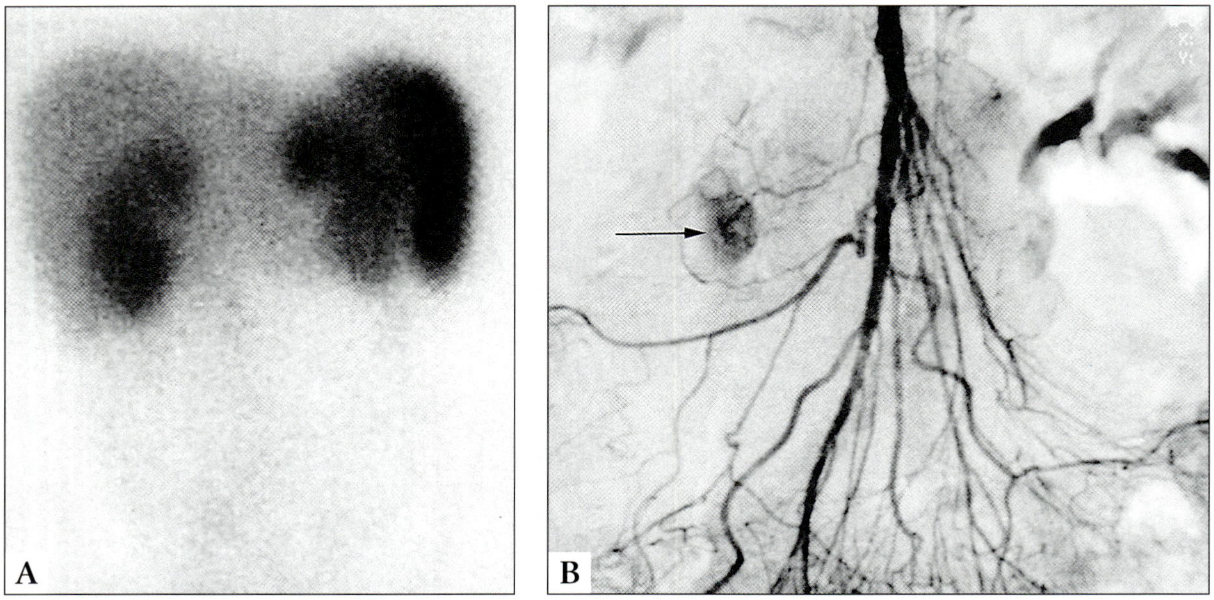

FIGURE 7-49.

A 75-year-old woman who was admitted to the hospital for the evaluation of syncope and mental status changes was noted to have inappropriately elevated levels of plasma insulin. **A**, An Indium (In)-111 pentetreotide planar anterior view and SPECT images of the upper abdomen were normal. Computed tomography image of the upper abdomen did not reveal any abnormality involving the pancreas. **B**, Angiography demonstrated a hypervascular focus (*arrow*) in the head of the pancreas. The lesion was enucleated at surgery and proved to be a 1.3 cm insulinoma by immunohistology.

Approximately 50% of patients with insulinoma will have normal results with In-111 pentetreotide scintigraphy. These insulinomas may express a subtype of somatostatin receptor that does not concentrate the radiopharmaceutical adequately for imaging purposes. It is also possible that some insulinomas may have either no receptors or may have an inadequate number of receptors to allow for their detection by scintigraphy.

CYSTIC FIBROSIS OF THE PANCREAS (*SEE* CHAPTER 8)

REFERENCES

1. Venu RP, Greenen JE, *et al.*: Idiopathic recurrent pancreatitis: an approach to diagnosis and treatment. *Dig Dis Sci* 1989, 34:55–60.
2. Lee SP, Nicholls JF, *et al.*: Biliary sludge as a cause of acute pancreatitis. *N Engl J Med* 1992, 326:589–593.
3. Ros E, Navarro S, Bru C, *et al.*: Occult microlithiasis in "idiopathic pancreatitis": Prevention of relapses by cholecystectomy or ursodeoxycholic acid therapy. *Gastroenterology* 1991, 101:1701–1709.
4. Steinberg WM, Tenner S: Acute pancreatitis. *N Engl J Med* 1994, 330:1198–1210.
5. Steinberg WM, Goldstein SS, Davis ND, *et al.*: Diagnostic assays in acute pancreatitis. *Ann Intern Med* 1985, 102:576–580.
6. Ranson JHC, Rifkind KM, Turner JW: Prognostic signs and nonoperative lavage in acute pancreatitis. *Surg Gynecol Obstet* 1976, 143:209–213.
7. Ranson JHC: Etiological and prognostic factors in human acute pancreatitis. *Am J Gastroenterol* 1982, 77:177–181.
8. Bradley EL, Murphy F, *et al.*: Prediction of pancreatic necrosis by dynamic pancreatography. *Ann Surg* 1990, 210:495–504.
9. London NJM, Lesse T, *et al.*: Rapid bolus contrast enhanced dynamic computed tomography in acute pancreatitis: a prospective study. *Br J Surg* 1991, 78:1452–1456.
10. Freeny PC, Lawson TL: *Radiology of the Pancreas.* New York: Springer-Verlag; 1982:334.
11. Fölsch UR, Nitsche R, Lüdtke R, *et al.*: Early ERCP and papillotomy compared with conservative treatment for acute biliary pancreatitis. *N Engl J Med* 1997, 336:237–242.
12. Layer P, Yamamoto H, Kalthoff L, *et al.*: The different courses of early- and late-onset idiopathic and alcoholic chronic pancreatitis. *Gastroenterology* 1994, 107:1481–1487.
13. Neiderau C, Grendell JH: Diagnosis of chronic pancreatitis. *Gastroenterology* 1985, 88:1973–1995.
14. Vitas GJ, Sarr MG: Selected management of pancreatic pseudocysts: operative versus expectant management. *Surgery* 1992, 111:123–130.
15. Yeo CJ, Bastidas JA, Lynch-Nyhan A, *et al.*: The natural history of pancreatic pseudocysts documented by computed tomography. *Surg Gynecol Obstet* 1990, 170:411–417.
16. Freedman SD, Waxman I: Biology of pancreatic cancer. In *Gastrointestinal Cancers: Biology, Diagnosis, and Therapy.* Edited by Rustgi AK. Philadelphia: Lippincott-Raven; 1995:315–323.
17. Trede M, Carter DC: Clinical evaluation and preoperative assessment. In *Surgery of the Pancreas.* Edited by Trede M, Carter DC. Edinburgh: Churchill Livingstone; 1993:423–431.
18. Trede M: The surgical options. In *Surgery of the Pancreas.* Edited by Trede M, Carter DC. Edinburgh: Churchill Livingstone; 1993:433–442.
19. Geer RJ, Brennan MF: Prognostic indicators for survival after resection of pancreatic adenocarcinoma. *Am J Surg* 1993, 165:68–72.
20. Moertel CG, Frytak S, Hahn RG, *et al.*: Therapy of locally unresectable pancreatic carcinoma. *Cancer* 1981, 48:1705–1710.
21. Kalser MH, Ellenberg SS: Pancreatic cancer: Adjuvant combined radiation and chemotherapy following curative resection. *Arch Surg* 1985, 120:899–903.

Chapter

8

Pediatric Gastroenterologic and Hepatic Disorders

EDITOR

Paul E. Hyman

CONTRIBUTORS

Carol Lynn Berseth
Anupama Chawla
Fredric Daum
Carlo Di Lorenzo
Peter R. Durie
Jacob C. Langer
Susan R. Orenstein
Philip Rosenthal
Vasundhara Tolia
Jon A. Vanderhoof

NECROTIZING ENTEROCOLITIS OF INFANCY

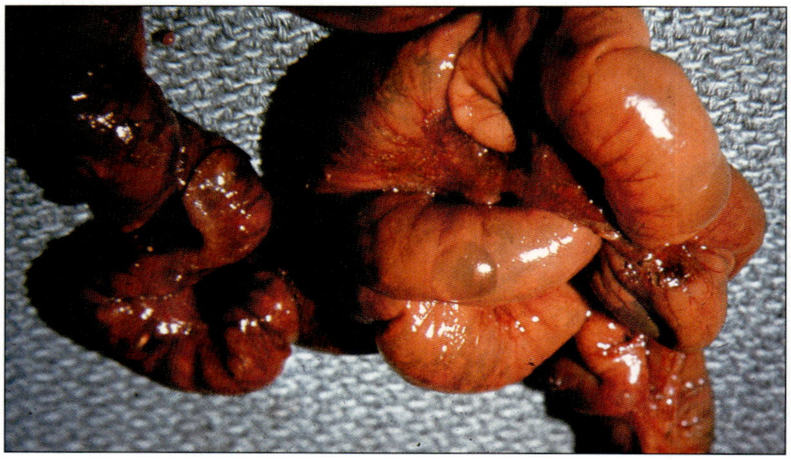

FIGURE 8-1.

Currently no single cause of necrotizing enterocolitis (NEC) has been scientifically established. The most common features of NEC are the presence of intramural bubbles of gas and large areas of necrosis. It is currently thought that the cause of NEC is multifactorial. Many infants who develop NEC have had episodes of asphyxia, hypotension, or both. Thus, poor splanchnic bed perfusion may contribute to NEC. Several inflammatory mediators have been shown to be abnormal in infants who develop NEC, and many episodes of NEC are associated with specific bacteria, such as clostridia and klebsiella. Thus, bacterial gut flora may predispose an infant to developing NEC. Finally, the incidence of NEC is 10-fold higher among infants who have been fed, suggesting that the metabolic stress of feeding or specific characteristics of formulas (*ie*, osmolarity) contribute to NEC.

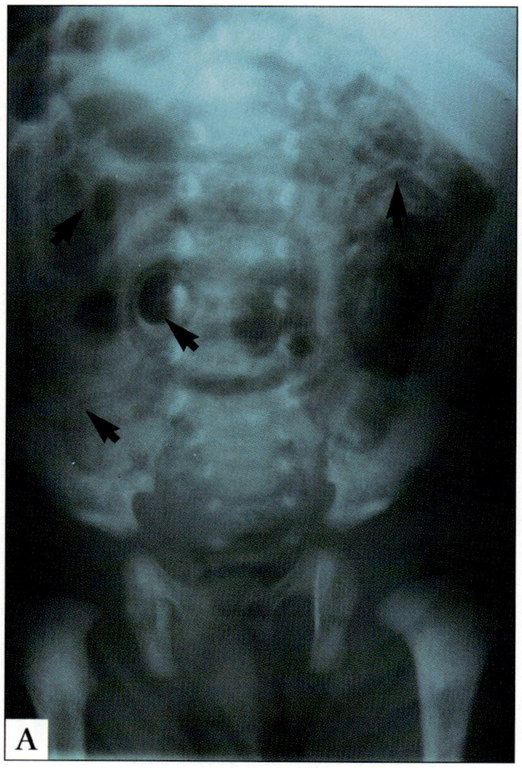

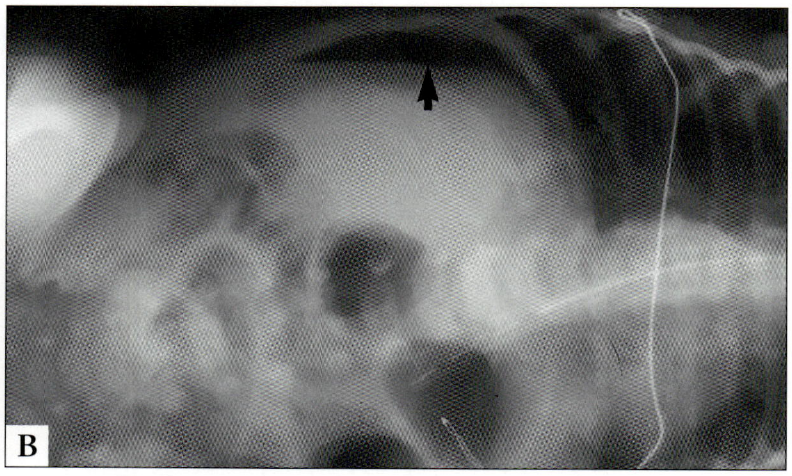

FIGURE 8-2.

Not all infants who present with symptoms of necrotizing enterocolitis (NEC) develop radiographic findings of NEC. Therefore Bell's criteria are used to designate whether an infant has Stage I (suspect), Stage II (definite), or Stage III (advanced) disease. Infants who lack radiographic findings for NEC are designated to have Stage I disease. **A**, Infants with Stage II or III disease radiographically demonstrate pneumotosis intestinalis (*arrows*) with or without air-fluid levels. **B**, In Stage III, infants are critically ill and may exhibit frank bowel perforation or presence of air tracking into the biliary tree or persistent dilation of a single bowel loop. Here there is free abdominal air (*arrow*) seen in the lateral view.

PHYSIOLOGIC JAUNDICE AND BREAST MILK JAUNDICE

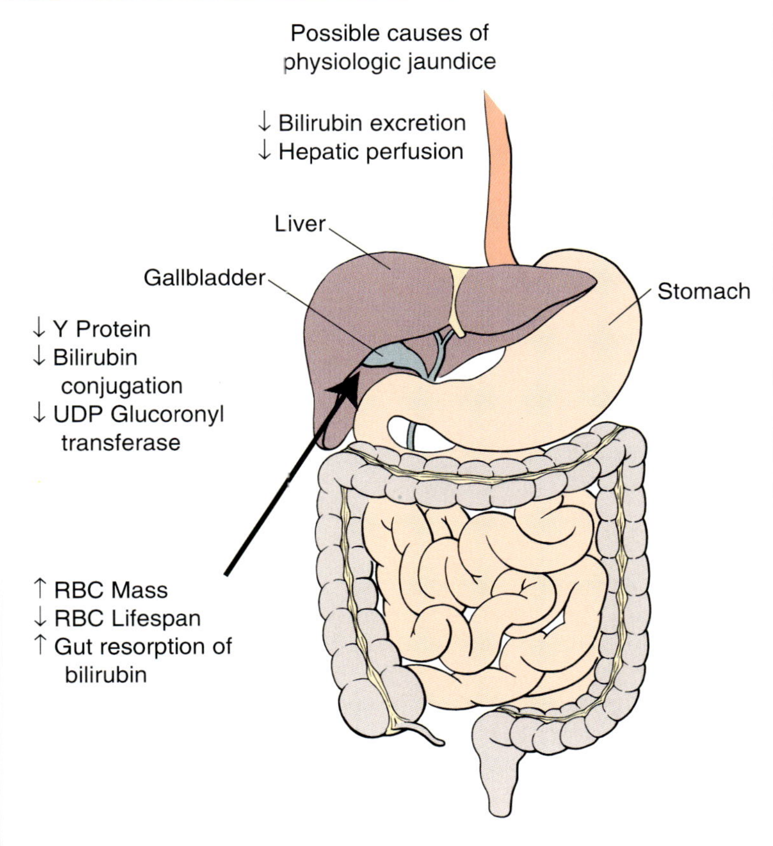

FIGURE 8-3.

The transient postnatal rise in serum bilirubin is thought to result from multiple factors. The amount of bilirubin delivered to the neonatal liver for conjugation is increased compared with that seen in the adult. This increased delivery results from the presence of an increased circulating red cell mass (normal hemoglobin in the newborn ranges 15 to 21 g/dL) and a shortened red cell life span (90 vs 120 days in the adult). There is defective uptake of bilirubin by the liver as a result of decreased levels of Y protein, and conjugation of bilirubin is decreased in that UDP-glucuronyl transferase activity is decreased in the neonate compared with the adult. Bilirubin excretion is also limited in the neonate compared with the adult. Finally, the enterohepatic circulation in the neonate is increased in the neonate, contributing to an additional increased load presented to the neonatal liver. In addition to these factors, increased bilirubin is also associated with ethnic factors, perinatal events such as birth asphyxia and maternal diseases such as diabetes. RBC—red blood cell.

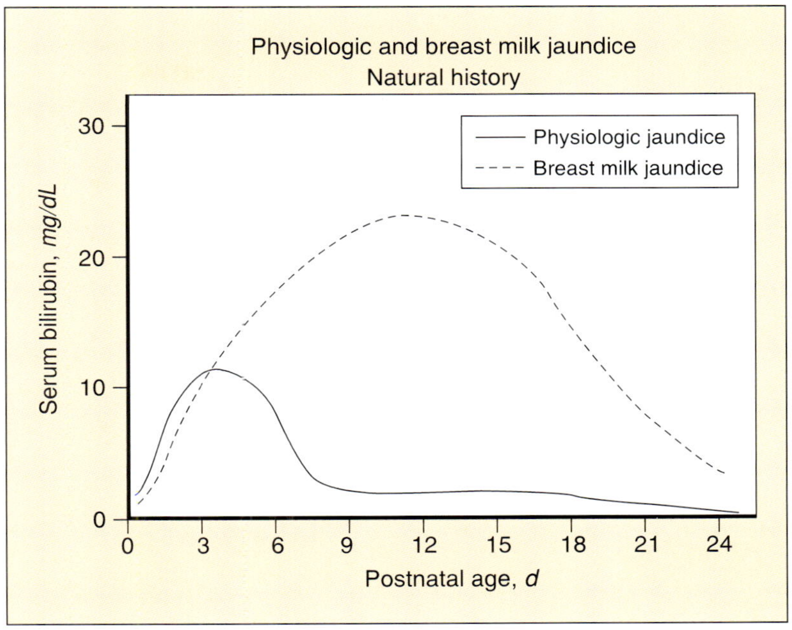

FIGURE 8-4.

Two types of nonpathologic transient jaundice occur in the newborn. Physiologic jaundice is defined as a transient increase in serum unconjugated bilirubin during the first postnatal week. Serum concentrations in the healthy newborn rise rapidly from birth to peak at a level of 7 to 10 mg/dL by postnatal day 3 to decline quickly by postnatal days 5 to 7 to a level of 2 mg/dL. This lower serum value persists for 2 weeks and then decreases to a normal adult value. Breast milk jaundice typically occurs after the third postnatal day. Serum bilirubin concentrations may increase to 20 to 25 mg/dL by the end of the second postnatal week and gradually decline over 1 to 4 months [1,2].

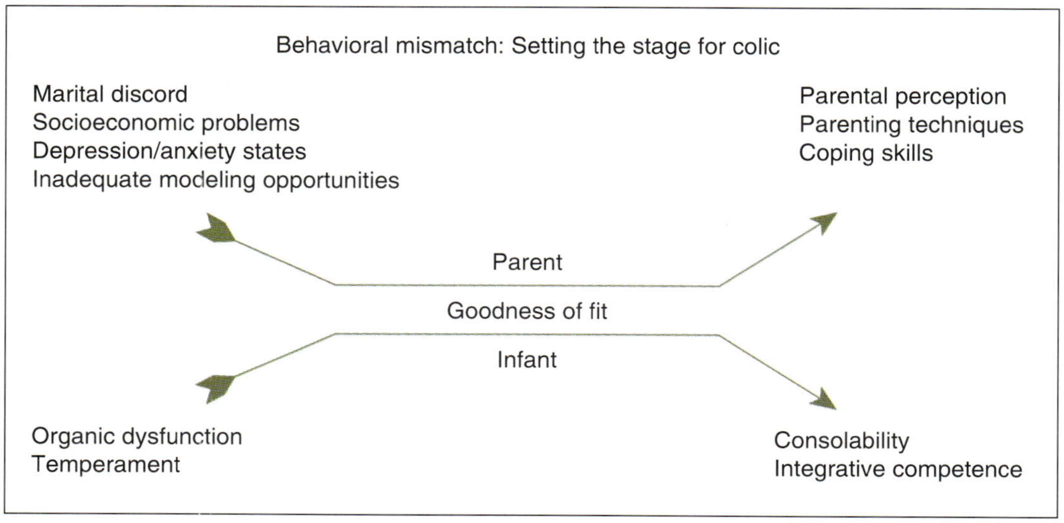

FIGURE 8-5.

The interactions that occur between the newborn and a parent represent a composite of complex interrelationships of processes occurring within the parent, processes occurring with the infant, and the interactions between the infant and the parent [3]. Both the parent and the infant arrive at the point of their interaction with predisposing characteristics. For the parent, the presence of marital discord, psychiatric issues such as depression, distraction by socioeconomic issues, or lack of adequate modeling for parenting behavior may alter parental perceptions, attentiveness, or coping abilities. In turn, infants may bring temperament-related problems, real organic disease, or normal physiologic development to the interaction. In addition, parental deficiencies and skills must match infant deficiencies and skills to optimize the interaction. All of the determinants shown in this figure have been studied in families whose infants have colic, and all have been shown to play a contributing role to colic, but none has been shown to have an independent causal relationship [3]. Most treatment strategies for colic are focused on the parent. This is not to say that the cause of colic necessarily resides in the parent, and it is important that the physician alleviate the parent of unnecessary guilt and feelings of inadequacy of parenting skills [3a]. Some parents may require additional education concerning the natural history of crying and the transient nature of colic. They also require reassurance that they did not cause their baby's colic and empathetic support for coping with a difficult situation. Strategies often employ redefinitions for parents in an attempt to alter their perception or threshold for excessive crying and encouragement to have respite from caring for the infant. Parents may need advice or observe actual role modeling to be taught appropriate coping strategies. A small number of infants may have bovine protein sensitivity, and exclusion of that protein from the nursing mother's diet or the formula-fed diet may alleviate symptoms. Numerous trials have shown little effectiveness for multiple changes in the formula fed to the infant or the use of medications.

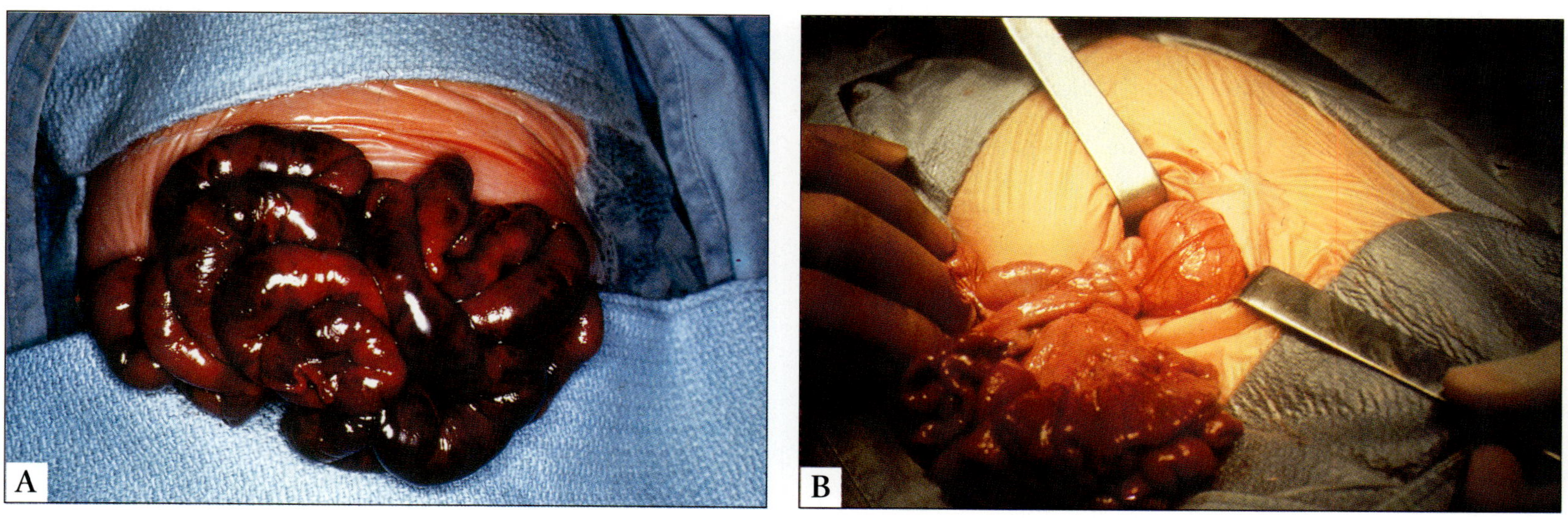

FIGURE 8-6.

Midgut volvulus with ischemia (**A**) and without ischemia (**B**). This condition can occur in children at any age who were previously well. The bowel (and the patient) can be salvaged only by immediate recognition, laparotomy, and detorsion. For this reason, immediate surgical consultation should be obtained in all children who present with bilious or protracted vomiting.

CAUSES OF PERITONITIS IN CHILDHOOD

Gastrointestinal	Genitourinary	Other
Appendicitis	Pyelonephritis	Trauma
Gastroenteritis	Ovarian cyst	Rectus hematoma
Inflammatory bowel disease	rupture	Primary bacterial peritonitis
Meckel's diverticulitis	torsion	Sickle cell crisis
Torsion of omental cyst	hemorrhage	Porphyria
Intestinal obstruction with ischemic bowel	Ovarian tumor with torsion	Henoch-Schönlein purpura
Midgut volvulus	Mittelschmerz	Familial Mediterranean fever
Acute cholecystitis	Pelvic inflammatory disease	
Pancreatitis		
Necrotizing enterocolitis		
Intestinal perforation		

FIGURE 8-7.

Causes of peritonitis in childhood. Peritonitis may be caused by a large number of disease processes involving several different organ systems.

DIAGNOSTIC CRITERIA FOR APPENDICITIS

History
- Periumbilical pain migrating to the right lower quadrant
- Nonbilious vomiting
- Anorexia
- Pain on walking, jumping, and driving over bumps

Physical examination
- Flushed face
- Low-grade fever (fever usually higher with perforation)
- Lies on side with hips flexed
- Localized peritoneal signs in right lower quadrant (may have diffuse peritonitis if perforated)
- Referred rebound tenderness to right lower quadrant

Laboratory
- Mild elevation in leukocyte count, usually higher with perforation
- May have mild hematuria or pyuria from bladder or ureteral irritation

Radiologic
- Local ileus in right lower quadrant (may have diffuse ileus if perforated)
- Appendicolith in right lower quadrant
- Scoliosis to right side
- Loss of psoas shadow on right side

Ultrasound
- Noncompressable, thick-walled tubular structure with localized tenderness
- May see appendicolith with acoustic shadow
- No evidence of ovarian pathology to explain symptoms

Computerized tomography
- Thick-walled structure with surrounding inflammation in right lower abdomen
- May show localized appendiceal abscess if perforated

FIGURE 8-8.

Diagnostic criteria for appendicitis. The diagnosis is made clinically, and not all these criteria need to be satisfied. It is important to remember that "not every child with appendicitis has read the textbook."

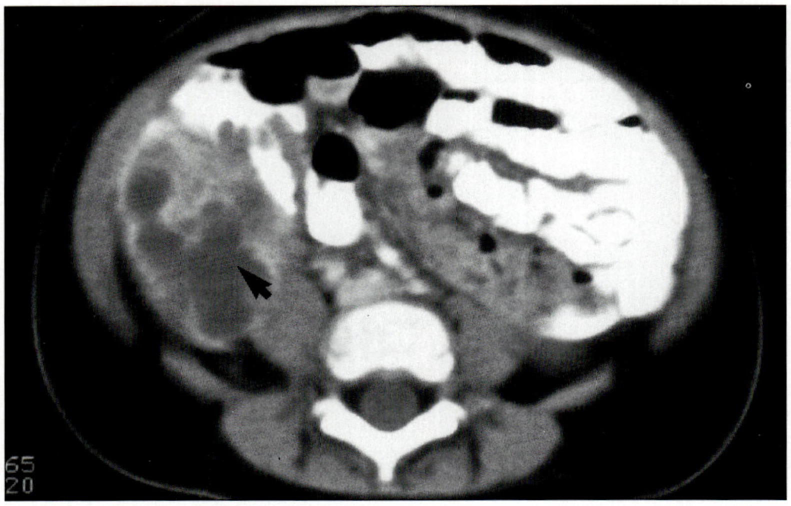

FIGURE 8-9.

Radiologic studies in the diagnosis of acute appendicitis. CT scan showing localized appendiceal abscess in right lower abdomen (*arrow*). (*Courtesy of* Dr. M. Siegel, St. Louis, MO.)

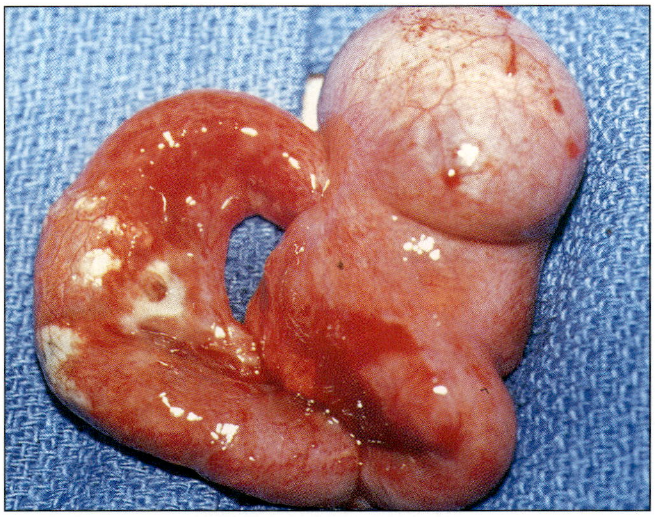

FIGURE 8-10.

Intraoperative photograph of an inflamed appendix during open appendectomy. It remains controversial whether laparoscopic appendectomy results in a shorter hospital stay, fewer wound infections, or faster return to normal activity than open appendectomy. In the pediatric population, the laparoscopic approach is reserved for adolescents, particularly girls in whom ovarian pathology may be causing the problem.

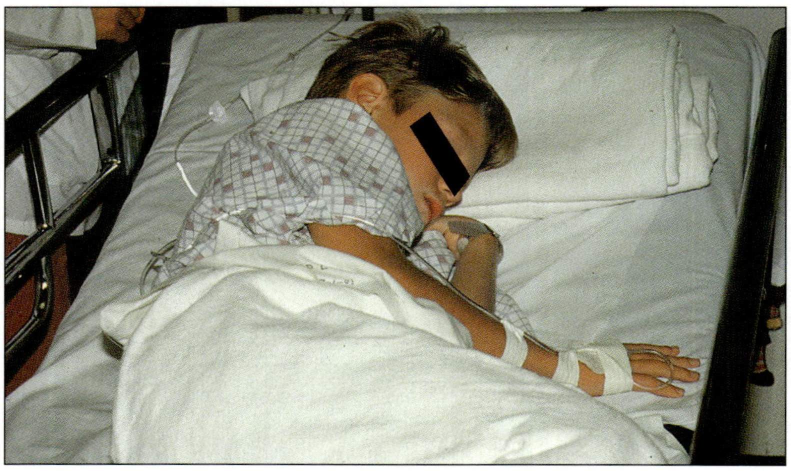

FIGURE 8-11.

Typical position of a child with appendicitis. The child lies quietly with hips flexed. The clinician should also note the facial flushing.

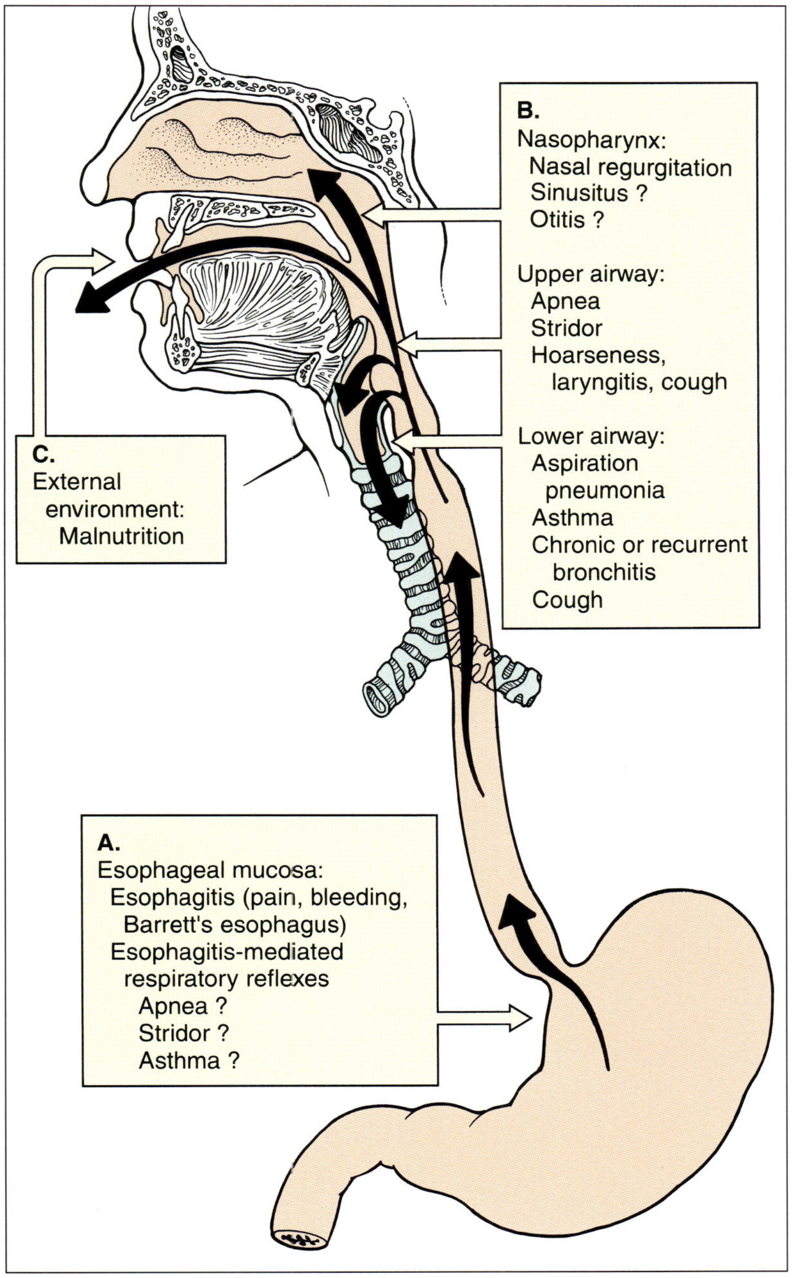

FIGURE 8-12.

A–C, Harmful destinations of the refluxate. Perhaps because of immature protective reflexes or other factors, the destination of the refluxate plays a larger role in young children than in adults with gastroesophageal reflux disease. The classic destination of refluxate—the esophagus—is responsible for esophagitis and its diverse esophageal sequelae (*eg*, pain, bleeding, stricture, Barrett's esophagus, and malignancy). An esophageal destination may also provoke respiratory symptoms through reflex mechanisms. Other hazardous targets of the refluxate are the lower and upper airways, including the nasopharynx. Finally, the external environment is indirectly a harmful destination because of implied caloric loss.

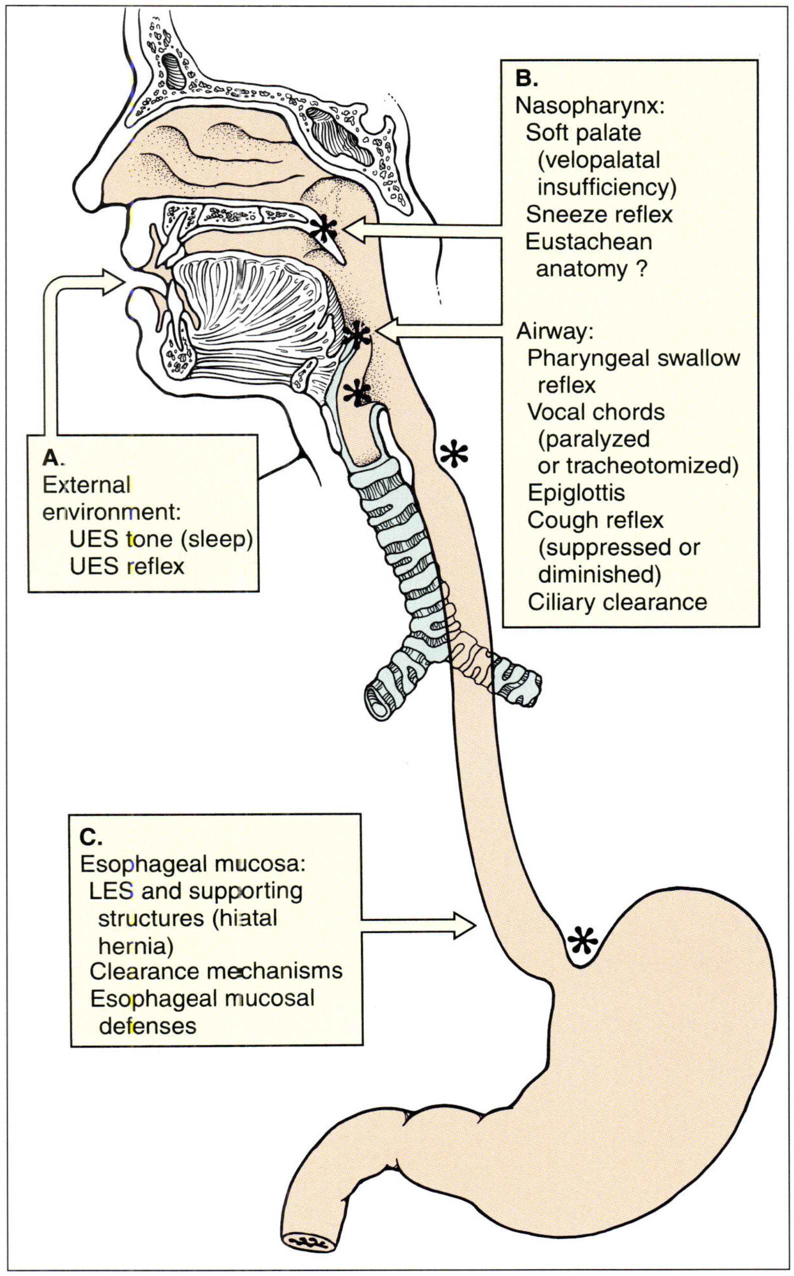

FIGURE 8-13.

A–C, Protection of vulnerable targets of the refluxate. Although the lower esophageal sphincter (LES*) and its supporting structures represent the primary first-line defense against harmful effects of reflux, these are reinforced by the clearance mechanisms previously discussed and by esophageal mucosal defenses against injury [4]. Protection against reflux-related tissue damage proximal to the esophagus is provided first by the upper esophageal sphincter (UES*)—and its reflexively augmented tone during gastroesophageal reflux—and then by the structures that protect the airway during either swallowing or reflux—the epiglottis*, vocal cords*, and soft palate* [5–10]. The swallow reflex, which occurs when the pharynx is stimulated, is an elaborate mechanism that removes refluxate from a dangerous location at the crossroads of the airway and the gastrointestinal tract. The cough and sneeze reflexes clear the lower airway and nasal passages when matter does enter the respiratory tract. In parentheses are some factors that may impair these protections, such as sleep state, velopalatal insufficiency, cough suppression, and tracheotomy.

DIFFERENTIAL DIAGNOSIS OF REGURGITATION AND VOMITING BY LOCUS OF STIMULUS

- Stimulation of central vomiting center:
  - Drugs; toxins
  - Metabolic disease
    - Diabetic ketoacidosis, diabetes insipidus, lactic acidosis, adrenal insufficiency
    - Phenylketonuria, maple-syrup-urine disease, methylmalonic acidemia
    - Hereditary fructose intolerance, galactosemia, tyrosinemia
    - Hyperammonemia, Reye's syndrome, fatty acid oxidation disorders
    - Uremia, renal tubular acidosis
- Stimulation of supramedullary receptors:
  - Improper feeding and psychobehavioral problems
    - Overfeeding, air feeding, baby bouncing
    - Psychogenic, volitional
  - Vestibular disease, "motion sickness"
  - Increased intracranial pressure
    - Subdural effusion or hematoma
    - Hydrocephalus
    - Cerebral edema or tumor
    - Meningoencephalitis, Reye's syndrome
- Stimulation of peripheral receptors:
  - Pharyngeal: gag reflex sinusitis post-nasal drip
  - Esophageal (nonreflux)
    - Obstruction—stricture, ring, stenosis, foreign body
    - Dysmotility—esophageal body dysmotility, achalasia
  - Gastric
    - Obstruction—pyloric stenosis, web, foreign body, bezoar
    - Dysmotility—impaired gastric emptying
    - Peptic ulcer disease
  - Intestinal
    - Infection, enterotoxin, appendicitis
    - Allergy—cow's milk, soy, eosinophilic gastroenteritis
    - Obstruction
      - Web, stenosis, superior mesenteric artery syndrome
      - Volvulus, Intussusception
      - Adhesions
      - Meconium ileus, meconium plug, Hirschsprung's disease
  - Hepatobiliary: hepatitis, cholecystitis
  - Pancreatic: pancreatitis
  - Urinary: urinary infection, pyelonephritis
  - Generalized: sepsis, peritonitis

FIGURE 8-14.

Differential diagnosis of regurgitation and vomiting. Although regurgitant reflux is often recognized clinically, caution must be exercised to avoid missing other causes for the vomiting. (*Adapted from* Orenstein *et al.* [11].)

INFANTS WITH AN ACUTE LIFE-THREATENING EVENT (1983 TO 1990; *N* = 3799)

Diagnosis	*N*	%
Known cause		
Digestive	1107	47
Gastroesophageal reflux	770	20
Infection	152	
Aspiration	105	
Malformations	75	
Dumping syndrome	5	
Neurologic	683	29
Vasovagal syndrome	376	
Epilepsy	150	
Infection	150	
Subdural hematoma	5	
Malformation	2	
Respiratory	353	15
Infection	275	
Airway abnormality	74	
Alveolar hypoventilation	4	
Cardiovascular	82	3.5
Infection	35	
Cardiomyopathy	18	
Arrhythmia	18	
Congenital malformation	11	
Metabolic and Endocrine	59	2.5
Hypoglycemia	23	
Hypocalcemia	12	
Food intolerance	10	
Reye's syndrome	6	
Hypothyroidism	2	
Nonesterified fatty acid metabolism deficiency	2	
Leigh's syndrome	1	
Carnitine	1	
Menke's syndrome	1	
Fructosemia	1	
Miscellaneous	71	3
Accidents	39	
Sepsis	11	
Munchausen's syndrome	8	
Nutritional error	7	
Drug effect	6	
Total	2355	62
Unknown cause		
Apparently minor incident	874	23
Apparently severe incident (idiopathic ALTE)	570	15
Total	1444	38

FIGURE 8-15.

Differential diagnosis of infantile apnea or an acute life-threatening event (ALTE). Because the diagnosis of apnea caused by reflux is usually presumptive, care must be taken to keep the broad differential diagnosis in mind. This table gives the relative frequencies of etiologies in 3799 infants who were carefully and systematically evaluated. Gastroesophageal reflux figures prominently. (*Modified from* Kahn *et al.* [12].)

PEPTIC ULCER IN CHILDREN

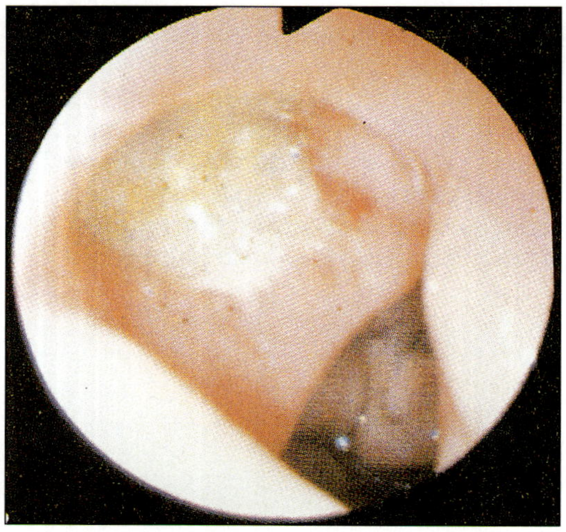

FIGURE 8-16.

Diagnosis of peptic disease. Studies comparing radiologic and endoscopic techniques in children have shown that radiology identifies 50% to 90% of duodenal ulcers demonstrated by endoscopy [13]. In addition, there is a high risk of false-positive and false-negative radiologic diagnoses in children. Although the double-contrast barium studies are superior to single-contrast studies in demonstrating mucosal lesions, these tests are uncomfortable to patients, and overinterpretation of nonspecific findings, such as pylorospasm and thickened folds, may lead to erroneous diagnoses.

Endoscopy is safe and accurate in the hands of an experienced gastroenterologist. It offers the advantage of obtaining targeted mucosal biopsies from different areas for histology and other special tests. Endoscopic visualization cannot reliably detect mucosal disease; therefore, biopsies are an integral part of the endoscopic exam [14]. This figure shows a duodenal ulcer with sharp edges in the duodenal bulb. Most peptic ulcers in children are associated with the *Helicobacter pylori* infection.

PRESENTING SYMPTOMS OF PEPTIC ULCERS AT DIFFERENT AGES

Symptoms	Newborn	1 month to 6 years	> 6 years
Vomiting	+	+	±
Feeding problems	+	+	-
Irritability	+	+	-
Abdominal pain	-	±	+
Gastrointestinal bleeding	+	+	+
Association of pain with meals	-	-	+

FIGURE 8-17.

The presenting symptoms of primary peptic ulcer vary with the age of the child [15–17]. In the neonates, the most common symptoms of peptic disease include vomiting, feeding difficulty, irritability, failure to thrive, gastrointestinal bleeding, pyloric outlet obstruction, and perforation. In infants and young children, between a month to 6 years of age, vomiting, unexplained crying, feeding problems, and occult or overt bleeding are the major symptoms. When abdominal pain occurs in infants who cannot speak, their behavior may change. Intractable fussiness, food refusal, and failure to thrive may be caused by abdominal pain. In older children and adolescents, the symptoms are similar to those in adults. Epigastric or periumbilical pain with nocturnal awakening, a temporal association to meals, nausea, vomiting, and heartburn can occur with different degrees of severity.

Tomomasa and coworkers [18] analyzed 13 ulcer-related symptoms and signs in children 6 to 15 years of age; they concluded that a combination of epigastric pain associated with meals, positive family history of peptic ulcer, vomiting, and bleeding were most suggestive of ulcers in children. Stress or secondary ulcers present with catastrophic events like massive hemorrhage or perforation.

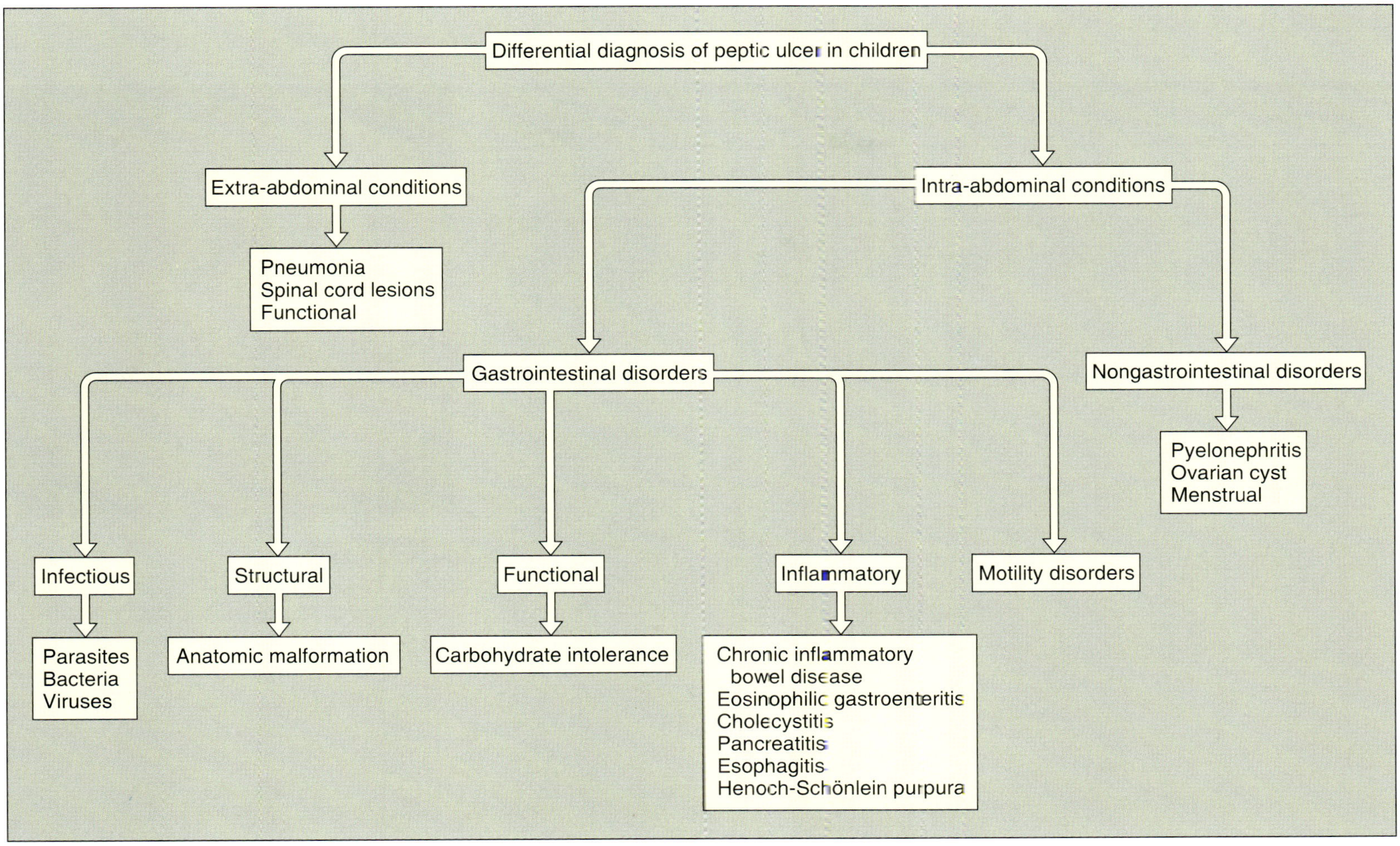

FIGURE 8-18.

Many conditions mimic some or all of the symptoms of peptic disease. These can be broadly classified into extra-abdominal and intra-abdominal disorders. The intra-abdominal category can be further subdivided into gastrointestinal and nongastrointestinal diseases. Special consideration needs to be given to differentiating the very common functional recurrent abdominal pain of childhood from peptic disease. Long duration of symptoms is not a reliable distinguishing factor. In a study of 100 children with ulcers, the mean interval between the onset of symptoms and diagnosis was 1.8 years. A delay of 4.8 years for diagnosis has been reported for symptoms beginning of early childhood [19].

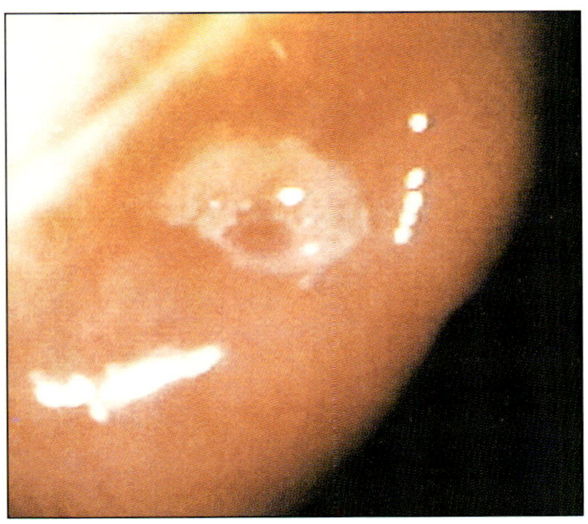

FIGURE 8-19.

Bleeding gastric ulcer with protruding vessel.

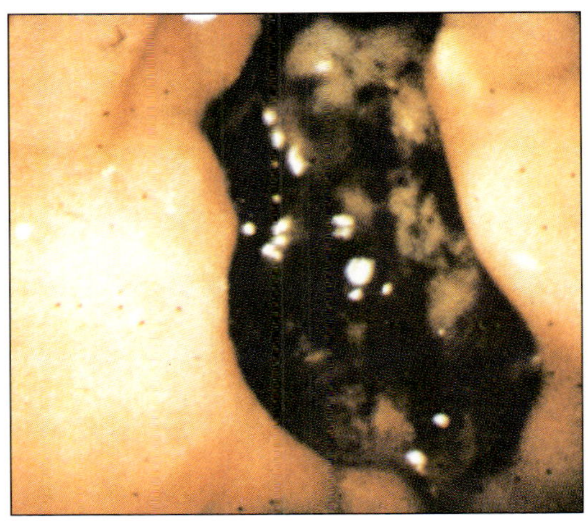

FIGURE 8-20.

Duodenal ulcer with black slough adhering to the ulcer base.

DIFFERENTIAL DIAGNOSIS OF UPPER GASTROINTESTINAL BLEEDING		
Age group	**Common causes**	**Less common causes**
Neonates (0–30 days)	Swallowed maternal blood Gastritis Duodenitis Peptic ulcer	Coagulopathy Vascular malformations Gastric/esophageal duplication Leiomyoma
Infants (30 days–1 year)	Gastritis and gastric ulcer Esophagitis Duodenitis	Esophageal varices Foreign body Aortoesophageal fistula
Children (1–12 years)	Esophagitis Esophageal varices Gastris and gastric ulcer Duodenal ulcer Mallory-Weiss tear Nasopharyngeal bleeding	Leiomyoma Salicylates Vascular malformation Hematocelia
Adolescents (12 years–adult)	Duodenal ulcer Esophagitis Esophageal varices Gastritis Mallory-Weiss tear	Thrombocytopenia Dieulafoy's lesion Hemobilia

FIGURE 8-21.

Differential diagnosis of upper gastrointestinal bleeding. The etiology of upper gastrointestinal bleeding can vary according to the age of the patient. The differential diagnosis at different ages is outlined in this table. Both common and rare etiologies are included. Diseases associated with coagulopathy or thrombocytopenia can lead to bleeding secondary to any interruption of mucosal integrity.

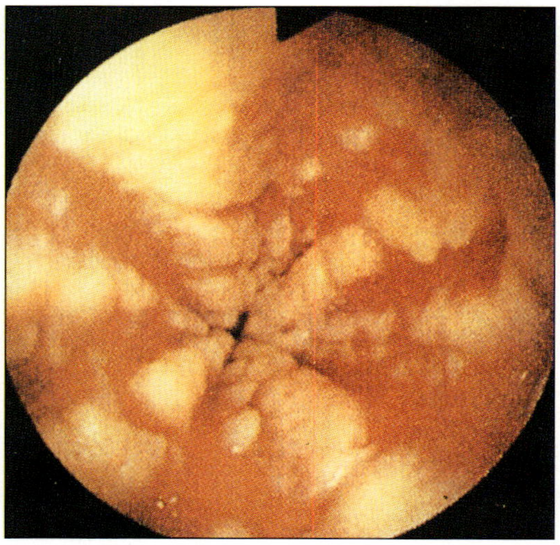

FIGURE 8-22.

Severe candida esophagitis with erosions and exudates, causing upper gastrointestinal bleeding.

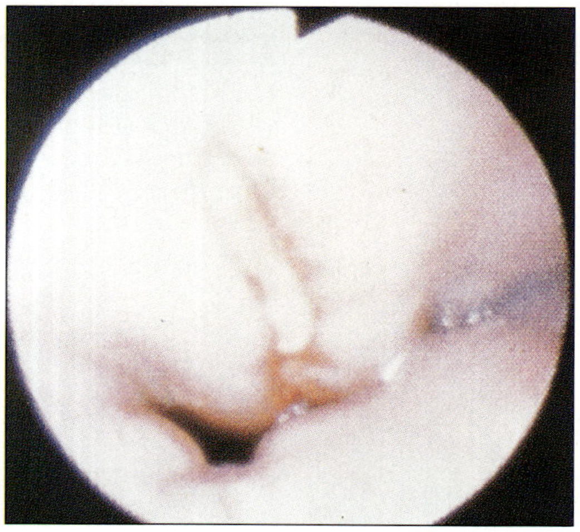

FIGURE 8-23.

Mallory-Weiss tear seen as a healing vertical deep erosion at gastroesophageal junction.

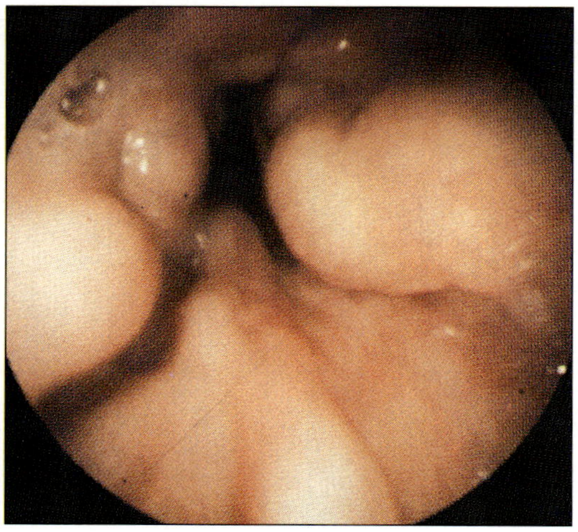

FIGURE 8-24.

Esophageal varices seen as beaded tortuous prominences along distal esophagus.

Celiac disease

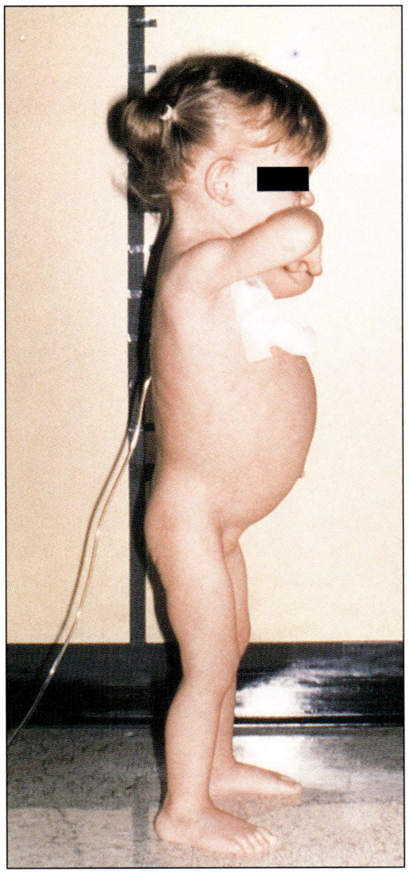

FIGURE 8-25.

Child with celiac disease. Note the protuberant abdomen and the marked muscle wasting and evidence of malnutrition. Children with celiac disease may exhibit no unusual findings on physical examination and rarely are as severely affected as this girl. This photograph was selected to demonstrate the physical findings. This child responded very well to a strict gluten-free diet that she must follow for the rest of her life.

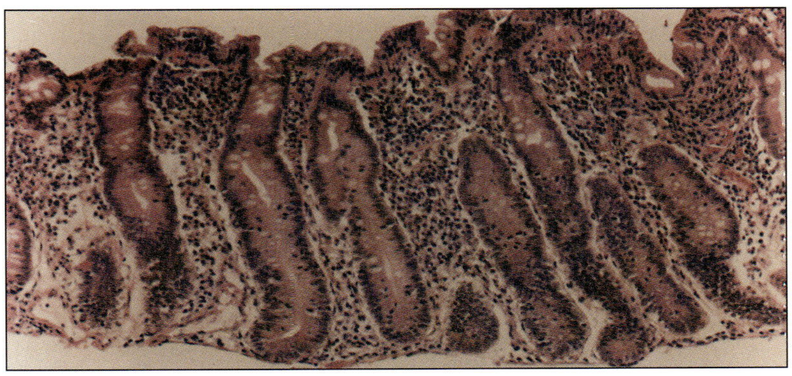

FIGURE 8-26.

Biopsy specimen obtained from a patient with celiac disease. This is the classic flat lesion of celiac sprue. No villi are visible because the epithelium is totally flat. An intense inflammatory infiltrate is present in the lamina propria, primarily mononuclear cells. A marked increase in mitotic epithelial cell activity is present in the crypts, another hallmark of celiac disease. The surface epithelium has lost its polarity, with the normal basal orientation of the nuclei disturbed. Although these findings are common in celiac disease, they are also nonspecific and may occur, in extreme cases, from a variety of small intestinal disorders. (*Courtesy of* Robert Kruger, MD, Children's Hospital, Omaha, NE.)

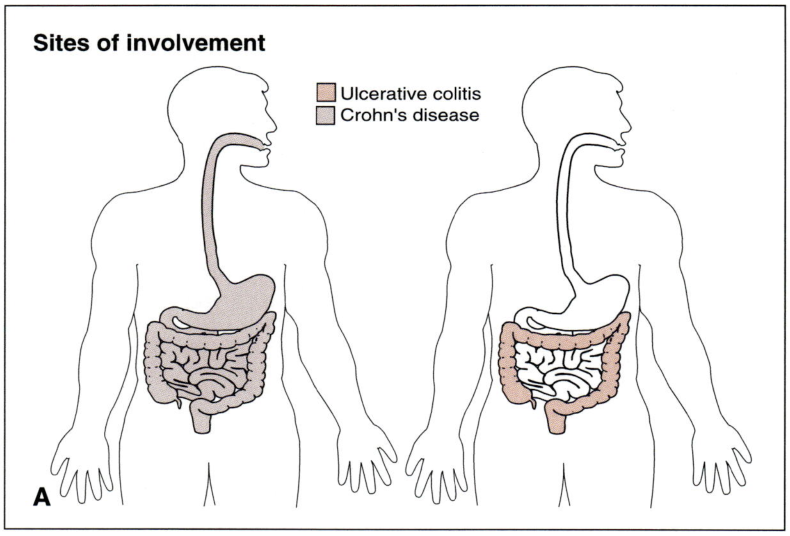

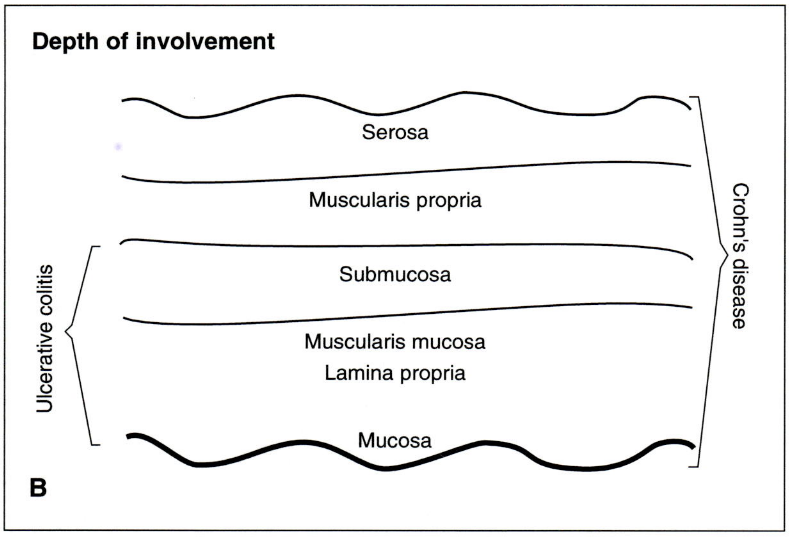

FIGURE 8-27.

Inflammatory bowel disease comprises two distinct diseases—ulcerative colitis and Crohn's disease. In both, there is chronic inflammation of the gastrointestinal tract. **A**, Although ulcerative colitis involves only the colon, Crohn's disease can involve any part of the gastrointestinal tract from the mouth to the anus, including the perianal region. In Crohn's disease, ileocolonic involvement is the most common. In ulcerative colitis presenting in adults, proctitis is the most common initial presentation (46.5%), 23% presenting with more extensive left-sided colitis and about 10% to 15% with total colitis. The extent of inflammation in children at presentation is still uncertain. Of patients with proctitis, 50% to 60% progress to left-sided or total colitis [20]. **B**, In Crohn's disease, the inflammation is transmural, whereas in ulcerative colitis the inflammation is limited to the mucosa and submucosa.

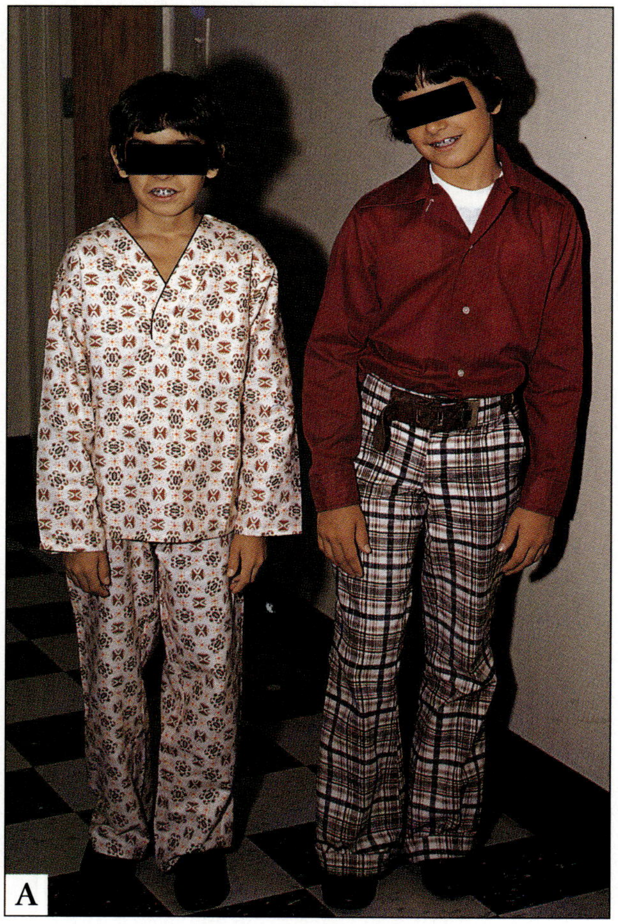

FIGURE 8-28.

Growth failure in Crohn's disease. Monozygotic twins at 12 years of age. The patient on the left was 3 inches shorter and 15 pounds lighter at presentation than his monozygotic twin brother.

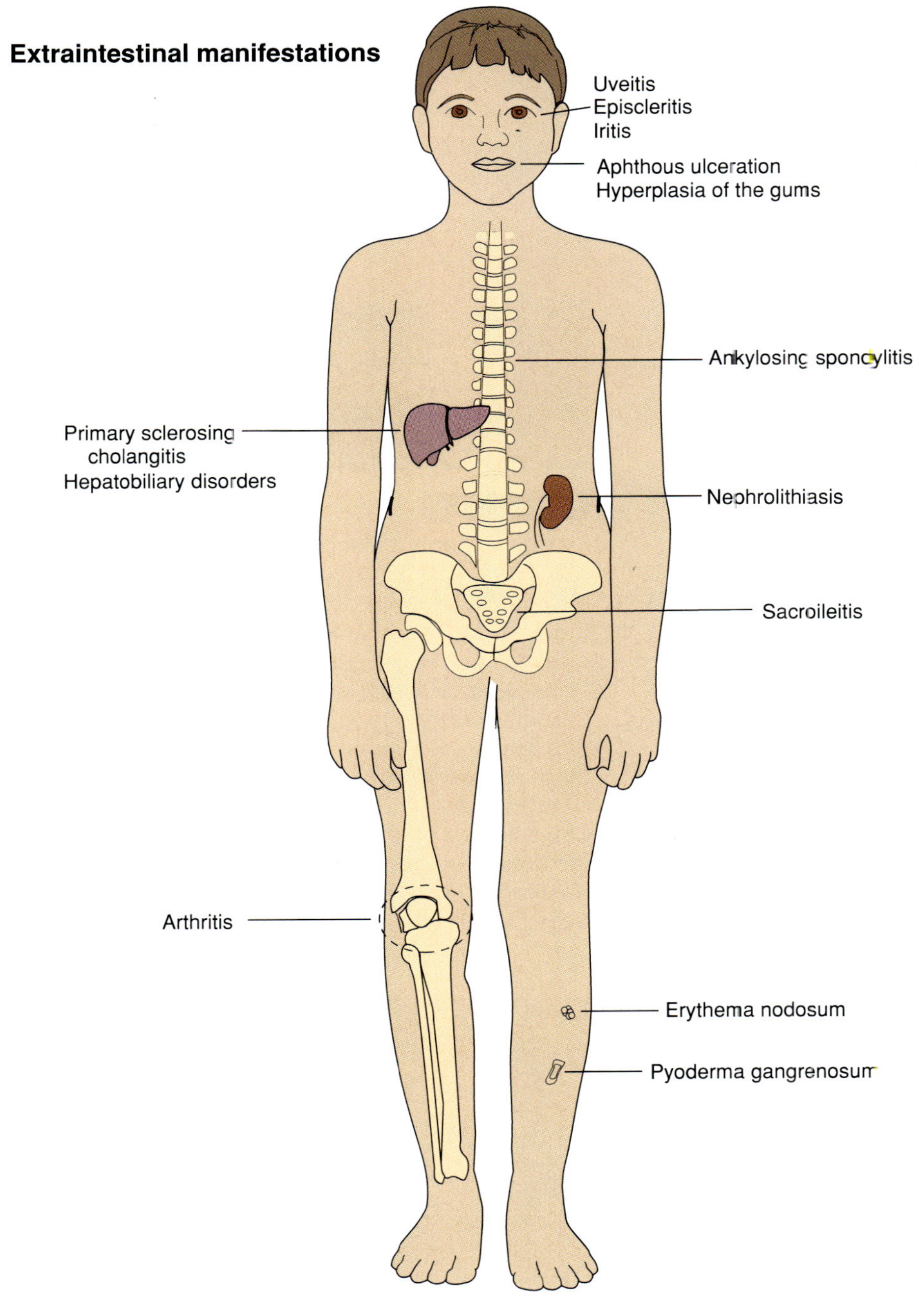

FIGURE 8-29.

Extraintestinal manifestations (EIMs). EIMs occur frequently in inflammatory bowel disease and may precede overt bowel symptoms [21–24]. Primary EIMs are those that seem to share the pathogenesis of the disease involving the skin, eyes, liver, joints, and mucous membranes. Secondary EIMs are those secondary to long-standing disease (*eg*, kidney stones, obstructive uropathy, and gallstones). Secondary EIMs appear to occur more often in patients with Crohn's disease.

Arthralgias are probably the most common EIM in inflammatory bowel disease. Arthritis is uncommon. When arthritis occurs, it presents most commonly as peripheral arthritis, is asymmetric, and involves the lower extremity joints. Axial arthropathies consisting of sacroileitis with ankylosing spondylitis occur in patients with inflammatory bowel disease 10 to 30 times more often than in the general population [25,26]. Severity of peripheral arthritis correlates with the severity of inflammatory bowel disease, whereas the symptoms of axial arthropathies do not. Axial arthropathies are rarely seen in childhood.

Dermal manifestations associated with inflammatory bowel disease are also frequently seen; the most frequent are erythema nodosum, vasculitic skin changes, and pyoderma gangrenosum [27]. Psoriasis is also seen with increased frequency in patients with Crohn's disease [28]. Ocular manifestations include uveitis, episcleritis, iritis, and marginal corneal ulcerations. Crohn's disease patients with disease limited to the large bowel have a higher incidence of eye abnormalities [29–31].

A relatively common hepatobiliary disorder seen in association with inflammatory bowel disease is sclerosing cholangitis [32,33]. Sclerosing cholangitis can occur alone or in association with inflammatory bowel disease. It is more frequently seen in association with ulcerative colitis than with Crohn's disease [34,35]. Incidence of inflammatory bowel disease in sclerosing cholangitis is reported to be from 25% to 74% [36,37]. Sclerosing cholangitis is seen in 1% to 4% of patients with inflammatory bowel disease.

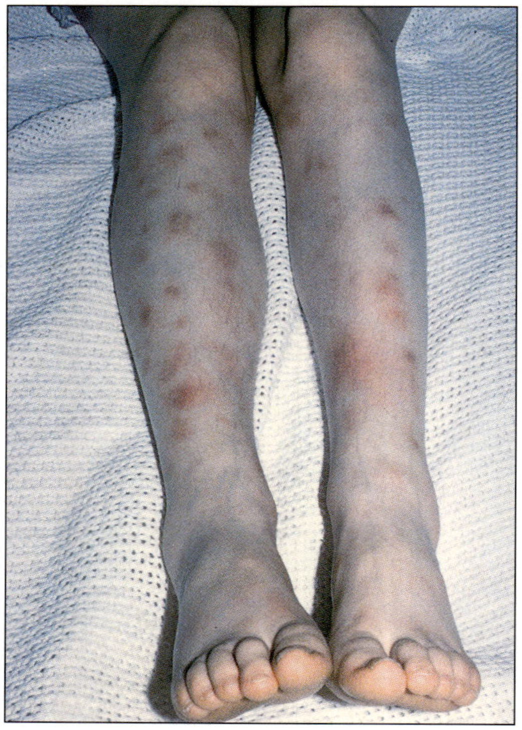

Figure 8-30.

Erythema nodosum. Erythema nodosum is the most common dermatologic manifestation of inflammatory bowel disease [38]. The incidence of erythema nodosum ranges from 0.5% to 9% among patients with ulcerative colitis and 2% to 15% among patients with Crohn's disease [39,40]. Erythema nodosum often appears with active disease.

The lesions, usually multiple, are characterized by very tender, warm, red subcutaneous nodules on the pretibial region of the lower extremities. Erythema nodosum has been noted with pregnancy, use of oral contraceptives, and in association with several systemic conditions, including streptococcal infection, tuberculosis, sarcoidosis, viral illness, and certain drug eruptions [41–44]. The nodules of erythema nodosum associated with inflammatory bowel disease often respond rapidly to treatment of the bowel disease, especially if corticosteroids are prescribed.

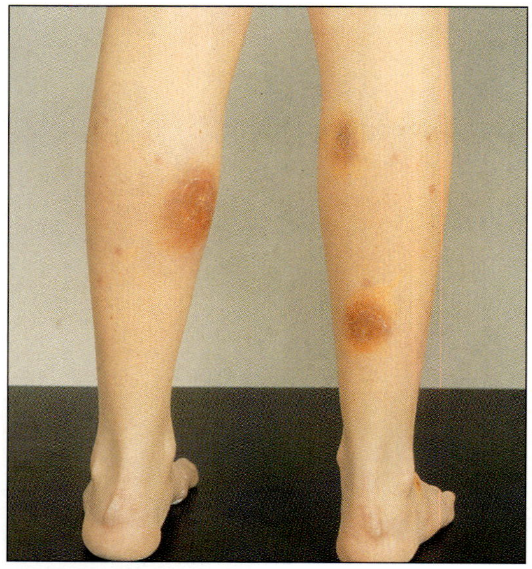

Figure 8-31.

Pyoderma gangrenosum in Crohn's disease. Not all of the inflammation in inflammatory bowel disease occurs in the gastrointestinal tract. A small percentage of patients with ulcerative colitis or Crohn's disease develops extraintestinal manifestations of the disease, including arthritis, uveitis, or, as in this patient, skin lesions. Erythema nodosum and pyoderma gangrenosum are most common. Here, the deep ulcerated lesions of pyoderma gangrenosum on the legs are shown. Prednisone or cyclosporin heal these lesions. (*Courtesy of* David R. Mack, MD, University of Nebraska, Omaha, NE.)

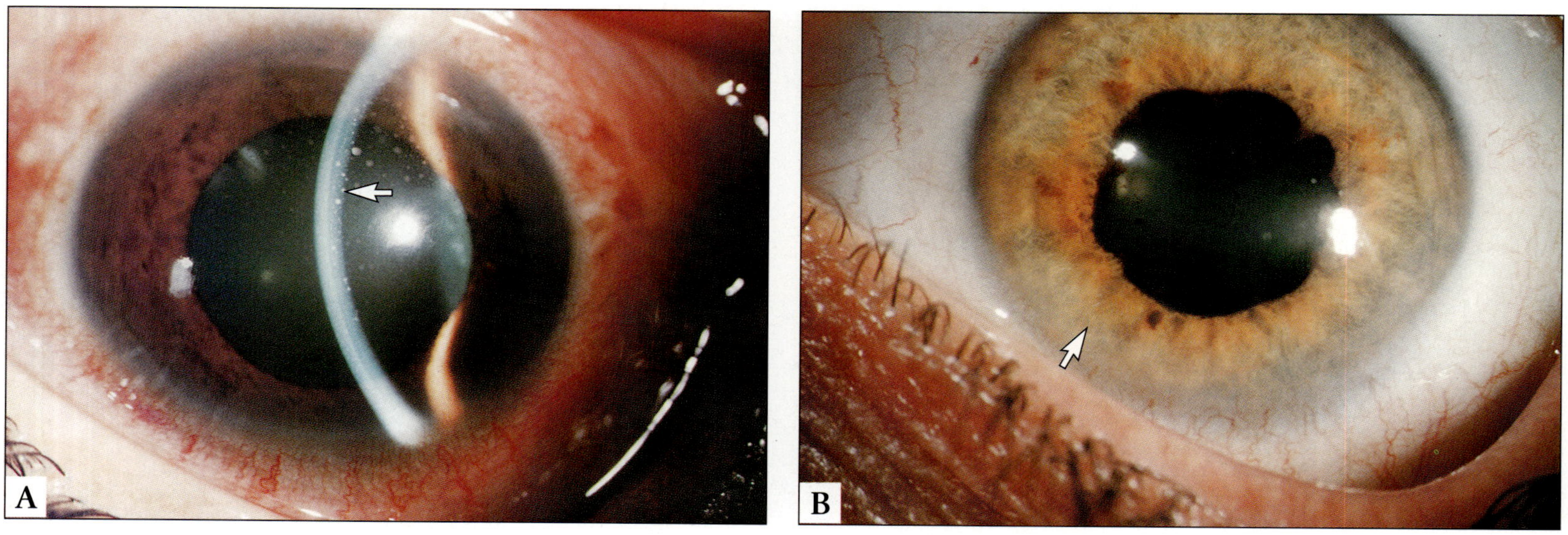

Figure 8-32.

Ophthalmologic findings. A multiplicity of eye problems are seen in both Crohn's disease (5%–10%) and ulcerative colitis (5%), including episcleritis and scleritis, optic neuritis and uveitis. Iritis and iridocyclitis are types of uveitis seen in inflammatory bowel disease. **A**, Iridocyclitis in one or both eyes is the most common finding in patients with ulcerative colitis. Characteristic peripheral keratitic precipitation on the cornea is seen on slit-lamp examination (*arrow*). **B**, Patient with Crohn's disease with acute iritis and typical posterior synechiae (*arrow*) reflecting inflammatory adhesions of the iris to the lens capsule. (*Courtesy* of Jeffrey L. Willig, MD, Manhasset, NY.)

CROHN'S VERSUS ULCERATIVE COLITIS

CROHN'S COLITIS	ULCERATIVE COLITIS
Rectum spared in 20% to 30% of children	Rectum almost always involved
Inflammation	Inflammation
Patchy	Continuous
Early	Early
Aphthous ulcers in normal mucosa	Granular mucosa
	Friable mucosa
Late	Late
Linear deep ulcers in normal mucosa	Diffusely inflamed mucosa with ulceration
Pseudopolyps	Pseudopolyps
Sinuses, fistulas, and strictures	Strictures (rule out malignancy)

FIGURE 8-33.

Crohn's colitis versus ulcerative colitis. Despite the differences enumerated in 10% of cases, it still is impossible to distinguish between Crohn's colitis and ulcerative colitis. Endoscopic biopsies, which only include the mucosa and muscularis mucosa, often do not distinguish between the two conditions. Rectal sparing, patchy involvement, and aphthous ulceration, features that are considered pathognomonic of Crohn's disease, have been seen in endoscopic and surgical specimens of ulcerative colitis [45]. Inflammatory infiltration of mucosa and submucosa associated with crypt distortion, crypt abscesses, and Paneth's cell metaplasia can be seen in both. However, in Crohn's disease, granulomas may be present in up to 28% of rectal biopsies if serially sectioned [46,47], a feature not seen in ulcerative colitis.

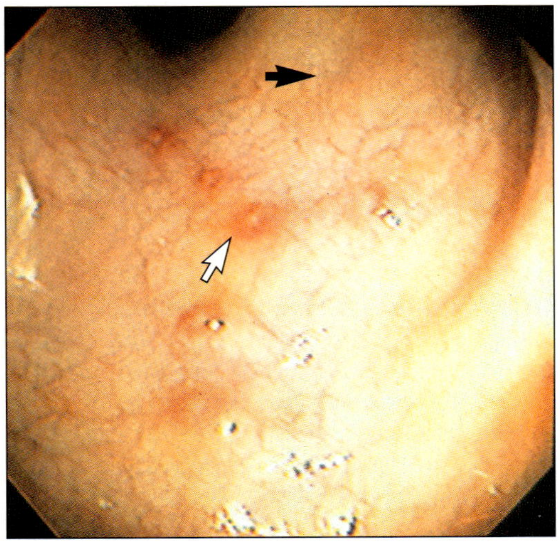

FIGURE 8-34.

Crohn's colitis—aphthous ulceration. Aphthous ulcers are tiny, pinpoint lesions with exudate (*open arrow*) surrounded by an erythematous margin. Microscopically, these are tiny foci of mucosal ulceration often overlying enlarged lymphoid follicles. Normal mucosa (*closed arrow*) is seen adjacent to the inflamed mucosa.

Aphthous ulcers may be the earliest recognizable lesion of Crohn's disease, but infiltration by lymphocytes, polymorphonuclear cells, and plasma cells probably precedes the development of the aphthous ulcer [48]. Aphthous ulcers can occur anywhere from the mouth to the anal area. These lesions may also be seen by air-contrast barium enema.

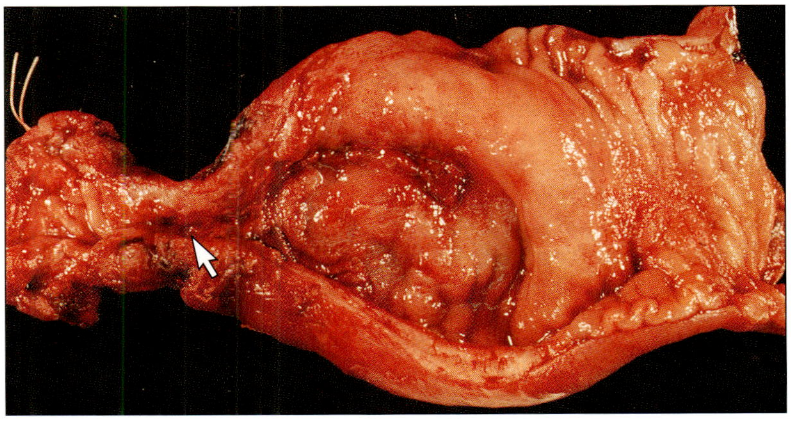

FIGURE 8-35.

Crohn's ileitis—stenosis. Stenosis of the distal portion of the specimen (*arrow*) associated with marked thickening of the bowel wall and proximal dilatation with mucosal ulceration. Classically, such patients present with symptoms of obstruction and a "string sign" radiologically. Histologic sections of the strictured intestine demonstrate muscularis mucosa, markedly expanded by hyperplasia of the smooth muscle cells and the presence of large amounts of collagen. The muscularis propria is also expanded. (*Courtesy of* E. Kahn, Manhasset, NY.)

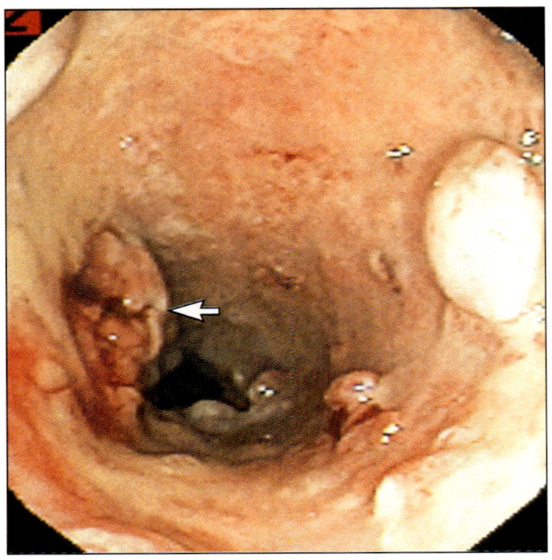

FIGURE 8-36.

Ulcerative colitis—mass lesion. Adenomatous polyps are extremely rare in the pediatric population. Endoscopically, adenomas (*arrow*) are indistinguishable from pseudopolyps. Adenocarcinoma is a well-known complication of ulcerative colitis; an increased incidence is also being reported in Crohn's disease [49]. Consensus is that in disease present over 10 years and with pancolitic involvement, there is a greater risk of colon cancer, even in the pediatric population [50].

DRUG THERAPY—AMINOSALICYLATE PREPARATIONS IN INFLAMMATORY BOWEL DISEASE

Drug	Formulation	Site/Activation
Oral		
Sulfasalazine	Sulfapyridine linked to 5-ASA by azo bond	Colon; bacterial cleavage of azo bond
Rowasa (Solvay Pharmaceuticals, Marietta, GA)	5-ASA coated with acrylic resin L 100	Distal ileum and colon; pH > 6
Asacol (Proctor & Gamble, Cincinnati, OH)	5-ASA coated with acrylic resins	Distal ileum and colon; pH > 6
Pentasa (Marion Merrell Dow, Kansas City, MO)	5-ASA in ethyl cellulose microgranules	Small intestine; time release
Dipentum (Kabi Pharmacia, Piscataway, NJ)	5-ASA dimer linked by azo bond	Colon; bacterial cleavage of azo bond
Rectal		
Foam	5-ASA	Rectum/sigmoid
Enemas	5-ASA suspension	Rectum/sigmoid and left colon
Suppositories	5-ASA	Rectum/sigmoid ? Left colon

FIGURE 8-37.

Aminosalicylate preparations. Sulfasalazine has been used for almost 50 years in the treatment of inflammatory bowel disease. It is used in mild to moderate ulcerative colitis and Crohn's colitis. Intolerance and allergic reactions have limited its use [51]. Sulfasalazine interferes with the absorption of folic acid, thus requiring folic acid supplementation. Most of the drug's toxicity has been attributed to the sulfa portion, which serves as a vehicle for transport of 5-aminosalicylic acid (5-ASA) to the colon. Because of possible toxicity, mesalamine preparations have been formulated using a variety of carrier systems. Various vehicles used require bacterial cleavage, a pH higher than 6, or are time-released, therefore making the active ingredient available in the distal ileum and/or colon. Eighty percent to 90% of patients intolerant or allergic to sulfasalazine can tolerate the newer agents [52].

Rectal 5-ASA therapy has proven to be efficacious in patients with distal ulcerative colitis. A dosage of 2 to 4 g per day of 5-ASA in enema form has been shown to achieve a 93% clinical and sigmoidoscopic remission rate [53,54]. 5-ASA in suppository form given in doses of 200 mg to 1 g, 2 to 3 times daily, has also proven to be effective in patients with proctitis and distal colitis [55,56]. Recently, a foam preparation has also become available.

Mode of action of these 5-ASA preparations remains unclear. 5-ASA has an inhibitory effect on the lipoxygenase pathway of arachidonic-acid metabolism and thus decreases the production of leukotrienes that cause the inflammation inherent in inflammatory bowel disease [57]. 5-ASA has also been shown to be an effective scavenger of oxygen-derived free radicals implicated in the pathogenesis of a variety of inflammatory states [58].

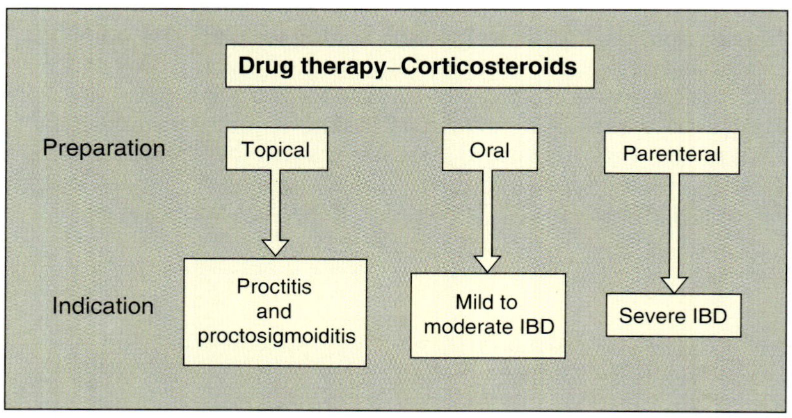

FIGURE 8-38.

Corticosteroids. Topical preparations are often used in children with mildly active ulcerative colitis or Crohn's colitis with symptoms predominantly of distal left-sided colitis (tenesmus and urgency). In the asymptomatic child, rectosigmoid pathology is not an indication in itself for corticosteroid therapy [59]. For the moderately ill child with inflammatory bowel disease (IBD), oral prednisone is effective in a dose ranging from 0.2 to 2 mg/kg per day (to a maximum of 50 to 75 mg/d). For more severe symptoms, intravenous hydrocortisone is the treatment of choice (0.2 to 1.0 mg/kg/dose every 6 hours). It is unclear whether steroids have a role in maintenance therapy. There are no dose-dependent studies based on clinical, laboratory, endoscopic, or histologic data to indicate the daily dosage required to induce remission.

In children treated with steroids, there are two side effects that are of great concern: cosmetic side effects and linear growth suppression. The cosmetic side effects of steroids are very disturbing, especially to adolescent patients. These include a moonlike facies, acne, hirsutism, and striae. In children with IBD, it has been shown that daily steroid therapy for 7 days can decrease serum procollagen levels, a biochemical marker for linear bone growth [60]. Steroids taken every second day have been shown to be beneficial in limiting these effects while maintaining reduced disease activity [61].

Rectal enemas and foam preparations, although efficacious, may lead to considerable absorption and systemic side effects. Glucocorticoid derivatives have been developed that act locally on the mucosa but have little or no systemic activity. Beclomethasone dipropionate [62], tixocortol pivalate [63,64], budesonide [65,66], and fluticasone propionate [67] have proven to be effective topical therapies that do not severely depress plasma cortisol levels. They all undergo a rapid first-pass metabolism in the liver, thereby limiting their systemic side effects. Oral budesonide has led to remission in 50% to 60% of patients with Crohn's disease. Fluticasone propionate is poorly absorbed (<50%) and whatever is absorbed is rapidly metabolized during its first pass through the liver, thus making it more attractive for the treatment of small-bowel Crohn's disease. These newer steroids have been used only rarely in the pediatric population, and their efficacy has not yet been determined.

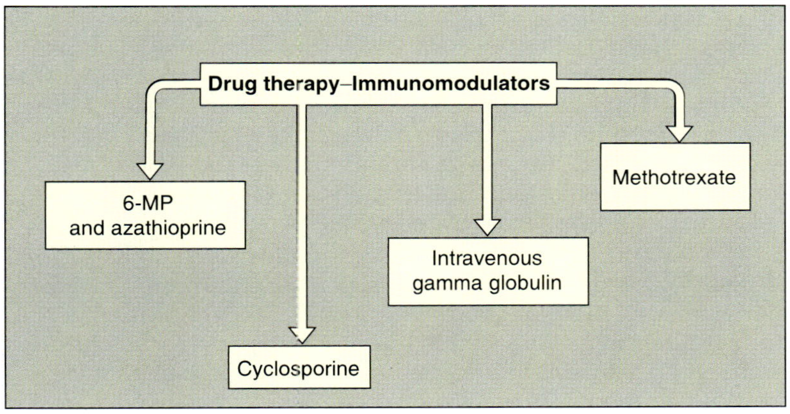

FIGURE 8-39.

Immunomodulators. Azathioprine and 6-mercaptopurine (6-MP) (a major metabolite of azathioprine) both appear effective in the treatment of Crohn's disease and ulcerative colitis. 6-MP is being used increasingly in adolescents with steroid-dependent and intractable Crohn's disease. Clinical trials in adults with Crohn's disease have demonstrated marked improvement in symptoms and lessened disease activity when these agents have been used for at least 3 to 6 months [68]. Data from clinical experience in adolescents with intractable Crohn's disease indicate that two thirds of these patients experienced remission of disease and that 80% were able to discontinue corticosteroid treatment completely when 6-MP was used for at least 1 year [69].

In limited observations, cyclosporine [70,71] has been effective pharmacotherapeutically in about 40% to 50% of children with acute fulminant ulcerative colitis. Further data are needed to determine the actual efficacy of cyclosporine in both the short-term and long-term treatment of children with ulcerative colitis. Cyclosporine has little role in the treatment of Crohn's disease, but it may be effective in the treatment of fistulas complicating Crohn's disease [72].

Intravenous gamma globulin therapy is an alternative medical therapy proposed for Crohn's disease and ulcerative colitis. Experience indicates that selected patients with intractable Crohn's disease may respond favorably to intravenous gamma globulin infusion [73]. There are no data to indicate the efficacy or adverse side effects of methotrexate in children with inflammatory bowel disease.

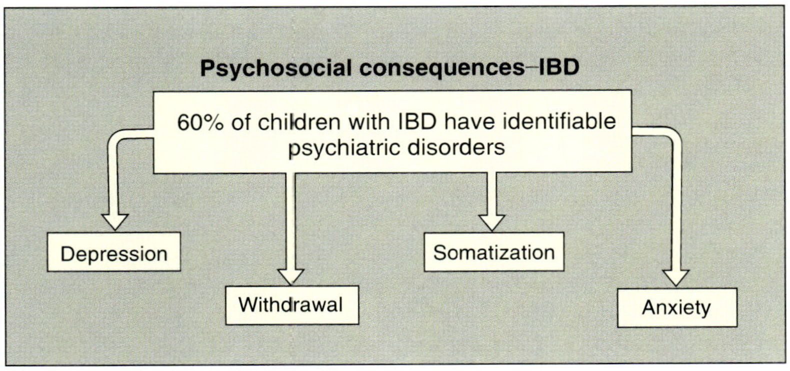

FIGURE 8-40.

Psychosocial consequences—inflammatory bowel disease (IBD). Comorbid psychiatric illnesses have been reported in children and adolescents with IBD. In one study, 60% of children and adolescents with either Crohn's disease or ulcerative colitis had an identifiable psychiatric disorder [74]. Adolescents with IBD have psychologic styles characterized by depression, anxiety, withdrawal, and frequent somatization. These traits appear to be at least in part the sequelae of having chronic intestinal disease. Studies have shown these adolescents have abnormal coping skills in dealing with stressful life events [75].

FUNCTIONAL BOWEL DISORDERS IN CHILDREN

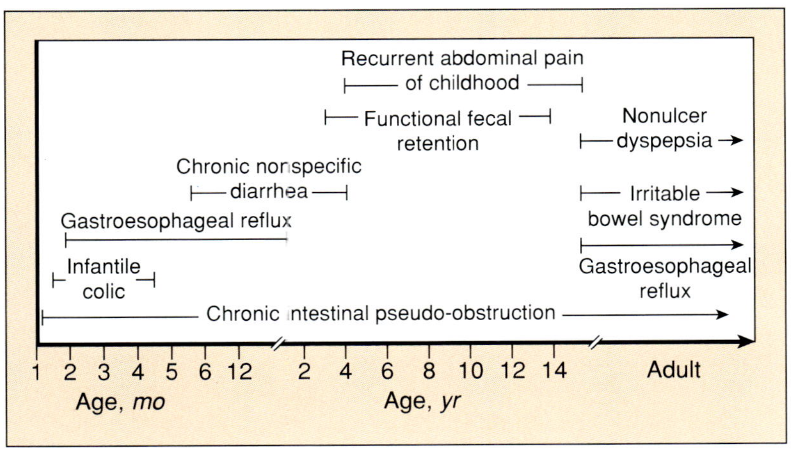

FIGURE 8-41.

Functional bowel disorders in children. There is an age-specific vulnerability to different functional bowel diseases. Sometimes different functional complaints arise at different ages in the same patient. A colicky infant may present later in life with chronic nonspecific diarrhea followed by recurrent abdominal pain and symptoms typical of irritable bowel syndrome. Other diseases, such as gastroesophageal reflux, present with different symptoms in infancy or late childhood.

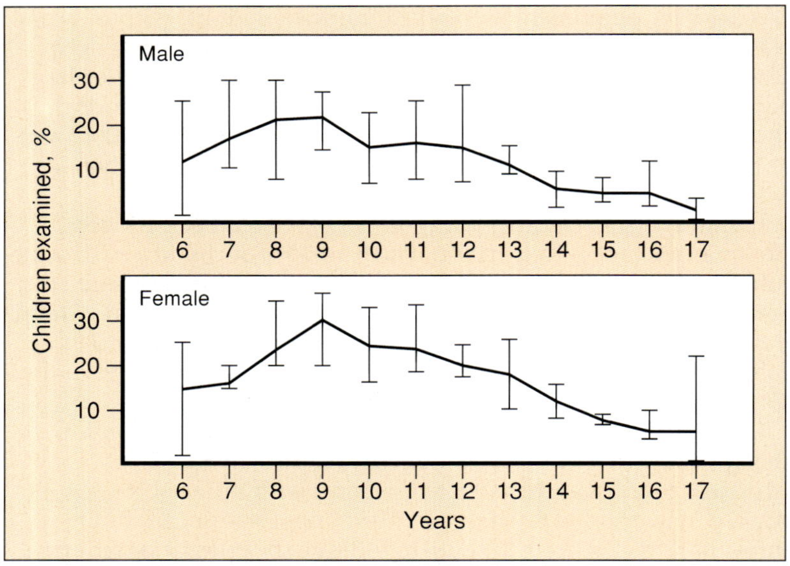

FIGURE 8-42.

Abdominal pain is one of the most common symptoms in childhood and adolescence. *Chronic* or *recurrent abdominal pain* (RAP) is defined as the presence of at least three episodes of abdominal pain occurring over a period of at least 3 months. Recurrent abdominal pain is also called *functional abdominal pain of childhood* because up to 90% of children have no organic cause for their pain. The pain usually begins gradually and is located in the periumbilical or midepigastric region. Characteristically, there is no correlation with meals, exercise, or position. The pain often interrupts daily activities but only rarely awakens the child. Description of the pain is vague, although the pain is more often reported as constant rather than colicky. It is common for the child with RAP to complain of headache, dizziness, or fainting, symptoms that have suggested a systemic autonomic nervous system vulnerability. Children with RAP often undergo extensive medical investigation aimed at finding an organic cause for their symptom. Although often described as if they encompass a homogenous population, children with RAP represent a heterogeneous group, with symptoms often overlapping those of nonulcer dyspepsia or irritable bowel syndrome.

This figure shows prevalence of RAP in school age boys and girls [76]. The *vertical bars* indicate the standard deviation calculated from observations repeated every year during an 8-year period. Approximately 5% of all pediatric outpatient visits are due to RAP. Both Apley, in his survey of 1000 English children [77], and Øster, who surveyed 2500 Danish children [76], reported that the prevalence of RAP seems to peak at 9 years of age. Another later peak for girls aged 13 to 14 was reported by Apley. Abdominal pain presenting before age 4 requires an in-depth evaluation to rule out organic causes. Age of onset in children older than 13 to 14 years demands a thorough evaluation of systemic inflammatory conditions and gynecologic disorders. (*Modified from* Øster [76].)

FINDINGS SUGGESTING ORGANIC DISEASE IN CHILDREN WITH RAP

- Pain away from the umbilicus
- Pain that awakens patient from sleep
- Radiation of pain to back, shoulder, lower extremities
- Weight loss or failure to thrive
- Bilious or bloody emesis
- Fever
- Jaundice
- Dysuria
- Positive family history of peptic disease, inflammatory bowel disease
- Elevated sedimentation rate
- Anemia
- Guaiac-positive stools

FIGURE 8-43.

Findings suggesting the presence of organic disease in children with recurrent abdominal pain (RAP). The presence of these features signals the need for a more extensive evaluation for organic disease. The most likely organic cause for abdominal pain is a disease involving either the genitourinary tract or the gastrointestinal tract [78]. Laboratory evaluation at the time of the first visit should include complete blood count, erythrocyte sedimentation rate, serum lipase, urinalysis and urine culture, stool examination for occult blood, ova, and parasites. When these tests yield negative results and the history and physical examination are compatible with a diagnosis of RAP, the physician should not embark in any additional invasive testing that will only reinforce in the child and the family the concept that something is seriously wrong with the child's health. The physician should instead make diagnosis of RAP and provide a thorough explanation to the patient and family of what RAP means.

CONSTIPATION IN CHILDREN

CONSTIPATION

CHILDREN	ADULTS
More common in boys	More common in women
Resolves at puberty	Begins at puberty
Withholding behavior	Straining behavior
Fecal incontinence very common	Fecal incontinence less common
High-fiber diet rarely helpful	High-fiber diet helpful
Surgery never indicated in functional constipation	Surgery successful in selected patients
Better prognosis	Worse prognosis

FIGURE 8-44.

Comparison between childhood and adulthood constipation. In childhood, constipation is more common among boys than girls. In adulthood, it is more common among women [79]. Constipation is the chief complaint in 3% of all pediatric outpatient visits and up to 25% of children referred to pediatric gastroenterologists have a disorder of defecation [80,81]. As illustrated in the figure, the ratio of females to males varies along the life span. Childhood constipation is equally distributed among different social classes with no relation to family size, ethnic background, or age of the parents [82]. The incidence of childhood constipation increases when a parent, a sibling, or a twin is constipated. Constipation in children differs significantly from constipation in adults. Diagnostic and therapeutic approaches need to be adjusted to patient's age. (*Adapted from* Devroede [79].)

CAUSES OF CONSTIPATION IN CHILDREN

- Functional
- Anatomic
  - Anorectal malformations
  - Strictures
  - Tumors
- Neurogenic conditions
  - Hirschsprung's disease
  - Cerebral palsy and developmental retardation
  - Myelodysplasia
  - Spinal cord trauma
  - Neurofibromatosis
  - Intestinal neuronal dysplasia and other visceral neuropathies
  - Botulism
- Systemic and metabolic disorders
  - Electrolyte abnormalities (hypokalemia, hypercalcemia)
  - Hypothyroidism
  - Cystic fibrosis
  - Diabetes mellitus
  - Malabsorption
  - Multiple endocrine neoplas a type 2B
- Drugs
  - Opiates, anticholinergics, anticonvulsants, tryciclic antidepressants, antacids, sucralfate, iron, vitamin D intoxication, and lead ingestion
- Diet

FIGURE 8-45.

Causes of constipation in children. Many organic disorders can cause constipation, but only a minority of children have organic or anatomic causes for the condition. In neurologically devastated children, constipation is common and the cause may be multifactorial. The absence of normal skeletal muscle tone and coordination may result in a poor defecatory effort. When tube feedings are used, the absence of dietary fiber may be constipating. Sensory or motor abnormalities may exist due to affected enteric neurons, just as there are abnormalities in the central nervous system. Anticonvulsant drugs often cause constipation. In children with spinal cord injury or dysraphism, the external anal sphincter and levator ani muscles, which depend on sacral nerves 2, 3, and 4, may be impaired. Children with myelomeningocele have both constipation and fecal incontinence [82].

CONSTIPATION AND HIRSCHSPRUNG'S DISEASE

FEATURE	FUNCTIONAL CONSTIPATION	HIRSCHSPRUNG'S DISEASE
Delayed passage of meconium	Rare	Common
Symptoms from birth	Rare	Common
Soiling	Common	Rare
Obstructive symptoms	Rare	Common
Withholding behavior	Common	Rare
Large caliber stools	Common	Rare
Enterocolitis	Never	Possible
Rectal ampulla	Enlarged	Narrowed
Stool in ampulla	Common	Rare
Male predominance	Yes	Yes

FIGURE 8-46.

Differentiating features between functional constipation and Hirschsprung's disease. The incidence of Hirschsprung's disease is 1 in 5000 live births and is found in fewer than 1% of children presenting for the first time with constipation. There are sufficient differences between these two entities so that in most cases rectal biopsy, anorectal manometry, and radiologic tests are unnecessary. When the clinical presentation is consistent with functional constipation, it is wise to treat the child before embarking on a series of tests to "rule out Hirschsprung's disease" or other colonic neuromuscular diseases.

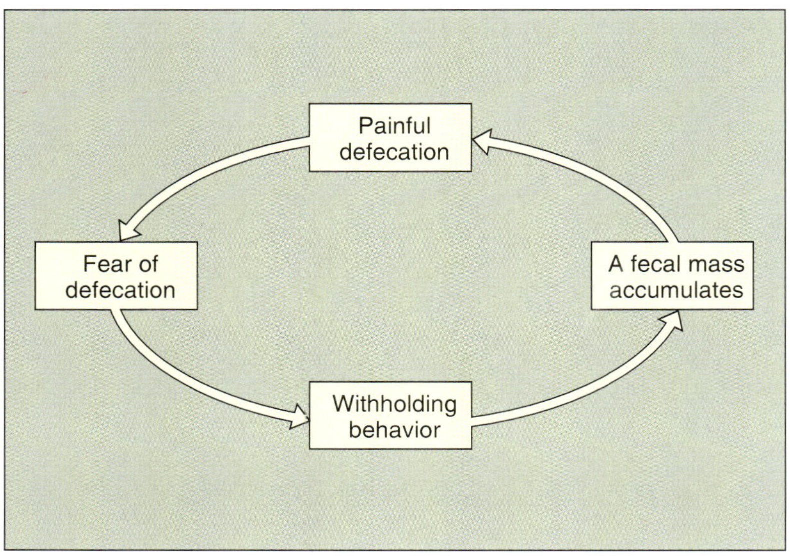

FIGURE 8-47.

Treatment of childhood functional constipation. In functional fecal retention the physician needs to provide reassurance that the condition will most likely resolve and must prescribe stool softeners to ensure painless defecation. The child needs to understand that responding to the defecatory urge and not holding back is key for the success of the treatment. There are two phases to treatment: passage of the rectal mass and maintenance. Almost every fecal mass can be softened and liquefied with sufficient quantity and duration of cathartics. Enemas are avoided because they are often interpreted by the child as a punishment [83]. After elimination of the rectal mass, treatment should be continued for several months with lower doses of cathartics. Agents commonly used in this phase include lubricants such as mineral oil, osmotic agents such as lactulose or milk of magnesia, and stimulants such as senna derivatives. The dosage of the drug is titrated to obtain the desired response. After a few months of painless and soil-free defecation, the patient is slowly weaned from the medication.

CYSTIC FIBROSIS

THE PATHOLOGY OF CYSTIC FIBROSIS

Organ	Physiologic Changes	Pathology
Lung	Distal airway obstruction, glandular hyperplasia, mucous hypersecretion	Early—terminal bronchiolar plugging, peribronchiolar inflammation Late—mucus casts, atelectasis, bronchiectasis, emphysema, cor pulmonale
Pancreas	Decreased volume and increased concentration of secretions	Early—duct plugging, dilatation, acinar atrophy Late—fibrous and fatty replacement, and loss of islets
Intestine	Concentrated secretions, mucus altered—hyperglycosylated and hypersulfated	Meconium plug, distal ileum; crypt dilatation; meconium peritonitis; distal intestinal obstruction syndrome; constipation
Liver	Reduced bile salt secretion, increased circulating bile salt concentration	Early—bile ductular hyperplasia, eosinophilic plugging of intrahepatic bile duct, focal biliary cirrhosis Late—multilobular cirrhosis
Gallbladder	Reduced bile salt pool, lithogenic bile	Cystic duct occlusion, hypoplastic gallbladder, gallstones
Salivary glands	High calcium concentration	Inspissated mucus in intercalated ducts, mild inflammation
Epididymis and vas deferens	Reduced secretions	Absent—fibrous replacement

Figure 8-48.

Pathology of cystic fibrosis (CF). Nearly all lesions in the disease have an obstructive element whereby a duct or air passage is blocked by mucus and/or other proteins. The airway and pancreatic lesions have the most adverse effects on health, but hepatic, intestinal, and reproductive tissues are also significantly affected pathologically. The pathologic changes closely mirror CF transmembrane conductance regulator (CFTR) expression on the epithelial cell surface of the respective organs.

The lung is not affected until after birth. Mucous plugging of small bronchioles and local inflammation are the earliest features. There is impaired clearance of airway secretions, which allows chronic infections to develop in the small airways, giving rise to chronic inflammation and progressive damage.

In contrast to the lung, the pancreas is affected in utero. At birth, intralobar ducts are plugged with proteinaceous material. Acinar cells show progressive atrophy. In time, both acini and proximal ducts atrophy and are replaced by fibrous tissue and fat. In the early stages, endocrine elements are relatively preserved, but islets also begin to disappear during adolescence. CF-associated diabetes mellitus is a common problem among adolescents and adults.

The intestine may also be affected in utero because of the low flow rate of intestinal contents. Rubbery masses of meconium may accumulate and obstruct the terminal ileum, giving rise to meconium ileus. After birth, predominantly in adolescence and adulthood, intermittent subacute intestinal obstruction with inspissated mucofeculent material is common.

CF-associated liver disease is characterized by small biliary ducts obstructed by eosinophilic material. This produces a patchy form of liver disease, focal biliary cirrhosis. In a small percentage of affected individuals, more extensive multilobular cirrhosis develops. The gallbladder is frequently atrophic and filled with mucus. The cystic duct and the intrahepatic and extrahepatic ducts may be filled with mucus and sludge.

The vas deferens is occluded in almost all males with CF. Thus, virtually all males with CF are sterile. In females, increased viscosity of cervical mucus has been described. Pathology is minimal, however. Healthy females with CF successfully conceive and are capable of carrying pregnancies to term. (*From* Forstner and Durie [85]; with permission.)

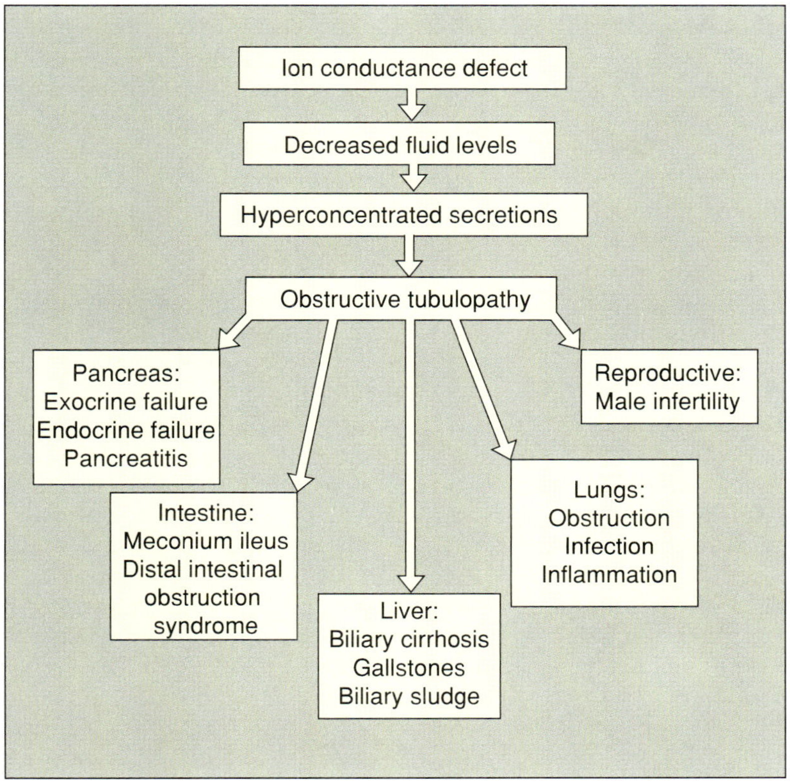

FIGURE 8-49.

Pathophysiology of cystic fibrosis. The ion conductance defect in epithelial tissues almost always results in reduced fluid flow within epithelia of organs normally possessing cystic fibrosis transmembrane conductance regulator (CFTR) expression. Absent or dysfunctional CFTR would be expected to lead to functional consequences in organs with a high concentration of macromolecules in the lumen of the ducts. A variety of organs listed in this figure are affected pathologically when proteins or other macromolecules precipitate, form plugs, slow ductal flow, and lead to blockage. (*Adapted from* Forstner and Durie [84].)

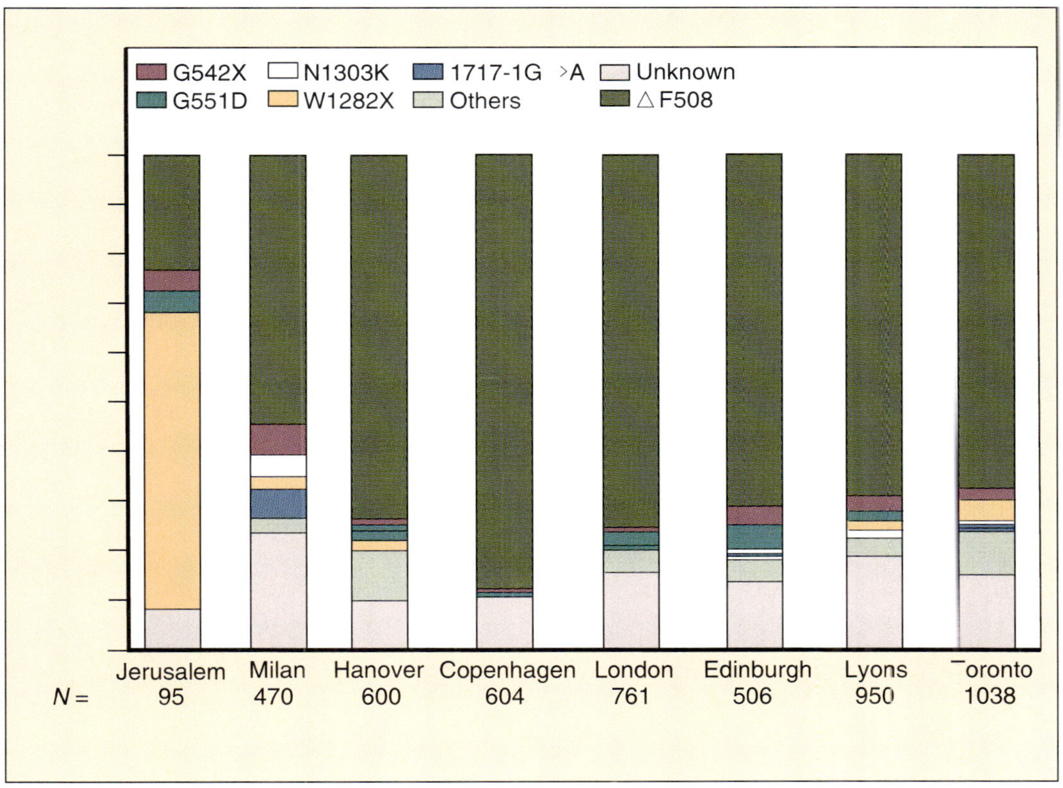

FIGURE 8-50.

The relative frequencies of the common cystic fibrosis transmembrane conductance regulator (CFTR) gene mutations in selected population centers are shown. A founder effect is apparent for some of the more common mutations. For example, ΔF508 accounts for almost 90% of CFTR mutations detected in the Danish population, suggesting that this mutation originated in Northeastern Europe. In contrast, ΔF508 accounts for only 22% of the cystic fibrosis chromosomes in the Ashkenazi Jewish population living in Israel. In that population, the nonsense mutation W1282X is common. It should be noted that a number of mutations remain unknown. (*Adapted from* Tsui [85]; with permission.)

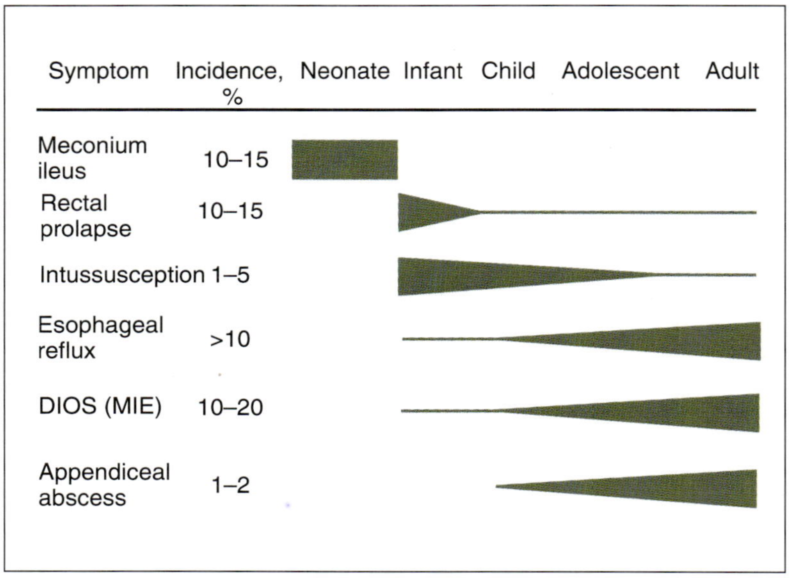

FIGURE 8-51.

Gastrointestinal manifestations vary with age and disease progression. Approximately 10% to 15% of cystic fibrosis (CF) patients present at birth with signs and symptoms of intestinal obstruction. The cause is a plug of meconium in the terminal ileum that is acquired in utero. Half the cases are complicated by volvulus and atresia with or without attendant meconium peritonitis. Rectal prolapse occurs in almost 20% of patients, usually between 1 and 2.5 years of age [86]. In almost half these cases, episodes of prolapse precede diagnosis. Rectal prolapse has a tendency to resolve spontaneously.

Gastroesophageal reflux that may cause severe esophagitis and esophageal stricture increases in frequency with age, being more common in older children or adults with chronic pulmonary disease [87]. Distal intestinal obstruction syndrome (DIOS) or meconium ileus equivalent (MIE) occurs mainly in patients with pancreatic insufficiency [88]. It results from inspissated fecal masses that adhere tightly to the intestinal mucosa, particularly in the ileocecal area. An abdominal mass can be palpated in the abdomen. Complete bowel obstruction is rare; more often it causes partial bowel obstruction with intermittent abdominal pain that may result in loss of appetite and weight loss. Classical symptoms of acute appendicitis seem to be relatively rare in CF. More frequently, patients develop an appendicial abscess that is frequently misdiagnosed as DIOS.

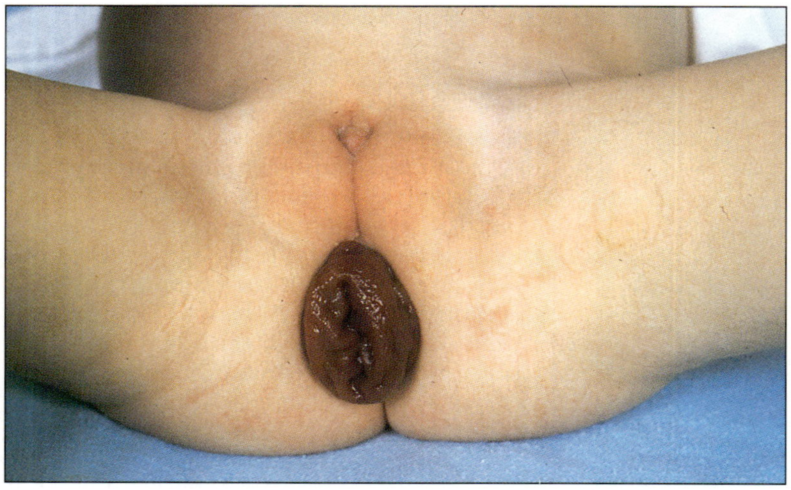

FIGURE 8-52.

Rectal prolapse, which usually occurs during passage of a large bowel motion, can be a frightening condition for parents of young children with cystic fibrosis. It is hardly ever associated with major medical complications and is easily reduced manually. This condition usually resolves spontaneously by 3 to 4 years of age. Surgical intervention is not advocated, unless the condition is persistent.

LIVER AND BILIARY TRACT COMPLICATIONS IN CYSTIC FIBROSIS

LOCATION	COMPLICATION	INCIDENCE, %
Liver	Steatosis	20–66
	Focal biliary cirrhosis	10–72
	Multilobular biliary cirrhosis	<1–24
	Portal hypertension	<5–28
Gallbladder	Nonvisualized gallbladder	12–40
	Microgallbladder	30
	Distended gallbladder	3–20
	Atretic cystic duct	16
	Cholelithiasis	0–33
Common bile duct	Distal stenosis	10–33
	Sclerosing cholangitis	1
	Cholangiocarcinoma	Rare

FIGURE 8-53.

Hepatobiliary disorders associated with cystic fibrosis (CF) in childhood. Various complications are observed in the liver and biliary tract of children with CF. With improved management of the respiratory, pancreatic, and nutritional complications, an increasing incidence of hepatobiliary disorders in CF has been seen. CF is an autosomal recessive disorder affecting 1 in 2500 live births in the white population. It is characterized by thick, tenacious secretions that obstruct the pulmonary, pancreatic, intestinal, and biliary systems. The presence of an elevated sweat chloride concentration aids in diagnosis. The CF gene encodes a protein, the CF transmembrane conductance regulator (CFTR), which is a cyclic adenosine monophosphate–dependent chloride channel. In the liver, CFTR has been localized to biliary epithelial cells but not to hepatocytes. Although over 100 mutations of the gene have been recognized, Δ F508 is a frequently encountered mutation. (*Adapted from* Suchy [89].)

CLINICAL SIGNS OF MALNUTRITION IN CYSTIC FIBROSIS	
In infancy and childhood	**In late childhood and adolescence**
Growth retardation	Growth retardation
Delayed bone age	Weight deficit
Weight deficit	Muscle wasting
Muscle wasting	Delayed puberty
Pot belly	Hepatomegaly
Rectal prolapse	Hypoalbuminemia
Hypoalbuminemia	Osteopenia
Edema	Ataxia
Anemia	Ophthalmoplegia
Bruising	
Bleeding	
Skin rash	
Hepatomegaly	
Developmental delay	

FIGURE 8-54.

Clinical features of malnutrition. Signs and symptoms of malnutrition vary according to the patient's age, but most are related to a protein-calorie deficit or malabsorption of essential nutrients [84]. Most patients with cystic fibrosis (CF) and pancreatic insufficiency present in infancy with some manifestations of maldigestion and are often malnourished. The abdomen is distended and muscles appear wasted, particularly in the buttocks and thighs. Growth failure is an early sign. The appearance of edema, hypoalbuminemia, and anemia herald severe protein-calorie malnutrition; this generally occurs in infants under the age of 6 months. Growth retardation is a variable feature during childhood. In general, patients improve rapidly with adequate attention to caloric requirements, vitamin needs, and pancreatic enzyme supplementation. In most CF centers, nutritional support is now viewed as an integral part of the multidisciplinary care of patients with CF. Aggressive programs have been instituted to prevent malnutrition. It is now generally accepted that the primary objective of nutritional management is to achieve normal nutrition and growth for children of all ages.

CHOLESTATIC DISORDERS IN PEDIATRICS

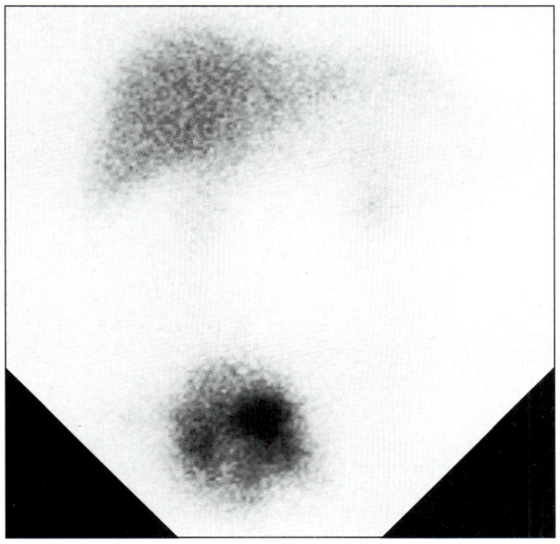

FIGURE 8-55.

Extrahepatic biliary atresia. This disorder is characterized by necroinflammatory progressive destruction of the biliary tree, including both the extrahepatic and intrahepatic bile duct. In spite of numerous proposed mechanisms, its etiology and pathogenesis remain unknown. With continued cholestasis, portal and periportal fibrosis develop, proceeding to bridging fibrosis and cirrhosis if uncorrected. Hepatobiliary scan of a 2-month-old child with conjugated hyperbilirubinemia and acholic stools. The scan demonstrates good uptake of tracer by the liver, but no excretion of isotope into the intestine. Instead, there is excretion of isotope through the kidneys into the urinary bladder. The evaluation of this child should proceed with a liver biopsy and an intraoperative cholangiogram to assess the patency of the extrahepatic biliary tree.

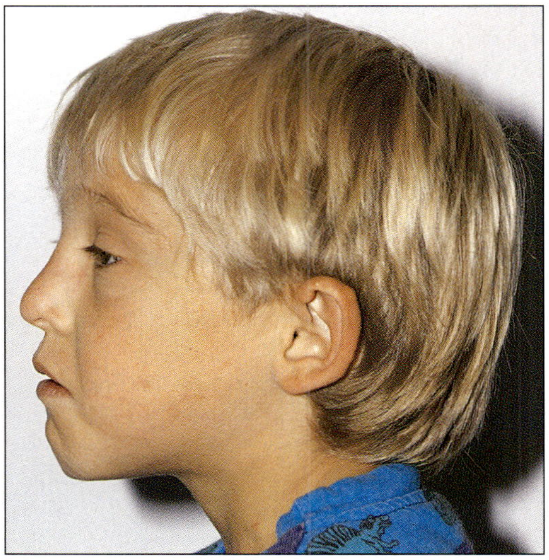

FIGURE 8-56.

Alagille's syndrome (arteriohepatic dysplasia). Typical facies associated with chronic cholestasis include frontal bossing, deep-set eyes, bulbous tip of nose, and a pointed chin. The classic syndrome includes chronic cholestasis usually presenting in infancy with significant pruritus, xanthomas, and hypercholesterolemia. Liver biopsy reveals a paucity of the interlobular bile ducts. The usual cardiac abnormality in Alagille's syndrome is peripheral pulmonic stenosis, though other cardiac anomalies, including tetralogy of Fallot and coarctation of the aorta, have been reported. The typical bone defect is *butterfly vertebrae*. Other bone defects reported include hemivertebrae, a lack of the normal progressive widening of the interpedicular distance down the lumbar spine, shortening of the distal phalanges, and an abnormally short ulna. Ophthalmologic findings in Alagille's syndrome include posterior embryotoxon (a thickening of Schwalbe's line) and retinal pigmentary changes. Recent reports suggest an association of Alagille's syndrome with small deletions on the short arm of chromosome 20 (*ie*, 20p deletion).

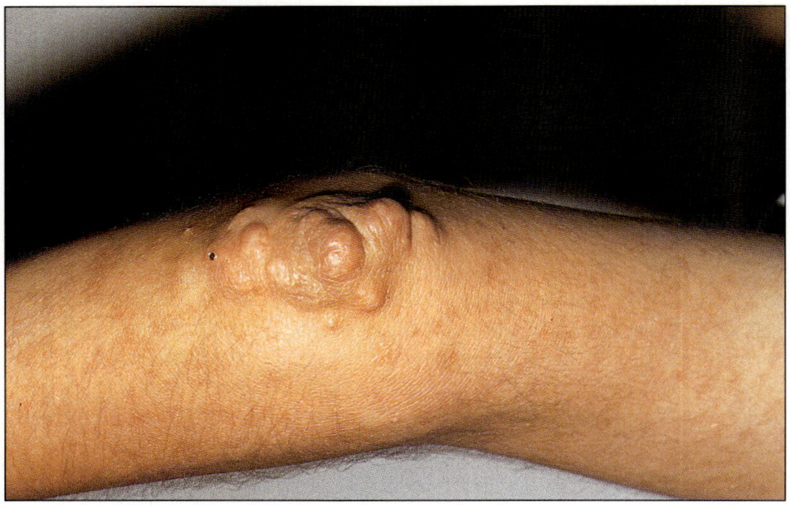

FIGURE 8-57.

Xanthomas. This slide depicts severe cutaneous xanthomas in a 7-year-old boy with Alagille's syndrome whose serum cholesterol level is approximately 1 g/dL. Severe intrahepatic cholestasis is associated with hypercholesterolemia, the deposition of cholesterol in skin, mucous membranes and arteries, and the development of xanthomas.

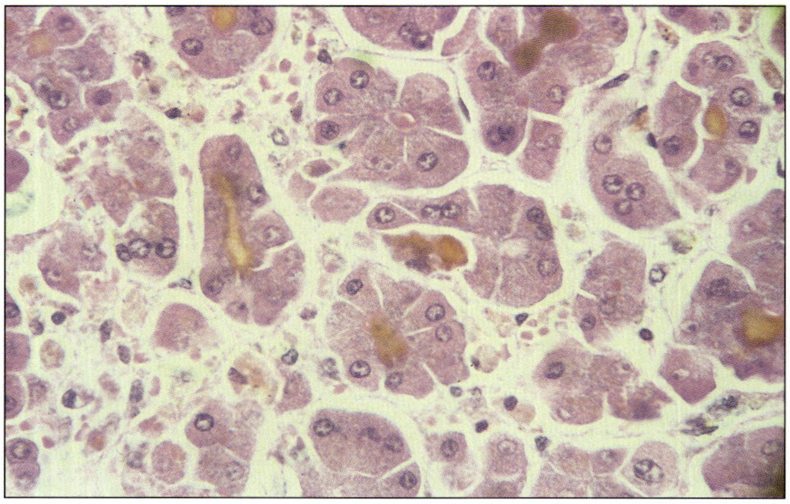

FIGURE 8-58.

Total parenteral nutrition (TPN)–associated cholestasis. Significant cholestasis, inflammation, and fibrosis in the liver of a premature infant who developed necrotizing enterocolitis and received total parenteral nutrition for 3 months before this biopsy specimen was taken. Cholestatic liver disease associated with the administration of TPN in preterm infants is a well-recognized clinical entity that occurs much more frequently in infants than adults. Despite numerous efforts to establish its mechanism, the origin of TPN–associated cholestasis remains undefined and no specific therapy exists. Continuation of TPN may further exacerbate the cholestasis and result in significant hepatocellular injury with the development of fibrosis and cirrhosis, but cessation of TPN in an infant with a dysfunctional gastrointestinal tract may itself result in starvation, malnutrition, and death. (Hematoxylin and eosin stain, original magnification × 450.)

REFERENCES

1. Gardner LM, Auerbach KG: Breast milk and breastfeeding jaundice. *Adv Pediatr* 1987, 34:249.
2. Oski FA: Disorders of bilirubin metabolism. In *Diseases of the Newborn*. Edited by Taeusch HW, Ballard RA, Avery ME. Philadelphia: WB Saunders; 1991.
3. Popoulsek H, Papoulsek M: Biological basis of social interactions: Implications of research for an understanding of behavioral deviance. *J Child Psychol and Psychiatry* 1983, 24:117–129.

3a. Weissbluth M: Colic. In Current Pediatric Therapy. Edited by Gellis SS, Kagan BM. Philadelphia: W.B. Saunders; 1993:233–236.

4. Orlando R: Esophageal epithelial defenses against acid injury. *Am J Gastroenterol* 1994, 89:S48–S52.
5. Kahrilas P, Dodds W, Dent J, *et al.*: Effect of sleep, spontaneous gastroesophageal reflux, and a meal on upper esophageal sphincter pressure in normal human volunteers. *Gastroenterology* 1987, 92:466–471.
6. Lang I, Shaker R: An update on the physiology of the components of the upper esophageal sphincter. *Dysphagia* 1994, 9:229–232.
7. Shaker R, Ren J, Kern M, *et al.*: Mechanisms of airway protection and upper esophageal sphincter opening during belching. *Am J Physiol* 1992, 262:G621–G628.
8. Sondheimer JM: Upper esophageal sphincter and pharyngoesophageal motor function in infants with and without gastroesophageal reflux. *Gastroenterology* 1983, 85:301–305.
9. Staiano A, Cucchiara S, De VB, *et al.*: Disorders of upper esophageal sphincter motility in children. *J Pediatr Gastroenterol Nutr* 1987, 6:892–898.
10. Winship D: Upper esophageal sphincter: does it care about reflux? *Gastroenterology* 1983, 85:470–472.
11. Orenstein SR, Cohn JF, Shalaby TM, Kartan R: Reliability and validity of an infant gastroesophageal reflux questionnaire. *Clin Pediatr* 1993, 32:472–484.
12. Kahn A, Rebuffat E, Franco P, *et al.*: Apparent life-threatening events and apnea of infancy. In *Respiratory Control Disorders in Infants and Children*. Edited by Beckerman R, Brouilette R, Hunt C. Baltimore: Williams and Wilkins; 1992:178–189.
13. Drumm B, Rhoads JM, Stringer DA, *et al.*: Peptic ulcer disease in children: etiology, clinical findings and clinical course. *Pediatrics* 1988, 982:410–414.
14. Carpenter HA, Talley NJ: Gastroscopy is incomplete without biopsy: clinical relevance in distinguishing gastropathy from gastritis. *Gastroenterology* 1995, 108:917–926.
15. George DE, Glassman M: Peptic ulcer disease in children. *Gastrointest Endosc Clin North Am* 1994, 4:23–37.
16. Sherman P: Peptic ulcer disease in children: diagnosis, treatment, and the implication of Helicobacter pylori. *Gastroenterol Clin North Am* 1994, 23:4:707–725.
17. Tolia V, Dubois RS: Peptic ulcer disease in children and adolescents: a ten-year experience. *Clin Pediatr* 1983, 2:665–669.
18. Tomomasa T, Hsu JY, Shigeta M, *et al.*: Statistical analysis of

symptoms and signs in pediatric patients with peptic ulcers. *J Pediatr Gastroenterol Nutr* 1986, 5:711–715.

19. Murphy MS, Eastham EJ, Jimenez M, *et al.*: Duodenal ulceration: review of 100 cases. *Arch Dis Child* 1987, 62:544–558.
20. Perenboom RM, Rijk MC, Rikken GH, Van Tongeren JH: The course of illness in ulcerative colitis. *Ned Tijdschr Geneeskd* 1990, 134:438–442.
21. Fiasse R, Lurhuma AZ, Favaro S, *et al.*: Circulating immune complexes and disease activity in Crohn's disease. *Gut* 1978, 19:611–617.
22. Jewell DP, Machennun I: Circulating immune complexes in inflammatory bowel disease. *Clin Exp Immunol* 1973, 14:219–226.
23. Doe WF, Booth CC, Brown DC: Evidence for complement-binding immune complexes in adult coelaic disease, Crohn's disease, and ulcerative colitis. *Lancet* 1973, 1:402–403.
24. Mayer I, Meyers S, Janowitz H: Cryoproteins in Crohn's disease: an etiology of extraintestinal manifestations. *J Clin Gastroenterol* 1981, 3(suppl. 1):17.
25. Levine JB: The arthropathies of IBD: more than meets the eye. *IBD News* 1990, 11:1.
26. McEwen JC, Ling C, Kirsner JB: Arthritis accompanying ulcerative colitis. *Am J Med* 1962, 33:923–941.
27. Paller AS: Cutaneous changes associated with inflammatory bowel disease. *Pediatr Dermatol* 1986, 3:439–445.
28. Lee FI, Bellary SV, Francis C: Increased occurrence of psoriasis in patients with Crohn's disease and their relatives. *Am J Gastroenterol* 1990, 85:962–963.
29. Hopkins DJ, Horan E, Burton IL, *et al.*: Ocular disorders in a series of 332 patients with Crohn's disease. *Br J Ophthalmol* 1974, 58:732–737.
30. Calkins BM, Reed JF, *et al.*: The occurrence of extraintestinal complications in IBD patients by location of lesion and family history of IBD. *Lit Rev Ther Inflam Bowel Dis* 1990, 56:531.
31. Ellis PP, Gentry JH: Ocular complications of ulcerative colitis. *Am J Ophthalmol* 1964, 50:779–785.
32. LaRusso NF, Wiesner RH, Ludwig J, MacCarty RL: Primary sclerosing cholangitis. *N Engl J Med* 1984, 310:899–903.
33. Warren GH, Kern F: The biliary tract in inflammatory bowel disease. *Clin Gastroenterol* 1983, 12:255–268.
34. Helzberg JH, Petersen JM, Boyer JL: Improved survival with primary sclerosing cholangitis: a review of clinicopathologic features and comparison of symptomatic and asymptomatic patients. *Gastroenterology* 1987, 92:1869–1875.
35. White TT, Hart MJ: Primary sclerosing cholangitis. *Am J Surg* 1987, 153:439–443.
36. Wiesner RH, LaRusso NF: Clinicopathologic features of the syndrome of primary sclerosing cholangitis. *Gastroenterology* 1980, 79:200–206.
37. Kern F: Hepatobiliary disorders in inflammatory bowel disease. In *Progress in Liver Disease*. Edited by Popper H, Schaffner F. New York: Grune & Stratton; 1976, 5:575–589.
38. Johnson ML, Wilson HT: Skin lesions in ulcerative colitis. *Gut* 1969, 10:255–263.
39. Basler RSW: Ulcerative colitis and the skin. *Gut* 1980, 64:941–954.
40. Monsen U, Hellers G, Johansson C: Extracolonic diagnoses in ulcerative colitis: an epidemiologic study. *Am J Gastroenterol* 1990, 85:711–716.
41. Anderson PC: Erythema nodosum. In *Clinical Dermatology*. Edited by Demis DJ. Philadelphia: Harper and Row; 1990:1–8.
42. Moreno AJ, Weisman I, Kenney RL, *et al.*: Concurrence of erythema multiforme and erythema nodosum. *Cutis* 1983, 31:275–278.
43. Lofgren S: Primary pulmonary sarcoidosis: early signs and symptoms. *Acta Med Scand* 1992, 26:259–260.
44. Debois J, Vandepitte J, Degreef H, *et al.*: Yersinia enterocolitica as a cause of erythema nodosum. *Dermatologica* 1978, 156:65.
45. Tanaka M, Riddell RH: The pathological diagnosis and differential diagnosis of Crohn's disease. *Hepatogastroenterology* 1990, 37:18–31.
46. Surawicz CM, Meisel JL, Ylvisaker T, *et al.*: Rectal biopsy in the diagnosis of Crohn's disease: value of multiple biopsies and serial sectioning. *Gastroenterology* 1981, 81:66–71.
47. Surawicz CM: Serial sectioning of a portion of a rectal biopsy detects more focal abnormalities: a prospective study of patients with inflammatory bowel disease. *Dig Dis Sci* 1982, 27:434–436.
48. Dourmashkin RR, Davies H, Wells C, *et al.*: Epithelial patchy necrosis in Crohn's disease. *Hum Pathol* 1983, 14:643–648.
49. Stahl TJ, Schoetz DJ, Roberts PL, *et al.*: Crohn's disease and carcinoma: increasing justification for surveillance? *Dis Colon Rectum* 1992, 35:850–856.
50. Schmitz-Moormann P, Pittner PM: The granuloma in Crohn's disease: bioptical study. *Pathol Res Pract* 1984, 178:467–476.
51. Das KM, Eastwood MA, McManus JP, Sircus W: Adverse reactions during salicylazosulfapyridine therapy and the relation with drug metabolism and acetylator phenotype. *N Engl J Med* 1973, 289:491–495.
52. Rao SS, Cann PA, Holdsworth CD: Clinical experience of the tolerance of mesalazine and olsalazine in patients intolerant of sulphasalazine. *Scand J Gastroenterol* 1987, 22:332–336.
53. Campieri M, Lanfranchi GA, Bazzochi G, *et al.*: Treatment of ulcerative colitis with high dose 5-aminosalicylic acid enemas. *Lancet* 1981, 2:270–271.
54. Campieri M, Lanfranchi GA, Brignoa C, *et al.*: 5-Aminosalicylic acid for the treatment of inflammatory bowel disease (Letter). *Gastroenterology* 1991, 89:701–703.
55. van Hees PA, Bakher JH, van Tongeren JH: Effect of sulphapyridine, 5-aminosalicylic acid and placebo in patients with idiopathic proctitis: a study to determine the active therapeutic moiety of sulphasalazine. *Gut* 1980, 21:632–635.
56. Williams CN, Hader G, Aguino JA: Double-blind placebo-controlled evaluation of 5-ASA suppositories in active distal proctitis and measurement of extent of spread using Tc-labelled 5-ASA suppositories. *Dig Dis Sci* 1987, 32:718–755.
57. Nielsen OH, Bukhave K, Elmgreen J, Ahnfelt-Ronne I: Inhibition of 5-lipoxygenase pathway of arachidonic acid metabolism in human neutrophils by sulfasalazine and 5-aminosalicylic acid. *Dig Dis Sci* 1987, 6:577–582
58. Craven PA, Pfanstiel J, Saito R, DeRubertis FR: Actions of sulfasalazine 5-aminosalicylic acid as reactive oxygen scavengers in the suppression of bile acid-induced increases in colonic epithelial cell loss and proliferative activity. *Gastroenterology* 1987, 92:1998–2008.
59. Daum F, Markowitz J, Rosa J, *et al.*: Does proctosigmoiditis in inflammatory bowel disease presage the imminent onset of symptoms? *J Pediatr Gastroenterol Nutr* 1989, 8:339–342.
60. Hyams J, Moore R, Leichtner A, *et al.*: Relationship of type I procollagen to corticosteroid therapy in children with inflammatory bowel disease. *J Pediatr* 1988, 112:893–898.
61. Whittington PF, Barnes HV, Bayless TM: Medical management of Crohn's disease in adolescence. *Gastroenterology* 1977, 72:1338–1344.
62. Kumana CR, Seaton T, Meghji M, *et al.* Beclomethasone dipropionate enemas for treating inflammatory bowel disease without producing Cushing's syndrome or hypothalamic-pituitary-adrenal suppression. *Lancet* 1982, 1:579–583.
63. Brattsand R: Overview of newer glucocorticosteroid preparations for inflammatory bowel diseases. *Can J Gastroenterol* 1990, 407–414.
64. Larochelle P, DuSouich P, Bolte E, *et al.*: Tixocortole pivalate, a corticosteroid with no systemic glucocorticoid effect after oral, intrarectal and intranasal application. *Clin Pharmacol Ther* 1983, 33:343–350.
65. Lofberg R, Danielsson A, Salde L: Oral budesonide ileocecal Crohn's disease: an initial experience (Abstract). *Gastroenterology* 1991, 100:A226.
66. Roth M, Ueberschaer B, Ewe K Gross V: Scholmerich slow release budesonide includes remission in active disease with little effect on adrenal function (Abstract). *Gastroenterology* 1992, 102:A688.
67. Carpani de Kaski M, Peters AM, Lavender JP: Fluticasone propionate

in Crohn's disease. *Gut* 1991, 32:657–661.

68. Present DH, Korelitz BI, Wisch N, *et al.*: Treatment of Crohn's disease with 6-mercaptopurine. *N Engl J Med* 1980, 302:981–987.
69. Markowitz J, Rosa J, Grancher K, *et al.*: Long term 6-mercaptopurine (6-MP) in adolescents with Crohn's disease. *Gastroenterology* 1991, 100:1156–1157.
70. Treem WR, Davis PM, Hyams JS: Cyclosporine treatment of severe ulcerative colitis in children. *J Pediatr* 1991, 119:994–997.
71. Benkov KF, Rosh JR, Schwersenz AH, *et al.*: Cyclosporine as an alternative to surgery in children with inflammatory bowel disease. *J Ped Gastroenterol Nutr* 1994, 19:290–294.
72. Hanauer SB, Smith MB: Rapid closure of Crohn's disease fistulas with continuous intravenous cyclosporin A. *Am J Gastroenterol* 1993, 88:646–649.
73. Rohr G, Kusterer K, Schille M, *et al.*: Treatment of Crohn's disease and ulcerative colitis with 7S-immunoglobulin. *Lancet* 1987, 1:170.
74. Strobel CT, Byren WJ, Ament MF: Home parenteral nutrition in children with Crohn's disease: an effective management alternative. *Gastroenterology* 1979, 272–279.
75. Gitlin K, Markowitz J, Pelcovitz D, *et al.*: Stress mediators in children with inflammatory bowel disease. In *Advances in Child Health Psychology: Proceedings of the Florida Conference.* Edited by Johnson J, Johnson S. Gainesville, Florida: University of Florida Press; 1990:54–62.
76. Øster J: Recurrent abdominal pain, headache and limb pains in children and adolescents. *Pediatrics* 1972, 50:165–170.
77. Apley J, Naish N: Recurrent abdominal pain: a field survey of 1000 school children. *Arch Dis Child* 1958, 33:165–170.
78. Rappaport L: Recurrent abdominal pain: theories and pragmatics. *Pediatrician* 1989, 16:78–84.
79. Devroede G: Constipation. In *Gastrointestinal Disease: Pathophysiology, Diagnosis, Management.* Edited by Sleisinger MH, Fordran JS. Philadelphia: WB Saunders; 1989:331–368.
80. Hyman PE, Fleisher D: Functional fecal retention. *Practical Gastroenterology* 1992, 16:29–37.
81. Loening-Baucke VA, Younoszai MK: Abnormal anal sphincter response in chronically constipated children. *J Pediatr* 1982, 100:213–218.
82. Anthony EJ: An experimental approach to the psychopathology of childhood: encopresis. *Br J Med Psychol* 1957, 30:146.
83. Gleghorn EE, Heyman MB, Rudolph CD: No-enema therapy for idiopathic constipation and encopresis. *Clin Pediatr* 1991, 30:669–672.
84. Forstner C, Durie PR: Cystic fibrosis. In *Pediatric Gastrointestinal Disease: Pathophysiology, Diagnosis, Management.* Edited by Walker WA, Durie PR, Hamilton JR, *et al.* Philadelphia: BC Decker; 1991:1179–1197.
85. Tsui L-C: The spectrum of cystic fibrosis mutations. *Trends Genet* 1992, 8:392–398.
86. Stern R, Izanti RJ, Boat TF, *et al.*: Treatment and prognosis of rectal prolapse in cystic fibrosis. *Gastroenterology* 1986, 82:707–710.
87. Scott RB, O'Laughlin EV, Gall DG: Gastroesophageal reflux in patients with cystic fibrosis. *J Pediatr* 1985, 106:223–227.
88. Koletzko S, Stringer DA, Cleghorn GJ, Durie PR: Lavage treatment of distal intestinal obstruction syndrome in children with cystic fibrosis. *Pediatrics* 1989, 83:727–733.
89. Suchy FJ: Liver Disease in Children. St. Louis: CV Mosby; 1994.

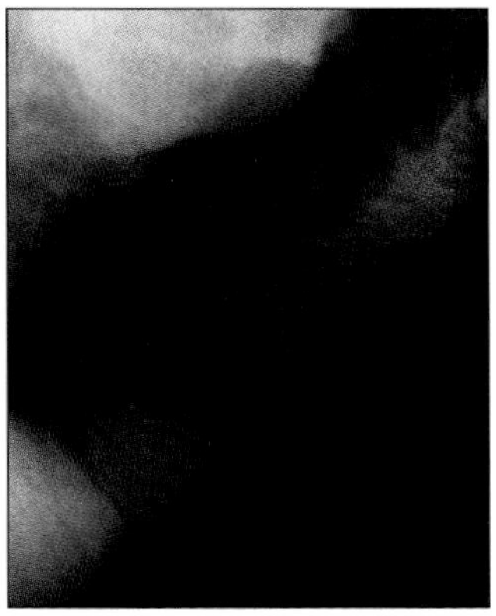

Index

Page numbers followed by *t* or *f* indicate tables or figures, respectively.

C

D

E

F

G

H

I

J

K

L

M

N

O

P

R

S

T

U

V

W